TEXTBOOK OF
MEN'S HEALTH

Published in association with

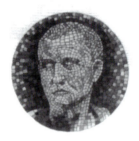

The International Society
for the
Study of the Aging Male

TEXTBOOK OF
MEN'S HEALTH

Editors-in-Chief
Bruno Lunenfeld, MD, and
Louis Gooren, MD, PhD

The Parthenon Publishing Group
International Publishers in Medicine, Science & Technology

A CRC PRESS COMPANY
BOCA RATON   LONDON   NEW YORK   WASHINGTON, D.C.

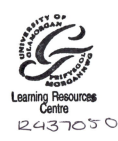
Library of Congress Cataloging-in-Publication Data

Textbook of men's health / edited by Bruno
Lunenfeld and Louis Gooren.
   p. ; cm.
   Includes bibliographical references and index.
   ISBN 1-84214-011-6 (alk. paper)
   1. Men--Health and hygiene. 2. Men--
Diseases. 3. Andrology. I. Lunenfeld,
Bruno. II. Gooren, Louis.
   [DNLM: 1. Health. 2. Men. 3. Health Status.
4. Risk Factors. 5. Sex Factors.
WA 300 T355 2001]
RC48.5 .T495 2001
616′.0081--dc21
                                    2001052034

British Library Cataloguing in Publication Data

Textbook of men's health
   1. Men - Health and hygiene 2. Men - Diseases
   I. Lunenfeld, Bruno II. Gooren, Louis
613′.04234

   ISBN 1842140116

Published in the USA by
The Parthenon Publishing Group
345 Park Avenue South, 10th Floor
New York, NY 10010, USA

Published in the UK and Europe by
The Parthenon Publishing Group
23–25 Blades Court
Deodar Road
London SW15 2NU, UK

Copyright © 2002
The Parthenon Publishing Group

Typeset by Siva Math Setters, Chennai, India
Printed and bound by Bookcraft (Bath) Ltd.,
Midsomer Norton, UK

Contents

List of principal contributors

Murad Alam, MD
Dermsurgery Associates
7515 Main, Suite 240
Houston, TX 77030
USA

Peter Alexandersen, MD
Center for Clinical and
   Basic Research A/S
Orla Lehmansgade 1, 4. sal
DK-7100 Vejle
Denmark

Nir Barzilai, MD
Divisions of Medicine & Endocrinology
Albert Einstein College of Medicine
Belfer Bld. 701
1300 Morris Park Avenue
Bronx, NY 10461
USA

Marc R. Blackman, MD
National Center for Complementary
   and Alternative Medicine
National Institutes of Health
8 West Drive, MSC 2669
Bethesda, MD 20892
USA

Steven Boonen, MD, PhD
Centre for Metabolic Bone Diseases
University Hospital Gasthuisberg
Herestraat 49, 3000 Leuven
Belgium

Mike A. R. Bosschaert, MD
St Antonius Hospital
R & D Cardiology
Nieuwegracht 12
3512 LP, Utrecht
The Netherlands

Simon R. J. Bott, FRCS
Trustees of The London Clinic Ltd
20 Devonshire Place
London, W1G 6BW
UK

Adrian R. Cassidy, MSc
Cambridge University Boat Club
Kimberly Road
Cambridge, CB4 9NJ
UK

Paul Clayton, PhD
UniVite Health
50 Aylesbury Road
Aston Clinton
Bucks, HP22 5AH
UK

Peter Collins, MD, FRCP, FESC, FACC
Cardiac Medicine
National Heart & Lung Institute
Imperial College School of Medicine
Dovehouse Street
London, SW3 6LY
UK

David Crook, PhD
Cardiovascular Biochemistry
St Bartholomew's & Royal London
   School of Medicine
Charterhouse Square
London, EC1 6BQ
UK

Leif Dahlberg, MD, PhD
Institute of Orthopedics
Universitetssjukhuset MAS
20502 Malmo
Sweden

Greta Dereymaeker, MD, PhD
Department of Orthopedics
University Hospital Gasthuisberg
Herestraat 49, 3000 Leuven
Belgium

Ali R. Djalilian, MD
National Eye and Health Institute
31 Centre Drive
Bethesda, MD 20892
USA

Dariush Elahi, PhD
Geriatric Research Laboratory
Massachusetts General Hospital
GRBSB-0015, 55 Fruit Street
Boston, MA 02114
USA

Ian F. Godsland, PhD
Endocrinology & Metabolic Medicine
Imperial College School
    of Medicine
Norfolk Place
London, W2 1PG
UK

Louis Gooren, MD, PhD
Department of Endocrinology
Vrije University Medical Center
Postbus 7057
1007 MB, Amsterdam
The Netherlands

Axel Heidenreich, MD
Department of Urology
Klinikum der Philipps-Universität
    Marburg
Baldingerstrasse
35043 Marburg
Germany

Jerome M. Hershman, MD
Department of Endocrinology
West Los Angeles VA Medical Center
11301 Wilshire Blvd
Los Angeles, CA 90073
USA

Jens O. L. Jørgensen, MD, DMSc
Medical Department
Åarhus Kommunehospital
DK-8000 Århus C
Denmark

Hosam K. Kamel, MB, BCh, FACP
Geriatric Evaluation
    and Management Unit
Clement J. Zablocki VAMC
5000 West National Avenue
Milwaukee, WI 53295
USA

Derek Le Roith, MD, PhD
Clinical Endocrinology Branch
National Institutes of Health
Building 10, Room 8D12
10 Center Drive, MSC 1758
Bethseda, MD 20892
USA

Anthony R. Leeds, FIBiol
Department of Nutrition
    and Dietetics
Kings College UCL
150 Stamford Street
London, SW1 8WA
UK

Guy Lloyd, MBBS, MRCP
Cardiothoracic Center
Guy's and St Thomas' Hospital Trust
Lambeth Palace Road
London, SE1 7EH
UK

Bruno Lunenfeld, MD
Professor Emeritus
Faculty of Life Sciences
Bar Ilan University
Israel

Per Mårin, MD, PhD
Department of Heart and
    Lung Diseases
Sahlgrenska University Hospital
SU/Ostra, CK, Plan 2
418 85 Goteborg
Sweden

John Marks, MA, MD, FRCP
Life Fellow of Girton College
University of Cambridge
Cambridge, CB3 0JG
UK

Jan Mievis, MD
Department of Orthopedics
University Hospital Gasthuisberg
Herestraat 49, 3000 Leuven
Belgium

Francesco Montorsi, MD
Department of Urology
University Vita e Salute - San Raffaele
Via Olgettina 60
20132 Milan
Italy

Alvaro Morales, MD
Department of Urology
Queen's University
Victory 4
Kingston General Hospital
Kingston, ON K7L 2V7
Canada

John E. Morley, MB, BCh
Division of Geriatric Medicine
St. Louis University Health Sciences Center
1402 S. Grand Boulevard, M-238
St Louis, MO 63104
USA

Robert A. Norman, DO
Department of Dermatology
Nova Southeastern University
Tampa, Florida 33615
USA

Acke Ohlin, MD, PhD
Department of Orthopedics
Malmo University Hospital
205 02 Malmo
Sweden

Frank Ondrey, MD, PhD
University of Minnesota School of Medicine
Department of Otolaryngology
Box 396, 420 Delaware Street
Minneapolis, MN 55455
USA

Vincent Ravery, MD
Department of Urology
Hospital Bicat
46 Rue Henri Huchard
75877 Paris Cedex 18
France

Janet L. Roberts, MD
Department of Dermatology
Oregon Health Sciences University
2222 NW Lovejoy, Suite 419
Portland, OR 97210
USA

Claude C. Schulman, MD
Department of Urology
University Clinics Brussels
Hospital Erasme
Route de Lennik 808
B-1070 Brussels
Belgium

Colette Shortt, PhD
Yakult UK Ltd
12–16 Telford Way
Westway Estate, Acton
London, W3 7XS
UK

Anne M. Spungen, EdD
Rehabilitation Medicine
Mount Sinai School
    of Medicine
Spinal Cord Damage
    Research Center
VA Medical Center
130 West Kingsbridge Rd, IE-02
Bronx, NY 10468
USA

Ronald S. Swerdloff, MD
Division of Endocrinology
Department of Medicine
Martin Research Building
Harbor-UCLA Medical Center
1124 West Carson Street
Torrance, CA 90502
USA

Syed H. Tariq, MD
Division of Geriatric Medicine
St Louis University School of Medicine
1402 S. Grand Boulevard, M-238
St Louis, MO 63104
USA

Koichiro Tatsumi, MD
Department of Respiratory Medicine
Chiba University School of Medicine
1-8-1 Inohana, Chuo-ku
Chiba 260-8670
Japan

Jos H. H. Thijssen, PhD
Department of Endocrinology
University Medical Center Utrecht
PO Box 85090
3508 AB Utrecht
The Netherlands

Randall J. Urban, MD
Department of Internal Medicine
University of Texas Medical Branch
301 University Blvd
Galveston, TX 77555
USA

Dirk Vanderschueren, MD, PhD
Internal Medicine, Department
  of Endocrinology
Catholic University of Leuven
Herestraat 49, B-3000 Leuven
Belgium

Alex Vermeulen, MD
Professor Emeritus
Department of Endocrinology
University Hospital Ghent
De Pintelaan 185
B-9000 Ghent
Belgium

Adrian Wagg, MBBS, FRCP
Department of Geriatric Medicine
University College London Hospital
25 Grafton Way
London, WC1E 6AU
UK

Ken W. Watkins, PhD
Health Promotion and Education
University of South Carolina
Columbia, SC 29208
USA

Christina Wang, MD
Division of Endocrinology
Department of Medicine
Harbor-UCLA Medical Center
1124 West Carson Street
Torrance, CA 90502
USA

Carolyn M. Webb, PhD
Cardiac Medicine
National Heart & Lung Institute
Imperial College School of Medicine
Dovehouse Street
London, SW3 6LY
UK

Wolfgang Weidner, MD
Department of Urology
Center for Surgery, Anesthesiology and Urology
Justus-Liebig University of Giessen
Klinikstrabe 29
D-35385 Giessen
Germany

Margaret-Mary G. Wilson, MRCP
Division of Geriatric Medicine
St. Louis University Health Sciences Center
1402 S. Grand Boulevard, M-238
St. Louis, MO 63104
USA

Ulrich H. Winkler, MD
Department of Obstetrics and Gynecology
Wetlar Clinic
35578 Wetlar
Germany

Joel Zonszein, MD, FACE, FACP
Montefiore Clinical Diabetes Center
Albert Einstein College of Medicine
1825 Eastchester Road
Bronx, NY 10461
USA

Preface

This volume breaks new ground in the medical care and management of men, particularly as they progress through the inevitable aging process. Whilst women's health care has been a specific focus of scientific and clinical attention for at least two centuries, comparatively little attention has been given to the gender-specific needs of men. Of course, certain specialties – urology in particular – have focused on men, but there has been very little recognition that the bodily, endocrinological, psychological, and other changes that take place in male physiology throughout life have an impact on men's health that warrants and requires an integrated understanding and approach to medical management.

The International Society for the Study of the Aging Male was formed in 1998 to increase clinical awareness of this need and to encourage gender-specific research and practice designed to improve the medical care of men from maturity to old age. Since its foundation 4 years ago, the development of the Society has been meteoric. It has established a peer-review journal for the field and has organized a series of Regional, Local, and World Congresses. In addition, not only has it attracted a rapidly growing world-wide membership but it has encouraged the development of a number of local, national societies affiliated to it – and this process is continuing apace.

This new textbook is the latest initiative of *The International Society for the Study of the Aging Male*. It represents an attempt to draw together relevant gender-specific knowledge across the whole field of men's health and to establish the outline of a curriculum for those clinicians concerned to develop their knowledge of, and expertise in, the subject. The range of topics covered by the textbook is wide; musculoskeletal disorders, cardiovascular disease, androgen-related conditions, central nervous system and cognitive disorders, endocrine disease, genitourinary problems, sensory organ degeneration, gastroenterology, dermatology and other age-related conditions are all discussed by an impressive international team of expert contributors. The book does, therefore, provide a unique overview of male health as an entity and offers valuable insights for improved management and clinical care.

Of course, this is only the start of an ongoing process of education and development – but it is a very important start. It is hoped that this volume will provide a foundation from which clinicians in many parts of the world can develop their own studies and which will also provide a basic framework from which specialist courses and learning programs can be planned and developed.

New and expanded editions of this textbook are envisaged on a regular basis and with each new edition we hope to expand its coverage and depth, based on the practical experience gained from the use of this initial volume. In due course we hope to provide a fully tested and truly comprehensive clinical guide that will serve the ongoing needs of all clinicians anxious to expand their knowledge of this gender-specific field. This first edition does, therefore, represent a major milestone in the important road that lies ahead.

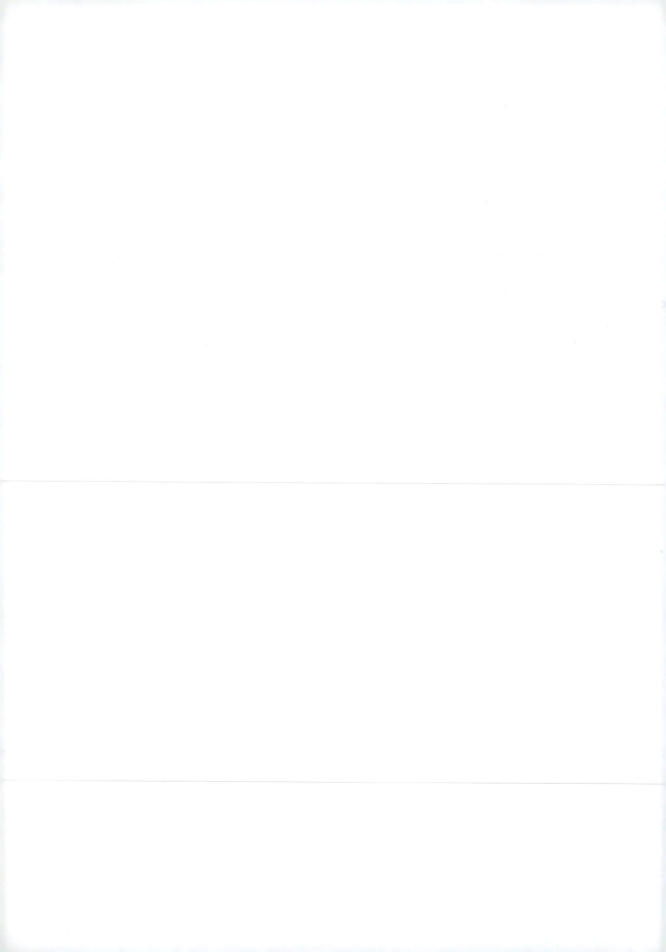

Section I

Diagnostics and primary assessment

Bruno Lunenfeld, MD, and Louis Gooren, MD, PhD

1 Aging men – challenges ahead

Bruno Lunenfeld, MD, and Louis Gooren, MD, PhD

AN AGING WORLD

First we were obsessed with the challenge of 'population explosion', then we shifted our concern to the problems of global ageing, and only now do we start to grasp the future consequences of a rapid fertility decline. E. Diczfalusy, 2000

The human race entered the 19th century with a global population of 978 million people, the 20th century with 1650 million people and the 21st century with a worldwide population of 6168 million. The estimates and projections of the United Nations indicate that between 1900 and 2100, the world population will increase seven-fold, from 1.65 billion to 11.5 billion: an increase of almost 10 billion people. This rapid increase in world population is regardless of the fact that effective family planning has significantly reduced fertility rates. In 1970 there were 22 countries with a total fertility rate at or below the replacement of 2.1. In the year 1999 there were 68 countries, and it is projected that by 2020, 121 countries representing 75% of the global population will have birth rates below the replenishment level (Tables 1 and 2).

Life expectancy for humans was about 30 years until the past hundred years or so. Today more than 75% of all human deaths in developed countries occur after the age of 75. The last century has been marked by the triumph of partially preventing the premature termination of life. During the past 50 years, infant mortality rates declined from 155/1000 to 52/1000

Table 1 Fertility rates in Europe in 1995

European Union (15 countries)
    Population 370 million
    Fertility rate 1.51

Other European countries
    Population 355 million
    Fertility rate 1.65

live births worldwide and from 72/1000 to 11/1000 in Europe[1]. During the same time-frame, a significant decline in overall mortality rates was also seen. This decline was mainly due to the development of antibiotics, vaccines, safer water, better sanitation and personal hygiene[2]. These events were responsible for the decrease of the appearance of epidemics and the control of most infectious diseases. Acute disease is no longer the major cause of death. Today one dies from chronic illnesses, degenerative diseases, metastatic cancer, immune deficiencies and other diseases which prolong disability, immobility and dependency. Dying has become in most instances a long, painful and expensive procedure[2].

The global increase in mean life expectancy and the drastic reduction of fertility rates has resulted in a rapidly aging world population (Figure 1). The effect of decreased fertility rates and increased life expectancy in selected Asian countries on the increase of its population above the age of 65 is demonstrated

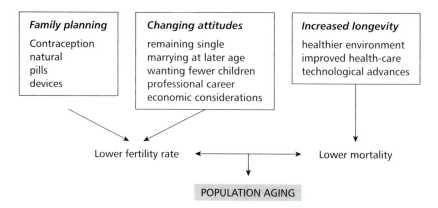

Figure 1 Factors contributing to a global increase in aging populations

Table 2 The effect of decrease in fertility rates and increase in mean life expectancy in selected Asian countries on their rising population (> 65 years)[12]

Country	Fertility rate		Life expectancy (years)		Percentage > 65 years	
	2000	2025	2000	2025	2000	2025
Singapore	1.2	1.5	80.1	82.5	9.7	18.4
Japan	1.4	1.6	80.7	82.9	17.1	27.6
S.Korea	1.7	1.7	74.4	79.2	10.8	23.4
China	1.8	1.8	71.4	77.4	10.2	19.7
Taiwan	1.8	1.7	76.4	80.4	12.6	24.1
Thailand	1.9	1.7	68.6	75.3	9.7	19.9
Vietnam	2.0	2.0	69.3	75.8	7.6	13.1
Burma	2.4	1.7	54.9	63.4	7.1	12.6
India	3.1	2.2	62.5	70.9	7.0	11.8
Malaysia	3.3	2.6	70.8	76.9	6.5	12.2
Philippines	3.5	2.4	67.5	74.6	5.7	10.1

in Table 2. It is projected that in general, the elderly population (above 65 years) will increase within the next 25 years by 82%, whereas the newborn rates will increase by only by 3% and the working-age population will increase by only 46%. The UN projects (in their 1998 revision) that by 2050, the proportion of persons above 60 years will for the first time exceed the proportion of children below 15 years, and in 13 countries more than 10% of the population will be made up of the oldest old (> 80 years old). Italy will have the dubious honor of leading with 14% of the population of the oldest old > 80 years. By the year 2050 Asia will be inhabited by almost 1 billion people

aged 65 and above. China, Japan, Singapore, Hong Kong and Macao will have become members of the 'club of 14' with more than 10% of their population aged 80 and above.

Since the last years of life are accompanied by an increase of disability and sickness, the demands on the social and health services will increase immensely. The high costs in relation to these services will strain the potential ability of health, social and even political infrastructures to the limit. The marked increase of the elderly population in relation to the working-age population will be compounded by a simultaneous decrease in the population of children, who make up the 'workers' of the next

Table 3 Life expectancy of men at different ages

Year of birth	Life expectancy at birth (years)	Expected number of years remaining at age (total lifespan)		
		15 years	45 years	65 years
1888	43.9	43.9 (58.9)	22.6 (67.6)	10.8 (75.8)
1988	70.5	56.4 (71)	28.2 (73.2)	13.0 (78)

Table 4 Disability-free life expectancy in the developing world[12]

Country		Life expectancy at birth (years)	Years of disability-free life expectancy at birth	Disability (years)
1	Japan	81	74.5	6.5
2	Australia	79.5	73.2	6.3
30	Singapore	78	69.3	8.7
51	S.Korea	72.8	65	7.8
59	Brunei	77.2	64.4	12.8
81	China	69.7	62.3	7.4
89	Malaysia	68.8	61.4	7.4
99	Thailand	68.2	60.2	8.0
113	Philippines	66.7	58.9	7.8
134	India	60.4	53.2	7.2
145	N.Guinea	55	47	8
148	Cambodia	53.8	45.7	8.1

generation. Thus a declining labor force will have to support an increasing number of elderly[3].

Although the mean life expectancy at birth has been prolonged by more than 25 years within the last century, life expectancy at the age of 65 increased by less than 3 years during the same time-frame (Table 3). Moreover, despite the enormous medical progress during the past few decades, 25% of life expectancy after age 65 is spent with some disability, and the last years of life are accompanied by a further increase of incapacity and sickness.

For a long time, life expectancy, the rate of infant mortality and causes of death were enough data to assess a population's health status and to determine national public health priorities. These indicators remain indispensable, as important mortality inequalities remain between different countries, populations and socioeconomic categories. With the lengthening of life expectancy at birth, non-communicable

diseases and associated disability receive increasing importance. Consequently the need for a new type of indicator, namely 'health expectancies: disability-free life expectancy, healthy life expectancy or active life expectancy' became necessary. The introduction of the concepts of the International Classification of Impairments, Disabilities and Handicaps[4] allowed the efficient use of health expectancy indicators. The recent Jakarta Declaration on leading health promotion into the 21st century confirms that 'the ultimate goal is to increase health expectancy and to narrow the goal in health expectancy between countries and groups'[5]. Today the first estimate of health expectancy (in most cases 'disability-free life expectancy') is available in most developed countries and increasingly also in developing countries (Table 4). Calculations on gains, differences or losses in health expectancy, (disability-free life expectancy, disease-free life expectancy, and dementia-free life expectancy) make it

Table 5 Difference between the highest and lowest income levels in disability-free life expectancy in Canada

Income level	Life expectancy (years)	Health expectancy (years)
Lowest	67.1	50
Second	70.1	57.9
Fourth	72.0	62.6
Highest	73.4	64.3
Total	70.8	59.5
Difference between richest/poorest	6.3	14.3

Adopted from Wilkins & Adams 1983[6]

possible to define public health priorities, assess health strategies, social inequalities, life-styles and therapeutic interventions. This kind of indicator demonstrates that not only do the poorest and least educated live less long, but they also experience a greater part of their life affected by disability or disease. In Canada, for example, the difference in life expectancy between the highest and lowest income levels was 6.3 years; the difference in disability-free life expectancy was 14.3 years (Table 5)[6].

The majority of older men today reside in developing countries. As the demographic transition gathers pace in the poorer regions of the world, an even greater proportion of the world's older men will live in countries and regions that have the least resources to respond to their needs. The communication revolution with globalization as its consequence, which started at the end of the last century, will peak during this century. But if we do not learn to share the resources and wealth of the earth, poverty will remain the biggest threat to mankind. It must be our aim that every human being on this earth should be able to age in reasonable health and with dignity.

The cost of caring for the increasing population of senior citizens will become prohibitive with its attendant socioeconomic consequences. To the prudent health-care administrators, the establishment of preventive measures, rather than concentration on interventive care, is an important strategic thrust in overall management of the aging population[3]. The ability for men to age gracefully and maintain independent living, free of disability, for as long as possible is a crucial factor in aging with dignity and would furthermore reduce health service costs significantly. To achieve this objective, a holistic approach to the management of aging has to be adopted[3].

The promotion of healthy aging and the prevention or drastic reduction of morbidity and disability of the elderly must assume a central role in the formulation of the health and social policies of many, if not all, countries in the next century. It must emphasize an all-encompassing life-long approach to the aging process, beginning with pre-conceptual events and focus on appropriate interventions at all stages of life. Life-history studies of childhood and adolescence demonstrate clearly that social factors probably operate in a cumulative fashion. There are significant social class differences in attainment of height, growth and other aspects of physical development, as well as in incidence of infectious and other diseases and risk of injury. For example, the nutritional status of the mother is now known to influence intrauterine growth rates, birth weights and the later life risks of several important health problems. In addition, a whole host of factors influence growth and development and in turn these factors influence the health status of men in the latter decades of their lives. Vulnerability to physical ill health in childhood and later adult life is associated with poor parental socioeconomic circumstances and low levels of parental education and concern. Cross-sectional studies show differences in mortality and morbidity as a function of socioeconomic status, across various disease categories throughout the life span. Poverty has a significant impact on both life and health expectancy. It should not only be measured in terms of property, employment, wages and income, but also in terms of basic education, health-care, nutrition, water and sanitation. Educational attainment and marital status have also been shown in several longitudinal studies to be powerful predictors of morbidity, health expectancy and mortality. In addition, age, gender and socioeconomic status influence disability-free life expectancy. The economic consequences of retirement place many older citizens in positions of financial vulnerability. As populations age, in both the developing and the developed worlds, the issue becomes how to keep older persons economically viable within their respective societies. No community is exempt from the financial hardships experienced by aging populations.

The life course perspective leads to important policy and strategy decisions. Firstly, it is clearly possible and desirable to improve the health status of men when they are old, although this approach is still not fully implemented. Secondly, a complementary approach to improving the health of older men would focus on appropriate interventions at all stages of their lives. The determinants of 'aging' and of 'life expectancy' extend from genetic and molecular determinants to the increasingly powerful forces of environmental, economical, technological and cultural globalization. Specific measures for the promotion of healthy aging should include:

(1) the promotion of a safe environment;

(2) healthy life-style including proper nutrition;

(3) appropriate exercise;

(4) avoidance of smoking;

(5) avoidance of drug and alcohol abuses;

(6) social interactions to maintain good mental health; and

(7) medical health-care, including the control of chronic illnesses.

If the program is implemented effectively, it should result in a significant reduction of the costs of health and social care, reduce pain and suffering, increase the quality of life of the elderly and enable them to remain productive and contribute to the well-being of society. The medical and socioeconomic implications of the demographic reality of this new world will be very different from all preceding epochs in history, indeed so new that most people, governments, national and private pension funds, as well as most health insurers, pharmaceutical and health industries, are not yet prepared for the emerging markets. An increase in the quality of life with a delay, decrease or prevention of disabilities will increase length of productive life of aging populations, will decrease dependency, and will decrease health costs related to expensive curative and palliative services.

MEN, AGING AND HEALTH

'Before a thing has made its appearance; order should be secured before this order has begun'
Lao Tzu

It is impossible to understand aging and health without a gender perspective. Both from a physiological and from a psychosocial point of view, the determinants of health as we age are intrinsically related to gender. There is increasing recognition that unless research and programs – on both clinical science and public health – acknowledge these differences, they will not be effective. While women experience greater burdens of morbidity and disability, men die earlier, yet the reasons for such premature mortality are not fully understood. The rapidity with which the global population is aging will require a sharp focus on gender issues if meaningful policies are to be developed. Yet so often gender in the health context is taken as being synonymous only with women's issues[7].

In contrast to the recent and much needed attention to the social position and health status of women, male health concerns have been relatively neglected. Men continue to have a higher morbidity and mortality rate[7] and life expectancy for men is significantly shorter than that for women in most regions of the world[2]. The course of disease, response to disease and public response to illness exhibit gender differences and often result in different treatments and different access to health-care. The conventional approach of the medical, behavioral and social sciences to the problem of male aging has been for a long time subject to oversight, disconnection and lack of interdisciplinary collaboration.

The major causes of morbidity and mortality all take effect over extended periods. For example, DNA is constantly being damaged and repaired, bones are in a constant process of cellular loss and replacement and atheromas are constantly accumulating inside arteries, which may or may not be removed. If the rate of decay is faster then the rate of repair, healthy tissue will be lost until the damage produces symptoms and finally results in disease. Therefore, primary prevention strategies will be most effective when initiated at the earliest opportunity. Ischemic heart disease, hypertension, stroke and lung cancer are diseases whose primary prevention needs to be addressed. When diseases are more prevalent at older ages (e.g. prostate and colorectal cancers, or osteoporosis) early diagnostic tests (e.g. PSA) and screening procedures play an important role in secondary prevention and self-care strategies[8].

A significant number of male related health problems, such as changes in body constitution, fat distribution, muscle weakness, urinary incontinence, loss of cognitive functioning, reduction in well-being, depression and sexual dysfunction, could be detected and treated in an earlier stage if both physicians and public awareness of these problems was more pervasive. This could effectively decrease morbidity, frailty and dependency, increase quality of life and reduce health service costs. Women visit the doctor 150% as often as men, enabling the detection of health problems in their early stages. However, usually men cost the health services more than women since they seek medical services at a more advanced stage of disease. While women are geared to preventive care, men generally come for 'reparation'.

When discussing age-related problems, it is often difficult to separate and to distinguish between; (1) the natural aging process, primarily genetically determined (which today cannot be changed); (2) aging amplifiers determined by environmental and developmental factors (which can be modified), and (3) an acute or chronic illness or intercurrent diseases (which can be prevented delayed or cured). It must not be forgotten that aging by itself is associated with reduced productivity, decreased general vigor, as well as with increased incidence of defined diseases. These include:

(1) cardiovascular diseases;

(2) malignant neoplasm;

(3) chronic obstructive pulmonary diseases;

(4) degenerative and metabolic diseases (arthrosis, diabetes, osteoporosis);

(5) visual loss (macular degeneration, cataract);

(6) hearing loss;

(7) anxiety, mood, depression and sleep disorders;

(8) sexual dysfunction;

(9) various dementias (i.e. Alzheimer's disease); and

(10) endocrine deficiencies.

Five out of six men in their sixties have one or more of these diseases. The chronic degenerative diseases have a long latency period before symptoms appear and a diagnosis is finally made. Once the diagnosis is made, drugs may alleviate symptoms, but are not very effective in altering the underlying disease, which unfortunately usually continues to deteriorate.

Cardiovascular disease

Heart disease and stroke are the major causes of death and disability in aging men. Approximately

52 million deaths occur worldwide each year, 39 million occurring in developing countries. About one-quarter of all deaths in developing countries and half of all deaths in developed countries are attributed to cardiovascular disease (CVD). Globally, there are more deaths from coronary heart disease (5.2 million) than from stroke (4.6 million). Death rates from CVD increase dramatically with age. Within each country, age specific death rates for all CVD increase at least twofold between the age groups 65–74 years and 75–84 years in both sexes, with at least 50% higher rates for elderly men than for women. Morbidity and disability from these diseases are also high; for example, the Global Burden of Disease project estimates that by 2020, coronary heart disease and stroke will be the first and second leading causes of death. Lack of exercise, smoking and obesity are recognized risk factors for CVD. A significant relationship exists between body fat mass and both CVD and overall mortality in men. The increased mortality as observed in obese men was inversely related with physical fitness.

Malignancy

Worldwide, more than nine million people developed cancer in 1997 and more than six million died of cancer. Cancer deaths increased from 6% to 9% of total deaths from 1985 to 1997 in developing countries, but remained constant at about 21% of total deaths in developed countries. The highest mortality rate was observed for lung cancer with approximately 790 000 deaths in 1997, followed by stomach, liver, colorectal, esophageal and prostate cancer.

Prostate cancer is the most prevalent malignancy and the third leading cause of cancer death in men. In 1990, worldwide there were 193 000 deaths from prostate cancer, with 127 000 of those deaths occurring amongst men aged 70 years and over and 51 000 amongst those aged 60–69 years. Since prostate cancer is primarily a disease affecting men over 50, the global trend towards an aging population means

that the number of prostate cancer deaths is predicted to increase markedly. In the year 2020, a global increase of 393 000 deaths is expected with 359 000 of those deaths among men > 70 years and 103 000 deaths among men aged 60–69 years.

Chronic obstructive pulmonary diseases and lung cancer are not only among the most frequent problems in men, but are the most preventable. In men, 90% of all cases are attributable to cigarette smoking. These data suggest that almost every male lung cancer patient could have prevented his disease. Strategies to promote smoking cessation should be a top public priority, especially in those developing countries where aggressive marketing by the tobacco industry is not counterbalanced by adequate public health information advertisements.

Osteoporosis

Osteoporotic fractures are also becoming more frequent in men. It has been estimated that 19% of men over the age of 50 years in the USA will have one or more fragility fractures in their lifetime, also more than four million men in the USA have low bone mass and are at risk for fractures[9]. Skeletal fractures diminish quality of life, advance dependency and constitute an important public health problem. Hip fractures in men result in a higher morbidity and mortality than in women. Secondary causes such as gastrointestinal diseases with malabsorption, alcoholism and malignant diseases are common. Etiologies such as hypogonadism and/or decrease of growth hormone (GH) are frequently not diagnosed, as clinical signs are subtle. The first sign of osteoporosis is often a spontaneous fracture of the lumbar spine, proximal femur, or distal forearm after a fall. Elderly persons are at a higher risk of falling, which can be attributed to use of certain medications, alterations in balance, poor vision, loss of muscle strength and prolonged reaction times. Preventive measures should target reducing bone loss and factors that contribute to falling. One of the most cost-effective prevention strategies is an adequate intake of calcium and vitamin D, and a physical exercise program which maximizes bone mass and muscle strength[10]. Hormone replacement therapy (HRT) together with proper nutrition and targeted physical activity may postpone the appearance of osteoporosis and delay or prevent bone fractures. The loss of vision, hearing and other senses should be recognized as more than physical problems. Such conditions have profound effects on social and personal interactions, economic viability and mental health of those affected, and should be treated seriously.

Depression

Depression is the most common functional mental disorder affecting aging males, and is underdiagnosed and undertreated. It has a high rate of recurrence and is associated with significantly increased mortality. Depression is closely linked in this group with physical illness and atypical or disguised altered presentations can make diagnosis difficult. Thorough holistic assessment and good communication skills are of utmost importance. Nurses and medical professionals can improve the mental health of these patients with therapeutic attitudes and actions. It must be remembered that about 90% of older men who attempt or complete suicide have had depression either undiagnosed or inadequately treated. If men continue to underreport depression, the morbidity of this condition will continue to increase. Proper identification and treatment of depression will have significant public health implications.

Cognitive decline

Cognitive decline with age is inevitable but the overall global impairment of the higher cortical functions can be delayed. Estrogen specifically maintains verbal memory in women and may prevent or forestall the deterioration in short- and long-term memory that occurs with normal aging. There is also evidence that estrogen decreases the incidence of Alzheimer's disease, delays its onset or both[11]. The delayed onset of Alzheimer's disease in men may be due to the fact that estrogen levels are significantly higher in aging men than in postmenopausal women. In women HRT has been shown to delay the onset of Alzheimer's disease and there is an urgent need to obtain equivalent information in men. Dementia is a major public health issue accounting for significant morbidity, loss of independence, loss of dignity and eventual institutionalization. The prevalence of severe dementia increases from 1% at ages 65–74, 7% at ages 75–84 up to 25% after the age of 85. Thirty-seven per cent of patients with Alzheimer's disease live in institutions compared with 1.7% of subjects without dementia.

Sexual dysfunction

Sexual desire, arousal, performance and activity decrease significantly with age with a striking increase in the prevalence of impotence in men over 50 years. Reasons for decreased sexual activities include loss of libido (partially due to decreased androgen production), lack of partner, chronic illness and/or various social and environmental factors, as well as erectile dysfunction (ED). It has been shown that sexual information significantly and independently, contributes to sexual enjoyment and satisfaction. Persistent interest in sexual activity results in positive mental and physical health benefits. The frequency, duration and degree of nocturnal penile tumescence decreases significantly with age. These events are concomitant with a significant decrease in bioavailable testosterone and a compensatory increase in luteinizing hormone, showing that aging is associated with decreased gonadal activity.

Worldwide more than 100 million men are estimated to have some degree of ED. Erection is a neurovascular phenomenon under hormonal control and includes arterial dilatation, trabecular smooth muscle relaxation and activation of the corporeal occlusive vein mechanism. Some of the major etiologies of ED are hypertension, diabetes, depression and heart disease. It should also be remembered that genitourinary and colon surgery very often cause ED. Nerve sparing surgery, which may reduce the incidence of ED, should be used whenever possible. Patients should be counseled prior to such interventions. Many drugs, particularly anti-hypertensive, antidepressant and psychotropic drugs may cause various degrees of ED. Therefore the treatment/therapy should be carefully considered, weighing the cost and benefit for each product and each individual patient. When focusing on the maintenance of quality of life among aging men, efforts to maintain, restore or improve sexual function should not be neglected. Recent advances in basic and clinical research have led to the development of new treatment options for ED, including new pharmacological agents for intracavernosal, intraurethral and oral use. Orally acting preparations with either central action (apomorphine) or peripheral action (sildenafil) alone/or in concert with androgens have significantly improved the fate of men with erectile and or sexual dysfunction. The management of ED should only be performed following proper evaluation of the patient and only by physicians with basic knowledge and clinical experience in diagnosis and treatment of ED.

Endocrine deficiencies

Partial endocrine deficiencies of aging are associated with a decrease in the peripheral levels of testosterone, dehydroepiandrosterone (DHEA) and its sulfate (DHEAS), GH, insulin-like growth factor I (IGF-I) and melatonin. With the decline of testosterone there is a concomitant increase in LH and follicle-stimulating hormone (FSH). In addition, sex hormone-binding globulin (SHBG) levels increase with age, resulting in further lowering of the concentrations of free biologically active testosterone. With aging there is a loss of circadian rhythmicity of testosterone. These changes are associated with a decrease in;

(1) general well-being;

(2) sexual pilosity and libido;

(3) cognitive function;

(4) red blood cell volume;

(5) muscle strength;

(6) bone mass (osteoporosis) with an increased fracture risk; and

(7) immune-competence;

(8) an increase of fat mass, with a change in fat contribution and localization;

(9) an increase in cardiovascular accidents;

(10) an increase in mood and sleep disorders.

With prolonged life expectancy men and women live one-third of their life with some hormone deficiency. In cases of endocrine deficiencies, irrespective of age, traditional endocrinology aims to replace the missing hormone or substances with hormone-like action. The decision to start HRT in men should only be taken after obtaining objective evidence of hormone deficiencies, with exclusion of secondary causes of endocrine dysfunction and after making the balance of risks and expected benefits of the replacement therapy. When data from long-term well-controlled studies become available, long-term substitution therapy with one or more hormonal preparations will most probably, if used correctly, improve the quality of life of aging men and may even delay the aging process. It is probably not unrealistic that in the future HRT in men will become as common as it is in women today. It has been demonstrated that interventions, such as HRT, the use of antioxidant drugs, proper and personally tailored nutrition, with vitamin supplements whenever necessary, as well as individually adjusted regular physical activity (aerobic, anaerobic and stretching) has significant physiological, psychological and social benefits for the elderly and may favorably influence some of the symptoms of aging as well as some of the pathological conditions in aging men.

Strategies to improve and maintain aging men's health

Das Altwerden kann kein Arzt verhindern. Aber er kann- ist er gut- viel dazu beitragen die Beschwerdlichkeiten zu mildern. Johann Wolfgang von Goethe#

(Aging no physician can stop. But he can if he is good do a lot to reduce the suffering and aches of aging)

The correct strategies in the management of aging should permit men to age in health and dignity, improving their quality of life by preventing the preventable and to delay and decrease the pain and suffering of the inevitable.

Educating both the public and health-care providers about the importance of early detection of male health problems will result in reduced rates of morbidity, mortality, as well as health costs, for many age-related diseases. Many men are reluctant to visit their health center or physician through fear, lack of information and psychological reasons. For more than 100 years, gynecologists have been specialized physicians for the medical care of the woman. About 50 years ago, gynecologists understood that the women's health physician is more than an obstetrician and an 'oncology oriented surgeon', and slowly the medically oriented gynecologist evolved, trained in reproductive endocrinology, perineonatology, ultrasound, family planning and recently in assisted reproductive procedures. The training curricula (especially in the USA and UK) are constantly modified and adapted to the needs of 'women's health'. The modern gynecologist is not only cure-oriented, but has been trained in preventive strategies and in the maintenance of health and well-being, from adolescence to menopause.

The present day surgically oriented urologist has also arrived at the same crossroad gynecologists reached 50 years ago. Urologists today are highly specialized surgeons for the prostate, kidney, bladder and the urinary tract. They have become highly specialized oncologists and

diagnosticians and many have also specialized in the diagnosis and treatment of ED. Others have become nephrologists or specialists in transplantation, or andrologists specializing in gonadal physiology and pathology, and in the treatment of infertility, in collaboration with gynecologists, extracting sperm from testis or epididymis or diagnosing and managing varicoceles. Training in urology is extremely long. With surgical procedures decreasing and being replaced by medical interventions the idea of medical urologists has evolved. The number of urologists worldwide today is far too low to take care of all men. To become the 'man's health physician' they will have to receive sufficient training in endocrinology, internal medicine especially cardiology, psychology/psychiatry, they will have to be trained to give guidance on nutrition and exercise and have a solid understanding of gerontology. The International Society for the Study of the Aging Male (ISSAM) is working together with the diverse urological and andrological associations to obtain this goal.

However, until this goal is achieved and sufficient urologists/andrologists have been trained, a 'gate keeper' will be required to serve and manage male health. Those who aspire to take the role of 'gate keeper' for male health will depend on the specific training, culture and the medical services of each geographical area and country.

Male health could be managed by an interdisciplinary group practice or by the primary health worker, the family physician, the endocrinologist or a specialist in internal medicine or gerontology. Each member of this profession can be trained to become a 'gate keeper' for male health and learn to screen men for their most probable risk factors, advise them on life-style and whenever necessary refer them to the specialist they need. When a man attends his family doctor for a common cold, a gastrointestinal disorder or any other acute infection the physician should, on the basis of the family history, body constitution, life-style and risk factors, advise the patient on preventive strategies or refer him to consult the correct specialist.

CONCLUSION

Men who are educated about the value of preventative health-care in prolonging their life span, quality of life and their role as productive family members will be more likely to participate in health screening. To obtain this goal it will be necessary to:

(1) make available a group of trained medical professionals who can understand, guide, educate and manage the problems of the aging men;

(2) provide more information about the normal male aging process and to advertise and promote aging in a positive and active way. Men should receive education and be prompted to take on teaching roles themselves, leading self-help groups and advocating on behalf of their aging communities;

(3) establish programs empowering men to become well-informed, active managers of their own health and the health of their surrounding society;

(4) obtain essential epidemiological data and to intensify basic and clinical research on aging men;

(5) assess age-related nutritional needs;

(6) develop strategies for physical exercise (aerobic for maintaining cardiac function, anaerobic, targeted to specific muscle groups, and stretching); and

(7) develop and assess new and improved drugs for prevention and treatment of pathological changes related to aging.

To this end, the efforts of all governmental and non-governmental organizations to promote aging men's health on local, national and international levels must be strongly encouraged. A holistic approach to this new challenge of the 21st century will necessitate a quantum leap in multidisciplinary and internationally coordinated research efforts, supported by a new partnership between industry and governments, philanthropic and international organizations. This collaboration we hope will enrich us with a better understanding of male health and aging, permit us to help to improve the quality of life, prevent the preventable, and postpone and decrease the pain and suffering of the inevitable.

References

1. United Nations Secreteriat Department of Economic and Social Affairs Population Division. *World Population Prospects, The 1998 Revision.* ESA/P/WP 150 New York: United Nations, 1998
2. Lunenfeld B. Aging male. *The Aging Male* 1998;1:1–7
3. Lunenfeld B. Hormone replacement therapy in the aging male. *The Aging Male* 1999;2:1–6
4. World Health Organization. *International Classification of Impairments, Disabilities and Handicaps.* Geneva: WHO, 1980
5. World Health Organization. *Jakarta Declaration on Leading Health Promotion Into the 21st Century.* Geneva: WHO, 1997
6. Wilikins R, Adams OB. Health expectancy in Canada, demographic, regional and social dimensions. *Am J Public Health* 1983;73:1073–80
7. Kalache A, Lunenfeld B. Health and the aging male. *The Aging Male* 2000;3:1–36
8. Tremblay RR, Morales AJ. Canadian practice recommendations for screening, monitoring and treating men affected by andropause or

partial androgen deficiency. *The Aging Male* 1998;1:213–21

9. Jones G, Nguyen T, Sambrook PN, *et al.* Symptomatic fracture incidence in elderly men and women: The Dubbo Osteoporosis Epidemiology Study (DOES). *Osteoporosis Intern* 1994;4:277–82

10. Rudman D, Drinka PJ, Wilson CR, *et al.* Relations of endogenous anabolic hormones and physical activity to bone mineral density and lean body mass in elderly men. *Clin Endocrinol* 1994;40:653–61

11. Sherwin BB. Can estrogen keep you smart? Evidence from clinical studies. *J Psychiatry Neurosci* 1999;24(4):315–21

12. United Nations. *World Population Prospects, The 1998 Revision*. New York: United Nations, 1999

2 Screening of the aging male

Louis Gooren, MD, PhD, and Bruno Lunenfeld, MD

The traditional role of the physician is to diagnose, treat and manage disease processes. Preventive medicine has largely been the domain of public health, but over recent decades individuals have increasingly experienced a need for preventive medicine in their lives. So, an additional role for the physician emerges: the screening and counseling of subjects who are asymptomatic, without (yet) signs or symptoms of disease. The motivation of individuals to seek medical screening may vary. Some will have a family history of disease. These people expect medical examination to reveal their propensity to develop this disease, and they are prepared to take early measures to prevent or ameliorate the course of the disease. Examples are cardiovascular disease and its risk factors hypertension, lipid disorders or diabetes mellitus type 2. Others expect that early diagnosis of conditions such as cancer promise a better outcome, or even a cure of the disease. Some people feel that information about a health-risk profile permits them to plan their life better, enabling them to make important decisions before it is too late. By contrast, there are others who do not wish to have this information since it would sap the joy of their life. This group will avoid screening opportunities.

Screening usually implies physical examination, laboratory tests and sometimes basic radiological tests, with the aim of discovering or reasonably excluding subclinical disease. A positive result usually leads to a more extensive diagnostic work-up. It is impossible to screen a person for all ailments, even if this would lead to early and meaningful preventive interventions. Screening will be more or less guided by the probability of certain risks in this individuals life.

Preventive medicine can be categorized as primary, secondary and tertiary.

Primary prevention refers to general measures to prevent disease, such as cessation of smoking and dietary and exercise recommendations, in non-diseased people. It is non-individualized. Secondary prevention is the (early) detection of pathology in individuals, so as to reverse or slow the course and improve prognosis of (highly prevalent) diseases, for example by routine measurement of blood pressure or the lipid profile. Tertiary prevention includes efforts to minimize the future negative health effects of factors operating in a disease already present, for example improving lipid profiles in patients with cardiovascular disease.

VALUE OF SCREENING TESTS

Interpretation of the results of diagnostic tools in screening requires an understanding of some basic principles of epidemiology.

The sensitivity and specificity of a test are important principles in diagnostic work-ups of patients and in screening of asymptomatic individuals. The sensitivity of a test represents the proportion of patients actually having the disease who will test positive in this test (true-positive rate). The specificity of a test equals the proportion of non-diseased patients who will have a negative outcome on testing (true-negative rate); in other words, will the test miss cases who actually have the disease? In the medical practice of screening there is great interest in the predictive value of a test. This does not refer so much to the ability of a test to confirm a disease, but the ability of that test to predict the disease. Similar to the sensitivity and specificity of a test, there is a positive predictive value, or the proportion of patients with a positive test who actually (will) have the disease; and the negative predictive value of a test equals the proportion of patients with a negative test result who indeed do not have the disease; again, in other words, what is the chance that actual cases will be overlooked? The predictive value of the test is influenced by the prevalence of the disease or condition of concern.

GUIDING PRINCIPLES OF SCREENING

It goes without saying that screening can never cover all diseases and conditions from which a human being can suffer. The resources for screening all potential diseases are simply not available. So, the question arises, what principles should guide the physician in the decision to screen? Naturally, the personal and family history provide information on an individual's health risks. There are a number of general principles directing the decisions. Is the morbidity and mortality of the condition serious? Does the condition screened have an important impact on health and life expectancy of the person in question? Will it save years of life and will these years have a reasonable quality of life? The disease should be sufficiently common. It is not cost-effective to screen for very rare conditions. The disease should also have a long enough preclinical duration before it becomes clinically manifest. Disease with a rather sudden onset, such as certain forms of leukemia, are difficult to screen. There should be a certain outlook regarding an available and efficacious treatment, which can positively change the

outcome and course of the disease. The screening procedure should have a very reasonable sensitivity, specificity and predictive value. The screening tests must be acceptable to the individual. Painful and tedious diagnostic procedures are less acceptable. The procedures should also be reasonably safe. And the costs of the screening should be affordable.

INTERPRETATION OF RESULTS OF SCREENING

As indicated above, for the interpretation of the results of screening an understanding of the epidemiology and the natural course of the disease, with and without therapeutic intervention, is required. The basic tenet of screening is to do more good than harm. The test result can be a reason to refer the subject to the relevant medical specialty, but the person in question will always undergo an initial evaluation of the screening results with the physician who performed the screening. The implications of specificity, sensitivity and predictive value are indicated above. How certain can the individual be that he does not suffer from the disease if he tests negative? If tested positive, how sure is the patient that he actually suffers from the disease, and how much reason is there to undergo additional testing? Needless to say, a positive result of screening is anxiety-provoking. It is difficult to cope emotionally with the statistical data of disease probability and disease course once one has tested positive in a screening procedure. The physician who embarks on screening should have a sound understanding of the diseases screened, so he/she can counsel the patients if they test positive.

GENERAL SCREENING TESTS

It is difficult to assess infirmity associated with the aging process. Part of it will be due to 'natural aging' and part of it to emerging disease processes, which will occur increasingly with aging. 'Natural aging' and emerging diseases affect individuals to varying degrees. For instance, hormone deficiencies do not affect all men to the same degree; and hypertension and diabetes mellitus range from mild to severe. Therefore, it is useful to have tools that provide a 'grip' on signs and symptoms of aging. Such an instrument also allows assessment of the successes of interventions in this population.

Developing rate scales is a difficult venture. The validation of questionnaires is an arduous process. Translation into another language implies a new validation in that language, to test whether questions are understood and interpreted linguistically and culturally in the same way as in the original language. A recently developed instrument is the 'aging males' symptoms' (AMS) rating scale[1]. This scale measures somatic, sexual and psychological aspects of an aging male's life. Originally developed in the German language, it has now been validated for English[2] (see Appendix), while validations for other European languages are well under way. Validations in other languages and in other geographical areas are welcomed.

The androgen deficiency in aging males (ADAM) scale developed by Morley and colleagues[3] tests whether certain symptoms are more likely to be present in aging men with declining levels of bioavailable testosterone (see Appendix).

UROLOGICAL SCREENING

Lower urinary tract symptoms

Many aging men will experience urinary problems ranging from nocturia, increased frequency of micturition, urgency, hesitancy, poor stream and postmicturition dribbling to loss of bladder control resulting in incontinence, and retention. Many of these complaints were previously referred to as 'prostatism'. However, these complaints may not be caused by prostatic disease and, therefore, the term 'lower urinary tract symptoms' (LUTS) is now preferred to describe these voiding problems. The correct nomenclature may avoid premature conclusions

that the etiology of the symptoms is prostatic in origin. Polyuria, for instance, may be a symptom of diabetes mellitus.

LUTS may have a considerable impact on the quality of life of the patient. The degree of bothersomeness rather than the objective magnitude of LUTS is the indication for diagnostic and therapeutic interventions.

LUTS may be subdivided into voiding and storage problems. Voiding problems are usually due to bladder outlet obstruction or detrusor dysfunction. The storage capacity of the bladder and the detrusor contractility decrease with age. In many cases, storage complaints are related to detrusor instability.

Population studies show a frequency of moderate-to-severe LUTS of 8–31% in men in their 50s, increasing to 27–44% of men in their 70s. But many men experience LUTS much earlier in life!

Several symptom scores have been developed as tools to quantify LUTS. The best known are the Symptom Index[4] and the International Prostate Symptoms Score (IPSS)[5], both produced by task forces of the Amercian Urological Association. The specificity of these is rather low because of the non-specificity of LUTS itself as a complaint. The IPSS has therefore been criticized as lacking specificity, and also as lacking usefulness for screening, and not including symptoms such as dribbling and incontinence. Therefore, bothersomeness and disease-specific or non-specific quality-of-life indices have been added as a tool in the management of LUTS and benign prostatic hypertrophy in Barry's Impact Index (BII)[6].

Patient screening for LUTS

Physicians screening for LUTS must be aware of the heterogeneity of the condition, but the first responsibility of the physician is to exclude serious life-threatening conditions such as prostate carcinoma or carcinoma *in situ* of the bladder.

Patients with LUTS usually show few signs of disease on inspection. Palpation of the abdomen may disclose a renal mass, and palpation of the suprapubic area may reveal bladder dilatation.

Digital rectal examination

Digital rectal examination provides clues regarding signs of prostate cancer, but it includes only the posterior aspect of the prostate. Nodularity, induration or asymmetry of the prostate may be indications of cancer. But small tumors and thsoe deep in the prostate gland may go unnoticed. It also provides information on the size of the prostate, although digital rectal examination tends to underestimate prostate volume[7].

Urine analysis

A simple dipstick test to rule out urinary tract infection and hematuria is recommended. It has a low predictive value, but is simple and cheap. Also, a urine sediment test may provide valuable information on the presence of leukocytes and erythrocytes, and protein cylinders.

Measurement of serum creatinine level is indicated to rule out renal insufficiency, which may be secondary to LUTS.

Prostate-specific antigen

Prostate-specific antigen (PSA) is a serine protease released by prostatic tissue. Healthy prostate tissue produces low levels, but prostatic conditions with elevated cellular proliferation, such as benign prostatic hyperplasia (BPH) and cancer, are associated with higher levels. Also, inflammatory conditions of the prostate may be associated with (even strong) elevations of PSA value. Since PSA is also produced by normal and benign hyperplastic prostatic tissue, it lacks specificity as a prostate cancer marker.

Various assays of PSA are available and the (arbitrary!) cut-off for normal values is above 4 ng/ml. Temporary elevations of PSA occur after prostate biopsy or prostate surgery as a result of an outpouring of PSA into the circulation. However, digital rectal examination of the prostate, or ejaculation, also has a limited effect on blood levels of PSA[8]. This is pertinent information. Usually, blood sampling for PSA takes place after physical examination of the patient, which may have included a digital rectal examination.

PSA values increase with age because of an age-related increase in prostate cellular growth. Furthermore, race is a factor in the distribution of normal PSA values. Therefore, age- and race-specific normal ranges have been proposed, but their clinical usefulness has not been validated.

Unfortunately, PSA characteristics lack specificity and sensitivity and predictive value, particularly when they are mildly elevated, for instance at 4–10 ng/ml. In men with PSA values above 10 ng/ml, approximately 1/3 will have a false-positive result. In men with PSA values between 4 and 10 ng/ml, the positive predictive value is only 28–35%. Consequently, about 2/3 men tested will have false-positive results. There are also (mainly small) prostate cancers associated with PSA values below 4 ng/ml.

Usefulness of PSA measurement to detect prostate cancer

Whether men should be screened for prostate cancer is currently hotly debated (for review see reference 9). Points in case are:

(1) PSA values lack sensitivity, specificity and predictive value. Men with small prostate tumors may still have normal PSA values. Conversely, the likelihood that a man with an elevated PSA value indeed has prostate cancer is relatively low but increases with the value of PSA.

(2) Digital rectal examination has only a limited capacity to diagnose cancers. Small tumors and those deep in the gland are not recognized. So, a negative digital rectal examination of the prostate is not grounds for reassurance. If the tumor is readily palpable, it is less likely to be confined to

the prostate capsule and already has an unfavorable prognosis. In other words, 'this tumor has been detected too late to be of great value for preventive medicine and belongs already to the domain of curative medicine'. On the positive side, digital rectal examination sometimes discovers tumors associated with normal PSA values.

(3) Men with elevated PSA levels will undergo additional testing. In a large proportion of these men, particularly when PSA levels are only mildly elevated, this testing will be redundant since PSA values above normal include a high percentage of false positives. Prostate biopsies carry a certain risk of bleeding and infection.

(4) If diagnosed with cancer, what will be the next step? Can the patient and/or his urologist accept a wait-and-see policy, many times justified, or will the patient be treated with one of the available treatment modalities, all associated with considerable potential morbidity such as incontinence and erectile dysfunction, with many times an enormous impact on quality of life?

(5) The conclusion must be that, currently, there is absolutely no consensus among experts that the benefits outweigh the harms, which is the basic tenet of screening.

Practical recommendations

Screening of the aging male should include a digital examination of the prostate, and most men will expect to have their PSA value determined. Finding a prostate nodule should lead to urological examination. Subjects who have an elevated PSA level should be monitored and followed up by digital rectal examination and PSA measurements. There is evidence that, in the normal range of PSA levels, the rate of change of PSA level over time provides useful information. An annualized rate of change (or the so-called PSA velocity) of > 0.75 ng/ml per year for 2 years should lead to urological evaluation and prostate

biopsy. If the first value of PSA was > 4.0 ng/ml, then an annualized rate increase of 0.4 ng/ml should be taken as a guideline[10]. Such guidelines allow the administration of androgens to individual hypogonadal aging men with due concern for adverse effects on the prostate[11]. When aging men receive androgens and/or growth hormone, it is thought to be reasonable to screen PSA levels every 3 months for the first 12–18 months and once per year thereafter.

ASSESSMENT OF BODY MASS INDEX AND FAT DISTRIBUTION

Body mass index (body weight in kilograms divided by the square of the height in meters) provides a better parameter than body weight itself to describe the degree of obesity. There is now solid evidence that fat distribution (a large visceral fat depot) is a strong predictor of cardiovascular disease and of the development of type 2 diabetes mellitus. Visceral fat is quantitatively most reliably assessed with computerized tomography or magnetic resonance imaging, which are too costly to become methods of mass screening, and probably redundant in assessing an individual case. A number of studies document that surrogate measures provide a reasonable indication of the amount of visceral fat accumulation. Waist/hip ratio > 0.95, waist circumference > 102 cm and sagittal diameter > 23 cm (measured with the patient supine) are all indications of visceral obesity. Thse patterns of body fat distribution are also linked to a negative biochemical cardiovascular risk profile[12]. So, it is possible by simple means to determine overweight and fat distribution patterns. The above values have typically been obtained in a Caucasian population.

The World Health Organization has recently proposed revised BMI guidelines for the Asia-Pacific region[13]. In Asians, a lower cut-off of > 23.0 kg/m^2 for overweight and > 25.0 kg/m^2 for obesity is recommended. This proposal has been made in the light of the fact that, in Asian populations, morbidity and mortality tend to occur in people with lower BMIs. Alongside their proposed revision of BMI, the WHO have also recommended that the upper limits for waist circumference in the Asia-Pacific region is > 90 cm for men and > 80 cm for women as Asians tend to accumulate intra-abdominal fat without developing generalized obesity.

SCREENING FOR CARDIOVASCULAR DISEASE

Cardiovascular disease continues to be a leading cause of death, with coronary heart disease accounting for more than 50% of its mortality. One in six deaths is explained by stroke. If patients survive stroke there is usually an impaired functional capacity. A large number of risk factors for cardiovascular disease have been identified. It has sometimes been difficult to establish whether the given variable constitutes a risk factor in itself, or whether the identified risk factor is merely a marker of cardiovascular risk (for an extensive review see reference 14). On the one hand, modification of that variable may reduce a person's cardiovascular risk but on the other hand, interventions to modify the surrogate marker may not benefit the individual. Interventions aimed at modifying surrogate markers of cardiovascular risk may be useless as long as the underlying risk is not modified. Many studies of interventions in cardiovascular disease have assessed their impact on risk factors (lipid levels, blood pressure values) without measuring their effects on clinical endpoints such as cardiovascular morbidity, its disease burden and its mortality. Admittedly, studies assessing cardiovascular morbidity and mortality are difficult and expensive, but the true value of interventions can only be convincingly demonstrated if and when this intervention reduces morbidity and/or mortality.

Unless present to an extreme degree, cardiovascular disease is rarely explained by one single risk factor. It is usually multifactorial. Risk factors are additive in their effects, and many risk factors are interdependently clustered,

for example visceral obesity and insulin insensivitity, and hypertension and hyperlipidemia (syndrome X). Not all risk factors carry equal weight in their potential harm to the cardiovascular system. Variables such as elevated blood pressure or hypercholesterolemia are continuous or graded, and therefore some risk factors cannot be categorized as simply present or absent. Sometimes the absolute value is less significant than the ratio of two variables, as is the case with the ratio of total cholesterol to high-density lipoprotein (HDL) cholesterol. Most risk factors have been identified in epidemiological studies, and carry a higher predictive value for populations than for individual subjects. In other words, it is often difficult to attribute the correct weight to the presence of a risk factor in an individual unless the magnitude of that risk factor is extreme, but most patients will have moderate magnitudes of risk factors such as a mildly elevated blood pressure and mild hypercholesterolemia.

Risk factors for cardiovascular disease

There are several risk factors whose control has been shown to reduce the risk of cardiovascular disease; in the case of others it is likely that their control contributes to cardiovascular health. Non-modifiable risk factors such as age, sex and family history are not addressed, or only indirectly.

Risk factors whose control reduces cardiovascular risk

Smoking Cigarette smoking is a serious threat related to cardiovascular disease, stroke and peripheral arterial disease in a dose-dependent fashion. Smoking is linked to myocardial infarction and sudden cardiac death.

Hypertension The relationship between hypertension and cardiovascular disease is graded; in other words, there is no cut-off value below which there is no increased risk. Therefore, it is desirable also to diagnose and treat mild-to-moderate hypertension. Since mild hypertension is much more prevalent in the general population than serious hypertension, many more people die of mild hypertension than of grossly elevated blood pressure. It is estimated that 35% of all cardiovascular events are related to hypertension. The protective effect of lowering blood pressure values in hypertensive subjects is well established. Obesity, particularly visceral obesity, is a major risk factor for hypertension. The notion that 'white coat hypertension' does not reflect a person's 'true' blood pressure, and is innocent, is no longer held by experts. The fact that the blood pressure rises to abnormally high values in situations of stress is not without significance for a person's cardiovascular health. If often forebodes 'fixed' hypertension.

There is a reasonable degree of consensus on what values of blood pressure constitute hypertension. There are different schools of thought with regard to interventions. Some will deem the need for treatment more pressing if elevated blood pressure in a person is associated with other risk factors, such as lipid disorders and/or diabetes mellitus. Others will take the value of blood pressure itself as the guiding principle. The blood pressure is considered to be elevated when systolic values above 160 mmHg and/or diastolic values above 90 mmHg are found. When additional risk factors are present, the upper level of the systolic value considered to be acceptable is 140 mmHg. The blood pressure is assessed during normal medical consultations. It may require three measurements during a couple of weeks or up to five measurements over 6 months before a verdict on the presence of hypertension can be made.

Thrombogenic factors   Endothelial function is of utmost importance for maintaining a non-thrombogenic state. Inhibition of platelet clotting and of fibrinogenesis is of great significance in the prevention of thrombosis. A large number of thrombogenic factors have been identified.

It has been established that circulating levels of fibrinogen impact on the occurrence of cardiovascular disease. Low-dose aspirin inhibits thrombogenesis and thereby cardiovascular events.

Diabetes mellitus   Diabetes is associated with both macrovascular and microvascular disease through a multitude of pathogenetic mechanisms. In all likelihood, strict glycemic control is helpful in slowing the development of atherosclerosis. Many risk factors of cardiovascular disease are cumulatively present in diabetics (insulin resistance, hypertension, dyslipidemia). The presence of diabetes is sufficient reason for the aggressive treatment of other risk factors. Diabetes mellitus is certainly a modifiable disease, and therefore well worth early diagnosis. The guidelines are straightforward. If fasting glucose levels are between 6 and 7 mmol/l there is an impaired glucose tolerance, warranting follow-up every 6 months. Values above 7 mmol/l represent clinical diabetes mellitus, requiring treatment.

Physical inactivity   The impact that lack of physical fitness has on cardiovascular disease is now well established. Even moderate levels of physical activity are beneficial. It leads to an improvement of virtually all known risk factors (body weight, blood pressure, glucose tolerance, lipid profile). A consensus meeting of the National Institutes of Health in the USA has recommended regular, moderately intense exercise (at least 30 min on most or all days of the week)[15].

Cholesterol   The causal relationship between total cholesterol, and even more so between low-density lipoprotein (LDL) cholesterol, and cardiovascular disease is well established. It is a graded relationship. Levels normally present in certain Western populations might already be in the 'danger zone'. Reduction of cholesterol and particularly of LDL cholesterol reduces the occurrence of cardiovascular disease, including stroke. Therefore, determination of cholesterol level is pivotal.

High-density lipoprotein cholesterol There is a graded, continuous, inverse relationship between the level of HDL cholesterol and cardiovascular risk. Several studies document that drug treatment to improve levels of HDL cholesterol have a beneficial effect on cardiovascular mortality. Smoking, being overweight and physical inactivity all have negative effects on HDL cholesterol levels.

Triglycerides Hypertriglyceridemia is often intertwined with other risk factors such as low HDL cholesterol, visceral obesity with its associated insulin resistance, and a prothrombotic state. Therefore, hypertriglyceridemia deserves attention but often requires more comprehensive diagnostic work-up and therapy, modifying the associated risk factors as well.

Measurement of lipids Assesssment of a lipid profile includes total cholesterol, HDL cholesterol, a calculated value of LDL cholesterol and triglycerides. There is a reasonable degree of consensus that total cholesterol should be < 5 mmol/l (< 200 mg/dl), HDL > 1.0 nmol/l (> 35 mg/dl), calculated LDL < 4.0 mmol/l (< 130 mg/dl) and triglycerides < 1.8 mmol/l (< 200 mg/dl). The ratio LDL/HDL should be < 4. In terms of clinical significance, and in decisions to undertake interventions, these results should be set against other cardiovascular risk factors such as hypertension, diabetes mellitus and family history.

Lipoprotein(a) Lipoprotein(a) is an LDL particle linked to apoliprotein(a). The gene for apolipoprotein(a) has a high degree of homology with the gene for plasminogen, which has led to the theory that lipoprotein(a) may displace plasminogen from its sites of action, thereby reducing its antithrombotic capacity. It is also similar in structure to LDL and may impair endothelial function. There are no known methods of modulating lipoprotein(a) levels.

Homocysteine Homocysteine levels have been linked to cardiovascular disease; it is probably an independent risk factor. Its pathogenetic mechanism is probably interference with endothelial nitric oxide production. Its levels can be reduced by administration of folic acid and vitamins B_6 and B_{12}, but the clinical efficacy of reduction has not been demonstrated.

Screening for coronary artery disease

Exercise electrocardiography for detection of coronary artery disease is the cornerstone. Ischemia manifests itself by ST segment depression. Its accuracy is greater when the ST segment depression is associated with angina pectoris in the test. Its accuracy is less for the posterior wall of the heart. The accuracy of the test ranges between 70 and 75%. Its cost is acceptable, but its value in persons with low risk is arguable.

There are a number of screening procedures such as stress nuclear perfusion imaging, the use of electron-beam computed tomography, or the measurement of intima media thickness and of brachial artery reactivity. These can only be done in specialized centers, and are beyond the scope of this contribution.

Primary hemochromatosis

Primary hemochromatosis is a genetically determined disease occurring in approximately 1/360 men and women. The disorder is characterized by an excessive storage of iron in tissues, leading to tissue damage. Its clinical manifestations may very. The symptoms are chronic fatigue, arthralgia, infertility, erectile dysfunction, cardiac disease, diabetes mellitus and an abnormal profile of liver enzymes, a series of complaints not rare in aging men. Patients have a normal hemoglobin level but increased serum ferritin and transferrin saturation.

OSTEOPOROSIS

Few men under the age of 60–70 will suffer from osteoporosis. If a man presents with severe osteoporosis, a number of diseases should be ruled out. Alcohol abuse, glucocorticoid treatment and hypogonadism account for 40–50% of male osteoporosis. Other causes important to rule out are: hyperthyroidism (either as a disease or an overdose of thyroid hormone replacement), multiple myeloma (Kahler's disease) and other malignancies, anticonvulsants, past or present chemotherapy, and gastrointestinal disorders impairing calcium absorption. The last may be subtle in their clinical manifestations, such as gluten enteropathy. Long-term hypogonadism, rheumatic disease, chronic use of corticosteroids, alcoholism, intestinal malabsorption, renal disease, dietary factors and heavy smoking may lead to premature loss of bone. A decrease in height and vertebral kyphosis, occurring in men mostly over 60 years of age, may be a sign of vertebral osteoporosis. History and clinical evaluation are factors in the decision whether to subject the patient to bone densitometry measurement.

The most widely used techniques to measure bone mineral density are dual-photon absorptiometry (DPA), dual-energy X-ray absorptiometry (DEXA) and quantitative computed tomography. Bone mineral density is measured usually at one or more of the following sites: lumbar spine (L_{2-4}), femoral neck, proximal femur and forearm. The measurements are absolute values but, for a more meaningful interpretation, values are often expressed as T scores (the number of statistical standard deviations of the mean of a general young population of that sex) or as Z scores (the number of statistical standard deviations of the mean of a population of that sex of similar age).

By definition a bone mineral density of more than −2.5 standard deviations (SD) below the mean is osteoporosis, requiring treatment and frequent follow-up at intervals of 6–12 months. Values between −1 and −2.5 SD below the mean represent osteopenia. The elimination of risk factors and preventive treatment are indicated. In the laboratory, the level of serum calcium plus serum albumin (to which it is largely bound) must be measured. Serum levels of alkaline phosphatase (if possible bone-specific)

and osteocalcin provide an insight into the degree of bone turnover. The excretion of calcium in the urine gives information about whether an abnormal amount of calcium is lost. Hydroxyproline or deoxypyridinoline, and collagen cross-links N-telopeptide are metabolic products of bone resorption. Calcium and hydroxyproline or deoxypyridinoline can be measured in a 24-h urine sample, but a reasonably good estimate is also obtained from a 2-h sample if values are related to creatinine values in this 2-h sample.

FUNCTIONALITY AND FUNCTIONAL DEPENDENCY

Screening of the aging male will be performed across a large age-range of men. For men in their 50s functional dependency is almost never an issue; with aging it becomes, however, increasingly relevant.

Several scales have been developed to measure independent functioning. They may be divided into basic, intermediate and advanced activities. The Katz scale[16] is widely used to assess basic activities of daily living (ADL), i.e. whether a person needs help with the following activities (see Appendix):

(1) Bathing;

(2) Dressing;

(3) Transferring within the home;

(4) Toileting;

(5) Maintaining continence;

(6) Feeding.

Less basic, intermediate ADL are usually measured by the Lawton and Brody instrumental ADL scale[17] (see Appendix) assessing the person's ability to perform the following activities:

(1) Shopping;

(2) Transportation;

(3) Using the telephone;

(4) Preparing meals;

(5) Taking medications;

(6) Managing money;

(7) Performing work around the house;

(8) Doing laundry.

Advanced ADL can be measured using the scale developed by Reuben and Colleagues[18] (see Appendix):

(1) Strenuous physical activity (such as hiking, bicycling);

(2) Heavy work around the house;

(3) Number of times walks 1 mile or more without rest;

(4) Number of times walks one-quarter of a mile or more without rest;

These scales may impress as simple tools, but several studies have documented that they are highly predictive of mortality, providing better indications than most laboratory-based tests.

Intervening variables in the actual performance of ADL are muscle weakness, particularly lower extremity weakness, and cognitive impairment. Lower extremity performance can be tested rather simply[19]:

(1) Chair stands: how often can a person within 30s, with the arms crossed over the chest, stand up from a chair?

(2) Tandem stand: can a person maintain balance for at least 3 s with one foot placed behind the other on a straight line?

(3) Timed walk: a subject is asked to walk approximately 3 m, turn 180°, and walk 3 m back in a straight line without staggering or stumbling within 90 s.

These relatively simple procedures have been validated as reliable measures of functionality[19].

COGNITIVE STATUS

The prevalence of dementia at age 65 is approximately 5–10%, rising progressively to 40–50% at age 85; it is worthwhile, therefore, having an assessment of cognitive status. The medical interview itself, probing into the patient's medical history, may already reveal defects in short-term memory. For more elaborate testing, the Mini-Mental State Examination[20] is available, and if the performance is poor on this test the Short Portable Mental Status Questionnaire[21] may be used (see Appendix). Age and education influence performance at these tests.

VISUAL IMPAIRMENT

Age-related visual changes affect central visual acuity, peripheral vision, contrast sensitivity and color vision. Two common conditions, cataract and glaucoma, are essentially preventable causes of blindness. Degeneration of the macula, which reveals itself by loss of central vision, is the leading cause of poor vision in elderly men. The medical history enquires whether the patient has an impairment of vision. The Snellen Eye Chart, which patients read from 5 m using their corrective lenses, provides an impression of visual acuity. Handheld cards such as the Rosenbaum Pocket vision screener are useful alternatives for near and distant vision. Inability to read better than 20/50 with correction is an indication for specialist assessment. The Amsler grid can be used to discover visual field defects, which may be related to macular degeneration or glaucoma.

HEARING IMPAIRMENT

Hearing impairment is present in 24% of individuals between ages 65 and 74 years, and increases to 40% in those older than 75 years. Hearing loss is associated with social dysfunction, and is to a large degree underdiagnosed. Hearing aids are, strangely enough, more negatively perceived as a sign of aging than corrective eye lenses. The 'whisper test' is simple, and provides a first indication of hearing loss. The examiner stands 5 m behind the patient, who covers alternately the left and right ears. Three words are whispered, which are to be repeated by the patient. Naturally, the acoustics of the room influence the result of the test.

DEPRESSION IN OLD AGE

Poor sleep, decrease in appetite, lethargy, fatigue and difficulty concentrating may be symptoms of depression. If accompanied by suicidal thoughts, this depression is to be taken very seriously. Depressions are often related to a recent unhappy but trivial event, experienced by the patient or his environment, which is then thought to account for the depressed mood, and this may lead to a delay in diagnosing depression. Naturally, in old age, organic factors may be responsible for depressed mood, such as impairment of brain function, cardiovascular disease, metabolic factors (diabetes mellitus, renal dysfunction, hypercalcemia), and the use of medical drugs and their side-effects on biological systems. As a rating scale, Beck's Depression Inventory[22] may be helpful (see Appendix).

SEXUAL FUNCTIONING IN OLD AGE

It is common knowledge that sexual functioning declines with aging. This is substantiated by several population surveys. The interindividual difference in degree of sexual problems encountered varies strongly. So is the willingness to ask for help. In aging men, it is primarily erectile function that shows a decline with aging. Normal sexual functioning including erectile capacity presupposes an integrity of the vascular, nervous and hormonal/metabolic systems, as well as a mindset ready to engage in sexual activity. So, in the work-up of aging men, these factors must be considered. Some drugs interfere with the above factors. A recently developed multidimensional self-administered scale, validated cross-culturally, assesses five domains of human sexuality: erectile function, orgasmic function, sexual desire, intercourse satisfaction and overall satisfaction[23] (see Appendix).

Physical examination includes: cardiovascular assessment, simple neurological testing (bulbocavernosus reflex, anal sphincter tone, testicular and penile sensitivity, perineal sensation), and primary and secondary sexual characteristics (testicular volume, sexual hair, gynecomastia).

HORMONAL DEFICIENCIES IN OLD AGE

Growth hormone

It is difficult to establish who is growth hormone (GH) deficient in adulthood or at an advanced age. The pulsatile nature of GH secretion and the large number of factors determining circulating levels of GH complicate the matter considerably, in the sense that a single measurement of GH does not provide meaningful information. A single measurement of insulin-like growth factor I (IGF-I) is a reasonable first indicator of one's GH status. In subjects under the age of 40 years, a normal level of IGF-I almost excludes GH deficiency. In subjects over the age of 40 years, things are more complicated. But measuring a IGF-I value of 15 nmol/l or higher excludes a deficiency of GH. So, the problem lies with patients with values below this level. It is amazing that some patients with proven GH deficiency (on the basis of extensive endocrine testing such as insulin-hypoglycemia, growth hormone-releasing hormone level and L-dopa stimulation test) still have normal IGF-I levels. IGF-binding protein-3 is another useful index of GH status. For the time being, the combination of signs and symptoms potentially attributable to GH deficiency and an IGF-I level and IGF-binding protein-3 in the lowest third provide a reasonable indication of (relative) GH deficiency. Once placed on GH administration, individual dose titration must be done on the basis of the IGF-I levels resulting from GH administration and the occurrence of side-effects. This is aimed to produce IGF-I levels in the normal range or only slightly above normal (0–1 SD above mean levels of IGF-I). Second, if side-effects occur (flu-like symptoms, myalgia, arthralgia, carpal tunnel syndrome, edema, impairment of glucose homeostasis), GH dosage is reduced in steps of 25%. Contraindications against GH use are: type 1 diabetes mellitus, active or a history of cancer, intracranial hypertension, diabetic retinopathy, carpal tunnel syndrome or severe cardiac insufficiency.

Dehydroepiandrosterone

There is an impressive decline of the adrenal androgens with aging; plasma levels are at their peak in the 20s, and subsequently decline by 10% per decade. By age 60 years, plasma levels may be down to 30–40% of young adult levels, and by age 80 years, levels are prepubertally low again, for which the term adrenopause has been coined. There is a considerable interindividual difference in plasma levels, up to three-fold or more, persisting with increasing age. There is no consensus by far on what levels of dehydroepiandroesterone (DHEA) represent a deficiency. Levels of DHEA sulfate found in patients with primary adrenal failure are in the order of $1.0–1.5\ \mu mol/l$. Reference values of DHEA sulfate for adults are not established, but values reported in the literature for aging populations lie in the order of $2–8\ \mu mol/l$. Most studies that have established the beneficial effects of DHEA (usually 50 mg/day) have not defined cut-off values for inclusion in the study.

Testosterone

There is no consensus on normal decreased values of testosterone in old age. Therefore, we are left with arbitrary criteria. On the basis of their large samples of healthy men, young, middle-aged and old, Vermeulen and colleagues have proposed accepting the same range of normal testosterone values for elderly men as for younger men. The proposed cut-off point for low testosterone values is arbitrarily 11 nmol/l for total testosterone and 0.255 nmol/l for free testosterone. Adopting these reference values, 1% of young men have values below this threshold, and more than 30% of men over 75 years of age will be hypogonadal by these criteria[24]. Until more data are collected, for the moment this is a reasonable approach

to the vexing question of who is testosterone deficient in old age.

Another variable that might be significant in assessing androgen status in old age is plasma level of sex hormone-binding globulin (SHBG). Its level increases with aging, possibly due to a decrease in GH production and an increase of the ratio of free estradiol to free testosterone[24]. The same group[25] demonstrated that the free testosterone value calculated by total testosterone/SHBG as determined by immunoassay appears to be a rapid, simple and reliable indicator of bioavailable testosterone, comparable to testosterone values obtained by equilibrium dialysis. So, without solid criteria for testosterone deficiency in old age, the determination of values of testosterone together with SHBG might provide a reasonable index of the androgen status of an aging person.

Hypothyroidism in the aged

Hypothyroidism may be overlooked in the elderly, since the symptoms are often attributed to the aging process with its associated asthenia, effects of drug use and loss of agility. The symptoms range from weakness, chronic fatigue and decreased heart rate to dry skin, hoarseness and slower tendon reflexes. Intolerance to cold, and weight gain, may be less pronounced in the elderly. Hypothyroidism should be suspected if there are occurrences of unexplained high levels of cholesterol and creatinine phosphokinase, severe constipation, congestive heart failure with cardiomyopathy and unexplained macrocytic anemia. The best diagnostic test for primary hypothyroidism is an increased serum thyroid-stimulating hormone (TSH) level, although TSH levels in the elderly who have hypothyroidism are lower than in younger patients with the same disease.

Hyperthyroidism in the elderly

Hyperthyroidism in the elderly may have a different presentation than in younger hyperthyroid subjects. Symptoms of hyperthyroidism in the young are signs of a hyperadrenergic state: nervousness, sweating, diarrhea, tremor, tachycardia and hyperactive reflexes. In older subjects, cardiac symptoms (atrial fibrillation, cardiac insufficiency) or mental symptoms (confusion, anorexia) may be the manifestations of thyroid hyperfunction. Weight loss with anorexia is more prevalent than increased eating. Treatment with amiodarone or iodine-containing radiocontrast agents may also evoke hyperthyroidism in the elderly. The diagnosis is based essentially on elevated levels of thyroxine and free tri-iodothyronine and suppressed levels of TSH.

References

1. Heinemann LAJ, Zimmerman T, Vermeulen A, et al. A new 'aging males' symptoms' rating scale. Aging Male 1999;2:105–14
2. Heinemann LAJ, Saad F, Thiele K, Wood-Dauphinees S. The aging males' symptoms (AMS) rating scale: cultural and linguistic validation into English. Aging Male 2001;4: 14–22
3. Morley JE, Charton E, Patrick P, et al. Validation of a screening questionnaire for androgen deficiency in aging males. Metabolism 2000; 49:1239–42
4. Barry MJ, Fowler FJ, O'Leary MP. The American Urological Association Symptom Index for benign prostatic hyperplasia. J Urol 1992; 148:1549–57
5. Abrams P, Blaivas J, Griffiths D. The objective evaluation of bladder outlet obstruction (urodynamics). In Cockett A, Houry S, Aso Y, et al., eds. The Second International Consultation on Benign Prostate Hyperplasia (BPH). Channel Islands: Scientific Communications International, 1993:115
6. Barry MJ, Fowler FJ, O'Leary MP. Measuring disease specific health status in men with benign prostatic hyperplasia. Measurement Committee of the American Urological Association. Med Care 1995;33(Suppl 4):145–55
7. Roehrborn CG, Girman CJ, Rhodes T. Correlation between prostate size estimated by digital rectal examination and measured by transrectal ultrasound. Urology 1997;49: 548–52
8. Crawford ED, Schutz MJ, Clejan S. The effect of digital rectal examination on prostate specific antigen. J Am Med Assoc 1992;267: 2227–8
9. Burack RC, Wood DP. Screening for prostate cancer; the challenge of promoting informed decision making in the absence of definitive evidence of effectiveness. Med Clin North Am 1999;83:1423–42
10. Snyder PJ. Development of criteria to monitor the occurrence of prostate cancer in testosterone clinical trials. In Bhasin S, Gabelnick HL, Swerdloff RS, Wang C, eds. Pharmacology, Biology, and Clinical Applications of Androgens. New York: Wiley-Liss, 1996:143–50
11. Morales A. Andropause, androgen therapy and prostate safety. Aging Male 1999;2:81–7
12. Turcato E, Bosello O, Francesco VD, et al. Waist circumference and abdominal sagittal diameter as surrogates of body fat distribution in the elderly: their relation with cardiovascular risk factors. Int J Relat Metab Disord 2000;24:1005–10
13. World Health Organization. The Asia-Pacific Perspective: Redefining Obesity and its Treatment. Health Communications Australia Pty Ltd, Australia, 2000:56
14. Frolkis JP. Screening for cardiovascular disease. Med Clin North Am 1999;83:1339–73
15. NIH Consensus Development Panel on Physical Activity and Cardiovascular Health. J Am Med Assoc 1996;276:241–6
16. Katz S, Ford AB, Moskowitz RW. Studies of illness of the aged. The index of ADL: a standardized measure of biological and psychological function. J Am Med Assoc 1963;185:914–18
17. Lawton MP, Brody EM. Assessment of older people: self maintaining and instrumental activities of daily living. Gerontologist 1969;9: 179–84
18. Reuben DB, Laliberte L, Hiris J. A hierarchical scale exercise scale to measure function at the advanced activities of daily living (AADL) level. J Am Geriatr Soc 1990;38:855–7

19. Ostchega Y, Harris TB, Hirsch R, Parsons VL, Kington R, Katzoff M. Reliability and prevalence of physical performance examination assessing mobility and balance in older persons in the US: data from the Third National Health and Nutrition Examination Survey. *J Am Geriatr Soc* 2000;48:1136–41

20. Folstein MF, Folstein SE, McHugh PR. 'Mini-Mental State': a practical method for grading the cognitive status of patients for the clinician. *J Psychiatr Res* 1975;12:189–94

21. Pfeiffer E. A Short Portable Mental Status Questionnaire for the assessment of organic brain deficit in elderly patients. *J Am Geriatr Soc* 1975;23:433–7

22. Beck AT, Ward CH, Mendelsohn M, *et al*. An inventory of measuring depression. *Arch Gen Psychiatry* 1961;4:561–71

23. Rosen RC, Riley A, Wagner G, *et al*. The International Index of Erectile Function (IIRF): a multidimensional scale for assessment of erectile dysfunction. *Urology* 1997; 49:822–30

24. Kaufman JM, Vermeulen A. Declining gonadal function in elderly men. *Baillière's Clin Endocrinol* 1997;11:289–98

25. Vermeulen A, Verdonck L, Kaufman JM. A critical evaluation of simple methods for the estimation of free testosterone in serum. *J Clin Endocrinol Metab* 1999;84:3666–72

APPENDIX
Office procedures

Personal data
Name
Date of birth
Occupation
Marital status
Employment status

Habits affecting health
Smoking
Alcohol consumption
Non-medical drug use
Balanced diet
Self-medication (painkillers/sleeping pills)
Sleep patterns
Mobility and exercise/recreation
Depressive feelings
Stress levels and coping mechanisms/relaxation

Medical history
Past medical conditions
Present medical conditions and their follow-up
Prescription drugs – continued use warranted?

Family history
Cardiovascular disease
    (hypertension/stroke/myocardial
    infarction/lipid disorders)
Parents alive? Age at death? Cause of death
Diabetes mellitus
Prostate cancer
Other cancers

Accidents
Accident-prone
Drunken driving
Risk taking

Psychosexual situation
Depressions?
Married
In a relationship
Sex-life satisfactory

Any specific concerns of the patient himself?

Specific history with regard to diseases of the aging male

Prostate disease
Frequency of micturition? Increased?
Nocturia
Dysuria/dribbling

Osteoporosis
Previous fractures
Family history
Rheumatic disease
Calcium intake
Thyroid disease
Intestinal disease
Corticosteroid use
Alcohol consumption
Risk factors warranting bone density
    measurement?

Cardiovascular disease
History of a cardiac event
Diagnosis/follow-up/medication

Hypertension/medication
Lipid profiles ever assessed?
Smoking
Exercise tolerance/dyspnea
Cardiac arrhythmia
Angina pectoris
Nocturia/edema
Signs of peripheral arterial disease

Impaired vision and hearing

Erectile function
Morning erections
Libido
Erectile problems (always/when tired/after
    alcohol consumption)

Physical examination
Routine
Special attention to the following

Height/weight and calculation of body mass index (BMI): BMI 25–30 obesity, 30–35 obesity requiring intervention, > 35 grossly obese

Waist circumference: if > 102 cm obesity

Sagittal diameter of the abdomen: if > 24 cm visceral obesity

Assessment of muscle strength: ask patient to get five times from his chair without using hands

Blood pressure

Rectal examination

Laboratory work-up
Hemoglobin/erythrocyte sedimentation rate
Creatinine

Fasting glucose/total cholesterol/triglycerides/ high-density lipoprotein

Prostate-specific antigen

Urine: glucose/protein

Testosterone

Simple office procedures
Peak expiratory flow rate
Hand-held dynamometer

More advanced procedures
Electrocardiogram/stress electrocardiogram
Prostate ultrasound
Bone densitometry

Activities of daily living[16]

Index of Independence in Activities of Daily Living

The Index of Independence in Activities of Daily Living is based on an evaluation of the functional independence or dependence of patients in bathing, dressing, going to toilet, transferring, continence and feeding. Specific definitions of functional independence and dependence appear below the index.

A. Independent in feeding, continence, transferring, going to toilet, dressing and bathing;

B. Independent in all but one of these functions;

C. Independent in all but bathing and one additional function;

D. Independent in all but bathing, dressing and one additional function;

E. Independent in all but bathing, dressing, going to toilet and one additional function;

F. Independent in all but bathing, dressing, going to toilet, transferring and one additional function;

G. Dependent in all six functions;

Other: Dependent in at least two functions, but not classifiable as C, D, E or F.

Independence means without supervision, direction or active personal assistance, except as specifically noted below. This is based on actual status and not on ability. A patient who refuses to perform a function is considered as not performing the function, even though he is deemed able.

Bathing (sponge, shower or tub)
Independent: assistance only in bathing a single part (as back or disabled extremity) or bathes self completely.
Dependent: assistance in bathing more than one part of body; assistance in getting in or out of tub or does not bathe self.

Dressing
Independent: gets clothes from closets and drawers; puts on clothes, outer garments, braces; manages fasteners; act of tying shoes is excluded.
Dependent: does not dress self or remains partly undressed.

Going to toilet

Independent: gets to toilet; gets on and off toilet; arranges clothes; cleans organs of excretion; (may manage own bedpan used at night only and may or may not be using mechanical supports).

Dependent: uses bedpan or commode or receives assistance in getting to and using toilet.

Transfer

Independent: moves in and out of bed independently and moves in and out of chair independently (may or may not be using mechanical supports).

Dependent: assistance in moving in or out of bed and/or chair; does not perform one or more transfers.

Continence

Independent: urination and defecation entirely self-controlled.

Dependent: partial or total incontinence in urination or defecation; partial or total control by enemas, catheters, or regulated use of urinals and/or bedpans.

Feeding

Independent: gets food from plate or its equivalent into mouth (precutting of meat and preparation of food, as buttering bread, are excluded from evaluation).

Dependent: assistance in act of feeding (see above); does not eat at all or parenteral feeding.

Evaluation form

Name .... Date of evaluation ....

For each area of functioning listed below, check description that applies (the word 'assistance' means supervision, direction of personal assistance).

Bathing

Either sponge bath, tub bath, or shower.

— Receives no assistance (gets in and out of tub by self if tub is usual means of bathing).
— Receives assistance in bathing only one part of the body (such as back or a leg).
— Receives assistance in bathing more than one part of the body (or not bathed).

Dressing

Gets clothes from closets and drawers, including underclothes and outer garments, and uses fasteners (including braces if worn).

— Gets clothes and gets completely dressed without assistance.
— Gets clothes and gets dressed without assistance except for assistance in tying shoes.
— Receives assistance in getting clothes or in getting dressed, or stays partly or completely undressed.

Toileting

Going to the 'toilet room' for bowel and urine elimination; cleaning self after elimination and arranging clothes.

— Goes to 'toilet room', cleans self and arranges clothes without assistance (may use object for support such as cane, walker or wheel-chair and may manage night bedpan or commode, emptying same in morning).

— Receives assistance in going to 'toilet room' or in cleansing self or in arranging clothes after elimination or in use of night bedpan or commode.
— Doesn't go to room termed 'toilet' for the elimination process.

Transfer
— Moves in and out of bed as well as in and out of chair without assistance (may be using object for support such as cane or walker).
— Moves in or out of bed or chair with assistance.
— Doesn't get out of bed.

Continence
— Controls urination and bowel movement completely by self.
— Has occasional 'accidents'.
— Supervision helps keep urine or bowel control; catheter is used, or is incontinent.

Feeding
— Feeds self without assistance.
— Feeds self except for getting assistance in cutting meat or buttering bread.
— Receives assistance in feeding or is fed partly or completely by using tubes or intravenous fluids.

Advanced activities of daily living[18]

Self-assessed current advanced social activities health status, and mental health score at entry, by group

Social Activities
Entertain at home:
1. At least weekly
2. At least monthly
3. At least yearly
4. Less than yearly or never

Visit others at their homes:
1. At least weekly
2. At least monthly
3. At least yearly
4. Less than yearly or never

Go out to eat:
1. At least weekly
2. At least monthly
3. At least yearly
4. Less than yearly or never

Work at a hobby:
1. At least weekly
2. At least monthly
3. At least yearly
4. Less than yearly or never

Travel out of town:
1. At least weekly
2. At least monthly
3. At least yearly
4. Less than yearly or never

Do you take longer trips?
1. Without help
2. With some help
3. Do not take longer trips

Health status
1. Excellent
2. Good
3. Fair
4. Poor

The Androgen Deficiency in Aging Males (ADAM) questionnaire, developed to detect the symptom complex related to decreased testosterone levels in older men[3]

1. Do you have a decrease in libido (sex drive)?
2. Do you have a lack of energy?
3. Do you have a decrease in strength, endurance, or both?
4. Have you lost height?
5. Have you noticed a decreased enjoyment of life?
6. Are you sad, grumpy, or both?
7. Are your erections less strong?
8. Have you noted a recent deterioration in your ability to play sports?
9. Are you falling asleep after dinner?
10. Has there been a recent deterioration in your work performance?

Any man answering yes to question 1 or 7 or any other questions has a high likelihood of having a low testosterone level.

Aging Male Symptoms (AMS) Questionnaire[2]

Which of the following symptoms apply to you at this time? Please, mark the appropriate box for each symptom. For symptoms that do not apply, please mark 'none'

		Score	None 1	Mild 2	Moderate 3	Severe 4	Extremely severe 5
					Symptoms		
1.	Decline in your feeling of general well-being (general state of health, subjective feeling)		□	□	□	□	□
2.	Joint pain and muscular ache (lower back pain, joint pain, pain in a limb, general back ache)		□	□	□	□	□
3.	Excessive sweating (unexpected/sudden episodes of sweating, hot flushes independent of strain)		□	□	□	□	□
4.	Sleep problem (difficulty in falling asleep, difficulty in sleeping through, waking up early and feeling tired, poor sleep, sleeplessness)		□	□	□	□	□
5.	Increased need for sleep, often feeling tired		□	□	□	□	□
6.	Irritability (feeling aggressive, easily upset about little things, moody)		□	□	□	□	□
7.	Nervousness (inner tension, restlessness, feeling fidgety)		□	□	□	□	□
8.	Anxiety (feeling panicky)		□	□	□	□	□
9.	Physical exhaustion/lacking vitality (general decrease in performance, reduced activity, lacking interest in leisure activities, feeling of getting less done, of achieving less, of having to force oneself to undertake activities)		□	□	□	□	□
10.	Decrease in muscular strength (feeling of weakness)		□	□	□	□	□
11.	Depressive mood (feeling down, sad, on the verge of tears, lack of drive, mood swings, feeling nothing is of any use)		□	□	□	□	□
12.	Feeling that you have passed your peak		□	□	□	□	□
13.	Feeling burnt out, having hit rock-bottom		□	□	□	□	□
14.	Decrease in beard growth		□	□	□	□	□
15.	Decrease in ability/frequency to perform sexually		□	□	□	□	□
16.	Decrease in the number of morning erections		□	□	□	□	□
17.	Decrease in sexual desire/libido (lacking pleasure in sex, lacking desire for sexual intercourse)		□	□	□	□	□

Have you got any other major symptoms?   Yes □   No □
If Yes, please describe:

THANK YOU VERY MUCH FOR YOUR COOPERATION

Short Portable Mental Status Questionnaire (SPMSQ)[21]

Instructions: Ask questions 1–10 in this list and record all answers. Ask question 4A only if patient does not have a telephone. Record total number of errors based on ten questions.

+	−

1. What is the date today? _____
                                    Month   Day   Year
2. What day of the week is it? _____
3. What is the name of this place? _____
4. What is your telephone number? _____
4A. What is your street address? _____
5. How old are you? _____
6. When were you born? _____
7. Who is the President of the US now? _____
8. Who was President just before him? _____
9. What was your mother's maiden name? _____
10. Subtract 3 from 20 and keep subtracting 3 from each new number, all the way down

_____   Total number of errors

To be Completed by Interviewer

Patient's name: _____   Date _____

        Sex: 1. Male   Race: 1. White
            2. Female   2. Black
                                         3. Other

Years of education: _____   1. Grade school
                                         2. High school
                                         3. Beyond high school

Interviewer's name: _____

Mini-Mental State[20]

.... Patient

.... Examiner

.... Date

Maximum score	Score	
		Orientation
5	(　)	What is the (year) (season) (date) (day) (month)?
5	(　)	Where are we: (state) (county) (town) (hospital) (floor)?
		Registration
3	(　)	Name three objects: 1 s to say each. (Then ask patient all three after you have said them. Give 1 point for each correct answer. Then repeat them until he learns all.) Count trials and record.
		Attention and calculation
5	(　)	Serial 7s: 1 point for each correct, stop after five answers. Alternatively spell 'world' backwards.
		Recall
3	(　)	Ask for the three objects repeated above. Give 1 point for each correct.
		Language
9	(　)	Name a pencil, and a watch (2 points). Repeat the following: 'No ifs, ands or buts' (1 point). Follow a three-stage command: 'Take a paper in your right hand, fold it in half and put it on the floor' (3 points). Read and obey the following: Close your eyes (1 point). Write a sentence (1 point). Copy design (1 point).
30	(　)	Total score

Assess level of consciousness along a continuum:

alert	drowsy	stupor	coma

Instructions for administration of Mini-Mental State Examination

Orientation
1. Ask for the date. Then ask specifically for parts omitted, e.g. 'Can you also tell me what season it is?' One point for each correct.
2. Ask in turn: 'Can you tell me the name of this hospital?' (town, county, etc.). One point for each correct.

Registration
Ask the patient if you may test his memory. Then say the names of three unrelated objects, clearly and slowly, about 1 s for each. After you have said all three, ask him to repeat them. This first

repetition determines his score (0–3), but keep saying them until he can repeat all three, up to six trials. If he does not eventually learn all three, recall cannot be meaningfully tested.

Attention and calculation
Ask the patient to begin with 100 and count backwards in steps of 7. Stop after five subtractions (93, 86, 79, 72, 65). Score the total number of correct answers. If the patient cannot or will not perform this task, ask him to spell the word 'world' backwards. The score is the number of letters in correct order, e.g. dlrow = 5, dlrow = 3.

Recall
Ask the patient if he can recall the three words you previously asked him to remember. Score 0–3.

Language
Naming: show the patient a wrist-watch and ask him what it is. Repeat for pencil. Score 0–2. Repetition: ask the patient to repeat the sentence after you. Allow only one trial. Score 0 or 1. Three-stage command: give the patient a piece of plain, blank paper and repeat the command. Score 1 point for each part correctly executed.

Beck's Depression Inventory[22]

A. (Mood)
   0. I do not feel sad.
   1. I feel blue or sad.
   2a. I am blue or sad all the time and I can't snap out of it.
   2b. I am so sad or unhappy that it is very painful.
   3. I am so sad or unhappy that I can't stand it.

B. (Pessimism)
   0. I am not particularly pessimistic or discouraged about the future.
   1a. I feel discouraged about the future.
   2a. I feel I have nothing to look forward to.
   2b. I feel that I won't ever get over my troubles.
   3. I feel that the future is hopeless and that things cannot improve.

C. (Sense of failure)
   0. I don't feel like a failure.
   1. I feel I have failed more than the average person.
   2a. I feel I have accomplished very little that is worthwhile or that means anything.
   2b. As I look back on my life all I can see is a lot of failures.
   3. I feel I am a complete failure as a person (parent, husband, wife).

D. (Lack of satisfaction)
   0. I am not particularly dissatisfied.
   1a. I feel bored most of the time.
   1b. I don't enjoy things the way I used to.
   2. I don't get satisfaction out of anything anymore.
   3. I am dissatisfied with everything.

E.   (Guilty feeling)
    0. I don't feel particularly guilty.
    1. I feel bad or unworthy a good part of the time.
    2a. I feel bad or unworthy practically all the time now.
    3. I feel as though I am very bad or worthless.

F.   (Sense of punishment)
    0. I don't feel I am being punished.
    1. I have a feeling that something bad may happen to me.
    2. I feel I am being punished or will be punished.
    3a. I feel I deserve to be punished.
    3b. I want to be punished.

G.   (Self-hate)
    0. I don't feel disappointed in myself.
    1a. I am disappointed in myself.
    1b. I don't like myself.
    2. I am disgusted with myself.
    3. I hate myself.

H.   (Self-accusations)
    0. I don't feel I am any worse than anybody else.
    1. I am very critical of myself for my weaknesses or mistakes.
    2a. I blame myself for everything that goes wrong.
    2b. I feel I have many bad faults.

I.   (Self-punitive wishes)
    0. I don't have any thoughts of harming myself.
    1. I have thoughts of harming myself but I would not carry them out.
    2a. I feel I would be better off dead.
    2b. I have definite plans about committing suicide.
    2c. I feel my family would be better off if I were dead.
    3. I would kill myself if I could.

J.   (Crying spells)
    0. I don't cry any more than usual.
    1. I cry more now than I used to.
    2. I cry all the time now. I can't stop it.
    3. I used to be able to cry but now I can't cry at all even though I want to.

K.   (Irritability)
    0. I am no more irritated now than I ever am.
    1. I get annoyed or irritated more easily than I used to.
    2. I feel irritated all the time.
    3. I don't get irritated at all at the things that used to irritate me.

L.   (Social withdrawal)
    0. I have not lost interest in other people.

    1. I am less interested in other people now than I used to be.
    2. I have lost most of my interest in other people and have little feeling for them.
    3. I have lost all my interest in other people and don't care about them at all.

M.   (Indecisiveness)
    0. I make decisions about as well as ever.
    1. I am less sure of myself now and try to put off making decisions.
    2. I can't make decisions any more without help.
    3. I can't make any decisions at all any more.

N.   (Body image)
    0. I don't feel I look any worse than I used to.
    1. I am worried that I am looking old or unattractive.
    2. I feel that there are permanent changes in my appearance and they make me look unattractive.
    3. I feel that I am ugly or repulsive looking.

O.   (Work inhibition)
    0. I can work about as well as before.
  1a. It takes extra effort to get started at doing something.
  1b. I don't work as well as I used to.
    2. I have to push myself very hard to do anything.
    3. I can't do any work at all.

P.   (Sleep disturbance)
    0. I can sleep as well as usual.
    1. I wake up more tired in the morning than I used to.
    2. I wake up 1–2 hours earlier than usual and find it hard to get back to sleep.
    3. I wake up early every day and can't get more than 5 hours sleep.

Q.   (Fatigability)
    0. I don't get any more tired than usual.
    1. I get tired more easily than I used to.
    2. I get tired from doing anything.
    3. I get too tired to do anything.

R.   (Loss of appetite)
    0. My appetite is no worse than usual.
    1. My appetite is not as good as it used to be.
    2. My appetite is much worse now.
    3. I have no appetite at all any more.

S.   (Weight loss)
    0. I haven't lost much weight, if any, lately.
    1. I have lost more than 5 pounds.
    2. I have lost more than 10 pounds.
    3. I have lost more than 15 pounds.

T.   (Somatic preoccupation)
    0. I am no more concerned about my health than usual.
    1. I am concerned about aches and pains *or* upset stomach *or* constipation *or* other unpleasant feelings in my body.
    2. I am so concerned with how I feel or what I feel that it's hard to think of much else.
    3. I am completely absorbed in what I feel.

U.   (Loss of libido)
    0. I have not noticed any recent change in my interest in sex.
    1. I am less interested in sex than I used to be.
    2. I am much less interested in sex now.
    3. I have lost interest in sex completely.

Self-maintaining and instrumental activities of daily living[17]

Physical Self-maintenance Scale

A.   *Toilet*
    1. Cares for self at toilet completely, no incontinence.
    2. Needs to be reminded, or needs help in cleaning self, or has rare (weekly at most) accidents.
    3. Soiling or wetting while asleep more than once a week.
    4. Soiling or wetting while awake more than once a week.
    5. No control of bowels or bladder.

B.   *Feeding*
    1. Eats without assistance.
    2. Eats with minor assistance at meal times and/or with special preparation of food, or help in cleaning up after meals.
    3. Feeds self with moderate assistance and is untidy.
    4. Requires extensive assistance for all meals.
    5. Does not feed self at all and resists efforts to others to feed him.

C.   *Dressing*
    1. Dresses, undresses and selects clothes from own wardrobe.
    2. Dresses and undresses self, with minor assistance.
    3. Needs moderate assistance in dressing or selection of clothes.
    4. Needs major assistance in dressing, but co-operates with efforts of others to help.
    5. Completely unable to dress self and resists efforts of others to help.

D.   *Grooming* (neatness, hair, nails, hands, face, clothing)
    1. Always neatly dressed, well-groomed, without assistance.
    2. Grooms self adequately with occasional minor assistance, e.g. shaving.
    3. Needs moderate and regular assistance or supervision in grooming.
    4. Needs total grooming care, but can remain well-groomed after help from others.
    5. Actively negates all efforts of others to maintain grooming.

E. *Physical ambulation*
   1. Goes about grounds or city.
   2. Ambulates within residence or about one block distant.
   3. Ambulates with assistance of (check one): a ( ) another person, b ( ) railing, c ( ) cane, d ( ) walker, e ( ) wheelchair.
      1. ( ) Gets in and out without help.
      2. ( ) Needs help in getting in and out.
   4. Sits unsupported in chair or wheelchair, but cannot propel self without help.
   5. Bedridden more than half the time.

F. *Bathing*
   1. Bathes self (tub, shower, sponge bath) without help.
   2. Bathes self with help in getting in and out of tub.
   3. Washes face and hands only, but cannot bathe rest of body.
   4. Does not wash self but is co-operative with those who bathe him.
   5. Does not try to wash self and resists efforts to keep him clean.

Instrumental Activities of Daily Living Scale

A. *Ability to use telephone*
   1. Operates telephone on own initiative. Looks up and dials numbers, etc.
   2. Dials a few well-known numbers.
   3. Answers telephone but does not dial.
   4. Does not use telephone at all.

B. *Shopping*
   1. Takes care of all shopping needs independently.
   2. Shops independently for small purchases.
   3. Needs to be accompanied on any shopping trip.
   4. Completely unable to shop.

C. *Food preparation*
   1. Plans, prepares and serves adequate meals independently.
   2. Prepares adequate meals if supplied with ingredients.
   3. Heats and serves prepared meals, or prepares meals but does not maintain adequate diet.
   4. Needs to have meals prepared and served.

D. *Housekeeping*
   1. Maintains house alone or with occasional assistance (e.g. 'heavy work-domestic help').
   2. Performs light daily tasks such as dishwashing, bedmaking.
   3. Performs light daily tasks but cannot maintain acceptable level of cleanliness.
   4. Needs help with all home-maintenance tasks.
   5. Does not participate in any housekeeping tasks.

E. *Laundry*
   1. Does personal laundry completely.
   2. Launders small items: rinses socks, stockings, etc.
   3. All laundry must be done by others.

F. *Mode of transportation*
1. Travels independently on public transportation or drives own car.
2. Arranges own travel via taxi, but does not otherwise use public transportation.
3. Travels on public transportation when assisted or accompanied by another.
4. Travel limited to taxi or automobile with assistance of another.
5. Does not travel at all.

G. *Responsibility for own medications*
1. Is responsible for taking medication in correct dosages at correct time.
2. Takes responsibility if medication is prepared in advance in separate dosages.
3. Is not capable of dispensing own medication.

H. *Ability to handle finances*
1. Manages financial matters independently (budgets, writes, checks, pays rent, bills, goes to bank), collects and keeps track of income.
2. Manages day-to-day purchases, but needs help with banking, major purchases, etc.
3. Incapable of handling money.

Individual items of International Index of Erectile Function Questionnaire and response options[23] (US version)

Question	Response options
1. How often were you able to get an erection during sexual activity?	0 = No sexual activity
	1 = Almost never/never
2. When you had erections with sexual stimulation, how often were your erections hard enough for penetration?	2 = A few times (much less than half the time)
	3 = Sometimes (about half the time)
	4 = Most times (much more than half the time)
	5 = Almost always/always
3. When you attempted sexual intercourse, how often were you able to penetrate (enter) your partner?	0 = Did not attempt intercourse
	1 = Almost never/never
	2 = A few times (much less than half the time)
4. During sexual intercourse, *how often* were you able to maintain your erection after you had penetrated (entered) your partner?	3 = Sometimes (about half the time)
	4 = Most times (much more than half the time)
	5 = Almost always/always
5. During sexual intercourse, *how difficult* was it to maintain your erection to completion of intercourse?	0 = Did not attempt intercourse
	1 = Extremely difficult
	2 = Very difficult
	3 = Difficult
	4 = Slightly difficult
	5 = Not difficult
6. How many times have you attempted sexual intercourse?	0 = No attempts
	1 = One to two attempts
	2 = Three to four attempts
	3 = Five to six attempts

4 = Seven to ten attempts
5 = Eleven+ attempts

7. When you attempted sexual intercourse, how often was it satisfactory for you?

0 = Did not attempt intercourse
1 = Almost never/never
2 = A few times (much less than half the time)
3 = Sometimes (about half the time)
4 = Most times (much more than half the time)
5 = Almost always/always

8. How much have you enjoyed sexual intercourse?

0 = No intercourse
1 = No enjoyment
2 = Not very enjoyable
3 = Fairly enjoyable
4 = Highly enjoyable
5 = Very highly enjoyable

9. When you had sexual stimulation *or* intercourse, how often did you ejaculate?

10. When you had sexual stimulation *or* intercourse, how often did you have the feeling of orgasm or climax?

0 = No sexual stimulation/intercourse
1 = Almost never/never
2 = A few times (much less than half the time)
3 = Sometimes (about half the time)
4 = Most times (much more than half the time)
5 = Almost always/always

11. How often have you felt sexual desire?

1 = Almost never/never
2 = A few times (much less than half the time)
3 = Sometimes (about half the time)
4 = Most times (much more than half the time)
5 = Almost always/always

12. How would you rate your level of sexual desire?

1 = Very low/none at all
2 = Low
3 = Moderate
4 = High
5 = Very high

13. How satisfied have you been with your overall *sex life*?

14. How satisfied have you been with your *sexual relationship* with your partner?

1 = Very dissatisfied
2 = Moderately dissatisfied
3 = About equally satisfied and dissatisfied
4 = Moderately satisfied
5 = Very satisfied

15. How do you rate your *confidence* that you could get and keep an erection?

1 = Very low
2 = Low
3 = Moderate
4 = High
5 = Very high

3 Laboratory tests in the endocrine evaluation of aging males

Jos H. H. Thijssen, PhD

INTRODUCTION

The demographic changes taking place in our society predict that the proportion of people over the age of 65 years will increase all over the world. The increase in average length of life has enormous consequences for all countries because of the increase of older people within a society. Although already many people of more than 65 years live in Western societies, the expectation is that in future more than one in four individuals will be over that age[1]. Therefore, the increasing interest in studies of aging can be well understood.

In general the endocrinology of aging is focusing on those hormonal systems that show age-related changes – decreases in circulating hormone concentrations[2]. There are three of these systems:

(1) Sex steroids, i.e. estrogens in women (menopause) and testosterone in men (andropause);

(2) Dehydroepiandrosterone (DHEA) and its sulfate (DHEAS) (adrenopause);

(3) Growth hormone (GH) and insulin-like growth factor I (IGF-I) (somatopause).

In this contribution attention will be given to hormones involved in the regulation of these three systems; no specific details will be given on other, clinically very important endocrine functions, such as those related to thyroid dysfunction or diabetes. Furthermore, sex steroids will be discussed extensively with the exception of estrone, progesterone and 17-hydroxy-progesterone, as these steroids hardly play a role in investigations in older males.

SEX STEROIDS

Androgens

Testosterone is not the only androgen in the male. Several other steroids have androgenic properties and they originate from different sources – the testis and the adrenal glands. Therefore, some relationships exist between the first two systems mentioned. Evidence has been presented that the secretion of hormones with androgenic activity by both of these two glands shows a major decrease with aging. Andro-stenedione is an exceptional steroid with androgenic activity, as it originates partly from the gonads and partly from the adrenals. Its production does not show the large age-related changes of DHEAS and/or testosterone. The production of cortisol, the most important hormone produced by the adrenals, does not show a decrease in its concentration in blood with aging.

DHEAS   DHT

↑↓   ↑

DHEA → Androstenedione ↔ Testosterone

Figure 1 Names and interconversions of the major androgens in the human. The arrows illustrate the peripheral interconversions of these steroids. Some of the reactions are reversible; others can proceed in both directions, as indicated by the arrows. DHEA, dehydroepiandrosterone; DHEAS, DHEA sulfate; DHT, dihydrotestosterone

After secretion from the producing gland, androgens can be converted peripherally into more or less active compounds. This is illustrated in Figure 1. One of the serious problems in attempting to gather information on the effective biological activity of androgens in an individual is the fact that part of the illustrated conversions can take place inside a target cell and the produced metabolite can have its action inside the same cell (so-called intracrine activity). For instance, the activation of testosterone to 5α-dihydrotestosterone (DHT) that takes place in cells of the prostate will not be reflected as a change in the concentration of DHT in the blood.

Dehydroepiandrosterone and its sulfate

Ample evidence has been published on the decrease of these adrenal androgens after the age of 30 years[3]. Based on its strong binding to albumin, the half-life of DHEAS in blood is very long and, as a consequence, its concentration in blood is very high; it is present in micromolar concentrations. The free DHEA is derived partly from the continuous conversion of the sulfate to the free form, a reaction occurring in many parts of the human body. Evaluation of the concentration of the adrenal androgens is most commonly performed by measurement of the concentration of DHEAS in blood. Because of its high concentration, measurement by immunoassay is relatively simple, whereas the specific determination of free DHEA requires an extensive chromatographic

pre-purification and therefore is labor intensive. There are no indications that the specific determination of the free DHEA has any advantage over measurement of DHEAS, except during dynamic studies when, for instance, the secretion of DHEA in the adrenals is stimulated. Then, the free DHEA shows an increase within a short period of a few hours, whereas DHEAS does not.

For the measurement of DHEAS, several sets of commercial reagents are available. Inspection of the reported results for DHEAS in external quality assessment schemes (EQAS) of several European countries shows that, during the year 2000, interlaboratory variation had a coefficient of variation of between 10.6 and 14.8% at concentrations between 3.7 and 15.6 μmol/l. Within one laboratory using one set of reagents, the coefficient of variation is smaller; variations of 5–8% can be expected. This indicates that the systematic differences in concentrations of DHEAS measured by different kits are reasonably acceptable.

The concentration of DHEA can be measured by competitive immunoassay only after extraction and chromatographic purification of the extract, necessitated by the much lower concentration of DHEA (nmol/l) in blood and the high concentrations of steroids that can interfere in the assay. No data are available of studies comparing the results of assays of DHEA as performed in different laboratories. In general, within the same laboratory a coefficient of variation of less than 10% can be expected.

Androstenedione

Less attention has been paid to the measurement of androstenedione, mainly because of its unknown role in male health. The concentrations of around 5 nmol/l can be measured by competitive immunoassays, and several kits are on the market. Data on the comparability of these kits are scarce, but during the year 2000 interlaboratory comparisons showed

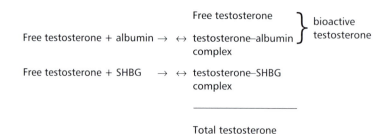

Figure 2 Different forms of testosterone in blood, and their relationships. SHBG, sex hormone binding globulin

a coefficient of variation of 13–18% at concentrations over 10 nmol/l and of 22–38% at physiological concentrations of 4–7 nmol/l. This indicates that interlaboratory comparisons show an unacceptable variation for this steroid.

Testosterone

The most important circulating androgen in the male is present in different forms because of its binding to two proteins, as illustrated in Figure 2. The most important binding protein is sex hormone binding globulin (SHBG), which has a high affinity for testosterone. In general, the hypothesis on the biological significance of the free hormones is supported by data for testosterone, indicating that the biological effects of testosterone bound to SHBG are much less than that of the free (i.e. non-protein-bound) hormone. The binding of testosterone to albumin is much less effective. Dissociation is supposed to occur rapidly, and therefore the expression 'bioactive testosterone' has been adopted, being the sum of free plus albumin-bound testosterone. Evaluation of the bioactive testosterone in individual subjects is of importance.

Some reagents have been developed for the measurement of the free or the bioactive testosterone, but in practice the results of these determinations have been disappointing because of insufficient specificity of the assays.

Free testosterone This can be measured with highly specific but time-consuming dialysis techniques. They have real value for the establishment of the 'true free testosterone'

concentrations in samples. As a more practical alternative for the determination of free testosterone, it has, for a long time, been calculated from the combined measurement of total testosterone, albumin and SHBG. Already 30 years ago, these three determinations allowed an accurate measurement of the 'true free testosterone'. A recent comparative study clearly showed that its calculation after measurement of total testosterone and SHBG was highly reliable[4], and that measurement of albumin was needed only occasionally, in patients with specific disorders affecting its concentration. In the Appendix a short description of the calculation of free testosterone from total testosterone and SHBG is given. In practice this formula is easy to program in any computer; in a spreadsheet the calculation can be performed in seconds.

Total testosterone This can be measured by competitive immunoassays, and many different sets of commercially available reagents have been developed. More recently developed assays utilize direct methods, without pre-purification of testosterone present in serum, but many investigators still rely on measurements after extraction of testosterone from serum and subsequent quantitative analysis. By the usually used extraction techniques, the possible interference of SHBG in the reaction can be prevented; in direct assays chemical blockers of testosterone binding to SHBG are being used.

A serious problem in clinical practice is the fact that the variation in results obtained

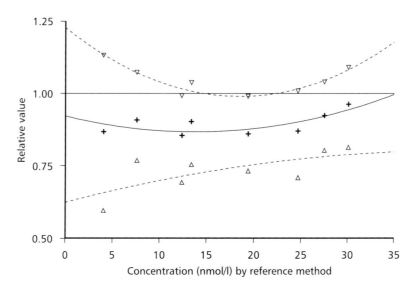

Figure 3 Median (+), 16th (Δ) and 84th (∇) centiles of results of testosterone measurements in external quality assessment schemes' samples during the year 2000. The results are compared with the 'true testosterone' values as measured by a reference method using gas chromatography mass spectrometry

with different methods is quite high, so that inter-laboratory variation is quite large[5]. Inspection of data recorded during the year 2000 for EQAS of testosterone shows that the coefficient of variation varies between 11 and 16% at concentrations, as in males, of more than 10 nmol/l, but it increases rapidly at lower concentrations, to reach more than 50% at levels of 2–3 nmol/l, as seen in children, women and hypogonadal males. Within one laboratory, the interassay variation can be lower than 5%, and therefore significant systematic variations in results as obtained by different sets of reagents are predictable. However, data on reproducibility do not give information on the accuracy of the different assays.

For information on the accuracy of testosterone determinations, results have been used of the EQAS as conducted by the German Society of Clinical Chemistry (Deutsche Geselschaft für Klinische Chemie, DGKC) during the year 2000. The reason for the use of these data is the fact that the samples distributed by the DGKC have been analyzed with a highly sophisticated 'reference method',

using gas chromatography mass spectrometry after extensive pre-purification and derivatization. This reference method gives results very close to the true concentrations of total testosterone. Figure 3 shows the results for testosterone as obtained in a varying number of laboratories (h = 229–535) that did report values for testosterone in the distributed samples. In this figure the median of the values reported is given for each of eight samples, together with the 16th and 84th centiles, similar to a standard deviation when the population has a Normal distribution. It can be concluded that a very large proportion of the reported results are lower than the true testosterone concentrations.

Separate analysis of the results obtained with the five most popular kits (each used by at least 20 laboratories) revealed that, in the concentration range of 5–30 nmol/l, the medians of the reported results were very slightly (< 5%) above the true concentrations in only three out of 40 results. However, 15 out of 40 median results were lower than 90% of the true values, indicating that indeed a large proportion of the available assays do have a negative bias, values reported being too low. Some of the popular kits show a negative bias of around 25% over the whole range of 5–30 nmol/l.

The reference values and the cut-off values for testosterone in the literature have often been obtained using older assays, which in practice give concentrations very close to the true testosterone values. The conclusions can only be that, for the interpretation of a reported testosterone concentration, it is necessary to obtain information on the performance of the reagents used to measure total testosterone. Therefore, reference values must be established locally, based on the technology used at each site. Extrapolation from data in the literature may be disadvantagous for the patient.

The second parameter needed to calculate free testosterone is SHBG. Measurement of SHBG is done by immunometric methods, utilizing two specific antibodies against different parts of the molecule. At concentrations of 30–50 nmol/l, interlaboratory variation was 9–12% over the year 2000, indicating that the agreement between laboratories is reasonable; at SHBG concentrations of more than 60 nmol/l a somewhat higher variation of about 15% was seen.

Taking the data on interlaboratory variation together, the conclusion is that the use of free testosterone values with concentrations obtained in one laboratory will probably be acceptable, with an interassay variation of < 10%, but that the use of data obtained from different sources should be avoided unless comparative results can be provided.

Measurement of salivary testosterone may become an alternative to free testosterone, because these testosterone concentrations in the male are supposed to be a close reflection of free testosterone values. The main problem is that no commercial reagents are available for the determination of testosterone in saliva, and therefore no data can be given on the comparability of the testosterone concentrations in saliva. In a research setting salivary testosterone may be very helpful, but results of further investigations are needed before salivary testosterone can become an alternative to the calculation of free testosterone on the basis of total testosterone and SHBG measurements.

Estrogens

Estradiol in the male attracts attention because there are some arguments for a specific role of estradiol, particularly in the elderly male. However, at least part of this possible role is played by estradiol generated inside some cells, the intracrine effects, and therefore there is less need for the determination of estradiol in blood. A serious problem exists in the measurement of estradiol, because of its very low concentrations in the blood of males, which means that none of the commercially available determinations is capable of measuring estradiol with an acceptable precision and with a reasonable degree of accuracy. To date, only assays using extraction and chromatographic purification prior to measurement by radioimmunoassay have given reliable information.

PROTEIN HORMONES

Luteinizing hormone

In a recent review[6] the measurement of luteinizing hormone (LH) is considered to be an important parameter in the investigation of patients with suspected hypogonadism. Measurement of LH takes place with immunometric assays and the EQAS data clearly show systematic differences between commercial assays. In particular, some of the assays based on chemiluminescence yield concentrations that deviate from other determinations. Overall, during the year 2000, interlaboratory variations of 11–27% were found at LH concentrations of 5–35 IU/l. There are indications of diverging standardization of some of the kits, although all of them declare results using the same International Reference Preparation. These data again point to the fact that extrapolated values from the literature can be used only after careful checking of the methods that have been used for the measurements.

For LH, no 'true values' are available, therefore it is impossible to give information on the accuracy of the determinations used in clinical practice. It is even possible that no 'true values' exist for the glycoprotein LH, as the measured 'total' LH is composed of several compounds, the so-called glycoforms of the polypeptide, differing in the amount and composition of the carbohydrate moieties attached to the peptide backbone. The immunoreactivity of these glycoforms probably shows variations in different methods. There are speculations that the composition of these glycoforms in blood differs between individuals and that this may change under certain pathophysiological conditions.

Follicle stimulating hormone

Determination of follicle stimulating hormone (FSH) is less important in the hormonal evaluation of aging males, but it does play a role. Similarly to the remarks on LH, EQAS data show that there are probably some differences in the standardization of different methods for the determination of this hormone as well. However, in general the problems are smaller for FSH; at concentrations of 6–42 IU/l, variations of 10–13% were found during the year 2000.

Prolactin

High prolactin levels have diagnostic value in the evaluation of hypogonadal males. This hormone is measured by immunometric assays that show systematic differences in the reported concentrations in blood. At the diagnostic level of about 0.6 IU/l, interlaboratory variation, as judged by EQAS data, is over 20%, partly dependent on differences in standardization of

the reagents. This means that extrapolation of data from the literature is not acceptable; the local laboratory should provide its own data on the performance of its determination.

Growth hormone and insulin-like growth factor I

As stated in the introduction, a decrease in the secretion of GH with age has been documented. Measurements of GH are mainly used in the clinical evaluation of children with short stature and in the diagnosis of acromegaly in adults. Nevertheless, it is realistic to consider determinations of GH in elderly subjects. The large circadian variations in the levels of GH preclude the use of single measurements. Stimulation tests are used to investigate the functioning of the GH axis. As an alternative, IGF-I can be measured because GH stimulates the liver to produce IGF-I and plasma levels of IGF-I reliably reflect the amount of stimulation by GH. Furthermore, IGF-I does not show a circadian rhythm, because of its significant protein binding to at least six different specific binding proteins.

The determination of GH is by immunometric assays that give systematic differences in results, especially at the very low levels of GH in children with a GH deficiency. Attempts have been made to improve the interlaboratory comparability; during the year 2000 the interassay variation was under 20% at levels of 5 mIU/l (2.5 ng/ml). IGF-I is also measured by immunometric assays using different substances to liberate IGF-I from its binding proteins. Few data are available on interlaboratory comparisons; available data show an appreciable variation of 20–25% at levels of 25 nmol/l, a normal concentration in adults. Again, this variation seems to be due to differences in standardization.

Additional hormones that may become of importance for the endocrine evaluation of aging males include determinations of inhibin-B[7], to evaluate Sertoli cell function, and melatonin[8]. However, no data on interlaboratory variation of these substances are available.

CONCLUSION

Hormonal evaluation in aging males will require determinations of several different hormones. The intention of this contribution has been to illustrate the problems arising from comparisons between results obtained in different laboratories. For some of the examples given, improvements in interlaboratory variation have been demonstrable over the past decade. It can be expected that continuous efforts will result in reliable determinations that are not only precise but also more accurate than the methods available at this time.

References

1. Diczfalusy E. The demographic revolution and our common future. *Maturitas* 2001;38:5–15
2. Lamberts SWJ, van den Beld AW, van der Lely A-J. The endocrinology of aging. *Science* 1997;278:419–24
3. Vermeulen A. Physiopathology of dehydroepiandrosterone and its sulfate. In Thijssen JHH, Nieuwenhuyse H, eds. *DHEA: a Comprehensive Review*. Carnforth, UK: Parthenon Publishing, 1999:13–35
4. Vermeulen A, Verdonck L, Kaufman JM. A critical evaluation of simple methods for the estimation of free testosterone in serum. *J Clin Endocrinol Metab* 1999;84:3666–72
5. Klee GG, Heser DW. Techniques to measure testosterone in the elderly. *Mayo Clin Proc* 2000;75(Suppl):S19–25
6. Kandeel FR, Koussa VKT, Swerdloff RS. Male sexual function and its disorders: physiology, pathophysiology, clinical investigations and treatment. *Endocr Rev* 2001;22:342–88
7. Mahmoud AM, Goemaere S, De Bacquer D, *et al.* Serum inhibin B levels in community-dwelling elderly men. *Clin Endocrinol* 2000; 53:141–7
8. Cornélissen G, Halberg F, Burioka N, *et al.* Do plasma melatonin concentrations decline with age? *Am J Med* 2000;109:343–5

APPENDIX

Calculation of free testosterone (FTe) from total testosterone (Te) and sex hormone binding globulin (SHBG) concentrations.

Concentrations of Te (= a) and SHBG (= b) in nmol/l.

Use the known association constant of Te to albumin at 37°C (3.6×10^4 l/mol), the concentration of albumin (43 g/l = 6.2×10^{-4} mol/l) and the association constant of Te to SHBG at 37°C (10^9 l/mol).

$$Te = FTe + [Te \times albumin] + [Te \times SHBG]$$
$$[Te \times albumin] = [3.6 \times 10^4] [6.2 \times 10^{-4}]$$
$$= 22 \times FTe$$
$$[Te \times SHBG] = FTe \times b / (1 + FTe)$$

Calculate first additonal factor D = (23 + b – a)

Calculate second additional factor E = SQRT ($D^2 + 92 \times a$)

FTe = 21.7 (E – D) in pmol/l.
Bioactive Te = FTe + [Te × albumin] = 23 × FTe in pmol/l (× 0.001 in nmol/l).

Example

At a Te concentration of 20 nmol/l and SHBG of 40 nmol/l this will result in a FTe of 390 pmol/l and bioactive Te of 8970 pmol/l = 8.97 nmol/l.

At 30 nmol/l for Te and 40 for SHBG, the FTe will become 630 pmol/l.

Section II

Genitourinary system

Claude C. Schulman, MD

Genitourinary diseases increase in prevalence with aging, and with the significant increase in life expectancy, the majority of men will probably be affected by a genitourinary disease during their lifetime. This has a major impact on public health resources.

In most Western countries men live an average of 5.8 years less than women. Education and awareness of male health problems for both the public and healthcare providers, and early detection of these problems, will eventually result in reduced rates of morbidity and mortality, as well as reduced health costs for these diseases. Indeed, men visit the doctor 150% less than women for a variety of reasons, including fear, lack of information, a greater emphasis on performance rather than longevity, and a natural tendency to be a 'risk taker'. Significant numbers of male health problems, such as prostate cancer (the most frequent cancer in men), benign prostatic hypertrophy, testicular cancer, incontinence, erectile dysfunction and various endocrine problems could be diagnosed and treated if men's awareness of these problems was greater.

Prostate cancer is the most common malignancy affecting men beyond middle age, and is the second most common cause of cancer death after lung tumours. This type of cancer usually has a slow growth rate; the lifetime risk of developing clinical cancer is about 10% and the risk of dying from the disease is about 3%. One out of eleven men will present with clinical prostate cancer. The widespread early detection programmes during the past decade have led to an absolute increase in the incidence of prostate cancer diagnosed at an earlier age and earlier stage. Hence, it is projected that more than one million men will be diagnosed with prostate cancer in the USA during the next 3 years. Age is the strongest predictor of the development of prostate cancer, and as a result of the world-wide trend towards an aging population, the incidence of clinical prostate cancer is predicted to increase very significantly.

Benign prostatic hypertrophy is one of the most common conditions affecting men after the age of 60 years, with about 40% of men showing symptomatic disease. Of these, about 17% between 50 and 59 years, 27% between 60 and 69 years, and 35% between 70 and 79 years, will need some form of treatment.

Erectile dysfunction has been shown in the last 20 years to be predominantly of organic etiology with a strong psychological impact. The probability of complete erectile dysfunction almost triples between the fifth and the seventh decade of life, affecting 5% of men over age 40, 10% of men in their sixties and 20% of men in their seventies. These figures suggest that some 20 million men in the USA may suffer from erectile dysfunction, with a similar prevalence among men in Europe. In the last couple of years, the treatment of erectile dysfunction has been revolutionized by new pharmacological approaches offering a simple and effective treatment for the vast majority of these men.

Testicular cancer is the most common cancer in men aged between 25 and 34 years. It is estimated that one man in 500 may develop testicular cancer by the age of 50. Provided that they are diagnosed at an early stage and treated adequately, the majority of these affected men will survive this disease due to successful combinations of different forms of treatment.

Incontinence which affects between 20–30% of women over the age of 60 years also affects men significantly after their seventies, and can be a severely dehabilitating condition.

In conclusion, education of both patients and healthcare providers on the importance of early detection of male health problems, and more specifically urological diseases, will result in reduced morbidity and mortality, as well as in a reduction of health costs and impact on the community.

4 Benign prostatic hyperplasia

Simon R. J. Bott, FRCS, and
Roger S. Kirby, MA, MD, FRCS (Urol), FEBU

INTRODUCTION

Benign prostatic hyperplasia (BPH) is the most common benign human neoplasm. Most men will live to an age where they have an 88% chance of developing histological BPH and a more than 50% chance of being symptomatic from benign prostatic obstruction (BPO)[1]. BPH seldom reduces the duration of a man's life, but it may impact heavily on his quality of life and on those closest to him.

The demand for medical intervention in BPH is increasing. The population of the Western world is aging such that, at birth, a man now has a life expectancy of over 73 years. Furthermore, the media and the Internet have heightened the awareness of BPO as a treatable condition, rather than an inevitability of old age as previously presumed.

While surgery remains the mainstay of treatment for symptomatic BPH, medical therapies are increasingly used, with proven effect. Patients often favor a tablet over an operation. Likewise, those that control the purse-strings perceive medical treatment as a cheaper alternative. This may or may not be true for two reasons. First, more men receive treatment than if surgery was the only treatment option. Second, some men start medical therapy that subsequently fails and then require a definitive surgical procedure, such as transurethral resection of the prostate (TURP). This phenomenon is termed the therapeutic cascade. Cost for medical treatment and the TURP must then be met rather than the cost of the TURP alone. From a health-care point of view, more men receiving treatment should reduce the incidence of lower urinary tract symptoms (LUTS) in the community as a whole. Furthermore, the therapeutic cascade is often favored by the patient who appreciates the stepwise approach to his care.

Prostate research is at an all-time high. Both the prevalence of BPH and its impact on men's quality of life have fueled the public's demand for newer, better treatments.

ETIOLOGICAL FACTORS

Inherited and environmental factors are implicated in the etiology of BPH. Prostatic enlargement appears to run in families, which suggests it is to some degree inherited[2]. Asian people have a lower incidence than white individuals, unless they migrate to the Western world where the incidence of BPH closely matches that of their white compatriots[3]. Furthermore, the incidence of BPH in Japan is rising as the Western diet becomes more popular there.

A large number of dietary components have been examined as causative agents for BPH. High-fat diets increase serum prolactin, which has a proliferative effect on the prostatic epithelium. Alcohol consumption of 25 oz or more per month may reduce the risk of surgery, as alcohol reduces serum testosterone[3].

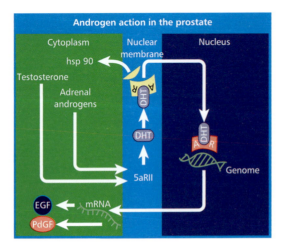

Figure 1 Androgen action in the prostate

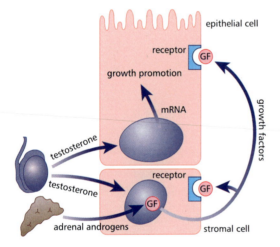

Figure 2 Growth factors promoting benign prostatic hyperplasia (BPH)

PATHOGENESIS

The development of BPH is a complex process that is not fully understood. What is clear is that aging and the hormone dihydrotestosterone (DHT) play a key role.

Dihydrotestosterone is a metabolite of the male sex hormone testosterone (Figure 1). Serum free testosterone levels fall with aging, whereas estrogen levels remain the same. This acquired endocrine imbalance may trigger BPH.

What is interesting is that if a man is castrated before puberty he will not develop BPH. However, if a man with BPH is castrated, the BPH does not necessarily regress, implying androgens have a role in initiating but not maintaining BPH.

The role of DHT in prostate development is elegantly demonstrated by a small population of men living in the village of Salinas in the Dominican Republic[4]. They have a congenital deficiency of the enzyme 5α-reductase that converts testosterone into DHT. They are capable of all the testosterone-dependent functions, such as the development of normal secondary sexual characteristics, but without DHT their prostates remain vestigial and they retain their hairline. Furthermore, they never develop BPH, unless DHT is administered.

Dihydrotestosterone binds to androgen receptors and stimulates the production of local growth factors (Figure 2). These include epidermal growth factor (EGF), fibroblast growth factor (FGF) and transforming growth factor (TGF). The precise role these factors play in BPH remains elusive. However, they normally control cell division and cell death (apoptosis); when an imbalance occurs, the rate of cell division exceeds the rate of cell death and this may lead to hyperplasia.

PATHOPHYSIOLOGY

The prostate lies between the neck of the bladder and the urogenital diaphragm, and in man (and in dogs) it surrounds the urethra. It is normally the size of a walnut but may grow 100–200% larger in BPH. It consists of three zones: the transition zone in which BPH develops, the peripheral zone where 70% of prostate cancers originate and the central zone (Figure 3).

The first histological sign of BPH may be evident in men in their twenties. Microscopic nodules appear in the periurethral glands around the verumontanum. These nodules are

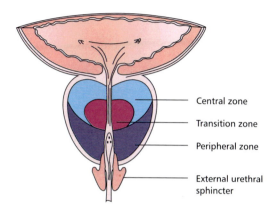

Figure 3 Anatomical zones of the prostate

- Central zone
- Transition zone
- Peripheral zone
- External urethral sphincter

composed of varying amounts of fibrous and smooth muscle cells as well as glandular hyperplasia, and may be a few millimeters to a few centimeters in diameter. As the prostatic adenoma enlarges it encroaches on the urethra, increasing resistance to urine flow by mechanical, or 'static', obstruction.

Interestingly, the overall size of the prostate does not correspond well with the degree of obstruction for two reasons. First, enlargement of the middle lobe of the prostate obstructs the bladder outflow but does not significantly affect the overall size of the prostate. Second, there is a 'dynamic' component to BPO exerted by the smooth muscle cells, contracting in response to sympathetic stimulation. The sympathetic nerves release norepiniphrine (noradrenaline), which binds to α receptors on the smooth muscle cells, initiating contraction.

The increased resistance exerted by the enlarged prostate causes the bladder muscle to undergo hypertrophy. Eventually, the detrusor muscle decompensates as collagen is deposited among the smooth muscle cells; this reduces the bladder compliance and renders the detrusor muscle atonic.

Furthermore, the bladder becomes 'irritable'. Recent research indicates that bladder irritability is due to transient ischemia of the autonomic nerves in the bladder at the time of voiding. A high intravesical pressure is required to expel the urine through the obstructing prostate; this pressure impedes blood flow. The impaired blood supply reduces oxygen delivery, damaging the nerves in the bladder wall. As the nerves are irreparably damaged, the bladder relies on its inbuilt myogenic, or muscle-generated, stimulation for bladder contraction. Myogenic stimulation is not under the control of higher nerve centers, and leads to more frequent bladder contraction as the bladder starts to fill. This gives rise to the symptoms of frequency, nocturia and urgency. The obstructing prostate impedes the flow of urine such that the patient observes a reduced stream. The bladder detrusor muscle taking longer to generate the higher pressure required to expel the urine results in hesitancy. This high pressure may be unsustainable, and the bladder tires before recovering and contracting again, giving rise to intermittency. Incomplete emptying occurs if the detrusor is unable to recover in a short time and residual urine remains in the bladder.

Benign prostatic hyperplasia progresses slowly with time, but patients' symptoms do not necessarily deteriorate. In one study looking at the symptoms of men with BPH in whom surgery was not warranted, 27% remaine stable, 15% improved and 58% deteriorated over 3 years without any other treatment[5].

PRESENTATION

Lower urinary tract symptoms are so common in the aging male that they are considered by many as part of growing older. Media coverage, heightened awareness of health-care professionals and the availability of medical therapy have meant that now more and more men are seeking treatment for their bothersome symptoms. Furthermore, as the profile of prostate cancer rises, patients are requesting assessment of their prostate to exclude malignancy; this inevitably draws attention to their outflow symptoms.

Table 1 Differential diagnosis of a man with lower-urinary tract symptoms

Malignancy
Prostate cancer
Carcinoma *in situ* (bladder)

Infection
Bacterial
Tuberculosis/bilharzia

Inflammation
Bladder stone
Interstitial cystitis

Neurological
Parkinson's disease
Cerebrovascular event
Multiple sclerosis
Bladder neck dysynergia

Mechanical
Urethral stricture
Severe phimosis

Drug-induced
Antidepressants, e.g. amitriptyline
Anticholinergics, e.g. oxybutynin
Diuretics, e.g. furosemide

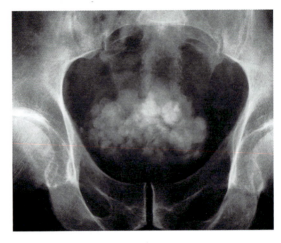

Figure 4 Pelvic radiograph showing multiple bladder stones

History

When assessing a man with LUTS, it is important to confirm the symptoms arise from the BPH rather than another pathology (Table 1), particularly prostate cancer. Second, it is essential to ensure the obstructing prostate has not given rise to complications including bladder stones (Figure 4), urinary tract infection or renal failure. A comprehensive history, a focused examination and the relevant preliminary investigation enable an accurate diagnosis to be made in the vast majority of cases. Those in whom uncertainty still exists can undergo further evaluation by transrectal ultrasound and biopsy, flexible cystoscopy and urodynamic studies.

Assessment of a man's LUTS is best achieved using a symptom score sheet (Figure 5); the most widely employed is the International Prostate Symptom Score (IPSS). This is used to assess the 'obstructive' and 'irritative' symptoms, and also asks how these symptoms affect the individual's quality of life. A score is given for each symptom, and these scores are totalled

to give a value that indicates whether a patient has mild, moderate or severe symptoms. These scores enable a quantitative assessment of symptoms; they do not enable the diagnosis of BPH to be made. Poor urinary flow and incomplete emptying are the most reliable indicators of prostatic obstruction, but this may be due to prostate cancer rather than BPH.

The irritative symptoms of frequency, nocturia and urgency are common in BPO. However, other pathologies give rise to an irritative picture: either as a complication of BPH such as a urinary tract infection or bladder stones, or as a separate bladder pathology such as carcinoma *in situ* of the bladder.

Medical conditions including diabetes mellitus and insipidus as well as treatment with diuretic agents can cause polyuria. The volumes of urine passed as well as the frequency are excessive. A time–volume chart in these men distinguishes polyuria from frequency. Neurological conditions can cause irritative bladder symptoms; Parkinson's disease, a history of strokes and multiple sclerosis can all alter bladder function.

A drug history especially pertaining to antidepressants such as amitriptyline or anticholinergic agents such as oxybutynin may be relevant, and a brief family history is prudent as

	Not at all	Less than 1 time in 5	Less than half the time	About half the time	More than half the time	Almost always	Patient score
• **Incomplete emptying** Over the past month, how often have you had a sensation of not emptying your bladder completely after you finished urinating?	0	1	2	3	4	5	
• **Frequency** Over the past month, how often have you had to urinate again less than 2 hours after you finished urinating?	0	1	2	3	4	5	
• **Intermittency** Over the past month, how often have you found you stopped and started again several times when you urinated?	0	1	2	3	4	5	
• **Urgency** Over the past month, how often have you found it difficult to postpone urination?	0	1	2	3	4	5	
• **Weak stream** Over the past month, how often have you had a weak urinary stream?	0	1	2	3	4	5	
• **Straining** Over the past month, how often have you had to push or strain to begin urination?	0	1	2	3	4	5	
• **Nocturia** Over the past month, how many times did you most typically get up to urinate from the time you went to bed at night until the time you got up in the morning?	0	1	2	3	4	5 +	
Total IPSS							

Figure 5 International Prostate Symptom Score (IPSS)

a first-degree relative with prostate cancer increases the patient's chance of acquiring the disease by 2–3-fold.

Clinical examination

A routine clinical examination should be performed. Abdominal examination may reveal a palpable bladder, indicating chronic retention of urine. A focused neurological examination will exclude neurological conditions that give rise to urinary symptoms. The digital rectal examination (DRE) is an essential component of the clinical examination of a man with LUTS. This includes assessment of the anal sphincter tone, palpation of the anal canal and rectal mucosa, and, finally, examination of the prostate. Prostate examination should concentrate on the size, shape and consistency of the gland (Table 2).

Although the DRE is not very sensitive, (fewer than 50% of cancers can be felt on

Table 2 Prostate examination

	Benign prostatic hyperplasia	Prostatitis	Prostate cancer
Size	enlarged	enlarged	enlarged or normal
Shape	smooth, symmetrical, central sulcus	smooth, symmetrical	nodular, asymmetrical loss of central sulcus, lateral and cranial extension
Consistency	rubbery	tender, firm or boggy, warm	hard

Table 3 Incidence of prostate cancer detected by prostate-specific antigen (PSA) and digital rectal examination (DRE)

	Incidence (%)		
	PSA < 4 ng/ml	PSA 4–10 ng/ml	PSA > 10 ng/ml
Normal DRE	9	20	31
Abnormal DRE	17	45	77

DRE), together with a prostate-specific antigen (PSA) result it can be used to improve detection of prostate cancer (Table 3).

INVESTIGATION

Urinalysis

Urinalysis may identify whether a patient's symptoms are as a result of another pathology, for example urinary tract infection or bladder cancer. Microscopic hematuria requires further investigation with urine culture and cytology. Upper-tract imaging and cystoscopy may also be requested to exclude conditions such as stones and bladder or renal tumors. If these investigations do not yield a diagnosis, there may be a 'medical' cause for microscopic hematuria. Glomerulonephritis, endocarditis and vasculitis can all produce dipstick-positive hematuria and require specialist investigation.

The presence of leukocytes implies infection, requiring formal urine microscopy and culture.

Blood tests

Serum creatinine levels are elevated in 10% of patients who present with LUTS. This is not always due to outflow obstruction, leading to back-pressure on the kidneys, but partly reflects the degree of comorbidity in the aging population tested. However, if the creatinine level is elevated further, investigation with upper-tract imaging may be required. Patients who have renal insufficiency have an increased risk of postoperative complications, and the mortality increases six-fold[6].

Acute and chronic retention can both impair renal function; overcoming the obstruction with a catheter or a TURP will improve the serum urea and electrolyte levels. Clearly, without relief of the obstruction, the renal function will continue to deteriorate; consequently, these cases are managed on an urgent basis.

PSA

The use of PSA testing as a screening tool remains controversial, and will continue to be until the results of large trials in Europe and North America are available. PSA testing in the symptomatic man is, however, recommended in the majority of cases. Patients should be counseled before undergoing the test. The merits and the drawbacks of the test, the possible need for a prostate biopsy and the therapeutic options if prostate cancer is diagnosed should be discussed. While PSA lacks prostate cancer tend to have a free/total ratio of less than 0.19, although they frequently have concomitant BPH that may distort the result.

Flow rate and residual volume

The urine flow test and post-void residual urine volume provide an objective assessment of a patient's symptoms. When performing a flow test, at least 150 ml must be passed to obtain an accurate result. For volumes smaller than 150 ml the bladder does not generate its maximum pressure, and therefore the achievable maximum flow rate is never reached. A maximum flow rate of less than 15 ml/s is considered significant for obstruction, although it is often helpful to repeat the test as a single result may not be representative. It should be remembered that factors other than BPH reduce the maximum flow rate, for example poor detrusor contractility or urethral strictures (Figure 6).

A significant residual volume, over 150 ml, is predictive of acute urinary retention and is a good indicator of whether a patient will ultimately require surgery for their LUTS. Again, more than one reading should be taken to minimize individual variation.

Urodynamics

Where the diagnosis is still in doubt, urodynamics studies can be undertaken. This involves passing a pressure transducer into the rectum and one into the bladder. The transducers record the change in pressure as the bladder is filled. The patient voids into a flow meter, and the pressures generated are again recorded (Figure 7). The rectal transducer records a change in abdominal pressure when the patient performs tasks, such as coughing, as this will also affect the intravesical pressure. The rectal pressure is subtracted from the intravesical pressure to give the pressure generated by the detrusor muscle: the detrusor pressure. This enables the specialist to distinguish between detrusor hypocontractility, where the detrusor

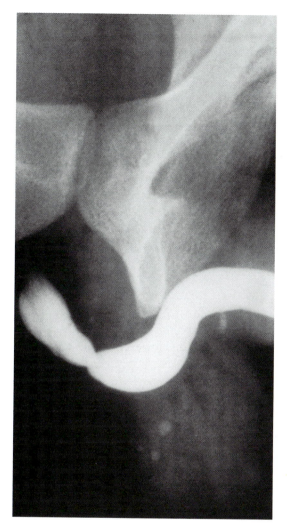

Figure 6   Ascending urethrogram demonstrating stricture in the bulbar urethra

specificity, it remains the most sensitive, simple test available to diagnose prostate cancer, especially when combined with DRE.

Attempts have been made to refine PSA testing to improve its sensitivity and specificity in detecting prostate cancer. Age-specific PSA correlates advancing age with increasing PSA; PSA velocity charts PSA over time to look at the rate of PSA rise; PSA density compares the PSA value with that expected for the size of the patient's prostate; and the free/total ratio relies on patients with BPH having a higher concentration of PSA in the free form. Patients with

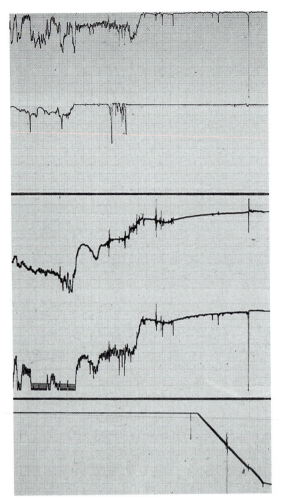

Figure 7 Urodynamic study (filling and voiding). Curve 1, bladder filled with saline; curve 2, intravesical pressure; curve 3, detrusor pressure: high pressure (> 100 cmH$_2$O) is required to overcome the obstruction; curve 4, intra-abdominal pressure, subtracted from intravesical pressure to give detrusor pressure: this patient is straining to overcome the obstruction; curve 5, urine flow rate: poor maximum flow with interruption (intermittency)

muscle is weak, dysynergia, where the detrusor contracts satisfactorily but the sphincter fails to relax appropriately, and outflow obstruction.

TREATMENT

The choice of treatment for a man with BPH depends on a number of issues: first, the degree to which he finds the symptoms bothersome;

second, the symptom score; and finally, the objective assessments of flow rate and residual volume.

Medical

Medical therapies offer a safe and effective treatment for patients who are troubled by their symptoms, and in whom complications have been excluded. Currently, the gold standard treatment for BPH is transurethral resection of the prostate (TURP); however, increasingly, medical options are used either as first-line treatment or as a definitive treatment over the longer term. The symptom score and flow rate improvements are less dramatic with oral medication; nevertheless, patients suffer less from side-effects.

Two classes of drugs are used: alpha-blockers reduce the dynamic component, and 5α-reductase inhibitors reverse the static component of BPO (Table 4). Using these together gives no significant advantage over monotherapy[7].

Alpha-blockers

Alpha$_1$ receptors are situated on smooth muscle cells found in the prostatic stroma, urethra and capsule, as well as the bladder neck. The stroma consists of smooth muscle and fibrous connective tissue. In normal individuals the stromal to epithelial component is 2 : 1; in BPH this becomes 5 : 1. Norepinephrine from sympathetic nerves binds to α receptors and stimulates smooth muscle contraction, leading to outflow obstruction (Figure 8).

Development Marco Caine and colleagues[8] first introduced alpha-blockers as a treatment for symptomatic BPH in 1978. They demonstrated an improvement in patient symptoms and voiding using the alpha-blocker phenoxybenzamine. Phenoxybenzamine binds nonselectively to both α$_1$ and α$_2$ receptors; the former are found in the lower urinary tract, and the latter are in nerve endings and are involved in the re-uptake of norepinephrine. As a result

Table 4 Alpha-blockers vs. finasteride

	Alpha-blockers	Finasteride
Onset of action	few hours	6–12 weeks
Symptom score improvement	40–60%	15%
Flow-rate improvement	1.0–4.0 ml/s	1.3–1.6 ml/s
Urinary retention/surgery	may reduce incidence	reduces incidence
Side-effects	postural hypotension drowsiness and headache, retrograde ejaculation	impotence, decreased libido, breast tenderness
Treatable prostate size	any	> 40 g
Effects on PSA	none	halves

PSA, prostate-specific antigen

of this non-selective alpha-blockade, a third of their patients suffered side-effects including dizziness, postural hypotension, tiredness and nasal congestion.

In 1978, the α_1-selective blocker prazosin, used as an antihypertensive agent, was shown to cause urinary incontinence[9]. Further studies identified the α receptor subtype α_1-adrenoceptor in prostate tissue[10]. Hedlund and colleagues[11] presented prazosin as the first selective α_1-adrenoceptor blocker to be used to treat BPO. They reported that prazosin improved symptoms and urine flow rate as well as reducing the post-void residual volume. Prazosin does not antagonize α_2 receptors; consequently, the side-effects were limited to 10–15% of cases. This resulted in the development of second-generation alpha-blockers, which include doxazosin, alfuzosin, terazosin and indoramin (Figure 9).

More recent research has uncovered further subclasses of α_1-adrenoceptors[12], and these are now the target of further pharmaceutical research. Drugs that reduce BPO with minimal side-effects, by selectively inhibiting the subtype of α_1-adrenoceptor found predominantly in the lower urinary tract are termed 'uroselective'. Tamsulosin is an α_{1A}-adrenoceptor antagonist and, as such, is uroselective.

Efficacy The alpha-blockers all have similar efficacy, despite the differing incidence of side-effects. Placebo controlled trials have reported symptom scores improve by 40–60%, and flow rates by 30–50%[13]. What is more, they have a rapid onset of action; alfuzosin produces an optimal flow rate improvement after a single dose, symptom improvement after 1 week and full therapeutic benefit after 3 months[14]. Furthermore, these improvements are maintained in open-label studies for at least 4 years. The risk of developing acute urinary retention and the need for surgical intervention is probably also reduced, although data from long-term, randomized, placebo-controlled trials are not yet available.

Side-effects Alpha-blockers are generally well tolerated. The main side-effects occur as a result of α_1-blockade in the brain and cardiovascular system. The most common adverse effects include tiredness, dizziness and headaches, which occur in 10–15% of patients. Less common side-effects (1–2%) include asthenia, palpitations and gastrointestinal disturbance such as nausea, vomiting, diarrhea and constipation.

Care is taken when prescribing these drugs for patients with orthostatic hypotension and in those using antihypertensive therapy, as they are prone to hypotensive collapse. The first and second generation of α_1-blockers may also give rise to hypotension after the first dose: the 'first dose effect'; therefore, a low initial dose is given and then subsequent doses are increased, titrating the therapeutic effect against any unwanted symptoms.

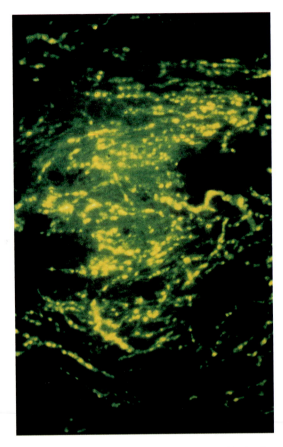

Figure 8 Section of prostate staining positively for norepinephrine

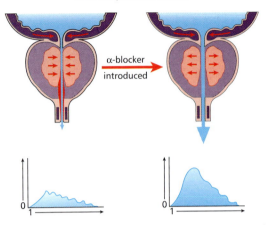

Alpha-adrenoceptor blockers relax the prostatic urethra

α-blocker introduced

Figure 9 Effect of alpha-blockers on the prostate and corresponding flow rate

The hypotensive effect of α_1-blockers can be used to treat hypertensive patients with BPO. Normotensive men do not experience a clinically significant fall in their blood pressure with doxazosin; however, hypertensive men achieve a significant reduction in mean arterial pressure[15]. One drug can therefore be given to improve compliance, limit drug interaction and reduce cost. Where the hypotensive effects would be detrimental, tamsulosin is a safer alternative. Tamsulosin may, however, cause retrograde ejaculation by relaxing the smooth muscle of the bladder neck.

5α-Reductase inhibitors

These act by blocking the enzyme-driven conversion of testosterone to dihydrotestosterone (DHT), and in doing so reverse the process of BPH. The enzyme responsible is 5α-reductase, which is also found in hair follicles of the skin. DHT plays a role in male-pattern balding, and patients taking a 5α-reductase inhibitor may notice some reversal of the balding pattern.

Background John Hunter, the Scottish surgeon, noted in 1786 that prostatic enlargement was related to the aging process and was dependent on normal testicular function[16]. J. W. White proposed bilateral orchidectomy as a treatment of BPH in the 19th century[17], and, although effective in 100 of his patients, not surprisingly castration was never popularized.

In 1963 it was reported that testosterone was metabolized in the prostate to DHT[18], and less than a decade later researchers identified DHT as the main androgen modulating prostate growth[19]. A frenetic search by the pharmaceutical industry resulted in the development of one drug: finasteride, which inhibits 5α-reductase and thereby reduces both prostate DHT levels by 90% and prostate size by an average of 30%[20]. Moreover, it does not affect the testosterone-dependent functions and is therefore better tolerated than the earlier antiandrogen treatments. Research is ongoing with dutasteride (GI198745), which inhibits two isoenzymes of 5α-reductase; this may in the future prove faster and more effective than finasteride.

Efficacy Finasteride, Proscar® 5 mg once daily, has been extensively investigated in a number of placebo-controlled trials. The SCARP trial (Scandinavian Reduction of the Prostate)[21], a large, double-blind, multicenter trial, compared the efficacy of finasteride with that of placebo over a 24-month period. The symptom score improved in the finasteride arm by 15%, compared with a 2% improvement in the placebo group, at 2 years. Likewise, the flow rate improved by 1.5 ml/s compared with a reduction of 0.3 ml/s in the controls. In the Proscar long-term efficiency and safety study (PLESS)[22], another randomized, placebo-controlled trial involving 3000 men in North America, finasteride was compared with placebo. This study showed that finasteride reduced the risk of urinary retention from 2.7% in the placebo group to 1.1% in the finasteride arm, and the need for surgical intervention from 6.5 to 4.2%.

It should be noted, however, that finasteride has been shown to be of little benefit over placebo for patients with smaller prostates (< 40 mg). Furthermore, as finasteride acts by reversing the disease process, it may take 3–6 months before an improvement in symptoms is seen. However, it has proven efficacy for at least 7 years.

Side-effects Finasteride is well tolerated. Approximately 3% of patients will suffer impotence, loss of libido and reduced ejaculatory volume, and patients should be warned of this before starting treatment. This is reversible if the treatment is discontinued. Breast enlargement or tenderness occurs in 1% of cases.

Proscar reduces serum PSA levels by 50% in patients with BPH, with or without prostate cancer. When evaluating the PSA of a patient who has been taking finasteride for 6 months or more, the PSA level should be doubled, to compare with the normal range for untreated men.

Phytotherapy

Phytotherapeutic agents are chemicals derived from plant extracts, and men have been taking a variety of these substances for their LUTS over many centuries. The fact that these 'natural remedies' have endured the test of time, and despite their expense are increasingly popular, is testament to their therapeutic potential, be this real or placebo. Evidence that these 'medicinal botanicals' are either safe or efficacious is difficult to obtain. Phytotherapies vary enormously, different plant extracts are incorporated into different tablets, the extraction process is not standardized, and there is even variation within the same plant species[23]. The active ingredients are often not known; therefore, combining the appropriate substances at a therapeutic, but non-toxic, dose is haphazard.

Trials that have been undertaken are either small or not placebo-controlled, or do not show a statistically significant difference from placebo. *Serenoa repens* (saw palmetto) is the most widely used phytotherapeutic for BPO. Its mechanism of action is probably similar to that of finasteride, i.e. it inhibits 5α-reductase, although it may have other effects. In a placebo-controlled trial, Permixon®, an extract of the American dwarf palm tree berry (*Serenoa repens*), improved symptom and flow rate scores compared with placebo; however, at the end of the trial neither patient nor clinician could show a difference in satisfactory response between Permixon and placebo[24]. Another trial compared Permixon with finasteride in over 1000 men; both treatments improved symptom scores by nearly 40% and peak flow improved in the finasteride group by 3.2 ml/s and by 2.7 ml/s in the Permixon group, a significant difference[25].

The trial was not placebo-controlled and lasted only 6 months, and therefore has less impact.

Undoubtedly though, in *in vivo* and *in vitro* studies[26,27], histological changes including prostate epithelial contraction and gland atrophy occur in response to Permixon treatment; furthermore, the incidence of side-effects is low. *Serenoa repens* may yet prove, in randomized placebo-controlled trials, to be a safe and effective treatment for BPO.

Other phytotherapies used for BPH include *Pygeum africanum* (African plum), *Urtica dioica* (stinging nettle) and *Secale cereale* (rye pollen). To date, no long-term placebo-controlled, double-blind trials have been performed to prove their efficacy and safety.

Surgical

Surgical treatments for BPH have been used since White performed bilateral orchidectomy on over 100 patients at the latter end of the 19th century. The first endoscopic prostatectomies were carried out in the 1930s, when the mortality from the procedure was 25%[28]. Since then, newer techniques have evolved: newer energy sources such as ultrasound, microwaves and lasers; newer modes of delivering the energy such as loops, bands, needles and transrectal probes, and, with the advent of fiberoptics, an improved light source. Despite these more recent developments, transurethral resection of the prostate (TURP) remains the gold standard with which all new technologies are compared.

TURP

In the National Health Survey of 1986, 96% of surgical procedures for BPH performed under the Medicare system in the USA were TURPs, and 350 000 TURPs were carried out that year. Despite an 80% increase in the diagnosis of BPH, fewer than 200 000 TURPs were performed a decade later[29]. This is because new guidelines were issued in the USA, recommending watchful waiting for patients with minimal symptoms, greater information for patients of the possible harmful effects of surgery, and a greater role for the patient in the decision-making process of which treatment modality should be adopted. Furthermore, alternative surgical treatments including vaporization, microwave and laser prostatectomies were under development, and newer, safer and more effective medical therapies became available. In Europe, although the number of TURPs performed is declining, the reduction is less dramatic. TURP can be performed under spinal, epidural or general anesthesia, and involves passing a resectoscope up the urethra. A diathermy loop is used to cut and cauterize the hyperplastic tissue, while irrigating fluid maintains a clear surgical field. The prostatic chips are flushed out and sent for histological examination.

Currently, 20% of patients with an obstructing prostate undergo TURP. TURP achieves a reduction in symptom score of 75%, an increased flow rate of 125% (absolute mean improvement of 9.7 ml/s) and a reoperation rate in the order of 2% per annum[30].

Morbidity and mortality of TURP   The mortality from the procedure has improved from 25% in Alcock's paper of 1932[28] to virtually zero today[30]. The morbidity likewise has decreased with advances in technology and experience. The transfusion rate is less than 8%[31] and frequency of surgery for urethral strictures and bladder neck stenoses is less than 5%. The transurethral resection syndrome remains a rare, but important complication. It is caused by absorption of irrigating fluid via the prostatic veins, and leads to hyponatremia and fluid overload resulting in fitting, coma and, ultimately, death. During an average TURP lasting 40 min, 1–2 l of irrigant is absorbed, but for larger prostates or in inexperienced hands the operating time is prolonged, increasing the amount of fluid absorbed and the risk of developing the syndrome.

Retrograde ejaculation occurs in 65% of men after TURP[30]. This is because the bladder neck sphincter is resected during TURP and so semen is able to reflux into the bladder during ejaculation, rather than pass down the urethra. TURP, however, does not affect potency: in a large study of American war veterans, potency was no different after TURP when compared with an age-matched population[32].

Open prostatectomy

Open prostatectomy is reserved nowadays for patients with large prostates in whom sufficient resection would not be achieved in the time available to perform a TURP. Likewise, patients who have a large bladder stone may also undergo this procedure, as the stone and BPH can be treated under one anesthetic. Open prostatectomy is an effective treatment, reducing the symptom score by 88% and increasing the flow rate by 230%. However, the morbidity and mortality associated with an open procedure and the prolonged hospital stay mean this is now used only for men with very large prostates (> 100 ml).

Transurethral vaporization of the prostate

Transurethral vaporization of the prostate was developed in an attempt to reduce blood loss. Vaporization employs a rollerball through which electric current passes to heat the prostate to over 100°C. This high temperature vaporizes intracellular water, and the cells explode leaving an immediate tissue defect. Blood loss and the incidence of transurethral resection syndrome are reduced, and it has follow-up symptom and flow rate scores equivalent to those of TURP in moderate-sized glands, after 3 years[33]. Some men suffer with prolonged irritative symptoms, particularly dysuria. Attempts are being made to combine the hemostatic properties of the electrovaporizing technique with the cutting abilities of the TURP loop – 'adding more gold to the gold standard'[34]. A resecting loop with similar cutting abilities to the TURP loop but with an increased contact area for coagulation is being developed. However, to date, the results of this band loop have failed to meet expectations, with no significant reduction in blood loss[35] when compared with TURP.

Lasers

Lasers are used more and more and in a greater variety of ways in the urinary tract, whether to treat ureteric stones, to resect bladder tumors or in surgery for BPH. They offer a precise cutting tool that is hemostatic; this makes them ideal for prostate surgery. They are used to heat the prostatic adenoma either under direct vision (visual laser ablation, VLAP), or with ultrasound guidance (transurethral laser incision of the prostate, TULIP). In both these prostate-ablating procedures the BPH undergoes coagulative necrosis and then sloughs off; tissue is not excised at the time of the procedure. Patients may therefore have prolonged periods of catheterization and frequently suffer from perineal and urethral pain.

Lasers are also used to excise prostatic tissue. Holmium laser resection and enucleation (HoLRP and HoLEP) involve cutting the prostate into wedges like the segments of an orange. The wedges are flushed into the bladder, fragmented with a tissue morcellater and removed. As the whole adenoma is excised, the symptom and flow rate improvements are even better than with TURP; furthermore, the hemostatic property of the laser not only reduces blood loss but also allows patients on anticoagulant therapy to continue their treatment. Although some fine-tuning is required before this kit is optimized, HoLEP is likely to replace TURP as the gold standard surgical treatment for BPH within the next decade.

High-intensity focused ultrasound

High-intensity focused ultrasound is a technique that, without any direct contact, ablates the prostate. A probe is passed into the rectum, and ultrasound waves are focused to heat the prostate to 80–200°C without damaging adjacent structures. There is no direct urethral trauma; this limits postoperative dysuria and theoretically urethral strictures. Early data were promising; significant improvements in both symptom score and flow rates were reported in the short term. The longer-term results, however, were disappointing; the symptoms and flow rate improvements were not sustained[36]. Consequently, this technique is no longer used in the treatment of BPH.

However, it is being adapted for use in prostate cancer for patients in whom radical treatment is inappropriate.

Transurethral microwave thermotherapy

Low- and high-energy microwave thermotherapy has been employed to heat the prostate either transurethrally or via a probe inserted through the rectum. The advantage of this technique is that it can be performed under local anesthesia as a day case, as there is minimal blood loss. It is therefore preferred for patients with significant comorbidity. The symptom score improvements are reasonable over the short term; however, two-thirds of patients require supplementary BPH treatment, the flow rate improvements are small and the duration of catheterization is often prolonged[30].

Transurethral needle ablation

Transurethral needle ablation (TUNA) involves inserting two antennae into the prostate transurethrally; these emit radiofrequency waves that heat the prostate to 60–90°C, without heating adjacent structures. As a result the pain-sensitive prostatic urethra is preserved, intraoperative pain is reduced and the

procedure can be performed under local anesthesia. Moreover, postoperative irritative symptoms and retention are also reduced.

The blood loss is negligible, although some patients complain of irritative symptoms; these usually resolve in a matter of a few weeks after surgery. In a recent paper, Roehrborn and colleagues[37] demonstrated that TUNA improved urodynamic parameters, although these improvements did not predict the degree of symptomatic response in either their TUNA or their TURP group. In an earlier study from the same institution, the authors demonstrated that TUNA was well tolerated, and provided substantive and lasting improvements in symptom score, flow rates and quality of life over 1 year[38].

SUMMARY

Benign prostatic hyperplasia (BPH) has a significant effect on men's quality of life in middle and old age. For some men the symptoms are of minor inconvenience, for others benign prostatic obstruction and its complications have a profound effect on their own lives and the lives of those around them.

In the future, research will improve our understanding of the pathophysiology, and with this knowledge will come progress in our pharmacological management of BPH. Advances in surgical techniques will reduce the incidence of complications and further improve symptom and flow rate scores. Improved patient education and a greater role for patients in the decision-making process will enable more men to obtain a better quality of life.

References

1. Carter HB, Coffey DS. The prostate: an increasing medical problem. *Prostate* 1990; 16:39–48
2. Abrams P, Schulman C, Vaage S and the European Tamsulosin Study Group. Tamsulosin, a selective α_{1C}-adrenoceptor antagonist; a randomised controlled trial in patients with benign prostatic 'obstruction' (symptomatic BPH). *Br J Urol* 1995;76:325–36
3. Chyou PH, Nomura AM, Stemmermann GN, Hankin JH. A prospective study of alcohol, diet and other lifestyle factors in relation

to obstructive uropathy. *Prostate* 1993;22: 253–64

4. Imperato-McGinley J, Guerrero L, Gautler T, *et al*. Steroid 5-α reductase in man: an inherited form of pseudohermaphroditism. *Science* 1974;186:1213–15

5. Birkoff J, Wiederhorn A, Hamilton M, Xinsser H. Natural history of benign prostate hypertrophy and acute urinary retention. *Urology* 1976;7:48–52

6. Holtegrewe HL, Valk WL. Factors influencing the mortality and morbidity of transurethral prostatectomy: a study of 2015 cases. *J Urol* 1962;87:450–9

7. Lepor H, Williford WO, Barry MJ, *et al*. The efficacy of terazosin, finasteride or both in benign prostatic hyperplasia. Veterans Affairs Co-operative Studies Benign Prostatic Hyperplasia Study Group. *N Engl J Med* 1996;335: 533–9

8. Caine M, Perlberg S, Meretyk S. A placebo controlled double-blind study of the effect of phenoxybenzamine in benign prostatic obstruction. *Br J Urol* 1978;50:551–6

9. Thien T, Delaere KP, Debruyne FM, Koene RA. Urinary incontinence caused by prazosin. *Br Med J* 1978;2:622–3

10. Caine M, Raz S, Ziegler M. Adrenergic and cholinergic receptors in the human prostate capsule and bladder neck. *Br J Urol* 1975;47: 193–202

11. Hedlund H, Andersson K-E, Ek A. Effects of prazosin in patients with benign prostatic obstruction. *J Urol* 1983;130:275–8

12. McGrath JC. Evidence for more than one type of postjunctional-adrenoceptor. *Biochem Pharmacol* 1982;31:467–84

13. Chapple CR. Pharmacotherapy for benign prostatic hyperplasia – the potential for α₁-adrenoceptor subtype specific blockade. *Br J Urol* 1998;81(Suppl 1):34–47

14. Jardin A, Bensadoun H, Delauche Cavallier MC, Attali P. Alfuzosin for treatment of benign prostatic hypertrophy. The BPH-ALF Group. *Lancet* 1991;337:1457–61

15. Kirby RS. Doxazocin in benign prostatic hyperplasia: effects on blood pressure and urinary flow in normotensive and hypertensive men. *Urology* 1995;46:182–6

16. Hunter J. *Observations on Certain Parts of the Animal Oeconomy*, 1st edn. London: Biblioteche Osteriana, 1786:38–9

17. White JW. Results of double castration on hypertrophy of the prostate. *Ann Surg* 1895; 25:1–59

18. Farnsworth WE, Brown JR. Testosterone metabolism in the prostate. *Natl Cancer Inst Monogr* 1963;12:323–5

19. Andersen KM, Liao S. Selective retention of dihydrotestosterone by prostatic nuclei. *Nature (London)* 1968;219:227–79

20. Stoner E and the Finasteride Study Group. The clinical effects of a 5 alpha-reductase inhibitor, finasteride, on benign prostatic hyperplasia. *J Urol* 1992;147:1298–302

21. Andersen J-T, Ekman P, Wolff H, *et al*. and the Scandinavian BPH Study Group. Can finasteride reverse the progress of benign prostatic hyperplasia? A two-year placebo-controlled study. *Urology* 1995;46:631–7

22. McConnell JD, Bruskewitz R, Walsh PC, *et al*. The effect of finasteride on the risk of acute urinary retention and the need for surgical treatment among men with benign prostatic hyperplasia. Finasteride Long-Term Efficacy and Safety Study Group. *N Engl J Med* 1998; 338:557–63

23. Dreikorn K, Borkowski A, Braeckman J, *et al*. Other medical therapies. In Denis L, Griffiths K, Murphy G, eds. *Proceedings of the Fourth International Consultation on Benign Prostatic Hyperplasia (BPH), July 1997*. Plymouth, UK: Health Publications, 1998:635–59

24. Descotes JL, Rambeaud JJ, Deschaseaux P, *et al*. Placebo-controlled evaluation of the efficacy and tolerability of Permixon® in benign prostatic hyperplasia after exclusion of placebo responders. *Clin Drug Invest* 1995; 9:291–7

25. Carraro JC, Raynaud JP, Koch G, *et al*. Comparsion of phytotherapy (Permixon®) with finasteride in the treatment of benign prostatic hyperplasia: a randomised international study of 1089 patients. *Prostate* 1996;29:231–40

26. Marks LS, Partin AW, Epstein JI, *et al*. Effects of saw palmetto herbal blend in men with

symptomatic benign prostatic hyperplasia. *J Urol* 2000;163:1451–6

27. Bayne CW, Donnelly F, Ross M, Habib FK. *Serenoa repens* (Permixon): a 5 alpha-reductase type I and II inhibitor – new evidence in a coculture model of BPH. *Prostate* 1999;40: 232–41

28. Alcock NG. Ten months' experience with transurethral prostate resection. *J Urol* 1932; 28:545–60

29. Mebust WK. Transurethral surgery. In Walsh PC, Retik AB, Vaughan ED, Wein AJ, eds. *Cambell's Urology*, 7th edn. Philidelphia: WB Saunders Co., 1998:Ch 49

30. Madersbacher S, Marberger M. Is transurethral resection of the prostate still justified? *Br J Urol* 1999;83:227–37

31. Horninger W, Unterlechner H, Stasser H, Bartsch G. Transurethral prostatectomy: mortality and morbidity. *Prostate* 1996;28: 195–200

32. Wasson JH, Reda DJ, Bruskewitz RC, *et al*. The Veterans Affairs Co-operative Study Group on transurethral resection of the prostate. A comparison of transurethral surgery with watchful waiting for moderate symptoms of benign prostatic hyperplasia. *N Engl J Med* 1995;332:75–9

33. Hammadeh MY, Madaan S, Singh M, Philp T. A 3-year follow-up of a prospective randomised trial comparing transurethral electrovaporization of the prostate with standard transurethral prostatectomy. *Br J Urol Int* 2000;86:648–51

34. Patal A, Fuchs GJ, Gutierrez-Aceves J, Andrade-Perez F. Transurethral electrovaporization and vapour-resection of the prostate: an appraisal of possible electrosurgical alternatives to regular loop resection. *Br J Urol Int* 2000;85(Suppl 2):202–10

35. Cynk M, Woodhams H, Mostafid H, *et al*. A prospective randomised controlled trial comparing Vaportome prostatic resection with TURP. *Br J Urol Int* 1999;83(Suppl 4):6

36. Madersbacher S, Schatzl G, Djavan B, *et al*. Long-term outcome of transrectal high intensity focused ultrasound therapy for benign prostatic hyperplaisa. *Eur Urol* 2000; 37:687–94

37. Roehrborn CG, Burkhard FC, Bruskewitz RC, *et al*. The effects of transurethral needle ablation and resection of the prostate on the pressure flow urodynamic parameters: analysis of the United States randomised study. *J Urol* 1999;162:92–7

38. Roehrborn CG, Issa MM, Bruskewitz RC, *et al*. Transurethral needle ablation for benign prostatic hyperplasia: 12-month results of a prospective, multicenter US study. *Urology* 1998;51:415–21

5 Prostate cancer

Michaël Peyromaure, MD, Vincent Ravery, MD, and Laurent Boccon-Gibod, MD, PhD

INTRODUCTION

Prostate cancer is the most common malignancy and the second leading cause of cancer mortality in males. Traditionally, prostate cancer was considered as a disease of the aging male, and this may be partly responsible for the delay in diagnosis and management. With the use of the digital rectal examination (DRE) and prostate-specific antigen (PSA) testing in screening programs, prostate cancer is being diagnosed at an earlier age and stage.

The increasing number of low-staged cancers in young men has led to the development of curative treatments. In males whose life expectancy is above 10 years, radical prostatectomy is the standard curative therapy when the tumor is organ-confined. However, impotence is a frequent long-term complication of surgery that impairs the patient's quality of life. Therefore, attention is focused on decreasing morbidity related to surgical treatment and developing alternative therapies. For locally advanced tumors various approaches, including combination treatments, are available that are still subject to debate. In metastatic disease the management remains palliative, and is based on hormonal therapy. In elderly men whose survival is not expected to be improved by curative therapy, watchful waiting and deferred treatment if necessary is the standard approach for localized tumors.

EPIDEMIOLOGY

In Europe and the USA, prostate carcinoma represents the most common cancer in males. Its incidence has rapidly increased since the 1970s because of the aging population and better diagnosis methods. There are national and racial differences in the incidence of prostate cancer. In Europe, the incidence is approximately 25 per 100 000 males per year[1]. The USA has the highest incidence of prostate cancer with 75 per 100 000 males per year, whereas Asia has the lowest with approximately 3 per 100 000[2]. In addition, the incidence and mortality rate of prostate cancer are 50% higher among African-Americans than among Caucasians in the USA.

The geographic differences in the incidence of prostate neoplasia may be explained by genetic factors. Heredity seems to be the most important risk factor. Indeed, the risk of developing prostate cancer is doubled when two first-line relatives (father or brother) have the disease[3]. Nevertheless, other findings suggest that prostate carcinogenesis depends partly on exogenous factors. When Asiatics move to the USA, their risk of having prostate cancer becomes that of Americans after one generation[4]. Some life-style factors are believed to play a major role in the occurrence of prostate cancer, but only few data, to date, are available in the literature. A high animal fat content in the diet may be one of the most important environmental factors related to prostatic carcinoma[5]. Even though only 3% of patients will die of their prostate cancer, the overall mortality of the disease is very important because of its high prevalence. After lung cancer, prostate carcinoma is the second leading cause of death by cancer in males. Since the 1990s, the mortality rate of prostate cancer has tended to decrease in Europe and the USA.

DETECTION

Since the 1980s, the wide use of the DRE and PSA testing has resulted in an increased detection of prostate cancer. A DRE abnormality leads to prostate carcinoma diagnosis in more than 20% of cases, regardless of the physician's specialty. When performed in a population of asymptomatic men, DRE allows the detection of prostate cancer in 0.1–4% of males submitted to screening[6].

The PSA level is a better independent predictor of prostate cancer than the DRE. Using monoclonal antibody assay, the overall predictive value of PSA testing is approximately 30% when the PSA level is between 4 and 10 ng/ml and more than 50% when the level is greater[7]. However, the threshold of PSA level to indicate a prostate biopsy remains uncertain. Some investigators suggest performing a prostate biopsy for PSA level lower than 4 ng/ml. Recently, a 24.5% rate of prostate cancer has been reported among patients with PSA levels between 2.5 and 4 ng/ml when systematic sextant biopsies were performed, regardless of DRE and ultrasound abnormalities[8].

Other PSA variables have been tested in an attempt to increase the predictive value of PSA, such as PSA density, PSA velocity, PSA doubling time and free PSA ratio. Free PSA ratio seems to be of particular interest when PSA is between 4 and 10 ng/ml[9]. Indeed, free PSA ratio has been proved to be significantly lower in prostate cancer than in benign prostatic hyperplasia. Many authors recommend the use of free PSA ratio when PSA is in the intermediate

range (4–10 ng/ml) and when the DRE is normal. However, the threshold value of free PSA ratio that may optimize the specificity of total PSA testing remains unknown[10].

Performing a prostate biopsy is the standard way to prove the presence of cancer and to obtain a cytological grading. The biopsy can be done under digital guidance when there is a DRE abnormality. Usually, biopsy cores are guided by ultrasound, and can be carried out without anesthesia in an out-patient setting. Bleeding complications occur in approximately 70% of patients[11]. Hematuria, hematospermia and rectal bleeding are the most common complications. The rate of acute prostatitis is less than 2% when an antibiotic and a rectal enema are given prior to the biopsy. Major complications requiring hospital admission are exceptional. The optimum number of biopsy cores for cancer detection is controversial. The standard number of cores is six, but several studies indicate that performing ten or 12 core biopsies may improve the detection rate of prostate cancer by 6.6–37%, without increasing the biopsy-related morbidity[12–14].

STAGING

Local staging (T-staging) of prostate carcinoma is of particular interest in patients with a life expectancy of 10 years or more. Indeed, the intent of treatment in these patients is curative only in the case of organ-confined disease. Although serum PSA level increases with local stage, its ability to predict the final pathological stage is limited when used as an individual parameter. In contrast, the combination of PSA, DRE, cytological grade and number of positive biopsy cores has been proved to be predictive of local extension[15]. Computed tomography (CT) and/or endorectal magnetic resonance imaging (MRI) may be useful in addition to clinical and cytological parameters to assess local invasion, particularly in cases of seminal vesicle involvement and significant capsular effraction.

Nodal staging (N-staging) should be performed only when curative treatment is planned. The combination of PSA and biopsy findings has a good predictive value for N-staging, whereas the sensitivity of CT and MRI is less than 70%[16]. Nodal metastases are better detected by surgical open or laparoscopic lymphadenectomy. A group of patients with low risk (< 10%) of nodal involvement has been defined: one lobe-confined cancer at DRE, PSA < 20 ng/ml and Gleason score < 7[17]. In the opinion of most authors, preoperative imaging by CT and/or MRI is not necessary in this group.

Metastasis staging (M-staging) is important in patients whose disease is suspected to be advanced. The gold standard for M-staging is bone scintigraphy, since bone metastases are the most frequent occurrence. The presence of bone metastases is associated with poor prognosis, and can generate skeletal complications that impair quality of life. Serum PSA level is the best predictive parameter of bone metastases. A PSA level greater than 100 ng/ml has been reported to have a positive predictive value of 100%[18]. In contrast, the negative predictive value of a PSA level below 20 ng/ml is approximatively 99%[19]. Bone scintigraphy is considered by most authors to be unnecessary when the pretreatment PSA level is < 10 ng/ml.

LOCALIZED PROSTATE CANCER

Definitions and general considerations

'Clinically localized prostate cancers' are stage T1 and T2 cancers. Stage T1a and T1b cancers are incidental histological findings after transurethral resection or open prostatectomy for benign prostatic hyperplasia. Stage T1a is defined as 5% or less of prostatic tissue involved in the cancer, while stage T1b is defined as more than 5% of tissue involved. The risk of tumor progression of untreated T1a prostate cancer is only 5% after 5 years, but increases up to 50% after 10 years[20]. The risk of tumor

progression of untreated T1b is more than 80% after 5 years. Stage T1c cancers are clinically undetectable, and diagnosed by needle biopsy for PSA abnormality. The incidence of T1c prostate cancer has increased since PSA testing has become widely used. One study showed that 30% of T1c prostate cancers had an extraprostatic extension (locally advanced cancers)[21]. Stage T2 cancers are clinically palpable and confined to the prostate. Stage T2a is defined as one abnormal lobe of the prostate, while T2b involves both lobes. Disease progression rates of untreated T2a and T2b carcinomas after 5 years are 40% and 75%, respectively[22].

Three treatments have been proved to be efficient in eradicating localized prostate cancer: surgical removal of the prostate and vesical vesicles (radical prostatectomy), external beam radiotherapy and interstitial radiotherapy. It is admitted that patients who will benefit from these treatments are those whose life expectancy exceeds 10 years. No benefit is expected in older patients who are likely to die from another disease.

Radical prostatectomy

Indications for radical prostatectomy are presumably curable tumors in patients whose life expectancy is above 10 years: localized tumors (T1, T2), PSA level < 10 ng/ml, Gleason score < 8, tissue core invaded by cancer ≤ 20% and number of positive biopsies ≤ 50%.

Many experts consider radical prostatectomy to be the gold standard treatment in young patients having organ-confined disease. Radical prostatectomy can be performed with a transperineal approach, but is usually performed retropubically. Compared with the perineal approach, the retropubic approach is associated with a lower rate of positive surgical margins, especially in stage T2 cases[23]. Moreover, the retropubic prostatectomy allows simultaneous removal of pelvic lymph nodes.

Radical prostatectomy is still associated with a high rate of morbidity. However, perioperative mortality has considerably decreased and is reported to be less than 1% in most series[24]. Major bleeding complications requiring blood transfusion and rectal injuries occur in approximately 5% of patients. The rate of persistent urinary incontinence is below 8%[25]. The most common and worrisome complication at long-term follow-up is impotence. At 18 months, more than 70% of patients complain of erectile dysfunction after radical prostatectomy.

Nerve-sparing techniques have been described to decrease the rate of postoperative impotence, leading to an impotence rate of 14% after 18 months[26]. However, one-third of potent patients need sildenafil[26]. Although it has not been clearly established, the risk for local recurrence after nerve-sparing surgery seems to be higher than after the standard procedure. Therefore, candidates for nerve-sparing radical prostatectomy should have low-staged and low-graded tumors.

Since the early 1990s, laparoscopic radical prostatectomy has been commonly performed in laparoscopy-specialized centers. The main difficulty of the laparoscopic procedure is its long learning curve. Compared with open surgery, the laparoscopic procedure has been reported to result in less morbidity, without increasing positive surgical margins and impotence[27]. However, further follow-up is needed to assess biological postoperative results.

Many studies have evaluated the results of radical prostatectomy, but only a few have been performed prospectively with a long follow-up. In most reports, surgical removal of the prostate has been shown to be curative in localized cancer, with an overall disease-free survival rate of greater than 60% within 10 years. In the largest series, the rate of 10-year PSA-free survival was between 52 and 77%[17,28]. Analyzing the results of radical prostatectomy performed in the Johns Hopkins Institute, Alexianu and Weiss[29] reported a 97.8% success rate after 7 years, defined as postoperative PSA level below 0.2 ng/ml.

Follow-up after radical prostatectomy is based on PSA monitoring and DRE. PSA is expected to be undetectable within 3 weeks after radical prostatectomy. An increasing PSA level may indicate local recurrence or systemic recurrence. When PSA is still detectable, three parameters will help to distinguish between local recurrence and distant metastases: pathology, time to PSA recurrence and delay of PSA elevation. Positive surgical margins and/or undifferentiated tumors increase the risk of residual cancer and pelvic disease recurrence. A delayed and slowly increasing PSA level is generally due to residual local disease, while a rapidly increasing PSA rather indicates distant metastases.

Neoadjuvant hormonal therapy prior to radical prostatectomy

To improve the results of radical prostatectomy alone in prostate cancer, some authors have proposed giving hormonal therapy prior to prostate removal. Most of the published studies report a lower rate of positive surgical margins after surgery associated with androgen suppression than after surgery alone. However, no difference in the incidence of nodal metastases is noted. Moreover, the rate of PSA failure at long-term follow-up is the same in both groups. Comparing radical prostatectomy alone with neoadjuvant complete androgen blockade followed by surgery for T2b tumors, Soloway and colleagues[30] found rates of PSA failure at 24 months of 21% in both groups. In patients with T1b–T2c tumors, Goldenberg and co-workers[31] reported an even higher rate of PSA failure at 24 months when hormonal therapy was administered before surgery (28% in the neoadjuvant hormonal therapy group versus 20% in the control group). Nevertheless, one study showed better local disease control achieved by neoadjuvant therapy. Evaluating the effects of a 3-month neoadjuvant treatment prior to radical prostatectomy, Schulman and associates[32] reported a decreased rate of positive surgical margins in the neoadjuvant hormonal therapy group, in T2 tumors as well as in T3 tumors. Moreover, when evaluating the local control rate at 4 years in T2 tumors, the local recurrence rate was significantly lower in the neoadjuvant therapy group than in the control group (3% versus 11%). This was not the case for T3 tumors.

Even though local control may be, in the opinion of some authors, improved by neoadjuvant androgen deprivation, the question remains whether or not survival may be increased. To date, it remains impossible to answer this question because of unsufficient published data.

External radiation therapy

The curative indication of external radiotherapy is similar to that of radical prostatectomy: organ-confined cancer in patients with a life expectancy above 10 years. Radiotherapy is considered to result in lower rates of incontinence and erectile dysfunction than with radical prostatectomy. In a recent study comparing both treatments, some authors found a statistically lower rate of impotence related to external radiation than after surgery (41–55% versus 80–91%)[33]. However, studies comparing sexual dysfunction after radiotherapy and nerve-sparing prostatectomy are lacking.

The major side-effects of conventional external radiotherapy are urinary irritative symptoms and bowel complications. Quality of life related to urinary problems was worse after radiation at 2 years of follow-up than after radical prostatectomy[34]. One year after external radiotherapy, the rates of rectal urgency and bowel incontinence were 40% and 10%, respectively[35].

To improve tumor targeting and to increase radiation intensity, three-dimensional conformal radiotherapy (3D-CRT) was developed in the mid-1990s. Bowel toxicity related to this technique has been reported to be significantly lower than that related to conventional radiotherapy. One year after radiation therapy, the rates of rectal urgency and bowel incontinence

were 22% and 0%, respectively[35]. Although intestinal complications occur less frequently, quality of life and urinary symptoms do not seem to be improved by 3D-CRT[35].

Oncological results of external radiotherapy are similar to those of radical prostatectomy. After radiation or radical prostatectomy, the survival rate depends on clinical stage, initial PSA level and Gleason score. For clinically localized cancer, the overall rate of disease-free survival after 10 years ranges between 43 and 66%[36,37]. Evaluating tumor response after 3D-CRT, Zelefsky and colleagues[38,39] reported that 93% of patients had no biochemical recurrence (PSA > 1 ng/ml) after 5 years, when the initial PSA level had been ≤ 10 ng/ml. This rate was 60% in patients with initial PSA level between 10 and 20 ng/ml and 40% in those with PSA level > 20 ng/ml. In some reports, results of 3D-CRT have been proved to be dose dependent, especially for an initial level of PSA < 10 ng/ml.

After radiation therapy, PSA monitoring is more difficult than after prostatectomy, because of residual PSA levels related to residual prostatic tissue. The DRE generally cannot distinguish between local disease recurrence and radiation-induced fibrosis. The level of PSA nadir seems to be of particular importance. It has been reported that a better negative value of tumor progression was obtained with a PSA nadir below 0.5 ng/ml. In a recent study, only 4% of patients having PSA nadir ≤ 0.5 ng/ml had tumor recurrence within 4 years[40]. However, the PSA nadir threshold remains controversial. For some authors, a PSA nadir below 1 ng/ml is associated with a low rate of disease recurrence within 5 years. Regardless of the actual PSA level, the kinetics of PSA levels seems to be informative. Most authors consider that three consecutive rises of PSA level after radiation are predictive of disease progression. PSA doubling time has been shown to be 13 months in patients with local recurrence and only 3 months in patients with distant metastases[41].

Interstitial radiotherapy (brachytherapy)

Interstitial radiotherapy consists of placing radioactive sources within the prostate, to deliver higher radiation doses without damaging surrounding tissues. Under anesthesia, radioactive seeds are placed using ultrasound guidance. Brachytherapy can be performed either with a high dose rate (HDR) for a short time or with a permanent low dose rate (LDR). HDR brachytherapy is usually used in combination with external radiotherapy in locally advanced tumors, while LDR brachytherapy may be indicated in organ-confined tumors (T1, T2). LDR brachytherapy is indicated in a curative intent. The most commonly used isotopes in LDR brachytherapy are iodine-125 and palladium-103. In some centers, the procedure is commonly performed on an out-patient basis. The operative time is about 2 h. Compared with prostatectomy, the major advantage of brachytherapy is its low morbidity rate. Although irritative bladder symptoms are frequent within the first week, major complications are exceptional. Rectitis is reported to occur in less than 2% of patients[42]. At 18 months of follow-up, the incontinence rate is reported to be 1–2%[38,43]. The impotence rate is reported to be around 30% in the largest series[38,44].

Previous transurethral surgery is a contraindication of interstitial radiotherapy because of an increased risk of postoperative incontinence.

Preliminary results of LDR brachytherapy are encouraging. In a recent series, a 9-year PSA-free survival rate above 80% was reported in patients with localized cancer[43]. Alexianu and Weiss[29] reported that, when a PSA level of 0.5 ng/ml is used as a threshold, the 7-year actuarial likelihood of disease-free progression is 79%. In the opinion of some authors, brachytherapy may be an alternative curative treatment to radical prostatectomy and external beam radiation in T1 and T2 prostate cancers. However, this new therapy must be evaluated in larger series, and requires comparison with standard treatments in prospective randomized trials. Today, most urologists remain cautious, and do not recommend the use of brachytherapy when the PSA level is above 10 ng/ml and/or the Gleason score is above 7.

PSA monitoring after brachytherapy is difficult because of the long half-life of the isotopes. Using iodine-125, the PSA nadir may be expected after 4 years[45]. A PSA threshold of 0.5 ng/ml is considered by most experts to be acceptable, but this threshold is still debated.

Watchful waiting

Watchful waiting/deferred treatment consists of a standpoint strategy until an active treatment may be required. Only patients with good compliance and easy access to health-care should be candidates for watchful waiting. The support for such management is based on the natural course of prostate cancer progression, which has been proved to be very slow. Commonly, deferred treatment is indicated in asymptomatic old patients (life expectancy < 10 years because of age or debilitating conditions) with localized or locally advanced cancer. However, it is now suggested by some experts that watchful waiting can also be indicated in younger patients in very selected cases. Only patients with stage T1a and well- or moderately differentiated tumors can benefit from deferred treatment. It is prudent to perform rebiopsy to avoid understaging of the tumor.

Chodak and colleagues[46] studied the results of watchful waiting in patients with clinically localized prostate cancer. The authors reported a correlation between survival rates and tumor grade. The overall 10-year disease-specific survival rate was 87% for grade 1 tumors, while it was 34% for grade 3 tumors. The 10-year metastasis-free survival rates for grade 1 and grade 3 were 81% and 26%, respectively. When analyzing the outcome of T1a patients, Chodak and colleagues found cancer-specific 10-year survival rates with grade 1 and grade 2 tumors to be 96% and 94%, respectively. These findings were confirmed by Albertsen and co-workers[47], who reported a correlation between Gleason score and the risk of dying from prostate cancer. In this study, the 15-year cancer-specific mortality rate was 8% when the Gleason score was < 5 versus 93% when it was > 7.

Although conservative treatment is admitted to be advantageous in elderly patients without symptoms, its indication in younger men remains controversial. Some studies evaluating watchful waiting in patients with a life expectancy exceeding 10 years concluded that the risk of dying from prostate cancer was higher than after curative treatment.

Prostatic intraepithelial neoplasia and 'clinically insignificant' prostate cancer

Performing prostate biopsies for PSA elevation among patients with a clinically unapparent tumor has led to the identification of premalignant abnormalities: prostatic intraepithelial neoplasia (PIN)[48]. Although patients with high-grade PIN have a 30% risk of developing a carcinoma within 5 years, PIN is not considered to be an indication for radical treatment. Most authors recommend a rebiopsy in males presenting with PIN because of its frequent association with prostate carcinoma. Indeed, in autopsy series, high-grade PIN is reported to be associated with prostate cancer in 50–100% of cases[49,50].

The wide use of prostate biopsy has also resulted in the discovery of small and low-cytological-grade tumors (less than 3 mm in only one biopsy core and Gleason score ≤ 6), considered by some authors to be 'clinically insignificant'. In the opinion of these experts, the treatment of such tumors should be curative in young patients but should be deferred in asymptomatic patients whose life expectancy is less than 10 years. The significance of such 'clinically insignificant' prostate neoplasms is still a matter of debate. Indeed, it has been shown that approximately 30% of prostate carcinomas are understaged by biopsy[51]. Therefore, it seems dangerous to defer treatment in patients whose tumor may contain pathological features more pejorative than those revealed by the biopsy.

LOCALLY ADVANCED PROSTATE CANCER

Definitions and general considerations

Locally advanced carcinomas are stage T3 and T4 cancers. Stage T3a is defined as capsular perforation and T3b as invasion of the seminal vesicles. T4 cancer is defined as extension to the surrounding organs (bladder and rectum). In the past, locally advanced cancers were more frequent than today and commonly treated by surgery. To date, it is universally admitted that patients with T4 tumors require palliative treatment. The management of T3 tumors is more controversial and may be curative in some patients without pejorative pathological features.

Radical prostatectomy for T3 tumors

Compared with prostatectomy for T1–T2 prostate cancer, surgical removal of T3 carcinoma is associated with a higher rate of intraoperative complications and an increased risk of local recurrence[52]. An overall PSA-free survival rate within 5 years after surgery has been reported to be only 20% in patients with T3 disease[53]. However, some authors have reported that only 8% of all T3 tumors are understaged, while about 15% are overstaged[52]. These findings support the curative intent of treatment in young patients with T3 cancer. In a recent series, a 5-year PSA-free survival rate exceeding 60% has been reported after radical prostatectomy in males with T3a prostate carcinoma and PSA level below 10 ng/ml.

Radical prostatectomy may be an option for patients with locally advanced cancer, but a selected group needs to be individualized. Until further reports are available, it seems reasonable in the opinion of most authors to limit indications to T3a tumors with PSA levels < 10 ng/ml[54].

As for localized cancer, neoadjuvant hormonal therapy prior to radical prostatectomy in T3 cancer has been recently proposed, but no advantage of such combined therapy has been noted.

Postoperative radiotherapy for T3 tumors

After radical prostatectomy for organ-confined cancer, approximatively 30% of specimens are found to contain foci of capsular effraction[55]. The risk of local recurrence without adjuvant therapy is considered to be 25–68%[56]. In such cases, postoperative radiotherapy has been proved to improve local disease control. In a study comparing radical prostatectomy alone and surgery plus adjuvant radiotherapy for T3 tumors, Valicenti and colleagues[57] reported rates of 5-year freedom from PSA relapse of 55% and 89%, respectively. In the opinion of some authors, radiation therapy should be delayed until the PSA level rises and becomes > 1 ng/ml[55]. Other authors consider that early adjuvant radiotherapy is more effective than salvage therapy for a rising PSA[58]. To date, no benefit at long-term follow-up has been shown in published series. Further data are required to assess the benefit of postoperative radiation therapy in terms of survival.

Hormonal manipulation alone

Hormonal manipulation is the standard therapy for T4 tumors and T3 tumors with high risk of recurrence (elevated PSA and/or unfavorable histological features). Many studies evaluating hormonal therapy alone in metastatic disease are available, but only a few with regard to locally advanced tumors. Consequently, the effectiveness of endocrine monotherapy in this latter indication remains unknown.

External radiotherapy combined with hormonal manipulation

In the past, radiation therapy alone was proposed not only for localized tumors but also for T3–T4 tumors. In stage T3 cancer, the overall 10-year survival rate and 10-year disease-free survival rate after radiotherapy alone have been reported to be 42% and 38%, respectively[59]. It is now admitted that radiation therapy alone is not the optimal treatment for locally advanced prostate cancer. Some authors suggest that hormonal therapy administered before and/or after radiation may improve the tumor response.

In a recent study, Bolla and associates[60] showed that 79% of patients with locally advanced prostate cancer treated by radiotherapy alone were local recurrence-free within 5 years, versus 97% of those treated by adjuvant hormonal blockade. The 5-year survival rate was 62% in the radiotherapy-alone group versus 78% in the combined group. In this study, the authors reported no increased morbidity when combination treatment was administered, even though hot flushes occured in 33% of patients in the combined-treatment group.

Lavardière and colleagues[61] analyzed local progression of T2b–T3 tumors treated either by androgen blockade 2 months before radiotherapy or by androgen blockade 3 months before, during and 6 months after radiotherapy. The authors reported rates of positive prostate biopsy at 2 years of 29% and 6%, respectively.

There is concern regarding the time when hormone therapy should be initiated. In another randomized study, Bolla and co-workers[62] compared the results of radiation therapy plus 3 years of adjuvant hormonal therapy with those of radiation therapy initially plus hormonal therapy only at disease recurrence, and found a better 5-year survival rate in the first group.

Deferred treatment

In the opinion of some experts, watchful waiting may be proposed in asymptomatic patients with locally advanced cancer and short life expectancy. This choice of therapy requires careful follow-up because of early occurrence of symptoms due to local disease progression.

PROSTATE CANCER WITH NODAL INVOLVEMENT OR DISTANT METASTASES

Hormonal therapy as first-line treatment

In the case of nodal involvement or distant metastases at diagnosis, treatment is palliative and comprises hormone therapy. Watchful waiting should be proposed only in exceptional cases of asymptomatic patients with very short life expectancy. Supported by the endocrine dependence of prostate cancer, hormonal therapy involves decreasing the level of testosterone. Hormonal manipulation is administered to reduce the tumor volume and the risk of progression, but it is not indicated for curative intent. Indeed, most prostate carcinomas become refractory to endocrine therapy after a median delay of 2 years. The mechanism of such hormonal resistance is not well known. Recent studies suggest that mutations of the androgen receptor gene may be responsible for the development of hormone independence[63].

Surgical castration (bilateral orchiectomy) is an efficient way to eliminate the circulating level of testosterone and cause the prostate to atrophy. Surgical castration used to be the gold standard of hormonal therapy before medical castration became available. To date, orchiectomy is still widely performed because of its simplicity and reduced cost. A benefit in terms of time to tumor progression is obtained in approximately 80% of patients, with a mean duration of 2.5 years[64]. The main complications of bilateral orchiectomy are hot flushes,

decreased libido and erectile dysfunction, which occur in more than 70% of patients. Long-term adverse effects of androgen blockade are muscle atrophy, osteoporosis, gynecomastia, depression and anemia[65].

Luteinizing hormone releasing hormone analogs (LHRHa) have also been proved to be efficient in advanced prostate cancer. LHRHa decrease the secretion of luteinizing hormone (LH) and follicle stimulating hormone (FSH) from the pituitary via a biofeedback mechanism, and thereby reduce the level of testosterone. However, the initial rise in LH and FSH results in a transient (3–5 days) increase of circulating testosterone levels. In patients with potential bone metastasis, this 'flare-up phenomenon' may worsen symptoms, and should be prevented by the administration of an antiandrogen during the first weeks of therapy. In practice, LHRHa are administered every 3 months or monthly by injection. The results for survival and complications of LHRHa have been shown to be similar to those reported after bilateral orchiectomy[66].

Estrogens represent an alternative hormone therapy. Estrogens block the secretion of LH and FSH by a feedback mechanism, and achieve medical castration. In the opinion of some investigators, decreased androgen synthesis may also be a direct effect of estrogen administration. In one of the largest series evaluating the effects of estrogen therapy on advanced prostate cancer, 5-year progression-free survival was 68%[67]. At a follow-up exceeding 60 months, the survival rate was 31%, and similar to that reported following orchiectomy. Estrogens can be administered either orally or parenterally. The major disadvantage of estrogen therapy is cardiovascular toxicity (venous thrombosis, pulmonary embolism, stroke and heart attack)[68]. The combined use of acetyl salicylic acid may reduce the rate of cardiovascular complications.

Antiandrogens block the action of androgens within intraprostatic cells. Antiandrogens can be administered either alone or in combination with surgical or medical castration (complete androgen blockade). Non-steroidal antiandrogens act only upon androgen receptors in cells, while steroidal androgens also have effects upon the pituitary gland. Non-steroidal androgens tend to increase the serum testosterone level, whereas steroidal antiandrogens lower levels of testosterone and LH, which may induce loss of libido and erectile dysfunction[69]. In patients with locally advanced cancer, there are no published data that support the advantage of complete androgen blockade compared with antiandrogen monotherapy. There are differences in side-effects with various antiandrogens when taken alone[70]. Flutamide induces mainly diarrhea, hepatic dysfunction and breast tenderness. The main side-effects of nilutamide are visual disturbances, respiratory disturbance and hepatic dysfunction. Gynecomastia and breast pain are noted using bicalutamide.

Few studies have evaluated results of androgen blockade with long-term follow-up. Because of the outcome of hormonal independence, progression-free survival rates at 5 years are estimated to be less than 70%. According to the literature, approximatively one-third of patients with advanced prostate cancer are still alive 5 years after the beginning of hormonal manipulation[67].

To prevent early androgen independence, some authors propose beginning hormonal therapy at the time of symptom presentation instead of at the time of diagnosis. To date, no randomized study has shown any benefit in terms of survival and quality of life from delayed versus early treatment.

Intermittent hormonal therapy

The goals of intermittent hormonal manipulation are to prolong survival by delaying progression to androgen independence and to improve quality of life by avoiding the side-effects of continuous androgen deprivation. Intermittent hormonal therapy has been evaluated in few studies either with LHRHa alone or with complete androgen blockade. Unfortunately, prospective randomized studies with long-term follow-up have not, to date, been published. This lack of data is responsible for controversies regarding intermittent androgen suppression. In the opinion of experts who recommend such intermittent treatment, periods of 6–9 months on therapy are usually necessary, and the mean off-therapy intervals are approximatively 50% of this duration. In a recent review of published series, the mean time to disease progression was reported to be 32 months[71]. Bouchot and colleagues[72] analyzed the outcome of 43 patients with metastatic prostate cancer treated by intermittent androgen suppression with a mean follow-up of 43.7 months. The mean off-therapy duration was 6.7 months after the first therapy period, while it was 3.8 months after the second therapy period. Seven patients became hormone-independent after the first therapy period, and ten after the second. Using the European Organization for Research and Treatment of Cancer (EORTC) quality-of-life questionnaire QLQ-C30, quality of life was reported to be similar for the on-therapy and the off-therapy periods. However, a rapid decrease in adverse effects related to hormonal deprivation was noted in all patients during the off-therapy periods.

After radical prostatectomy

In the opinion of most urologists, adjuvant treatment by androgen suppression may be advocated in patients who are found to have nodal involvement after radical prostatectomy. Although no prospective randomized study to date has evaluated the impact upon survival of such a treatment, it seems reasonable to propose androgen suppression when disease is found to have nodal involvement. Indeed, it has been proved that nodal involvement is associated with a high risk of local recurrence and distant metastases. Immediate adjuvant surgical castration has shown a 10-year cancer-specific survival rate of 80%[73]. Conflicting data exist regarding the time to initiate neoadjuvant hormonal therapy: some authors suggest that early hormone therapy should be advantageous, while others recommend delayed treatment.

Androgen-independent cancer

About 10% of prostate cancers are androgen-independent at diagnosis, and more than 80% become androgen-independent after a mean hormonal treatment period of 2 years[68]. When tumor progression occurs despite endocrine deprivation, it is essential to document the castration levels of testosterone.

If the serum testosterone level is not decreased, optimized hormonal therapy is indicated to improve castration. Incomplete androgen blockade should be completed by the combination of LHRHa or surgical castration and an antiandrogen. The dose of antiandrogen should be increased when using an antiandrogen that achieves a dose-dependent response.

If the serum testosterone is at a minimal level, there is evidence that the cancer has become hormone-independent and requires a second-line treatment. Some clinical and biochemical responses have been described with discontinued antiandrogen therapy. The mechanism of this phenomenon, called 'antiandrogen withdrawal syndrome' remains unknown, but androgen receptor mutations are suspected[74]. There are no published data dealing with the efficacy of discontinued antiandrogens. What is known is that a few patients with hormone-independent cancer will show a brief response when stopping antiandrogens. This suggests that discontinued treatment should be tested before proposing chemotherapy. Secondary hormonal therapy using estrogens with corticosteroids or antiandrogens at high dose is an alternative. However, there are no randomized studies evaluating secondary hormonal treatments, so therapeutics are chosen on an individual basis.

Chemotherapy may be indicated when prostate cancer becomes refractory to all other treatments. No single chemotherapeutic agent has been demonstrated to provide a survival benefit. On the contrary, several pilot studies have suggested a synergy effect when chemotherapy is combined with other drugs[75]. Several studies have evaluated the combination of mitoxantrone, vinblastine, etoposide, methotrexate, cisplatin or carboplatin with corticosteroids or estramucine. Some phase II trials have shown promising results, but such combined therapies remain to be tested in phase III trials[76,77]. Combinations of three drugs are being tested in phase II trials, for example estramucine plus etoposide and cisplatin. Taxanes are also being currently investigated, and preliminary evaluation shows promising results in combination with estramucine[78].

Recently, attention has been focused on new cytotoxic agents. Growth factor inhibitors such as suramin and flavopiridol have been proved to decrease the proliferation of prostate cancer cells *in vitro*, but further evaluation by clinical trials is required. The combination of suramin plus hydrocortisone has been shown to be advantageous when compared with placebo plus hydrocortisone in a multicenter double-blind phase III study[79].

Radioisotopes such as strontium-89 and samarium-153 may be useful in decreasing pain related to bone metastases. The use of parenteral radioisotopes is reported to achieve a clinical response in approximately 70% of patients[80].

PROSTATE CANCER AND THE AGING MALE

General considerations

In Europe, the mean age of patients at diagnosis of prostate cancer is above 72 years[81]. In the opinion of most authors, it is not suitable to perform prostate biopsies when localized cancer is suspected (PSA < 10 ng/ml) in elderly men, because the natural course of the disease without treatment is expected to be longer than the patient's life expectancy. Patients over 75 years old are considered to have a life expectancy below 10 years, and therefore to receive no benefit from curative therapies.

However, randomized studies dealing with quality of life and survival in elderly patients, comparing watchful waiting or hormonal manipulation versus curative treatment, have not been performed. With increasing longevity, it should be questioned whether elderly men should be diagnosed and treated like younger patients.

Deferred treatment

Deferred treatment is widely accepted, as it is felt that this approach may not compromise survival. Gronberg and colleagues[82] reported a direct influence of age on the loss of life expectancy. These authors also underlined the difference between relative survival and loss of life expectancy, the latter signifying the absolute effect of prostate cancer. In their series, relative survival was the same for all age groups if adjusted for cancer grade. However, the loss of life expectancy varied among age groups. For grade 1 tumors, the loss was 11 years for the younger group and only 1.2 years for the older group[83]. These authors suggest that patients with well- and moderately differentiated clinically localized prostate cancer, with a life expectancy of 10 years or less, can be safely monitored and treatment deferred until progression. Early treatment, usually hormonal, at the time of local or systemic progression results in a better quality of life than delaying treatment until symptomatic progression. Analysis of the literature suggests that deferred treatment may be appropriate in elderly patients with PSA < 10 ng/ml, Gleason score ≤ 6, good performance status and reasonable life expectancy, in whom the risk for having disease-related symptoms is particularly low.

Mortality data for the general population compiled by the insurance industry in the USA indicate that the proportion of men surviving 10 years from a patient age of 60, 70 and 80 years is 77.6%, 52.2% and 19.7%, respectively[81]. Additionally, 28% of men at age 70 years are expected to survive at least 15 years. Therefore, systematic, serial, potentially curative treatment of men 70 years old or older would exclude a significant subset of men whose life expectancy would afford them years of tumor-free survival. On the other hand, taking into account age only would lead to the treatment with curative intent of patients whose life expectancy, because of comorbidity, is much lower than that of same-age patients. This is why therapeutic decisions must be taken on an individual basis[84].

Radical prostatectomy

Kerr and Zincke[85] investigated the benefits of radical prostatectomy in men over 75 years old, by comparing two groups of patients (≤ 55 years and ≥ 75 years old) treated for clinically localized prostate cancer. In this series, elderly patients had higher-pathological-stage and higher-grade tumors. Significant urinary incontinence occurred in 16% of the elderly compared with 3% of the younger patients at 1 year. This study confirmed that if well selected, these patients can have excellent survival, but that it is difficult to recommend such a surgical procedure owing to the high rate of incontinence, which significantly impairs quality of life.

Andropause

Andropause, a syndrome in aging men, consists of physical, sexual and psychological symptoms that include weakness, reduced muscle and bone mass, sexual dysfunction, depression, anxiety, insomnia and reduced cognitive function[86]. Free testosterone levels begin to decline at a rate of 1% per year after age 40 years. It is estimated that 20% of men aged 60–80 years have levels below the lower limit of normal. Although the causal relationship between decreasing testosterone levels and the development of andropause symptoms is not firmly established, the administration of testosterone to this population results in clinical improvements. Most studies to date have focused on the physical benefits of testosterone replacement, and have failed to assess psychological symptoms rigorously. Preliminary data suggest that therapy may benefit elderly men with new-onset depression. However, the most worrisome problem of testosterone replacement is the potential risk for increased prostate cancer occurrence[86–88]. Despite this concern, a limited number of studies administered the hormone weekly for up to 2 years, with only mild increases in PSA level. It remains unclear at what age such therapy should start and what monitoring should be performed. Further clinical investigations are necessary to evaluate the risk for developing prostate cancer in men submitted to testosterone therapy.

References

1. Black RJ, Bray F, Ferlay J, Parkin DM. Cancer incidence and mortality in the European Union: cancer registry data and estimates of national incidence for 1990. *Eur J Cancer* 1997;33:1075–107

2. Carter HB, Piantadosi S, Isaacs JT. Clinical evidence for and implications of the multistep development of prostate cancer. *J Urol* 1990; 143:742–6

3. Steinberg GD, Carter BS, Beaty TH, *et al*. Family history and the risk of prostate cancer. *Prostate* 1990;17:337–47

4. Zaridze DG, Boyle P. Cancer of the prostate: epidemiology and aetiology. *Br J Urol* 1987; 59:493–502

5. Denis L, Morton MS, Griffiths K. Diet and its preventive role in prostatic disease. *Eur Urol* 1999;35:377–87

6. Pedersen KV, Carlsson P, Varenhorst E, *et al*. Screening for carcinoma of the prostate by digital rectal examination in a randomly selected population. *Br Med J* 1990;300: 1041–4

7. Haas GP, Montie JE, Pontes JE. The state of prostate cancer screening in the United States. *Eur Urol* 1993;23:337–47

8. Babaian RJ, Johnston DA, Naccarato W, *et al*. The incidence of prostate cancer in a screening population with a serum prostate specific antigen between 2.5 and 4 ng/ml: relation to biopsy strategy. *J Urol* 2001;165: 757–60

9. Morote J, Encabo G, De Torres IM. Use of free prostate-specific antigen as a predictor of the pathological features of clinically localized prostate cancer. *Eur Urol* 2000;38: 225–9

10. Ravery V, Boccon-Gibod L. Free/total PSA ratio – hope and controversies. *Eur Urol* 1997; 31:385–8

11. Rodriguez LV, Terris MK. Risks and complications of transrectal ultrasound guided prostate needle biopsy: a prospective study and review of the literature. *J Urol* 1998; 160:2115–20

12. Levine MA, Ittman M, Melamed J, Lepor H. Two consecutive sets of transrectal ultrasound guided sextant biopsies of the prostate for the detection of prostate cancer. *J Urol* 1998; 159:475–6

13. Naughton CK, Ornstein DK, Smith DS, Catalona WJ. Pain and morbidity of transrectal ultrasound guided prostate biopsy: a prospective randomized trial of 6 versus 12 cores. *J Urol* 2000;163:168–71

14. Ravery V, Goldblatt L, Royer B, *et al*. Extensive biopsy protocol improves the detection rate of prostate cancer. *J Urol* 2000;164:393–6

15. Partin AW, Yoo J, Pearson JD, *et al*. The use of prostate specific antigen, clinical stage and Gleason score to predict pathological stage in men with localized prostate cancer. *J Urol* 1993;150:110–14

16. Hricak H, Dooms GC, Jeffrey RB, *et al.* Prostatic carcinoma: staging by clinical assessment, CT and MR imaging. *Radiology* 1987; 162:331–6

17. Partin AW, Pound CR, Clemens JQ, *et al.* Prostate-specific antigen after anatomic radical prostatectomy: the Johns Hopkins experience after 10 years. *Urol Clin North Am* 1993;20:713–25

18. Rana A, Karamanis K, Lucal MG, Chisholm GD. Identification of metastatic disease by T category, Gleason score and serum PSA level in patients with carcinoma of the prostate. *Br J Urol* 1992;69:277–81

19. Oesterling JE. Prostate-specific antigen: a critical assessment of the most useful tumour marker for adenocarcinoma of the prostate. *J Urol* 1991;145:907–23

20. Lowe BA, Listrom MB. Incidental carcinoma of the prostate: an analysis of the predictors of progression. *J Urol* 1988;140:1340–4

21. Oesterling JE, Suman VJ, Zincke H, Bostwick DG. PSA detected (clinical stage T1c or B0) prostate cancer: pathologically significant tumours. *Urol Clin North Am* 1993;20:687–93

22. Graverson PH, Nielsson KT, Gasser TC, *et al.* Radical prostatectomy versus expectant primary treatment in stages I and II prostatic cancer. A 15 year follow-up. *Urology* 1990;36: 493–8

23. Boccon-Gibod L, Ravery V, Vordos D, *et al.* Radical prostatectomy for prostate cancer: the perineal approach increases the risk of surgically induced positive margins and capsular incisions. *J Urol* 1998;160:1383–5

24. Davidson PJ, Van den Ouden D, Schroeder FH. Radical prostatectomy: prospective assessment of mortality and morbidity. *Eur Urol* 1996;29:168–73

25. Hautmann RE, Sauter TW, Wenderoth UK. Radical retropubic prostatectomy: morbidity and urinary continence in 418 consecutive cases. *Urology* 1994;43:47–51

26. Walsh PC. Patient-reported urinary continence and sexual function after anatomic radical prostatectomy. *J Urol* 2000;164:242

27. Guillonneau B, Vallancien G. Laparoscopic radical prostatectomy: the Montsouris technique. *J Urol* 2000;163:1643–9

28. Zincke H, Oesterling JE, Blute ML, *et al.* Long-term (15 years) results after radical prostatectomy for clinically localized (stage T2c or lower) prostate cancer. *J Urol* 1994; 152:1850–7

29. Alexianu M, Weiss GH. Radical prostatectomy versus brachytherapy for early-stage prostate cancer. *J Endourol* 2000;14:325–8

30. Soloway MS, Sharifi R, Wajsman Z, *et al.* The Lupron Depot Neoadjuvant Prostate Cancer Study Group. Randomized prospective study comparing radical prostatectomy alone versus radical prostatectomy preceded by androgen blockade in clinical stage B2 (T2bNxM0) prostate cancer. *J Urol* 1995;154:424–8

31. Goldenberg SL, Klotz LH, Srigley J, *et al.* The Canadian Urologic Oncology Group. Randomized, prospective, controlled study comparing radical prostatectomy alone and neoadjuvant androgen withdrawal in the treatment of localized prostate cancer. *J Urol* 1996;156: 873–7

32. Schulman CC, Debruyne F, Forster G, *et al.* The European Study Group on Neoadjuvant Treatment of Prostate Cancer. 4-Year follow-up of a European prospective randomized study on neoadjuvant hormonal therapy prior to radical prostatectomy in T2–3N0M0 prostate cancer. *Eur Urol* 2000; 38:706–13

33. Madalinska JB, Essink-Bot ML, De Koning HJ, *et al.* Health-related quality-of-life effects of radical prostatectomy and primary radiotherapy for screen-detected or clinically diagnosed localized prostate cancer. *J Clin Oncol* 2001;19:1587–8

34. Lithin MS, Pasta DJ, Yu J, *et al.* Urinary function and bother after radical prostatectomy or radiation for prostate cancer: a longitudinal, multi-variate quality of life analysis from the Cancer of the Prostate Strategic Urologic Research Endeavor. *J Urol* 2000;164:1973–7

35. Hanlon AL, Natvinsbruner D, Peter R, Hanks GE. Quality of life study in prostate cancer patients treated with 3-dimensional conformal radiation therapy: comparing late bowel and bladder quality of life symptoms to that of the normal population. *Int J Radiat Oncol Biol Phys* 2001;49:51–9

36. Fowler JE, Braswell NT, Pandey P, Seaver L. Experience with radical prostatectomy and radiation therapy for localized prostate cancer at a Veterans Affairs medical center. *J Urol* 1995;153:1026–31

37. Kuban DA, El-Mahdi AM, Schellhammer PF. Prostate-specific antigen for pretreatment prediction and posttreatment evaluation of outcome after definitive irradiation for prostate cancer. *Int J Radiat Oncol Biol Phys* 1995;23:307–16

38. Zelefsky MJ, Wallner KE, Ling CC. Comparison of the 5-year outcome and morbidity of three-dimensional conformal radiotherapy versus transperineal permanent iodine-125 implantation for early-stage prostate cancer. *J Clin Oncol* 1999;17:517–22

39. Zelefsky MJ, Lyass O, Fuks Z, *et al.* Predictors of improved outcome for patients with localized prostate cancer treated with neoadjuvant androgen ablation therapy and three-dimensional conformal radiotherapy. *J Clin Oncol* 1998;16:3380–5

40. Crook JM, Bahadur YA, Bociek RG, *et al.* Radiotherapy for localized prostate carcinoma. The correlation of pre-treatment prostate specific antigen and nadir prostate specific antigen with outcome as assessed by systematic biopsy and serum prostate specific antigen. *Cancer* 1997;79:328–36

41. Hancock SL, Cox RS, Bagshaw MA. Prostate specific antigen after radiotherapy for prostate cancer: a reevaluation of long-term biochemical control and the kinetics of recurrence in patients treated at Stanford University. *J Urol* 1995;154:1412–17

42. Blasko JC, Ragde H, Luse RW, *et al.* Should brachytherapy be considered a therapeutic option in localized prostate cancer? *Urol Clin North Am* 1996;23:633–50

43. Blasko JC, Grimm PD, Sylvester JE, *et al.* Palladium-103 brachytherapy for prostate carcinoma. *Int J Radiat Oncol Biol Phys* 2000; 46:839–50

44. Ragde H, Blasko JC, Grimm PD, *et al.* Interstitial ^{125}I radiation without adjuvant therapy in the treatment of clinically localized prostate carcinoma. *Cancer* 1997;80:442–53

45. Kaye KW, Olson DJ, Payne JT. Detailed preliminary analysis of [125]Iodine implantation for localized prostate cancer using percutaneous approach. *J Urol* 1995;153:1020–5

46. Chodak GW, Thisted RA, Gerber GS, *et al.* Results of conservative management of clinically localized prostate cancer. *N Engl J Med* 1994;330:242–8

47. Albertsen PC, Hanley JA, Gleason DF, Barry MJ. Competing risk analysis of men aged 55 to 74 years at diagnosis managed conservatively for clinically localized prostate cancer. *J Am Med Assoc* 1998;280:975–80

48. Fowler JE Jr, Bigler SA, Lynch C, *et al.* Prospective study of correlations between biopsy-detected high grade prostatic intraepithelial neoplasia, serum PSA concentration, and race. *Cancer* 2001;91:1291–6

49. Haggman MJ, Macoska JA, Wojno KJ, Oesterling JE. The relationship between prostatic intraepithelial neoplasia and prostate cancer: critical issues. *J Urol* 1997;158:12–22

50. Zlotta AR, Raviv G, Schulman CC. Clinical prognostic criteria for later diagnosis of prostate carcinoma in patients with isolated prostatic intraepithelial neoplasia. *Eur Urol* 1996;30:240–55

51. Ravery V, Boccon-Gibod Li, Dauge-Geffroy MC, *et al.* Systematic biopsies accurately predict extracapsular extension of prostate cancer and persistent/recurrent detectable PSA after radical prostatectomy. *Urology* 1994;44:371–6

52. Lerner SE, Blute ML, Zincke H. Extended experience with radical prostatectomy for clinical stage T3 prostate cancer: outcome and contemporary morbidity. *J Urol* 1995;154: 1447–52

53. Morgan WR, Bergstralh EJ, Zincke H. Long-term evaluation of radical prostatectomy as treatment for clinical stage C (T3) prostate cancer. *Urology* 1993;41:113–20

54. Van Poppel H, Goethuys H, Callewaert P, *et al.* Radical prostatectomy can provide cure for well-selected clinical stage T3 prostate cancer. *Eur Urol* 2000;38:372–9

55. Ravery V. Lamotte F, Hennequin C, *et al.* Adjuvant radiation therapy for recurrent PSA after radical prostatectomy in T1–T2 cancer. *Prostate Cancer Prostatic Dis* 1998;1:321–5

56. Zietman AL. Locally advanced or recurrent prostate cancer. In Vogelzang NJ and Miles BJ,

eds. *Comprehensive Textbook of Genitourinary Oncology*. Baltimore: Williams & Wilkins, 1996:782–90

57. Valicenti RK, Gomella LG, Ismail M, *et al*. The efficacy of early adjuvant radiation therapy for pT3N0 prostate cancer: a matched-pair analysis. *Int J Radiat Oncol Biol Phys* 1999;45:53–8

58. Anscher MS. Adjuvant radiotherapy following radical prostatectomy is more effective and less toxic than salvage radiotherapy for a rising prostate specific antigen. *Int J Cancer* 2001;96:91–3

59. Perez CA, Hanks GE, Leibel SA, *et al*. Localized carcinoma of the prostate (stages T1B, T1C, T2, and T3). Review of management with external beam radiation therapy. *Cancer* 1993;72:3156–73

60. Bolla M, Gonzales D, Warde P, *et al*. Improved survival in patients with locally advanced prostate cancer treated with radiotherapy and goserelin. *N Engl J Med* 1997; 337:295–300

61. Lavardière J, Gomez JL, Cusan L, *et al*. Beneficial effect of combination hormonal therapy administered prior and following external beam radiation therapy in localized prostate cancer. *Int J Radiat Oncol Biol Phys* 1997;37:247–52

62. Bolla M, Collette L, Gonzales D, *et al*. Long term results of immediate adjuvant hormonal therapy with goserelin in patients with locally advanced prostate cancer treated with radiotherapy (phase III EORTC study). *Int J Radiat Oncol Biol Phys* 1999;45:147

63. Taplin ME, Bubley GJ, Shuster TD, *et al*. Mutation of the androgen-receptor gene in metastatic androgen independent prostate cancer. *N Engl J Med* 1995;332:1393–8

64. Veterans Administration Cooperative Urological Research Group. Treatment and survival of patients with cancer of the prostate. *Surg Gynecol Obstet* 1967;124:1011–17

65. Catalona WJ. Management of cancer of the prostate. *N Engl J Med* 1994;331:996–1004

66. Peeling WB. Phase III studies to compare goserelin with orchidectomy and with diethylstilboestrol in treatment of prostatic carcinoma. *Urology* 1989;33(Suppl 5):45–52

67. Haapiainen R, Ranniko S, Ruutu M. Orchiectomy versus oestrogen in the treatment of advanced prostate cancer. *Br J Urol* 1991;67:184–7

68. Byar DP, Corle DK. Hormone therapy for prostate cancer: results of the Veterans Administration Cooperative Urological Research Group Studies. *Natl Cancer Inst Monogr* 1988;7:165–70

69. Soloway MS, Matzkin H. Antiandrogenic agents as monotherapy in advanced prostatic carcinoma. *Cancer* 1993;71:1083–8

70. Pavone-Macaluso M, Pavone C, Serretta Y, Daricello G. Antiandrogens alone or in combination for treatment of prostate cancer: the European experience. *Urology* 1989;34:27–36

71. Van Cangh PJ, Tombal B, Gala JL. Intermittent endocrine treatment. *World J Urol* 2000;18:183–9

72. Bouchot O, Lenormand L, Karam G, *et al*. Intermittent androgen supression in the treatment of metastatic prostate cancer. *Eur Urol* 2000;38:543–9

73. Zincke H. Extended experience with surgical treatment of stage D1 adenocarcinoma of prostate. Significant influences of immediate adjuvant hormonal treatment (orchiectomy) on outcome. *Urology* 1989;33:27–36

74. Kelly WK, Scher HI. Prostate specific antigen decline after antiandrogen withdrawal syndrome. *J Urol* 1993;149:607–9

75. Kamradt JM, Pienta KJ. Etoposide in prostate cancer. *Expert Opin Pharmacother* 2000;1: 271–5

76. Ellerhorst JA, Tu SM, Amato RJ, *et al*. Phase II trial of alternating weekly chemohormonal therapy for patients with androgen-independent prostate cancer. *Clin Cancer Res* 1997;3:2371–6

77. Hudes GR, Greenberg R, Krigel RL, *et al*. Phase II study of estramucine and vinblastine, two microtubule inhibitors, in hormone-refractory prostate cancer. *J Clin Oncol* 1992; 10:1754–61

78. Smith DC, Esper PS, Todd RF, Pienta KJ. Paclitaxel, estramucine and etoposide in patients with hormone refractory prostate cancer (HRPC): a phase II trial. *Proc Am Soc Clin Oncol* 1997;16:310

79. Small EJ, Meyer M, Marshall ME, *et al*. Suramin therapy for patients with symptomatic hormone refractory prostate cancer: results of a randomized phase III trial comparing suramin plus hydrocortisone to placebo plus hydrocortisone. *J Clin Oncol* 2000;18: 1440–50

80. Porter AT, McEwan AJ, Powe JE, *et al*. Results of a randomized phase III trial to evaluate the efficacy of strontium-89 adjuvant to local field external beam irradiation in the management of endocrine resistant metastatic prostate cancer. *Int J Radiat Oncol Biol Phys* 1993;25:805–13

81. Vercelli M, Quaglia A, Marani E, Parodi S. Prostate cancer incidence and mortality trends among elderly and adult Europeans. *Crit Rev Oncol Hematol* 2000;35:133–44

82. Gronberg H, Damber JE, Jonsson H, Lenner P. Patient age as a prognostic factor in prostate cancer. *J Urol* 1994;152:892–5

83. Gronberg H, Berg HA, Damber JE, *et al*. Prostate cancer in Northern Sweden. Incidence, survival and mortality in relation to tumour grade. *Acta Oncol* 1994;33:359–63

84. Corral DA, Bahnson RR. Survival of men with clinically localized prostate cancer detected in the eighth decade of life. *J Urol* 1994;151: 1326–9

85. Kerr LA, Zincke H. Radical retropubic prostatectomy for prostate cancer in the elderly and the young: complications and prognosis. *Eur Urol* 1994;25:305–12

86. Comhaire FH. Andropause: hormone replacement therapy in the ageing male. *Eur Urol* 2000;38:655–62

87. Basaria S. Risks versus benefits of testosterone therapy in elderly men. *Drugs Aging* 1999;15:131–42

88. Lund BC, Bever-Stille KA, Perry PJ. Testosterone and andropause: the feasibility of testosterone replacement therapy in elderly men. *Pharmacotherapy* 1999;19:951–6

6 Erectile dysfunction

Francesco Montorsi, MD, Matteo Zanoni, MD,
Andrea Salonia, MD, and Patrizio Rigatti, MD

INTRODUCTION

Erectile dysfunction (ED) is defined as the persistent inability to attain and/or maintain a penile erection sufficient to complete a satisfactory sexual intercourse[1]. To become a matter of sufficient medical interest to lead to a search for the appropriate therapy, ED should cause personal distress either to the patient himself or to the couple; this is an important concept, especially when the aging man is considered, as it is notorious that, although erectile function deteriorates progressively with aging and a significant proportion of elderly men would report having some form of ED if asked, only a minority of them will finally request treatment[2].

However, as the average life span is progressively increasing, we should expect a corresponding increase in the number of men reporting ED. This implies a progressive increase in the demand for medical help that will be sustained by the availability of new, user-friendly forms of therapy for ED, including sildenafil, and other drugs for oral administration which will become available in the near future. The need for continuing education of family practitioners and non specialist physicians, especially those taking care of the aging patient population, is thus of paramount importance to guarantee an appropriately good level of medical assistance.

The aim of this chapter is to review the data currently available on the epidemiology, pathophysiology and management of ED.

EPIDEMIOLOGY OF ERECTILE DYSFUNCTION

An association between aging and male ED has been shown in several epidemiological studies. In 1948, Kinsey and colleagues[3] first demonstrated that there is a decline in sexual activity and erectile function with aging. This study, which involved more than 15 000 individuals aged 10–80 years, remains the largest population-based study to provide normative data on male sexual behavior. In that study, the incidence of ED was 25% in men 65 years old and 75% in men over 80 years. Likewise, Diokno and associates[4] studied the relationship between aging and sexual behavior in 296 men over 60 years, and found that the incidence of ED among married men increased from 29% when aged 60–64 years to 64% in men older than 80 years. Studies by Pearlman and Kobashi[5], Frank and colleagues[6] and others in the 1970s have shown ED-related age dependency. The Baltimore Longitudinal Study of Aging reported that, by the age of 55 years, ED was a problem in 8% of all healthy men, and that at ages 65, 75 and 80 years the prevalence increased to 25%, 55% and 75%, respectively[7]. Pfeiffer and Davis[8] observed in 261 men that age was negatively correlated with current sexual function. In 225 geriatric clinic patients, Mulligan and co-workers[9] found the rate of ED to be 26% at age 65 years and younger, and 50% at age 75 years and older. Keil and associates[10], studying self-reported sexual function in the Charleston Heart Study Cohort, found the rate of sexual inactivity to be 30% in men aged 60–69 years and 60% at age 80 years and older.

The most contributive epidemiological investigation was certainly represented by the Massachusetts Male Aging Study (MMAS), a community based, multidisciplinary survey of health and aging in men, including a private, self-administered questionnaire on sexual function and activity[11]. A total sample of 1290 men with ages ranging from 40 to 70 years completed the questionnaire and were considered for the final evaluation. In the total sample, the mean probability of some degree of ED was $52.0 \pm 1.3\%$ (standard error). Between subject ages of 40 and 70 years, the probability of complete ED tripled from 5.1 to 15%, while the probability of moderate ED doubled from 17 to 34%. Within the same age range, the probability of minimal ED remained constant at approximately 17%. An estimated 60% of the men were not impotent at age 40 years, with a decrease to 33% not impotent at age 70 years. Whenever age was tested by multivariate linear regression or multivariate analysis of variance in conjunction with another predictor of ED, age invariably proved to be statistically significant at $p < 0.0001$. No other variable, whether correlated with age or not, diminished the predictive power of simple age.

Heightening the importance of these epidemiological data is the projection that, by the year 2030, given current trends, 20% of the US population will be more than 65 years old[12]. Moreover, life expectancy for men attaining age 65 years increased substantially in the 20th century[13].

PATHOPHYSIOLOGY OF ERECTILE DYSFUNCTION

Penile erection is a neurovascular phenomenon under psychological control. Erections are usually classified as central, reflexogenic and nocturnal erections. In central erections, an initial stimulus starting from supraspinal centers travels through the spinal cord and reaches the corpora cavernosa, traveling ultimately along the cavernous nerves. Terminal branches of the cavernous nerves release several neurotransmitters, which are involved in initiating the erectile process. In addition, endothelial cells lining the walls of the cavernous sinusoids release active mediators. Nitric oxide (NO), vasoactive intestinal polypeptide, acetylcholine and a number of prostaglandins are considered the most important erectogenic neurotransmitters, which ultimately lead to relaxation of the smooth muscle cells within the walls of the penile arteries and sinusoids. Relaxation of the intracavernosal sinusoids leads to blood filling of the corpora cavernosa, with the subsequent compression of the subalbugineal venular plexus against the inner surface of the tunica albuginea, thus activating the veno-occlusive mechanism of the corpora cavernosa. When this mechanism is activated, blood is actually entrapped within the corpora cavernosa, which become an isovolumetric reservoir. Further arterial inflow then leads to an increase in intracorporeal pressure and to penile rigidity. When ejaculation and orgasm are achieved, norepinephrine is released by neural adrenergic fibers within the corpora cavernosa, and smooth muscle contraction is stimulated with subsequent penile detumescence. The same cascade of events is also seen with reflexogenic erections, in which the triggering event is produced by mechanical stimulation of the dorsal nerve of the penis, which sends signals to the lumbosacral cord where synapses with parasympathetic fibers traveling back to the corpora cavernosa take place. The continuous stimulation of the penis occurring naturally during sexual intercourse contributes to maintain activation of the descending neural pathways to the corpora cavernosa, thus sustaining penile rigidity until ejaculation or cessation of stimulation[14]. Nocturnal erections occur during rapid eye movement (REM) sleep from intrauterine life to late senescence, and are still poorly understood. They are believed to represent a spontaneous mechanism for oxygenating the corpora cavernosa and maintaining the viability of cavernosal tissue[15]; they are particularly at risk for deterioration in the aging male, as discussed below.

Abnormalities of erectile function have been traditionally classified as neurogenic (failure to initiate), arteriogenic (failure to fill) and venogenic (failure to store)[16]. However, the term venogenic ED should be viewed as mainly identifying abnormalities in the corpus cavernosum anatomy and histology, leading to alteration of the cavernous veno-occlusive mechanism. In addition, abnormalities of the sex-hormone milieu may significantly affect the quality of penile erections, and this aspect has attracted much interest with regard to its role in the aging population. The process of aging may affect all the pillars of the erectile process including nerves, arteries, veins, cavernous tissue and hormones; however, evidence in the literature of aging-induced damage to these structures has certainly been influenced by the availability of techniques for identifying certain types of damage, and this is why vascular and endocrinological abnormalities affecting the male erectile system seem to play a leading role in this regard.

Age-related smooth muscle dysfunction has long been recognized in the respiratory[17], gastrointestinal[18] and cardiovascular[19] systems. Aging also affects the genitourinary tract and is associated with lower urinary tract symptoms[20] and sexual dysfunction[3–11] in both men and women. How aging leads to smooth muscle dysfunction is, at best, poorly understood. Atherosclerosis-induced arterial insuffiency is a common clinical problem in the elderly, and remains the leading cause of death in the adult population[21,22]. The abdominal aorta and its branches, especially the bifurcation of the iliac arteries, is involved earliest and most severely by atherosclerotic lesions[22]. Atherosclerosis of the aortoiliac arterial bed can potentially compromise the blood supply of the lower

genitourinary tract. For example, atherosclerotic disease of the pudendal and cavernosal arteries has been shown to be a major cause of ED in the elderly patient[23]. Major risk factors for atherosclerosis such as hypertension, hypercholesterolemia, smoking and diabetes[21,22] have also been found to be associated with smooth muscle degeneration, for example impaired relaxation of vascular smooth muscle[24,25]. In animal models, atherosclerosis-induced pelvic ischemia can produce functional and structural alterations in detrusor[26] and corporal cavernosal smooth muscle[27], which parallel the age-related changes in bladder and cavernosal smooth muscle in humans. Therefore, there has been increasing interest in the possible role of atherosclerosis-induced ischemia in lower urinary tract symptoms and ED of the elderly.

There are numerous studies showing that atherosclerosis and subsequent tissue ischemia affect significantly both the arterial inflow to and the veno-occlusive mechanism of the corpora cavernosa[27,28]. The severity of arterial occlusion has also been correlated with the decreased proportion of smooth muscle in the corpus cavernosum. The decrease in smooth muscle content of the corpus cavernosum is associated with the impairment of cavernosal expandability and subsequent veno-occlusive dysfunction[29]. These animal studies have thus identified the association between veno-occlusive dysfunction of the corpora cavernosa and corporeal fibrosis. It is likely that hypoxia-induced overexpression of transforming growth factor-β_1 (TGF-β_1) may play a key role in the process of ischemia-induced damage. TGF-β_1 is a pleotropic cytokine, demonstrated to be an essential mediator of tissue fibrosis[30]. Overproduction of TGF-β_1 decreases the smooth muscle–connective tissue ratio by inducing the expression of collagen, fibronectin and proteoglycans, while inhibiting the growth of smooth muscle cells and the activity of collagenase[30,31]. Another important role of cavernosal oxygen tension appears to be the regulation of prostanoid production in the corpus cavernosum, as it has been shown that low oxygen tension decreases basal and stimulated production of prostaglandin-I$_2$, thromboxane-A$_2$, prostaglandin-2α and prostaglandin-E$_2$[32]. Decreased levels of PGE$_1$ also correlate with increased expression of TGF-β_1 mRNA in human corpus cavernosum smooth muscle cells, and it is thus likely that the effect of low oxygen tension on prostanoid production may also have a role in ischemia-induced cavernosal fibrosis[32].

The significant role of cavernosal oxygen tension in maintaining a normal smooth muscle–connective tissue ratio suggests a possible role for nocturnal penile tumescence (NPT) in oxygenation of the corpus cavernosum. Aging has been shown to decrease the frequency, duration and degree of these erections[33,34]. Although it has been widely accepted that impairment of NPT is caused by ED, it is known that a decrease of NPT can be found in potent men as a function of aging[34]. It is an interesting hypothesis that NPT may serve to oxygenate the corpus cavernosum periodically and that an age-related decrease in the quality and number of NPTs can indirectly affect erectile function by not exposing the penis to sufficient oxygen. Rather than ED leading to impaired NPT, a decreased frequency of NPT may compromise erectile function. We have recently demonstrated that the administration of 100 mg of sildenafil at bedtime in patients with ED of various etiologies produces a statistically significant increase in the nocturnal penile rigidity and tumescence activity units as measured by the RigiScan device compared to placebo[35]. These data have opened the door to further study investigating the possible role of the daily administration at bedtime of sildenafil in the prevention or treatment of ED in the aging patient.

The endocrine milieu plays a significant role in the regulation of erectile function. In men, several hormonal systems show gradual decline during aging, represented by a decrease in their bioactive hormone concentrations. Andropause is characterized by a gradual decline in serum total and bioavailable testosterone, owing to a decrease in testicular Leydig cell number and in their secretory capacity, as well as an age-related decrease in episodic and stimulated gonadotropin secretion[36]. Both cross sectional[36] and longitudinal[37] studies have shown that, in healthy males, mean serum total testosterone levels decrease by about 30% between ages 25 and 75 years, whereas mean serum free testosterone levels decerease by as much as 50% over the same period. The steeper decline of free testosterone levels is explained by an age-associated increase in sex-hormone binding globulin (SHBG) binding capacity[38]. It has recently become clear that not only testosterone decreases with age but also serum estradiol and estrone[39]; in addition circulating levels of dehydroepiandrosterone and its sulfate gradually decline with aging[40]. Finally, the third endocrine system that gradually declines in activity with aging is the growth hormone–insulin like growth factor axis[41]. The role of androgen deficiency with regard to sexual function is still poorly understood. Morley and colleagues[42] have suggested the clinical use of a screening checklist composed of ten items to identify the so-called low testosterone syndrome, which seems to be a more scientifically appropriate term to define andropause (Table 1). All men presenting with a low testosterone level and answering yes to at least two of the ten questions should be diagnosed as having a medical problem related to their hypogonadal status. Two questions investigate the levels of libido and erection, and, if both are found to be abnormal they should alert the physician to this potential etiology of the patient's ED.

In summary, it seems reasonable to hypothesize that the ED of aging is the result of atherosclerosis induced cavernosal ischemia, leading to cavernosal fibrosis and veno-occlusive dysfunction. Abnormalities in circulating levels of hormones controlling sexual organs, especially testosterone, most probably play a significant role at least in some patients. As the ED of

Table 1 St Louis University screening checklist for low testosterone syndrome[42]

(1) Do you have a decrease in libido (sex drive)?
(2) Do you have lack of energy?
(3) Do you have a decrease in strength or endurance?
(4) Have you lost height?
(5) Have you noticed a decreased 'enjoyment of life'?
(6) Are you sad or grumpy?
(7) Are your erections less strong?
(8) Are you falling asleep after dinner?
(9) Have you noted a recent deterioration in your ability to play sports?
(10) Has there been a recent deterioration in your work performance?

aging appears to be a slowly progressive disorder, it appears to be wise for the patient to seek medical intervention earlier rather than later, to minimize the development of veno-occlusive dysfunction.

ASSESSMENT OF THE PATIENT WITH ERECTILE DYSFUNCTION

As already mentioned in the 'introduction' to this chapter, it is relevant to stress that many aging men (and their partners) experience a sexual dysfunction but do not want (or seek) any form of treatment because they are not bothered by the dysfunction itself or not willing to disclose their concern. This was recently found in an epidemiological study in the Netherlands, where a representative sample of a city population ($n = 1215$, ages 40–80 years) were interviewed about the prevalence of ED and its impact on quality of life[43]. There was an age-related increase in the prevalence of ED, reaching a 37% rate in the 70–79 year age group and an age-related decrease in the proportion of men being bothered by the ED (73% in the 40–49 year age group vs. 46% in the 70–79 year age group).

This is essential to remember when interviewing an aging man who has requested medical help for any possible reason regardless of his sexual function, as the diffuse availability of easy to handle and self-administered questionnaires designed to investigate the patient's sexual function[44] has contributed towards ready evaluation of the patient's sexual health. History should be investigated to identify the sexual problem (for example, erectile dysfunction versus premature ejaculation versus loss of libido), as sometimes the patient himself may be confused while reporting his sexual problems, and identification of the real medical condition is not necessarily immediate. More important is identification of the risk factors for ED, which include serious medical conditions or life-style factors such as: ischemic heart disease, hypertension, diabetes, perineal–pelvic trauma, hyperlipidemia, depression, previous pelvic surgery, smoking, heavy drinking, and use of recreational or medically indicated drugs. Most of these risk factors are more frequently found in the aging population, and this is the reason they need to be investigated extensively when interviewing the patient. A psychosocial history is also important, to obtain information on the couple's relationship (if existing) and on the partner's health. This is of particular importance in the aging patient as in the present authors' experience, the partner will probably be in the menopause stage of life, and could potentially suffer some form of sexual dysfunction herself. For example, an aging patient who suffers mild worsening of his capacity to attain a rigid erection may have a partner who has severe problems with her vaginal lubrication (the so-called sexual arousal disorder) during the excitation phase, which precipitates the couple's problem, thus rendering sexual intercourse impossible[45].

Physical examination should investigate the patient at a systemic level and more specifically his genital apparatus. The general patient assessment includes determination of height and weight, and calculation of the body mass index, determination of blood pressure, identification of the peripheral vascular pulses (carotid, aortic, femoral and pedidial), determination of the peripheral reflexes (knee reflex, Achilles tendon reflex and bulbocavernosus reflex) and a brief evaluation of peripheral sensitivity. Digital rectal examination of the prostate gland should be always performed in the aging man, as this population is by definition at higher risk of developing prostate cancer.

Laboratory testing should be done in every aging patient presenting with an ED complaint. Serum glucose, lipids and prostate-specific antigen levels should be measured. In addition, total testosterone and prolactin should be evaluated in all patients[46]. Further tests should be performed if clinically indicated by the patient interview and physical examination.

At the end of the patient's interview and physical examination, and with the results of the blood tests, it is almost always possible to identify the etiology of the problem (psychogenic, organic or mixed) and to discuss the various treatment options with the patient. Further testing is seldom required at this stage, as it will rarely change the therapeutic strategy for the resolution of the patient's ED.

Guidelines for choice of therapy for patients with ED apply substantially to the aging male population; first line therapy includes oral drug therapy, the use of a vacuum device and sex therapy. The last is less frequently indicated in the aging patient, as the proportion of patients with pure psychogenic ED in this age group is certainly less than in younger patients. However, it has been the present authors' experience to see aging patients with ED for whom a couple-approach with sex

therapy has been necessary, and it has been useful to introduce into the couple's sexual life-style an oral drug aimed at improving the man's erectile function. The vacuum device is able to create a rigid erection in the majority of cases and regardless of the patient's age; however, its use is somewhat troublesome, and it is usually best accepted by patients living in a very close couple relationship and for whom patient–partner confidentiality is not a problem. The use of vacuum devices has been dramatically reduced by the advent of sildenafil in the clinical field.

Sildenafil has certainly revolutionized the therapeutic approach to ED in the aging patient. Penile erection depends on the relaxation of corpus cavernosum smooth muscle, which occurs when locally released NO induces an increase in cyclic guanosine monophosphate (cGMP) levels[47]. Nitric oxide-induced increases in cGMP levels in the corpus cavernosum are attenuated by phosphodiesterase type V (PDE5), which metabolizes cGMP[48]. Sildenafil, a selective inhibitor of PDE5, has been shown to be an effective and well-tolerated oral agent for treating ED in the general population of adult men with ED of broad spectrum etiology[49]. In a study recently conducted by one of the authors of this chapter[50] and specifically devoted to the assessment of sildenafil in the elderly population, efficacy and safety data were obtained from five major, double-blind, placebo-controlled studies of oral sildenafil taken as required (but no more than once daily) over a 12-week to 6-month period. Data for the elderly (aged > 65 years) patients enrolled in four studies (two fixed dose and two flexible dose studies in patients with broad-spectrum etiology ED) were pooled for analysis. The fifth study considered had enrolled only men with ED and a concurrent clinical diagnosis of diabetes of more than 5 years' duration for type I diabetes and more than 2 years' duration for type II diabetes. Patients using nitrates or NO donors were excluded from this study. A total of 411 elderly patients with ED of broad spectrum etiology and 71 elderly patients with ED and diabetes were randomized to treatment in these studies. The patients in the broad spectrum ED studies were randomized to receive either fixed- or flexible-dose sildenafil (from 25 to 100 mg) or placebo. In all five studies, patients were instructed to take the study drug 1 hour before sexual activity but not more than once daily.

At the end of treatment, 69% of the patients in the broad spectrum ED subgroup who received sildenafil reported that treatment had improved their erections, compared with 18% who had received placebo ($p < 0.001$). Similarly, a significant treatment effect was observed for the ED and diabetes subgroup patients who received sildenafil. Fifty per cent (50%) of these patients reported improvements in their erections, compared with 10% of those who received placebo ($p < 0.001$). Questions 3 and 4 of the International Index of Erectile Function (IIEF) were used to assess the effect of sildenafil and placebo on the capacity to attain and maintain an erection during sexual activity; scores for both questions were significantly improved by sildenafil, while placebo did not cause any significant change ($p < 0.001$). Sildenafil treatment was well tolerated by the elderly patients with ED (with or without concomitant diabetes) who were enrolled in these five studies. The most commonly experienced adverse events in the two subgroups were headache, flushing and dyspepsia, which occurred in 17%, 13% and 8%, respectively, of patients receiving sildenafil. Most of these adverse events were mild to moderate in nature. Altered vision was experienced by a small number of patients who received sildenafil (4%) and was usually described as a transient and mild color tinge in vision, increased sensitivity to light or blurred vision. Twenty-two (22) elderly patients enrolled in these studies experienced serious adverse events: 11 were patients receiving placebo and 11 were patients receiving sildenafil. None of these serious adverse events

were considered to be related to treatment. The rate of discontinuation owing to adverse events was low (3%) for patients receiving sildenafil and was similar to that in the placebo treatment group.

The results of this combined analysis show that sildenafil is an effective therapy in elderly men with ED of various etiologies and with concomitant illnesses. More than two-thirds of the men in the broad-spectrum ED subgroup and one-half of the men in the ED and diabetes subgroup reported improved erections with sildenafil treatment.

Newer agents have recently become available including apomorphine, a dopamine receptor agonist, and IC351 and vardenafil, two inhibitors of PDE5. Apomorphine is a centrally-acting agent which ultimately activates the cascade of events leading to smooth muscle relaxation within the corpus cavernosum and penile erection. It is available as a small tablet to be administered sublingually, 20 minutes prior to sexual activity. Doses that will become available include 2 and 3 mg; patients will be instructed to take the 2 mg dose first and titrate to the higher dose if 2 mg is ineffective. Large randomized studies on apomorphine have been completed in the USA and Europe, and show that nearly 50% of the attempts to have sexual intercourse were successful in patients with ED of broad-spectrum etiology[51]. Adverse events at these doses were rare and well tolerated and included nausea and vomiting in less than 2% of the cases. Syncope has been reported with higher doses but its rate of occurrence with the 2 and 3 mg doses is less than 0.5%.

Research in the field of new PDE5 inhibitors has led to the identification of IC351 and vardenafil, two agents currently under investigation in phase III clinical trials which should become available during the second quarter of the year 2002. IC351 has a long half-life and very important selectivity for PDE5. Large randomized studies have been completed both in the USA and Europe and have shown a 90% rate of positive responses to the general assessment question "Did treatment improve your erections?" Similar results have been achieved with vardenafil, an agent which has a pharmacokinetics very similar to sildenafil, although it shows a higher selectivity for PDE5.

Although sildenafil is clearly a reliable option for the majority of elderly patients with ED, extensive information about other therapeutic modalities, including intracavernous injection therapy, intraurethral drug therapy and placement of penile implants should be given to aging ED patients. Guidelines for treatment of ED include these treatment options as second- and third-line therapies. However, there are many patients who either do not want to or cannot be treated with sildenafil, and who would like to consider other possibilities. In addition, a certain proportion of patients are not totally satisfied by the erectogenic results obtained with sildenafil, and are willing to be treated in an alternative way.

Intraurethral administration of alprostadil using the Medicated Urethral System for Erection (MUSE) system has initially shown promising results which, unfortunately, have not been confirmed by subsequent studies based on the everyday use of the drug[52]. Intracavernosal injection of alprostadil or vasoactive drug mixtures is a reliable option for treatment of ED; the erectogenic effect of this treatment (in terms of achievement of penile rigidity) is usually superior to that of sildenafil[53]. Although some type of manual dexterity is needed to handle the intracorporeal injection, new injecting devices are now available that make this treatment readily usable by the aging population. Placement of a penile implant is usually considered for patients who do not respond to other less invasive forms of therapy. In the present authors' experience, it is uncommon to place a penile implant in patients older than 65 years as the sexual needs of these patients are usually well addressed by other therapeutic alternatives[54].

The use of hormones in the treatment of ED in the aging male remains controversial. Testosterone has long been known for its ana- bolic effects[55]. Muscle weakness, anemia, low- ered bone mass and mood disturbances rapidly normalize in mid-adult hypogonadal men during testosterone replacement therapy. It is not known whether testosterone therapy in older men has beneficial effects on muscle function, sexual function, sense of well-being and quality of life, and whether this can be done safely. Only prospective, double-blind, placebo-controlled studies evaluating the effect of the administration of testosterone in aging hypogonadal men with ED will answer the question of the potential beneficial use of this hormone in the management of these patients. A word of caution should finally be given when summarizing the therapeutic options for ED in aging patients. It has been shown that most of these patients suffer from diffuse vascular ath- erosclerotic disease which often affects the heart. As sexual activity should be viewed as any other form of physical activity that causes consumption of energy, it should be remem- bered that a sudden start or increase in sexual activity resulting from the use of any effective erectogenic treatment might cause some form of cardiac overload. Easy guidelines for the assessment of the baseline cardiac condition of the ED patient have recently been published by the Princeton panel and should be followed in all cases[56]. However, it should be clearly stated that in the correctly selected aging patient with ED, an effective therapeutic modality can always be identified.

In summary, management of ED in the aging male is first based on extensive evaluation of the patient's sexual and medical history and on the assessment of the patient's and couple's needs and expectations. Although several ther- apeutic options are currently available to treat the patient's symptoms, it seems that, in most patients, oral pharmacotherapy plays the major role because of its high efficacy and safety.

References

1. National Institutes of Health Consensus Development Panel on Impotence. *J Am Med Assoc*, 1993;270:83

2. Slob AK. Age, libido and male sexual function. *Prostate* 2000;10(Suppl):9

3. Kinsey AC, Pomeroy WB, Martin CE. Age and sexual outlet. In Kinsey AC, Pomeroy WB, Martin CE, eds. *Sexual Behaviour in the Human Male*. Philadelphia: WB Saunders Co., 1948:218–62

4. Diokno AC, Brown MB, Herzog R. Sexual function in the elderly. *Arch Intern Med* 1990;150:197

5. Pearlman CK, Kobashi LI. Frequency of intercourse in men. *J Urol* 1990;107:298

6. Frank E, Anderson C, Rubinstein D. Frequency of sexual dysfunction in 'normal' couples. *N Engl J Med* 1978;299:111

7. Morley JE. Impotence. *Am J Med* 1986; 80:897

8. Pfeiffer E, Davis GC. Determinants of sexual behaviour in middle and old age. *J Am Geriatr Soc* 1972;20:151

9. Mulligan T, Retchin SM, Chinchilli VM, Bettinger CB. The role of aging and chronic disease in sexual dysfunction. *J Am Geriatr Soc* 1988;36:520

10. Keil JE, Sutherland SE, Knapp RG, *et al*. Self-reported sexual functioning in elderly blacks and whites: the Charleston heart study experience. *J Aging Health* 1992;4:112

11. Feldman HA, Goldstein I, Hatzichristou D, *et al*. Impotence and its medical and psychosocial correlates: results of the Massachusetts Male Aging Study. *J Urol* 1994;151:54

12. United States Bureau of the Census. *Statistical Abstract of the United States 1992*, 112th edn. Washington DC: USBC, 1992:19

13. United States Bureau of the Census: *Historical Statistics of the United States, Colonial Times to 1970*, Bicentennial edn, part 2. Washington DC: USBC, 1975:56

14. Andersson KE, Wagner G. Physiology of penile erection. *Physiol Rev* 1995;75:191

15. Tarcan T, Azadzoi KM, Siroky MB, *et al*. Age-related erectile and voiding dysfunction: the role of arterial insufficiency. *Br J Urol* 1998; 82(Suppl 1):26

16. Benet AE, Melman A. The epidemiology of erectile dysfunction. *Urol Clin North Am* 1995;22:699

17. Rossi A, Ganassini A, Tantucci C, Grassi V. Aging and the respiratory system. *Aging* 1996;8:143

18. Geokas MC, Conteas CN, Majumdar AP. The aging gastrointestinal tract, liver and pancreas. *Clin Geriatr Med* 1985;1:177

19. Egashira K, Inou T, Hirooka Y. Effects of age on endothelium dependent vasodilation of resistance coronary artery by acetylcholine in humans. *Circulation* 1993;88:77

20. Diokno AC, Brown MB, Goldstein NG, Herzog AR. Urinary flow rates and voiding pressures in elderly men living in a community. *J Urol* 1994;151:1550

21. Rose G. Epidemiology of atherosclerosis. *Br Med J* 1991;303:1537

22. Bierman BL. Atherosclerosis and other forms of arteriosclerosis. In Wilson JD, Braunwald E, Isselbacher KJ, eds. *Harrison's Principles of Internal Medicine*, 12th edn. New York: McGraw-Hill, 1991;1:992–1001

23. Krane RJ, Goldstein I, Saenz de Tejada I. Impotence. *N Engl J Med* 1989;321:1648

24. Egashira K, Inou T, Hirroka Y. Impaired coronary blood flow response to acetylcholine in patients with coronary risk factors and proximal atherosclerotic lesions. *J Clin Invest* 1993;91:29

25. Johnstone MT, Creager SJ, Scales KM, *et al*. Impaired endothelium-dependent vasodilation in patients with insulin dependent diabetes mellitus. *Circulation*, 1993;88: 2510

26. Tarcan T, Siroky MB, Krane RJ, *et al*. Atherosclerosis-induced chronic ischemia causes bladder fibrosis and non compliance. The role of growth factors. *J Urol* 1998;159:135A

27. Azadzoi KM, Siroky MB, Goldstein I. Study of etiologic relationship of arterial atherosclerosis to corporeal veno-occlusive dysfunction in the rabbit. *J Urol* 1996;155:1795

28. Mulligan T, Katz PG. Why aged men become impotent. *Arch Intern Med* 1989;149:1365

29. Nehra A, Azadzoi K, Moreland RB. Cavernosal expandability is an erectile tissue mechanical property which predicts trabecular histology in an animal model of vasculogenic erectile dysfunction. *J Urol* 1998;159:2229

30. Border WA, Noble NA. Transforming growth factor β in tissue fibrosis. *N Engl J Med* 1994;331:1286

31. Morisaki N, Kawano M, Koyama N. Effects of TGF-β 1 on growth of aortic smooth muscle cells. Influences on interaction with growth factors, cell state, cell phenotype and cell cycle. *Atherosclerosis* 1991;88:227

32. Moreland RB, Traish AM, McMillin MA, *et al*. PGE1 suppresses the induction of collagen synthesis by TGF-β 1 in human corpus cavernosum smooth muscle. *J Urol* 1995;153:826

33. Karacan I, Williams R, Thornby J, Salis PJ. Sleep-related penile tumescence as a function of age. *Am J Psychiatr* 1975;132:932

34. Schiavi RC, Schreiner-Engel P, Mandeli J, *et al*. Healthy aging and male sexual function. *Am J Psychiatr* 1990;147:766

35. Montorsi F, Maga T, Ferini Strambi L, *et al*. Sildenafil taken at bedtime significantly increases nocturnal erections: results of a placebo-controlled study. *Urology* 2000;56:906

36. Vermeulen A. Clinical review 24: androgens in the aging male. *J Clin Endocrinol Metab* 1991;73:221

37. Morley JE, Kaiser F, Raum WJ, *et al*. Potentially predictive and manipulable blood serum correlates of aging in the healthy human male: progressive decreases in bio-available testosterone, dehydroepiandrosterone sulfate, and the ratio of insulin-like growth factor 1 to growth hormone. *Proc Natl Acad Sci USA* 1997;94:7537

38. Vermeulen A, Verdonck L. Some studies on the biological significance of free testosterone. *J Steroid Biochem* 1972;3:421

39. Ferrini RL, Barrett-Connor E. Sex Hormones and age: a cross-sectional study of testosterone and estradiol and their bioavailable fractions in community dwelling men. *Am J Epidemiol* 1998;147:750

40. Herbert J. The age of dehydroepiandrosterone (published erratum in *Lancet* 1995;345:1648). *Lancet* 1995;345:1193

41. Corpas E, Harman SM, Blackman MR. Human growth hormone and human aging. *Endocr Rev* 1993;14:20

42. Morley JE, Kaiser FE, Sih R, *et al*. Testosterone and frailty. *Clin Geriatr Med* 1997;13:685

43. Meuleman E, Donkers L, Kiemeney B. Erectile dysfunction: prevalence and quality of life. The Boxmeer study. *Aging Male* 2000;3(Suppl):12

44. Rosen RC, Riley A, Wagner G, *et al*. The International Index of Erectile Function (IIEF): a multidimensional scale for assessment of erectile dysfunction. *Urology* 1997;49:822

45. Goldstein I, Graziottin A, Heiman JR, *et al*. Female sexual dysfunction. In Jardin A, Wagner G, Khoury S, Giuliano F, Padma-Nathan H, Rosen R, eds. *Erectile Dysfunction*. Plymouth: Plymbridge Distributors Ltd, 1999:507–56

46. Meuleman E, Broderick G, Montorsi F, *et al*. Clinical evaluation and doctor–patient dialogue. In Jardin A, Wagner G, Khoury S, Giuliano F, Padma-Nathan H, Rosen R, eds. *Erectile Dysfunction*. Plymouth: Plymbridge Distributors Ltd, 1999:115–38

47. Burnett AL. Nitric oxide in the penis. Physiology and pathology. *J Urol* 1997;157:320

48. Boolell M, Allen MJ, Ballard SA. Sildenafil: an orally active type 5 cyclic GMP-specific phosphodiesterase inhibitor for the treatment of penile erectile dysfunction. *Int J Impot Res* 1996;8:47

49. Montorsi F, McDermott TED, Morgan R. Efficacy and safety of fixed-dose oral sildenafil in the treatment of erectile dysfunction of various etiologies. *Urology* 1999;53:1011

50. Wagner G, Montorsi F, Auerbach S, Collins M. Viagra (sildenafil citrate) improves erectile function in elderly patients with erectile dysfunction: a subgroup analysis. *J Gerontol* 2001;56A:M113

51. Heaton JPW. Apomorphine: an update of clinical trial results. *Int J Impotence Res* 2001;12:567–73

52. Shabsigh R, Padma-Natahan H, Gittleman M. Intracavernous alprostadil alfadex is more efficacious, better tolerated, and preferred over intraurethral alprostadil plus optional ACTIS: a comparative, randomized cross-over, multicenter study. *Urology* 2000; 55:109

53. Shabsigh R, Padma-Nathan H, Gittleman M, *et al*. Intracavernous alprostadil alphadex (Edex/Viridal) is effective and safe in patients with erectile dysfunction after failing sildenafil (Viagra). *Urology* 2000;55:477

54. Montorsi F, Rigatti P, Carmignani G, *et al*. AMS three-piece inflatable implants for erectile dysfunction: a long-term multi-institutional study in 200 consecutive patients. *Eur Urol* 2000;37:50

55. Brodsky IG, Balagopal P, Nair KS. Effects of testosterone replacement on muscle mass and muscle protein synthesis in hypogonadal men – a clinical research center study. *J Clin Endocrinol Metab* 1996;81:3469

56. Jackson G. Erectile dysfunction and cardiovascular disease. *Int J Clin Pract* 1999;53:363

7 Infertility in the aging male

Wolfgang Weidner, MD, Thorsten Diemer, MD, and Martin Bergmann, MD

INTRODUCTION

It is widely accepted and confirmed by longitudinal studies that serum testosterone levels decrease with age[1]. In healthy men, serum testosterone levels vary between 11 and 40 mmol/l; these levels decrease by about 30% between the ages of 25 and 75 years[2]. Most of the circulating serum testosterone is bound to albumin or sex hormone-binding globulin (SHBG). Only free testosterone and a part of the albumin-bound testosterone are readily biologically available. It has been established that with increasing age the bioavailable testosterone declines more steeply than total testosterone due to an age-associated increase in SHBG-binding capacity[3].

The decrease in serum testosterone is a result of primary testicular changes, altered neuroendocrine regulation of Leydig cell functions and an increase in SHBG. The testicular changes include a reduced secretory response to Leydig cells under human chorionic gonadotropin (hCG) stimulation due to a reduction in Leydig cell number and probably also due to changes in testicular steroid metabolism[1]. The decreased testicular activity is associated with a rise in luteinizing hormone (LH) secretion, but this modest increase is inadequate to compensate for the decreased testosterone levels in aging men. Furthermore, the circadian rhythmicity of LH is clearly disturbed in elder men[4]. The main cause for this seems to be a reduced mean LH pulse amplitude due to altered hypothalamic gonadotropin releasing hormone (GnRH) secretion[5]. There is also evidence of a primary testicular deterioration[6], documented by the decreasing concentration in blood of the Sertoli cell marker inhibin B and the gradual lowering of the inhibin B/follicle-stimulating hormone (FSH) ratio with age[6].

TESTICULAR CHANGES

Spermatogenesis is a life-long process which can be confirmed on testicular histology until late old age. However, spermatogenic efficiency estimated by the number of spermatozoa produced per day per gram of testicular parenchyma declines with age[7]. This decline is due to an increase of germ cell degeneration at all developmental steps throughout spermatogenesis, such as spermatogonia, spermatocytes and haploid spermatids. These degenerating cells are phagocytozed by the somatic Sertoli cells resulting in typical morphological alterations within the seminiferous epithelium. As a result of germ cell phagocytosis, Sertoli cells typically show an increased cytoplasmic storage of lipids after the fiftieth year of life (Figure 1). Focally, Sertoli cells can also show a re-expression of fetal characteristics such as cytokeratin 18 intermediate filaments[8]. Degenerative alteration of germ cells is obvious with the occurrence of (1) spermatogonia with large nuclei; (2) so-called 'megalospermatocytes', indicating a failure of the pairing of the homologous chromosomes, and (3) giant spermatids with numerous nuclei. In addition, maturation steps at the level of spermatogonia,

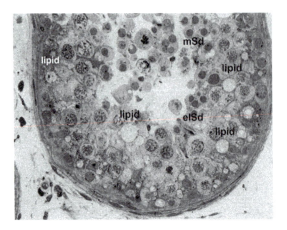

Figure 1 Seminiferous tubule showing qualitatively intact spermatogenesis with few elongated spermatids (elSd) together with intraluminal multinucleated spermatids (mSd), and typical Sertoli cell lipid inclusions (lipid). (semi-thin section, primary magnification: × 40)

primary spermatocytes or early round spermatids, or the total loss of germ cells leaving only Sertoli cells within the seminiferous tubules (Sertoli cell only) occur. Apoptosis was found to be one mechanism of germ cell degeneration, but is a somewhat rare event and does not seem to increase with age[9,10]. Concomitant with these alterations, seminiferous tubules show a reduction of the diameter and thickening of the lamina propria. After total atrophy of the seminiferous epithelium, only strands of fibrous tissue remain (tubular ghosts)[11].

Although these alterations are typical in elderly men, there is a great interindividual variation in degree. In addition, these alterations leading to the reduction of spermatogenic efficiency can also be observed in testes of adult young and middle-aged oligo- or azoospermic men[11].

LEYDIG CELL FUNCTION

The most obvious and interesting finding in human males is the slow decrease of serum testosterone, that appears to occur between the ages of 40 to 70 years[1,2,12]. The terms ADAM (androgen decline of the aging male), PADAM (partial androgen decline of the aging male),

and male andropause have been designed to reflect this circumstance. Between 10 and 15% of males are believed to have significant decreases of testosterone already by the age of 40 years and reveal symptoms that are typical or similar to those of manifest hypogonadism[13]. A variety of endocrine alterations have been discovered in aging males although the exact pathophysiology of these alterations is yet unclear and is probably complex due to significant cofactors[1,12,14]. However, the Brown Norway rat appears to offer the possibility of investigating the pathophysiology of the aging endocrinium in a very similar model to humans[15,16].

Aging of the Leydig cell: experimental data derived from aging Brown Norway rats

Aging Brown Norway rats (2–3 years old) display testosterone levels that are significantly different from serum levels of younger animals[15,16]. This appears to resemble situations that can also be found in aging human males, and interestingly the majority of rats seem to undergo this endocrine alteration. But what is the physiological basis of this alteration? Pathophysiologic models could explain such alterations on different levels of the endocrine axis. A couple of very well chosen and defined experiments have been designed to solve this problem[15,17,18]. Since LH levels do not change with aging in Brown Norway rats the responsible mechanisms seem to act decisively on the Leydig cell level[17]. When Leydig cells are isolated from young and aging animals and further stimulated *in vitro* by LH, young Leydig cells indicate a greater steroid output than aged cells, in part due to a reduction of LH receptors on the Leydig cell surface. In conclusion there is no doubt from these experiments that the alterations that lead to the reduction of serum testosterone in aging animals affect the Leydig cell itself rather than being a consequence of hypothalamic and pituitary regulation. Two impressive experiments have been designed to confirm this hypothesis: when terminally differentiated Leydig cells of aging Brown Norway rats with a reduced capacity to synthesize steroids are eradicated by administration of the specific cytotoxin ethane-1,2-dimethane-sulfonate (EDS), a new Leydig cell generation develops from mesenchymal stem cells in the interstitial spaces of the testis[16]. This well-established experimental tool has been used to show that a fresh Leydig cell generation gained the same steroidogenic power as Leydig cells from younger animals[16]. Moreover, if Leydig cell steroidogenesis is effectively suppressed by Silastic® testosterone implants that almost completely downregulate LH secretion from the pituitary for years, aged Leydig cells are as steroidogenic as Leydig cells of younger animals when the implants are finally removed[19]. On a molecular basis, distinct alterations in the expression of steroidogenic enzymes that are expressed in Leydig cells of the rat have been described. Most significantly, the StAR protein expression appears to be reduced as well as the expression of *P450scc* and *P450 c17*[18].

In conclusion, Leydig cells undergo a process of aging and an important part of this process is the act of steroidogenesis itself. An interesting concept to explain this phenomenon is that steroidogenesis is associated with permanent generation of reactive oxygen species (ROS), especially in the mitochondria, due to the activity of P450 oxygenase enzymes. This permanent generation of ROS could slowly damage enzymatic systems that are necessary for steroid biosynthesis, as has been demonstrated in other *in vitro* experiments with Leydig cells, and therefore build the foundation of decreased testosterone levels with age[20,21].

ADAM/PADAM IN HUMAN MALES

The molecular alterations described in rats are also evident in humans, but with certain differences. LH and FSH serum levels decrease with age, reflecting the reduction of Leydig cell steroidogenesis and alterations of the seminiferous epithelium with the reduction of Sertoli cells, respectively[1,3]. LH rhythmicity undergoes significant modulations in the elderly probably due to altered secretion of GnRH in the hypothalamus, but molecular concepts to explain this phenomenon are lacking[4,22]. The reduction of steroidogenesis in Leydig cells is amplified by the slow enhancement of SHBG resulting in an even sharper decrease in free testosterone (bioavailable) in the serum. Although there are technical problems concerning reliable techniques to estimate the free or non SHBG-bound testosterone, it is believed that bioavailable testosterone declines more steeply with increasing age than total serum testosterone, due to an age-dependent increase in SHBG binding of testosterone[2]. Dihydrotestosterone does not indicate a similar age-related decrease, and total estradiol levels remain largely unaffected by the aging process. The primary androgens of the adrenal gland, dehydroepiandrosterone and its sulfate (DHEA and DHEAS) also decrease with age, but the physiological relevance has yet to be elucidated.

Patients with decreased levels of testosterone due to aging usually complain about a variety of symptoms, of which erectile dysfunction (ED) is among the most mentioned. The Massachusetts Male Aging Study (MMAS) found an incidence of ED in 5–15% of males between the ages of 40 and 70. ED is not a direct consequence of the altered endocrine[13] situation, but is largely correlated to cofactors such as heart disease and medication. Loss of libido is an important symptom that correlates well to the loss of testosterone and is among those symptoms that respond well to hormone replacement therapy (HRT). Decline of bone density is another symptom that can be well explained from the endocrine deficiency and can be a strong argument for the use of HRT[6]. The loss of physical strength, reduction in muscle mass and enhancement of body fat have their origin in the reduction of testosterone, but

TEXTBOOK OF MEN'S HEALTH

Table 1 Chronic illness and reduced gonadal function[24]

Metabolic	Organ-defined	Iatrogenic
Severe obesity	Chronic obstruction airway disease (COAD)	Hemodialysis
Diabetes mellitus	Pulmonary fibrosis	Renal transplantation
Hypothyroidism	Cystic fibrosis	Chemotherapy
Cushing's disease	Rheumatoid arthritis	Irradiation
Uremia	Systemic lupus erythematosus	
Severe liver cirrhosis	Celiac disease	

are also heavily dependent on conditions of life-style and physical training. Change of mood and other psychological symptoms complete the picture of the variety of symptoms that are connected to the decline of testosterone in aging males.

CHRONIC ILLNESS AND REDUCED GONADAL FUNCTION

In this context it seems to be important to focus on the common determinants of aging, which must also be considered in relation to reproductive health[23]. Several forms of systemic chronic illness[24] (Table 1) may occur directly at the testicular level: reduced Leydig cell function will lead to androgen deficiency, while diseases affecting spermatogenesis may lead to male infertility. On the other hand there is no doubt that testosterone decline may also impair spermatogenesis. It is generally accepted that the testicular volume is correlated to the spermatogenetic quality. A decrease in testicular volume in older men could not be observed in two studies[25,26], although an influence of a chronic diseased status can not be ruled out with 100% certainty.

FURTHER LOCAL FACTORS

The impact of infections on decreasing gonadal function with age must be discussed etiologically[24]. Orchitis may contribute to decreasing sperm quality; lymphocytic and plasmacytic infiltrates have been identified in biopsy specimens in the peritubular tissue

indicating an age-dependent exposure to recurrent urogenital infections[27]. Others hypothesize that this effect may be blurred by a lower frequency of ejaculation in older men[26], although disorders of ejaculation are not evaluated in the literature according to age[28]. In addition to typical congenital and acquired causes, functional seminal emission problems such as side-effects due to the intake of drugs (especially antidepressants and alpha-blockers) may play a special role in increasing age. Of great importance for urologists in this context is the interference in sexual function caused by diseases of the prostate (for an overview see reference 29), which are generally not considered in the psychological and sexological literature. Undoubtedly, carcinoma of the prostate, whether untreated or under observation, has the greatest impact on sexuality, depending on the expectation of survival. In benign prostatic hyperplasia (BPH), about two-thirds of patients scheduled for operation still have erections and ejaculation[30], which will be hampered by conventional BPH therapy.

There are also some hints that premature ejaculation may often be associated with the 'increased' necessity of mechanical sexual stimulation in the case of erectile problems[30].

SPERM QUALITY AND AGING

As already detailed, the seminiferous tubules gradually become atrophic as a result of decreasing germinal epithelium, but these changes do not affect the entire testis volume due to their focal character[31]. Comparing the

Table 2 Semen parameters in young and elderly males[34]

Studies	Age (years)	Semen			
		Volume (ml)	Sperm count (millions/ml)	Motility (%)	Morphology (% normal)
Nieschlag et al, 1982[38]	24–37	4 +/– 1.7	77 +/– 51	68 +/– 14	52 +/– 13
	60–88	3.2 +/– 1.9	120 +/– 101	50 +/– 19	48 +/– 9
Haidl et al, 1996[41]	<35	3.23 +/– 1.5	115 +/– 103	30.4 +/– 14.5	26.5 +/– 13.9
	>45	3.22 +/– 1.7	66.9 +/– 66.6	23.1 +/– 13.7	20.7 +/– 16.2

daily sperm production of men aged 21–50 years with that of men aged 55–80 years, the younger group shows a 30% higher sperm production[32]. In contrast, men over 65 years show a highly significant decrease in daily sperm production[33]. This indicates a gradual decline of fertility with increasing age, although alterations in sperm quality may be minimal.

The question of whether semen parameters change with increasing age significantly, is difficult to answer due to lack of sufficient data and intraindividual variation of sperm measurements (Table 2)[34]. Leydig cell function of the human testis declines slowly but significantly with age[13,14,23]. Reproductive function seems to not be affected in the same manner[27]. In principle, spermatogenesis may be retained well into senescence. Although 50% of those over 80 years have been described as completely infertile[35], children have been fathered by men over 90 years of age[36]. Many authors demonstrated a decreasing sperm count and poorer sperm quality in older men[37–40]. However, the majority of studies underline the evidence of only minor differences in standard sperm parameters with age[27,38–40], with a decrease in motility and with normal morphology as the most important findings[38–40]. This is similar when functional sperm parameters in older fathers have been determined; no differences to those of younger men were found (see Table 2)[41].

FERTILITY AND AGING

Fertility usually persists well into old age. It is the age of the female partner, rather than the age

of the male partner that is the most important factor in determining the probability of reproduction of a couple presenting with infertility[31,39]. Interestingly, the number of pregnancies is not found to be different when comparing older males with a group of younger men with relatively old female partners[39]. Even in advanced male age, the reduced conceptive facility of the female partner is the more important factor than a reduced sperm quality of the male[26].

GENETIC RISKS IN AGING FATHERS

The effects of genetic factors on various components of health in aging are poorly understood[23], although in general the effect of hereditary influence on the incidence of chronic conditions seems to decrease with age[32]. There are many genetic syndromes that are associated with hypogonadism and which may also influence the fertility status, for example myotonic dystrophy, Kennedy's syndrome, some types of Down's syndrome, Prader-Willi syndrome, Kallmann syndrome and others[24]. All these syndromes affect primary androgen action and consequently also the spermatogenetic capacity.

It seems to be accepted that structural chromosomal anomalies in spermatozoa of aging men are detectable, but not significantly increased[26]. Theoretically, an age-dependent spontaneous mutation rate in aging fathers has to be discussed as a potential risk for future populations[33]; however, the real health risk remains incalculable[26].

Current opinion is that the increased age of the female partner, not the age of the male, is an indication for dedicated prenatal diagnostic management[26]. Nevertheless, although a negative influence of paternal age on pregnancy rates can not be demonstrated, an increase in structural abnormalities of aging spermatozoa has been reported and should be kept in mind. Furthermore, the questionable higher risk of autosomal dominant diseases has been discussed in relation to increased paternal age[42], a fact which has to be considered in the ongoing discussion.

CONCLUSIONS

Sexual health includes 'normal' libido, sexuality, erectile function and fertility. Sexual alterations in older men include libido disorders, decreasing sexual interest and possibly a decline in frequency of intercourse. These findings are significantly associated with typical hormonal findings which can be considered as the andropause. Although there are also characteristic alterations in the gonadal function, with many indications that a significant decrease in steroidogenesis in the Leydig cells is the most important factor in aging, healthy men remain fertile during their lifetime. Disturbed sperm parameters are frequently associated with chronic illness and concomitant diseases of the urogenital area. Although a negative influence of paternal age on pregnancy can not be demonstrated, the age of the female is the major factor in every infertile partnership. It is unclear whether increasing chromosomal abnormalities have to be discussed in relationship to the offspring. Finally it seems to be important not to view fertility problems in older men simply as a result of pathology while overlooking the effect of the natural process of aging.

References

1. Kaufmann JM. Hypothalamo-pituitary-gonadal function in aging men. *Aging Male* 1999;2: 157–65
2. Vermeulen A. Androgens in the aging male – clinical review 24. *J Clin Endocrinol Metab* 1991;73:221–4
3. Vermeulen A, Kaufmann JM, Giagulli VA. Influence of some biological indices on sex hormone binding globulin and androgen levels in the aging and obese male. *J Clin Endocrinol Metabol* 1996;81:1821–7
4. Bremner WJ, Vitiello MV, Prinz PN. Loss of circadian rhythmicity in blood testosterone levels with aging in normal men. *J Clin Endocrinol Metab* 1983;56:1278–81
5. Vermeulen A, Kaufmann JM. Role of the hypothalamo-pituitary function in the hypoandrogenism of healthy aging. *J Clin Endocrinol Metab* 1992;74:704–6
6. Comhaire FH. Andropause: hormone replacement therapy in the aging male. *Eur Urol* 2000; 38:655–62
7. Johnson L, Varner DD, Roberts ME, *et al.* Efficiency of spermatogenesis: a comparative approach. *Anim Reprod Sci* 2000;60–61: 471–80
8. Stosiek P, Kasper M, Karsten U. Expression of cytokeratins 8 and 18 in human Sertoli cells of immature and atrophic seminiferous tubules. *Differentiation* 1990;43: 66–70
9. Barnes CJ, Covington BW, Cameron IL, Lee M. Effect of ageing on spontaneous and induced mouse testicular germ cell apoptosis. *Aging* 1998;10:497–501
10. Brinkworth MH, Weinbauer GF, Bergmann M, Nieschlag E. Apoptosis as a mechanism of germ cell loss in elderly men. *Int J Androl* 1997;20:222–8
11. Holstein AF, Roosen-Runge EC, Schirren C. *Illustrated Pathology of Human Spermato-Genesis.* Berlin: Grosse Verlag Berlin, 1988
12. Hermann M, Untergasser G, Rumpold H, Berger P. Aging of the male reproductive system. *Exp Gerontol* 2000;35:1267–79
13. Gray A, Feldman HA, McKinlay HB, Longcope C. Age, disease and changing sex hormone levels in middle-aged men: results of the

Massachusetts Male Aging Study. *J Clin Endocrinol Metab* 1991;73:1016–25

14. Vermeulen A, Kaufman JM. Aging of the hypothalamic-pituitary-testicular axis in men. *Horm Res* 1995;13:25–8

15. Chen H, Hardy MP, Huhtaniemi I, Zirkin BR. Age-related decreased Leydig cell testosterone production in the Brown Norway rat. *J Androl* 1994;15:551–7

16. Chen H, Huhtaniemi I, Zirkin BR. Depletion and repopulation of Leydig cells in the testes of aging Brown Norway rats. *Endocrinology* 1996;137:3447–52

17. Grzywacz FW, Chen H, Allegretti J, Zirkin BR. Does age-associated reduced Leydig cell testosterone production in Brown Norway rats result from under-stimulation by luteinizing hormone? *J Androl* 1998;19:625–30

18. Luo L, Chen H, Zirkin BR. Are Leydig cell steroidogenic enzymes differentially regulated with aging? *J Androl* 1996;17:509–15

19. Chen H, Zirkin BR. Long-term suppression of Leydig cell steroidogenesis prevents Leydig cell aging. *Proc Natl Acad Sci USA* 1999;96:14877–81

20. Zirkin BR, Chen H. Regulation of Leydig cell steroidogenic function during aging. *Biol Reprod* 2000;63:977–81

21. Zirkin BR, Chen H, Luo L. Leydig cell steroidogenesis in aging rats. *Exp Gerontol* 1997;32:529–37

22. Veldhuis JD. Recent neuroendocrine facts of male reproductive aging. *Exp Gerontol* 2000;35:1281–308

23. World Health Organization. Men, aging and health. *Aging Male* 2000;3:3–36

24. Turner HE, Wass JAH. Gonadal function in men with chronic illness. *Clin Endocrinol* 1997;47:379–403

25. Handelsman DJ, Staraj S. Testicular size: the effects of aging, malnutrition and illness. *J Androl* 1983;6:144–51

26. Rolf C, Nieschlag E. Zeugungsfähigkeit und Fertilitätsrisiken alternder Männer. In Jocham D, Altwein J, Jünemann K-P, Schmitz-Dräger B-J, Weidner W, Wirth M, Kilian Marburg S, eds. *Aging Male* 2000:95–102

27. Krause W, Habermann B. No change with age in semen volume, sperm count and sperm motility in individual men consulting an infertility clinic. *Urol Int* 2000;64:139–42

28. Hendry WF. Disorders of ejaculation: congenital, acquired and functional. *Br J Urol* 1998; 82:331–41

29. Burger B, Weidner W, Altwein J. Prostate and sexuality: an overview. *Eur Urol* 1999;35:177–84

30. Weidner W, Altwein J, Hauck E, *et al*. Sexuality of the elderly. *Urol Int* 2001;66:181–4

31. Schill W-B, Köhn FM, Haidl G. The aging male. In Berg G, Hammar M, eds. *The Modern Management of the Menopause*. New York: Parthenon Publishing, 1993:545–65

32. Harris A, Cairns B. Health checks for people over 75. *Br Med J* 1992;305:1437

33. Crow JF. The high spontaneous mutation rate: Is it a health risk? *Proc Natl Acad Sci USA* 1997;94:8380–6

34. Plas E, Berger P, Hermann M, Pflüger H. Effects of aging on male fertility. *Exp Gerontol* 2001;35:543–51

35. Harman SM. Clinical aspects of aging of the male reproductive system. In Schneider EL, ed. *The Aging Reproductive System*. New York: Raven, 1978:29–58

36. Silber SJ. Effects of age on male fertility. *Semin Reprod Endocrinol* 1991;9:241–8

37. Merino G, Carranza-Lira S. Semen characteristics, endocrine profiles and testicular biopsies of infertile men of different ages. *Arch Androl* 1995;35:219–24

38. Nieschlag E, Lammers U, Freischem CW, *et al*. Reproductive functions in young fathers and grandfathers. *J Clin Endocrinol Metab* 1982;55:676–81

39. Rolf C, Behre HM, Nieschlag E. Reproductive parameters of older compared to younger men of infertile couples. *Int J Androl* 1996; 19:135–42

40. Schwartz D, Mayaux MJ, Spira A, *et al*. Semen characteristics as a function of age in 833 fertile men. *Fertil Steril* 1983;39:530–5

41. Haidl G, Jung A, Schill WB. Aging and sperm function. *Hum Reprod* 1996;11:558–60

42. Bordson BL, Leonardo VS. The appropriate uper age limit for several semen donors: a review of the genetic effects of paternal age. *Fertil Steril* 1991;56:397–401

8 Urinary incontinence

Adrian Wagg, MBBS, FRCP

The prevalence of bladder problems in men is lower than that in women at all ages (Table 1), but as in women, the prevalence of bladder problems increases in association with older age. Chronic infections, bladder stones, bladder tumors and primary bladder pathology such as detrusor overactivity may cause such problems in men, whether or not secondary to a neurological lesion. Incompetence of the urethral sphincter occurs rarely in men, and where it does occur it is usually due to trauma, surgery or nervous system disease. The elderly experience the same bladder problems as other adults. Where the elderly differ, though, is in their ability to respond and to compensate for problems which a younger adult may find trivial. Concomitant disease and drug therapy, in particular, may serve to render an elderly person incontinent.

The prevalence of incontinence also varies with the origin of the surveyed population (Table 1) and with the definition of incontinence employed in the study. In 1995, data from intensive testing of urinary tract function on normal, asymptomatic elderly people, half of them male, but without comparative controls were published, suggesting that normality was a rarity, only 18% of individuals falling into this category[1]. The problem with such research is that many 'age-related' studies have not used comparative samples of younger individuals and therefore it is difficult to ascribe their findings to age alone. However, it is certain that incontinence should never be

Table 1 Population estimates of prevalence of urinary incontinence in adults

	Percentage incontinent
Community dwelling women	
15–44 years	5–7
45–64 years	8–15
65 + years	10–20
Community dwelling men	
15–64 years	3
65 + years	7–10
Residential homes (men/women)	25
Nursing homes (men/women)	40
Hospital care (elderly and elderly mentally infirm) (men/women)	50–70

Reproduced with permission from Royal College of Physicians. *Incontinence: Causes, Management and Provision of Services*. London: Royal College of Physicians, 1995

viewed as a normal consequence of aging and that, worldwide, the expanding proportion of the population in late life will place an increasing burden on services delivering continence care. This article will review current understanding of the changes in lower urinary tract function and incontinence in men in later life.

AGE-RELATED EFFECTS

Much of the data relating to changes in lower urinary tract function are derived from studies of individuals with lower urinary tract symptoms who have undergone urodynamic studies. Data from community dwelling, continent individuals are sparse, but where they do exist, tend to

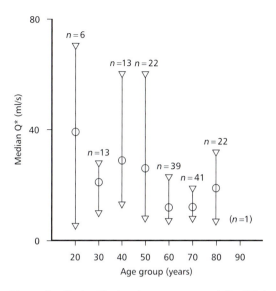

Figure 1 Contractile function as measured by Q* in association with greater age in men with lower urinary tract symptoms ($n = 157$)[2]

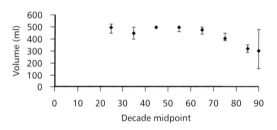

Figure 2 Increased age is associated with a reduction in bladder capacity (median ± 95% CI)[2]

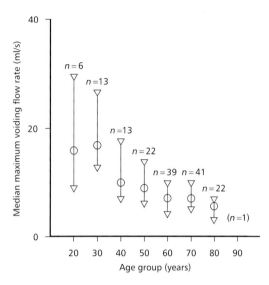

Figure 3 Median (± 95% CI) maximum flow rate for men in relation to greater age ($p < 0.001$)[2]

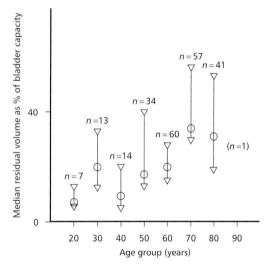

Figure 4 Post-void residual volume of urine related to increasing age in men with lower urinary tract symptoms. Figures 1–4 are all reproduced with permission from reference 2

confirm the associations identified by other means.

Detrusor contractile function (Figure 1), bladder capacity (Figure 2) and urinary flow rates (Figure 3) all appear to decline in association with greater age[2]. There is also an increase in the prevalence of incomplete emptying as demonstrated by the existence of a significant post-micturition residual volume of urine (Figure 4)[3]. In men, the progressive enlargement of the prostate with age tends to dominate the behavior of the urinary outflow tract, with up to half of all men suffering from outflow tract obstruction[4]. The changes in the bladder associated with prostatic hypertrophy, significant detrusor muscle hypertrophy[5], a reduction in

the number of acetylcholinesterase containing nerves[6], and an increase in the collagen to smooth muscle ratio[7] which causes the bladder to be less compliant, have all been demonstrated in association with age alone[8–10]. Thus it is unclear to what extent prostatic hypertrophy alone may contribute to the observed changes.

However, as obstruction increases, the bladder requires a greater contractile effort to overcome the effects of the obstruction. In a subgroup of men, this eventually leads to a chronically overdistended bladder, which fails to empty effectively; in others acute urinary retention may develop.

The evolution of detrusor instability is conventionally thought to be associated with the development of significant outflow tract obstruction and is present in 43–86% of patients[4]. This viewpoint has been reinforced by the fact that relief of the obstruction leads to bladder stability in a significant proportion[11]. However, once again, the incidence of detrusor instability increases in association with age *per se* and is similar in females. In men with lower urinary tract symptoms, the likelihood of detrusor instability being the cause of these reaches 85% in the eighth decade, regardless of the presence of significant outflow tract obstruction[2]. Detrusor instability will be discussed in more detail below.

CONSERVATIVE AND LIFE-STYLE MEASURES TO ADDRESS BLADDER PROBLEMS IN MEN

Smoking

One major study by Kosimaki and colleagues[12] has identified an association of bladder problems with cigarette smoking. The odds ratio of lower urinary tract symptoms was 1.47 for current smokers and 1.38 for former smokers when compared with men who had never smoked[12]. When adjusted for other risk factors associated with bladder problems, the risk associated with smoking still stood. As with other adverse effects of smoking, this association weakened following cessation of smoking and appeared to reach baseline after 40 years of abstinence. The association of smoking appeared to be strongest with the occurrence of detrusor instability. There are animal data which demonstrate an effect of nicotine upon the motor function of the bladder. There are, however, no prospective intervention trials of smoking cessation on improving bladder symptoms. However, there is little doubt that smoking should be discouraged in view of the cardiovascular risk, regardless of its effect upon lower urinary tract function.

Fluid advice

Fluid intake should be around 2–2.5 litres daily. Obviously an excessive fluid intake will lead to an increased urinary frequency. A daily average of 7–8 micturitions per 24 hours is considered the upper limit of normal. Limiting or reducing overall fluid intake is not effective for managing incontinence, and may lead to adverse effects, especially in the face of other medication, and particularly in the elderly, who already have a decrease in total body water. Judicious timing of fluid, especially at night, may be effective in reducing nocturnal urinary frequency.

The effect of caffeine on lower urinary tract function is hotly debated. Avoidance of excessive caffeine intake in teas, coffees and colas may exacerbate urinary frequency. However, there have been several short-term, urodynamic studies using oral caffeine which have shown no effect on the bladder[13]. Similarly in clinical trials no sustained benefit has been found[14]. However, recently a trial of caffeine reduction in a predominantly elderly group of women has been reported. A reduction in caffeine intake and maintenance of total fluid intake did lead to a reduction in urinary frequency[15]. Excess alcohol intake has a similar effect, in addition to the volume load, but there are no objective data from studies of alcohol reduction.

Weight reduction

In women, there is good evidence for a positive association of stress urinary incontinence and body mass, and some evidence that massive weight reduction (in a group of women who had undergone jaw wiring) reduces this[14,16]. Unfortunately, there is no such evidence for the male population and weight reduction should only be recommended as part of a management plan to maintain general health rather than for its putative effect upon continence status.

The 'lazy urethra'

Dribbling, which may occur late after micturition, is a significant problem in young men. The prevalence of this condition in one report ranged from 17% of men in their third decade to 27% when in their sixth[17]. This phenomenon is due to the retention of a column of urine in the bulbus urethra after voiding. The urine is voided at a later time and is often a cause of considerable embarrassment, due to staining of garments. There have been some studies which have examined this problem. The recommended treatment is to perform perineal massage following micturition to 'milk' the urethra of all urine prior to leaving the lavatory. This is a successful intervention but is not acceptable to some individuals because of the manipulation required. An alternative approach to the problem has been recently reported. This study demonstrated efficacy of the application of voluntary pelvic floor contraction, following taught pelvic floor exercises, in controlling the problem[18].

Overactive bladder (detrusor instability)

The overactive bladder is the commonest cause of urinary incontinence in the elderly regardless of gender. The conventional term for the condition, detrusor instability, fails to accurately reflect the true extent of the problem. This is because a diagnosis of detrusor instability, as defined by the International Continence Society, is based upon finding a spontaneous detrusor contraction whilst filling the bladder during urodynamic testing[19]. The difficulty

with this definition is that 25% of people with the classical symptoms of urgency, frequency with or without urge incontinence, will potentially be excluded from effective treatment for their condition by this criterion. In addition, up to 60% of normal, asymptomatic individuals exhibit spontaneous detrusor contractions during urodynamic investigations[20].

The true incidence of symptomatic detrusor instability is unknown due to the inherent difficulty of under-reporting but is estimated at between 10–15% of asymptomatic men and women between 10 and 50 years of age, rising to 35% of those aged over 75 years old[21].

In the vast majority of cases, the cause of detrusor overactivity is unknown. However, as noted above, it is commonly associated with bladder outflow obstruction in men, pelvic surgery in women and neurological injury or disease, such as spinal cord injury, multiple sclerosis, cerebrovascular disease, Parkinson's or Alzheimer's disease.

Patients' symptoms are extremely important in making a diagnosis of detrusor overactivity. Not all patients may experience all symptoms and many go to great lengths to avoid experiencing incontinence. Most often this is achieved either by restricting fluid intake or increasing urinary frequency. In addition to taking a relevant history, a patient-completed voiding diary is a useful aid[22]. The diary records urinary frequency and volumes passed as well as the number of incontinence episodes experienced.

Urinary tract infection and calculi may cause urinary urgency and urge incontinence, and should be excluded at an early stage. The simplest method to exclude infection is to use a rapid urinalysis dipstick. The leukocyte esterase and nitrite tests are an accurate method of assessing the absence of infection (combined negative predictive value 98%) and can enable early treatment. If recurrent infections or hematuria in the absence of infection is noted and subsequently confirmed then further investigation is needed.

TREATMENT INTERVENTIONS

The development of pharmacological treatment for bladder problems has been slow and it is only recently that drugs designed specifically with the bladder in mind have been developed. Antimuscarinic drugs are still the most widely used treatment in the UK. Data suggesting that such drugs can inhibit contractions of the detrusor are conflicting[23-25], however this does not appear to affect response to treatment. Trials which have utilized urodynamic studies to assess efficacy have normally shown that bladder capacity alone is significantly changed following treatment[26]. There are also data which suggest that those patients' symptoms respond as well to antimuscarinic agents regardless of the diagnosis being made by urodynamic or clinical characterization[27]. The chief drawback of these agents has been their side-effect profile, as the target receptor is ubiquitous in the body. Side-effects such as dry mouth, constipation, blurred vision and esophageal reflux have limited the tolerability of these agents.

The most commonly prescribed treatment for the overactive bladder in the UK is oxybutynin. Oxybutynin is both antimuscarinic, a direct muscle relaxant and a local anesthetic agent. Its chief metabolite, N-desethyl oxybutynin, is also pharmacologically active and occurs in higher concentrations than the parent compound. This metabolite is thought to be responsible for many of the adverse effects related to this drug. The efficacy of oxybutynin has been shown in both open and controlled trials[28,29]. The main drawback in trials of high dose oxybutynin (5 mg three times daily) has been the incidence of side-effects; the withdrawal rate has varied between 22–40% with up to 80% of those withdrawing suffering significant adverse reactions. More recent work using lower doses of the drug has also shown efficacy with a concomitant reduction in the adverse effects and an enhanced level of tolerability[30,31]. However, only 10–30% of patients will still be taking the drug one year after initiation[32].

Oxybutynin has been found to add little to the clinical effectiveness of a prompted voiding regimen in a nursing home population[33].

A modified release preparation with once daily administration has been recently approved for use in Europe. This preparation retains the efficacy of the standard release form but with up to 40% fewer reported side-effects[34]. Recent studies have concentrated upon comparing this compound to immediate release oxybutynin and have resulted in an equivalent efficacy in controlling urge incontinence. The incidence of dry mouth was similar, but with a reduced severity in one study by Versi and colleagues[35] and was reduced in incidence in a second study by Anderson and co-workers[36]. Approximately two-thirds of the patients prescribed extended-release oxybutynin for detrusor instability were still taking the medication 6 months later.

The side-effect profile of oxybutynin is also improved by other alternative methods of administration; both the rectal and intravesical route have been assessed[37,38]. Winkler and Sand[38] in a trial of 25 patients found a 48% response rate using the rectal route and 58% of responders were able to use the drug in the longer term. However, 48% of all patients suffered from dry mouth. Clearly the intravesical route has a limited acceptability to patients who are not routinely practicing intermittent catheterization.

Tolterodine is a newer, non-selective antimuscarinic competitive antagonist, which in the anesthetized cat model appears to have some functional selectivity for bladder muscarinic receptors over those in the salivary glands[39]. This appears to explain the lower incidence of dry mouth and the reduction in withdrawals due to severe dry mouth seen with use of the drug. Like oxybutynin it too has an active metabolite which appears to be responsible for some of the observed therapeutic effect[40]. Several randomized, double-blind placebo-controlled studies in patients with detrusor instability, detrusor hyper-reflexia, overactive bladder and specifically in the elderly have been performed[41-43]. In doses of 2 mg twice daily, tolterodine has consistently resulted in a reduction in urinary frequency and, in some trials, a reduction in the number of incontinence episodes. Where tolterodine has been compared to oxybutynin, the drug has been found equally efficacious. Tolterodine appears to have the advantage of greater tolerability and fewer withdrawals due to adverse effects, although there has been no direct comparison with the lower doses of oxybutynin used widely in UK practice. The proportion of patients continuing therapy for 6 months in one study comparing 500 patients taking either tolterodine or oxybutynin was statistically superior for tolterodine (32%) compared with oxybutynin (22%, $p < 0.001$). For those discontinuing either drug, oxybutynin was stopped significantly earlier[44].

Although tolterodine is more costly than oxybutynin, its use may allow treatment of a greater number of patients. What is not known, and not yet tested, is whether tolterodine has any other advantages, such as its effect upon cognitive impairment or other troublesome side-effects. In addition, the effect of bladder retraining with or without the drug has not been assessed.

The older antimuscarinic drug, imipramine, although not licensed for treatment of detrusor instability or overactive bladder, is commonly used for this indication. It is both a centrally- and peripherally-acting antimuscarinic agent, it blocks reuptake of serotonin (5-HT) and norepinephrine and has α-adrenergic agonist properties. There is also some evidence that the drug is an antidiuretic in mice. There is no evidence that imipramine can suppress unstable detrusor contractions but several small trials have shown the drug to be efficacious in the treatment of detrusor instability[45]. In the treatment of 10 elderly patients with detrusor instability the use of imipramine was efficacious in achieving continence (6/10 patients) in doses between 25–150 mg[46]. A commonly used antidepressant, doxepin, has also been assessed in a single-blinded cross-over study at a dose of either 50 mg at night or 50 mg nightly and 25 mg in the morning[47]. There was a significant decrease in nocturnal urinary frequency.

Propiverine hydrochloride has combined antimuscarinic and calcium channel blocking activity. It has several active metabolites and is rapidly absorbed orally where it undergoes significant first pass metabolism. There has been no cardiac toxicity associated with use of the drug to date. Clinical trials have demonstrated superiority to placebo in the treatment of detrusor hyper-reflexia in a 2-week double-blind placebo-controlled trial of oral treatment[48]. In comparative trials against flavoxate and placebo and oxybutynin and placebo, propiverine has demonstrated a similar efficacy to oxybutynin[49,50]. Madersbacher and colleagues[49], in a recent 4-week study comparing the use of propiverine against oxybutynin 5 mg twice daily and placebo, reported a similar efficacy in treatment of symptoms to oxybutynin, but with statistically significantly milder and less common incidence of dry mouth. Up to 20% of patients do, however, experience adverse effects which are mainly anticholinergic in nature. There are as yet no long-term data from European trials of the drug and its use has been confined to patients with urodynamically-confirmed detrusor instability, thus not including the 25% of patients with symptoms of bladder overactivity but normal urodynamics. In addition, there is no evidence regarding use of the drug in relation to behavioral intervention. The place of propiverine in the treatment of overactive bladder remains to be resolved but given its equal efficacy and apparent milder incidence of side-effects it is likely to remain as an alternative second-line treatment.

Trospium chloride, an antimuscarinic agent derived from atropine, has also recently been approved for use in Europe. This drug has been shown to be effective in the treatment of detrusor instability in several randomized controlled trials using urodynamic measures of diagnosis and extent of disease as well as clinical and quality of life outcomes[51,52].

The drug has been assessed in short-term studies versus placebo and standard release oxybutynin and has been found to be superior in effect to placebo and equivalent in efficacy to oxybutynin, when treating detrusor hyper-reflexia, at doses of 5 mg three times daily. The number of withdrawals due to side-effects in the trospium group was lower than the oxybutynin group[53].

The potential for antimuscarinic agents to cause a deterioration in cognition, especially in the elderly, has been well recognized in association with oxybutynin[54,55]. The effect of trospium chloride on electroencephalogram (EEG) activity has been assessed compared to oxybutynin administration in one study of 12 healthy volunteers. Trospium did not cause a significant reduction in EEG activity. The relationship of this to functional cognitive ability, however, is unknown and needs further study[56].

The drug flavoxate has been widely promoted for the treatment of the overactive bladder. Its possible mechanism of action in the treatment of bladder problems is unclear but it appears to have no anticholinergic properties[57]. Studies of its efficacy versus placebo have failed to show any beneficial effect of flavoxate[58,59], the reported reduction in urinary frequency ranging between − 21 and + 5%. In comparative, double-blind cross-over studies versus eme-promium or oxybutynin, flavoxate was found to be equally efficacious in achieving an improvement[60,61]. The use of flavoxate was associated with few side-effects. Given the lack of effect in placebo-controlled studies of flavoxate it is difficult to recommend its use.

Most drug therapy has conventionally been used in combination with bladder retraining. Bladder retraining was first described by Jeffcoate and Francis in 1966[62]. This technique involves the simple maxim 'hold on', which is simple to say but far from simple to perform, requiring much motivation and will-power. Even in the most motivated patient, bladder retraining can take months to achieve a lasting change in habit, and because of the difficulty

and continual attention required there is a high relapse rate. The regimen involves a gradual increase in the voiding interval, using frequency–volume charts as an objective reinforcement and guide. Data from trials of this method alone are conflicting and there have been few of sufficient methodological quality to allow firm conclusions to be drawn. Burgio and co-workers[63], in a recent study, showed that behavioral techniques alone may improve patients' experience of their disease to a similar extent to drug therapy when used alone, although the study was limited by its interpretation. There are data to suggest that a combination of pharmacotherapy and behavioral techniques may achieve results which are superior to either technique in isolation, although the number of patients in this study progressing to combination therapy was small. Where the patient is cognitively impaired or institutionalized, a progressive regular toilet-ting regimen may be employed[64]. There are no data to support the additional use of oxybutynin in this population[65], but tolterodine does have efficacy data as a sole treatment modality. Care has to be taken when introducing antimuscarinic medication to those with pre-existing cognitive impairment and to those already taking anticholinergic medication, as this may be exacerbated.

Surgery

Surgery is most applicable for those with detrusor overactivity associated with other conditions, such as outflow tract obstruction where the overactivity resolves in two-thirds of patients. For those with intractable disease uncontrollable by other means, the technique of clam ileocystoplasty or detrusor myomectomy (bladder autoaugmentation) is used. Both of these techniques aim to create a high capacity, low pressure and stable reservoir. The operation is effective, with abolition of the underlying instability in 50% of patients, in addition to an increase in bladder compliance and the functional capacity of the bladder. For between 15 and 75% of patients, the operation is associated with inefficient voiding so that self-catheterization is required to achieve complete bladder emptying. There is also concern about the metabolic effects due to the permeable endothelium of the small bowel being in contact with urine, the difficulty caused by intestinal mucus production and urinary tract infection.

Good results from surgery have been reported with variable time of follow-up and in patients up to the age of 80 years[66]. There is no evidence that denervation procedures, such as trigonal phenol injection, are efficacious. Likewise, data on the efficacy of repeated cystodistension in alleviating symptoms of overactive bladder are lacking.

Stress and post-prostatectomy incontinence

Men seldom suffer from stress urinary incontinence due to urethral sphincter insufficiency in the absence of surgery or trauma. Studies estimate the prevalence of this condition to be 4.6–9.2% of men[67,68].

There has been little, if any, systematic research of treatment of men with urethral incompetence. Two small studies of 20 and 7 men, six of whom in the latter were postoperative, have reported efficacy in terms of improvement of incontinence with ephedrine[69,70].

The incidence of incontinence following prostatectomy varies between 1–15% depending on the procedure used. The highest incidence is associated with radical prostatectomy. Periurethral procedures are associated with rates reported at from 0–8%[71,72].

The majority of these studies have followed patients in the short-term and are retrospective reviews, rather than prospective studies with the express intent to examine the phenomenon. There are also little data available in the reports to allow underlying diagnosis of incontinence to be established. There is clearly a requirement for a prospective study in this

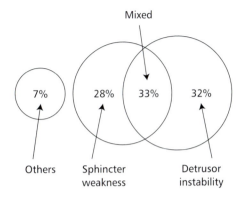

Figure 5 Causes of post-prostatectomy incontinence in 203 patients identified by urodynamic study

population of men post-surgery that pays attention to the degree and type of incontinence and its resolution in the longer term.

In late life, pre-existing bladder problems may co-exist (Figure 5), accounting for the observed underlying pathology. The integrity of the striated muscle sphincter is compromised in approximately 25% of incontinent patients[73]. Underlying detrusor instability accounts for the majority of cases either alone or in combination with sphincteric insufficiency. Factors that have been associated with an increased risk of incontinence following prostatectomy are an increased age[74], associated neurological disease or cognitive impairment[75,76]. Patients with pre-existing cerebrovascular disease or Parkinson's disease are at an increased risk of becoming incontinent following prostatic surgery[77]. Likewise, patients who have received radiotherapy are more likely to suffer from postoperative incontinence[78]. Where the prostatectomy has been for malignant disease, the risk of incontinence has been reported at between 2 and 5%[79,80].

When treated with artificial sphincters, the revision rate appears to be higher than when this technique is employed in patients who have not been exposed to radiotherapy, mostly due to a higher rate of erosion. There is some debate about the influence of prior surgery in more recent series, and it appears likely that there is no additional risk attributable to a repeat procedure. Poorer results from prostatic surgery are reported if there is co-existent detrusor instability and there are some reports of symptomatic worsening[81].

Treatment of post-prostatectomy incontinence should be targeted at the underlying pathology where appropriate. There is good evidence that the incidence of detrusor instability will rise in association with increasing age amongst the postoperative population and that this will lead to an increase in lower urinary tract symptoms which will require treatment[82]. There is good accumulating evidence that pelvic floor exercises should be the intervention of choice for post-prostatectomy incontinence, although there is an appreciable rate of spontaneous resolution. One recent short-term study of intensive pelvic floor therapy noted a significant reduction in incontinence[83]. Burgio and colleagues[84] reported the effective use of a combination of behavioral techniques to address this problem. There appears to be no additional benefit of electro-stimulation[85]. Periurethral injectable materials such as collagen, teflon paste and autologous fat have also been used in an attempt to treat stress incontinence in men. The reported results of this intervention have been contradictory and success in the short-term is followed by relapse[86,87]. However, once again, data with which to make an informed decision with respect to this treatment for stress incontinence are lacking. For patients with persistent stress incontinence following medical management, the implantation of an artificial urethral sphincter is a successful option: more than 70% of men will be either cured or significantly improved following the procedure. The presence of co-existent detrusor instability leads to a reduction in the success rate. Failure is mainly due to infection, urethral erosion or mechanical failure, although later devices are much less prone to this latter problem. In one report of long-term follow-up, 32.5% of patients required re-operation in the 3 years following the original operation[88].

Clean intermittent catheterization

In combination with antimuscarinic drugs, many elderly men with co-existent voiding inefficiency who would not be candidates for surgical treatment can be successfully managed by this technique[89]. Where a patient's dexterity is not good, a voluntary or statutory carer may be successfully employed if the frequency of intermittent catheterization required is not too high. There is still considerable debate (and little evidence) at what volume to intervene. Empirically, if the patient is continent and asymptomatic, then many would treat conservatively, some up to volumes in excess of 250 ml.

Nocturnal frequency, polyuria and enuresis

Nocturnal frequency is deemed to be excessive if greater than twice nightly. There is an increased incidence of frequent voiding in association with greater age. Prostatic hypertrophy and outflow tract obstruction is the commonest cause in men, the assessment and treatment of which is reviewed above. There are also several physiological changes which lead to an increasing likelihood of developing nocturnal frequency. Normally, adults produce two-thirds of their 24-h urine output by day and the other third by night. In older individuals this changes; renal concentrating ability falls and glomerular filtration rate increases in the supine position. There is a redistribution of fluid at night, particularly if the individual has venous insufficiency or is on medication, which predisposes to the development of peripheral edema. In addition, some older adults have a delayed diuresis in response to a fluid load and lose their diurnal rhythm of antidiuretic hormone (ADH) secretion[90]. When taken together, this means that the kidneys are working harder overnight to produce greater quantities of more dilute urine, the amount of which may be in excess of functional bladder capacity. All this is

Table 2 Concomitant diseases which may have an impact upon urinary incontinence

---

Diseases affecting mobility
Arthritis hip fracture
Contractures
Peripheral vascular disease
Stroke
Parkinson's disease

Nervous system disorders affecting cognition and neural control mechanisms
Dementia
Stroke
Parkinson's disease

Other medical conditions
Diabetes mellitus; causing polyuria and autonomic neuropathy
Congestive heart failure (CHF); leading to excess nocturnal urinary production
Venous insufficiency; a similar mechanism as CHF
Chronic lung disease; exacerbation of stress incontinence

---

in the absence of any pathology, such as heart failure, which may exacerbate the situation. Other diseases which perdispose to urinary incontinence are shown in Table 2. There is evidence for the efficacy of DDAVP[91] and early evening diuretic[92], and limited evidence for daytime recumbence[93], but these are not well tolerated by all. In particular, the usefulness of DDAVP may be limited to those individuals with true nocturnal polyuria – defined as producing > 50% of total daily urine output at night – rather than urinary frequency[94], and its use may be hampered by drug–drug interactions predisposing to hyponatremia or excessive secondary drinking habits.

Primary nocturnal enuresis may persist into adulthood. There is a genetic predisposition to primary nocturnal enuresis. In 1995, a Danish group reported finding a mutation on chromosome 13 that appeared to be partly responsible for nocturnal enuresis in some families[95]. Since then another gene, on chromosome 12, has been described[96]. These genes are known as *ENUR 1* and *2*, respectively. If both parents are enuretic then a child has a 70% chance of also being enuretic. This affects approximately

0.6–1% of all adults, 50% of whom will never seek help for the problem[97]. The majority of men with persistent nocturnal enuresis, up to the age of 65 years, appear to have underlying detrusor instability[98–100].

Treatment with imipramine has shown a marked antidiuretic effect on patients with nocturnal polyuria; this appears to be a vasopressin-independent effect, mediated by α-receptors in the proximal convoluted tubule. DDAVP is used although there are few data to support the intervention in patients other than those with neurological disease. A study comparing the use of DDAVP with the antimuscarinic medication oxybutynin showed no difference in improvement between the DDAVP group and combination treatment. For institutionalized, highly dependent men, the problem of nocturnal incontinence continues to require a major effort to manage effectively. The continuing developments in pad technology and the use of barrier creams can often minimize the disruption of sleep patterns. The use of electronic 'wet' alarms has also been advocated in the USA, but there has been little uptake in their use.

Containment

In most health economies, there is a massive expenditure on containment products. The most recent data for the UK suggest that in the region of £80 million is spent by the National Health Service annually. There is rationing of such products in many areas of England and Wales and, in addition, considerable spending on over-the-counter products. There are little up-to-date data on the efficacy of such products and even less comparative data upon which purchasing agencies may base their decisions, thus, for many, budgetary concerns dominate. However, a systematic comparison by the Continence Products Evaluation Network (all in one disposable bodywarm pads for heavy incontinence, 1998) demonstrated that the cheapest pads were not necessarily the

Table 3 Drug therapy which may potentially aggravate or predispose to urinary incontinence

Drug	Effect
Diuretics	increase urinary frequency and may precipiate urge incontinence in predisposed individuals
Calcium channel antagonists	associated with polyuria, especially at night when fluid redistribution occurs. Constipation
Anticholinergics (including antihistamines, antipsychotics, antipasmodics, anti-Parkinsonian agents)	may precipiate confusion, especially in those with pre-existing cognitive inpairment
α-adrenoreceptor agonists	may predispose to stress incontinence, due to relaxant effect on the external urethral sphincter
Non-steroidal anti-inflammatory drugs	salt and water retention
H₂ antagonists	confusion
Benzodiazepines and neuroleptics	any sedative medication with an appreciable hangover effect will exacerbate continence problems in those elderly people predisposed to problems

most effective and, for that matter, neither were the most expensive. There has been a trend for single supplier contracts in many areas of the UK, which has been cost driven. This denies more useful products to some patient groups. Likewise there is a shift away from single-use pads to washable products.

ADDITIONAL FACTORS IN THE ELDERLY MALE PATIENT

Concomitant disease and drug therapy, in particular, may serve to push an elderly person over the edge and become incontinent. The treatments for many bladder problems do not differ in elderly people and there is evidence to show that the elderly do just as well with treatment[101]. However, attention has to be paid to other factors which may limit the application of routine treatments.

Drug therapy

Many commonly used drugs may, through a variety of mechanisms, have an adverse effect upon the function of the lower urinary tract or the physical ability of an elderly person to cope with pre-existing urinary symptoms (see Table 3). The elderly are more likely to be taking a number of different drugs; interactions

between these and between any drug treatment for incontinence and pre-existing medication should be taken into account when prescribing for an elderly man.

Non-drug factors

Diabetes may certainly present incidentally as urinary incontinence in elderly people. Toxic confusional states and intercurrent illness may precipitate the problem, as can urinary retention. Whilst fecal impaction causes fecal incontinence and may cause urinary retention, the relationship between impaction and urinary incontinence is unclear, though often claimed. Other disease entities with an impact upon urinary problems are listed in Table 2.

Problems associated with physical disability

Physical problems with access to lavatory facilities and privacy also need to be considered, particularly in institutional settings. The provision of commodes or other urine collection devices, appropriate grab rails and raised toilet seats may be essential in maintaining continence for some people. Strategies aimed at maintaining mobility of elderly individuals also have a positive effect upon urinary incontinence[102].

Toiletting schedules

For those patients who are cognitively impaired, where there is little chance of active participation in behavioral methods of treatment, drug treatment may help in reducing the burden of incontinence. However, there is little evidence that use of oxybutynin in this scenario is effective[33]. There is no direct evidence of efficacy for tolterodine, but there are data for its effectiveness as a sole modality of treatment[103].

For many patients, strategies such as scheduled voiding (where patients are toiletted at regular intervals), individualized toiletting programs (where the toiletting is titrated to the patient's known voiding habits) and prompted voiding programs (where the patient is prompted to visit the toilet at regular intervals) are effective treatment options. The latter requires staff ability to ascertain whether the patient is wet or not and depends upon the ability of the patient to request toiletting. Neither regular or individual toiletting programs require this. All have been found to be effective in reducing incontinence episodes in nursing home patients[104,105]. All methods are very labor intensive, but there is evidence that, for regular toiletting regimens, a 4-hourly interval is as effective as a 2-hourly one[106]. For some elderly males, the only option available for the treatment of their urinary incontinence is containment, whether this is by virtue of physical or cognitive impairment. The main aims of containment devices are the protection of skin and clothing and the prevention of malodour. Such devices include condoms, clamps, absorbent underwear, single-use and reusable pads.

CONCLUSIONS

There is considerable debate about the contribution of outflow tract obstruction to the development of changes in bladder behavior leading to the development of detrusor instability. There is good evidence to suggest that this condition may develop in association with greater age alone. Detrusor instability accounts for the majority of cases of urinary incontinence in older males and can be successfully treated by behavioral techniques and pharmacotherapy. For men with post-prostatectomy incontinence, bladder overactivity accounts for over half of the observed cases of incontinence and thus is similarly amenable to treatment. There is much scope for further study of alterations in pathophysiology of the bladder in older men. This is especially pertinent given the increasing proportions of men who are likely to survive into late life.

References

1. Resnick NM, Elbadawi A, Yalla SV. Age and the lower urinary tract: what is normal? *Neurourol Urodyn* 1995;14:577–9
2. Malone-Lee JG, Wahedna I. Characterisation of detrusor contractile function in relation to old age. *Br J Urol* 1993;72:873–80
3. Bonde HV, Sejr D, Erdmann L, *et al*. Residual urine in 75-year-old men and women. A normative population study. *Scand J Urol Nephrol* 1996;30:89–91
4. Cockett ATK, Khoury S, Aso Y, *et al*. The second international consultation on benign prostatic hyperplasia. Proceedings 2: The effects of obstruction and ageing on the function of the lower urinary tract. Scientific communication International. Jersey C.I., 1993
5. Gilpin SA, Gosling JA, Barnard RJ. Morphological and morphometric studies of the human obstructed trabeculated urinary bladder. *Br J Urol* 1985;57:525–9
6. Gosling JA, Gilpin SA, Dixon JS, Gilpin CJ. Decrease in the autonomic innervation of human detrusor muscle in outflow obstruction. *J Urol* 1986;136:501–3
7. Cortivo R, Pagano F, Passerini G, *et al*. Elastin and collagen in the normal and

obstructed urinary bladder. *Br J Urol* 1981;
53:134–7

8. Holm NR, Horn T, Hald T. Detrusor in ageing and obstruction. *Scand J Urol Nephrol* 1995; 29:45–9

9. Gilpin SA, Gilpin CJ, Dixon JS, *et al*. The effect of age on the autonomic innervation of the urinary bladder. *Br J Urol* 1986;58: 378–81

10. Lepor H, Sunaryadi I, Hartanto V, Shapiro E. Quantitative morphometry of the adult human bladder. *J Urol* 1992;148:414–17

11. Abrams PH, Farrar DJ, Turner-Warwick R, *et al*. The results of prostatectomy: a symptomatic and urodynamic analysis of 152 patients. *J Urol* 1979;121:640–2

12. Kosimaki J, Hakama M, Huhtala H, Tammela TLJ. Association of smoking with lower urinary tract symptoms. *J Urol* 1998;159: 1580–2

13. Creighton SM, Stanton SL. Caffeine: does it affect your bladder? *Br J Urol* 1990;66: 613–14

14. Brown JS, Seeley DG, Fong J, *et al*. Urinary incontinence in older women: who is at risk? *Obstet Gynecol* 1996;87:715–21

15. Tomlinson BU, Dougherty MC, Pendergast JF, *et al*. Dietary caffeine, fluid intake and urinary incontinence in older rural women. *Int Urogynecol J Pelvic Floor Dysfunct* 1999; 10:22–8

16. Bump RC, Sugerman JH, Fantl A, McClish DM. Obesity and lower urinary tract function in women: effect of surgically induced weight loss. *Am J Obstet Gynecol* 1992;167:392–8

17. Furuya S, Ogura H, Tanaka M, *et al*. Incidence of post-micturition dribble in adult males from their twenties through fifties. *Acta Urol Japan* 1997;43:407–10

18. Paterson J, Pinnock CB, Marshall VR. Pelvic floor exercises as a treatment for post-micturition dribble. *Br J Urol* 1997;79:892–7

19. Abrams PH, Blaivas JG, Stanton SL, *et al*. Standardization of terminology of lower urinary tract function. *Neurourol Urodyn* 1988; 7:403

20. Robertson AS, Griffiths CJ, Ramsden PD, Neal DE. Bladder function in healthy volunteers: ambulatory monitoring and conventional urodynamic studies. *Br J Urol* 1994;73:242–9

21. Abrams PH. Bladder instability: concept, clinical associations and treatment. *Scand J Urol Nephrol* 1984;87:7

22. Abrams P, Klevmark B. Frequency volume charts: an indispensable part of lower urinary tract assessment. *Scand J Urol Nephrol* 1996; 179:47–53

23. Cardozo LD, Stanton SL. An objective comparison of the effects of parenterally administered drug in patients suffering from detrusor instability. *J Urol* 1979;122:58–9

24. Blaivas JG, Labib KB, Michalik J, Zayed AAH. Cystometric response to propantheline in detrusor hyperreflexia: therapeutic implications. *J Urol* 1980;124:259–62

25. Zorzitto ML, Jewett MAS, Fernie GR, *et al*. Effectiveness of propantheline bromide in the treatment of geriatric patients with detrusor instability. *Neurourol Urodyn* 1986; 5:133–40

26. Jonas U, Hofner K, Madersbacher H, Holmdahl TH. Efficacy and safety of two doses of tolterodine versus placebo in patients with detrusor overactivity and symptoms of frequency, urge incontinence and urgency: urodynamic evaluation. The International Study Group. *World J Urol* 1997;15:144–51

27. Hashimoto K, Ohnishi N, Esa A, *et al*. Clinical efficacy of oxybutynin on sensory urgency as compared with motor urgency. *Urologia Int* 1999;62:12–16

28. Cardozo LD, Cooper D, Versi E. Oxybutynin chloride in the management of idiopathic detrusor instability. *Neurourol Urodyn* 1987;6:256–7

29. Moisey CU, Stephenson TP, Brendler CB. The urodynamic and subjective results of treatment of detrusor instability with oxybutynin chloride. *Br J Urol* 1980;52:472–5

30. Bemelmans BL, Kiemeney LA, Debruyne FM. Low-dose oxybutynin for the treatment of urge incontinence: good efficacy and few side effects. *Eur Urol* 2000;37:709–13

31. Malone-Lee JG, Lubel D, Szonyi G. Low dose oxybutynin for the unstable bladder. *Br Med J* 1992;304:1053

32. Kelleher CJ, Cardozo LD, Khullar V, Salvatore S. A medium-term analysis of the subjective efficacy of treatment for women with detrusor instability and low bladder compliance. *Br J Obstet Gynaecol* 1997;104: 988–93

33. Ouslander JG, Schnelle JF, Uman G, *et al*. Does oxybutynin add to the effectiveness of prompted voiding for urinary incontinence among nursing home residents? A placebo controlled trial. *J Am Geriatr Soc* 1995;43: 610–17

34. Birns J, Lukkari E, Malone-Lee JG. A randomized controlled trial comparing the efficacy of controlled release oxybutynin tablets (10 mg once daily) with conventional oxybutynin tablets (5 mg twice daily) in patients whose symptoms were stabilized on 5 mg twice daily of oxybutynin. *Br J Urol Int* 2000; 85:793–9

35. Versi E, Appell R, Mobley D, *et al*. Dry mouth with conventional and controlled release oxybutynin in urinary incontinence. *Obstet Gynecol* 2000;95:718–21

36. Anderson R, Mobley D, Blank B, *et al*. Once daily controlled versus immediate release oxybutynin for urge urinary incontinence. *J Urol* 1999;161:1809–12

37. Collas D, Malone-Lee JG. The pharmacokinetic properties of rectal oxybutynin – a possible alternative to intravesical administration. *Neurourol Urodyn* 1997;16: 638–40

38. Winkler HA, Sand PK. Treatment of detrusor instability with oxybutynin rectal suppositories. *Int Urogynecol J* 1998;17:100–2

39. Nilvebrandt L, Hallen B, Larsson G. Tolterodine – a new bladder selective antimuscarinic agent. *Eur J Pharmacol* 1997; 327:195–207

40. Nilvebrandt L, Gillberg PG, Sparf B. Antimuscarinic potency and bladder selectivity of PNU-200577, a major metabolite of tolterodine. *Pharmacol Toxicol* 1997;81:169–72

41. Abrams P, Freeman R, Anderstrom C, Mattiasson A. Tolterodine, a new antimuscarinic agent: as effective but better tolerated than oxybutynin in patients with an overactive bladder. *Br J Urol* 1998;81:801–10

42. Millard R, Tuttle J, Moore K, *et al*. Clinical efficacy and safety of tolterodine compared to placebo in detrusor overactivity. *J Urol* 1999;161:1551–5

43. Malone-Lee JG. Proc International Continence Society. Int. Continence Society, Tokyo, Japan 1997; Abstract A188

44. Lawrence M, Guay DR, Benson SR, Anderson MJ. Immediate-release oxybutynin versus tolterodine in detrusor overactivity: a population analysis. *Pharmacotherapy* 2000; 20:470–5

45. Diokno AC, Hyndman CW, Hardy DA, Lapides J. Comparison of action of imipramine (tofranil) and propantheline (propanthine) on detrusor contraction. *J Urol* 1972;107:42–3

46. Castleden CM, Duffin HM, Gulati RS. Double blind study of imipramine and placebo for incontinence due to bladder instability. *Age Ageing* 1986;15:299–303

47. Lose G, Jorgensen L, Thunedborg P. Doxepin in the treatment of female detrusor overactivity: a randomised double blind cross over study. *J Urol* 1989;142:1024–6

48. Stohrer M, Madersbacher H, Richter R, *et al*. Efficacy and safety of propiverine in SCI-patients suffering from detrusor hyperreflexia – a double-blind, placebo-controlled clinical trial. *Spinal Cord* 1999; 37:196–200

49. Madersbacher H, Halaska M, Voigt R, *et al*. A placebo-controlled, multicentre study comparing the tolerability and efficacy of propiverine and oxybutynin in patients with urgency and urge incontinence. *Br J Urol* 1999;84:646–51

50. Halaska M, Dorschner W, Frank M. Treatment of urgency and incontinence in elderly patients with propiverine hydrochloride. *Neurourol Urodyn* 1994;13:428–30

51. Fuertes ME, Garcia Matres MJ, Gonzalez Romojaro V, *et al*. Ensayo clinico para evaluar la eficacia y tolerancia del cloruro de trospio (Uraplex) en pacientes con incontinencia por inestabilidad del detrusor y su repercusion en la calidad de vida. *Arch Esp Urol* 2000;53:125–36

52. Cardozo L, Chapple CR, Toozs-Hobson P, *et al*. Efficacy of trospium chloride in patients

with detrusor instability: a placebo-controlled, randomized, double-blind, multicentre clinical trial. *Br J Urol* 2000;85:659–64

53. Madersbacher H, Stohrer M, Richter R, *et al.* Trospium chloride versus oxybutynin: a randomized, double-blind, multicentre trial in the treatment of detrusor hyper-reflexia. *Br J Urol* 1995;75:452–6

54. Donnellan CA, Fook L, McDonald P, Playfer JR. Oxybutynin and cognitive dysfunction. *Br Med J* 1997;315:1363–4

55. Katz IR, Sands LP, Bilker W, *et al.* Identification of medications that cause cognitive impairment in older people: the case of oxybutynin chloride. *J Am Geriatr Soc* 1998;46:8–13

56. Pietzko A, Dimpfel W, Schwantes U, Topfmeier P. Influences of trospium chloride and oxybutynin on quantitative EEG in healthy volunteers. *Eur J Clin Pharmacol* 1994;47:337–43

57. Guarneri L, Robinson E, Testar R. A review of flavoxate: pharmacology and mechanism of action. *Drugs Today* 1994;30:91–8

58. Chapple CR, Parkhouse H, Gardener C, Milroy EJG. Double-blind, placebo-controlled cross-over study of flavoxate in the treatment of idiopathic detrusor instability. *Br J Urol* 1990;66:491–4

59. Dahm TL, Ostri P, Kristensen JK, *et al.* Flavoxate treatment of micturition disorders accompanying benign prostatic hypertrophy: a double-blind, placebo-controlled multi-centre investigation. *Urol Int* 1995;55:205–8

60. Stanton SL. A comparison of emepronium bromide and flavoxate hydrochloride in the treatment of urinary incontinence. *J Urol* 1973;110:529–32

61. Milani R, Scalambrino S, Milia R, *et al.* Double blind cross-over comparison of flavoxate and oxybutynin in women affected by urinary urge syndrome. *Int Urogynecol J* 1993;4:3–8

62. Jeffcoate TNA, Francis WJA. Urgency incontinence. *Am J Obstet Gynecol* 1966;94:604

63. Burgio KL, Locker JL, Goode PS, *et al.* Behavioral versus drug treatment for urinary urge incontinence in older women. A randomized controlled trial. *J Am Med Assoc* 1998;280:1995–2000

64. Burgio K, Locher JL, Goode PS. Combined behavioural and drug therapy for urge incontinence in older women. *J Am Geriatr Soc* 2000;48:370–4

65. Ouslander JG, Schnelle JF, Uman G, *et al.* Does oxybutynin add to the effectiveness of prompted voiding for urinary incontinence among nursing home residents? A placebo controlled trial. *J Am Geriatr Soc* 1995; 43:610–7

66. Chapple CR. Surgery for detrusor overactivity. *World J Urol* 1998;16:268–73

67. Kondo A, Saito M, Yamada Y, *et al.* Prevalence of hand washing urinary incontinence in healthy subjects in relation to stress and urge incontinence. *Neurourol Urodyn* 1992;11: 519–23

68. Malmsten UG, Milsom I, Moklander U, Norlen LJ. Urinary incontinence and lower urinary tract symptoms: an epidemiological study of men aged 45 to 99 years. *J Urol* 1997;158:1733–7

69. Diokno AC, Taub M. Ephedrine in the treatment of urinary incontinence. *Urology* 1975; 5:624–5

70. Awad SA, Downie JW, Kiruluta HG. Alpha adrenergic agents in urinary disorders of the proximal urethra. Part 1. Sphincter incompetence. *Br J Urol* 1978;50:332–5

71. Doll HA, Black NA, McPherson K, *et al.* Mortality, morbidity and complications following transurethral resection of the prostate for benign prostatic hypertrophy. *J Urol* 1992;147:1566–73

72. Kaplan SA, Laor E, Fatal M, Te AE. Transurethral resection of the prostate versus transurethral electrovapourisation of the prostate: a blinded, prospective comparative study with one year follow up. *J Urol* 1998;159: 454–8

73. Fitzpatrick JM, Gardina RA, Worth PHL. The evaluation of 68 patients with post prostatectomy incontinence. *Br J Urol* 1979;51:552–5

74. Steiner MS, Morton RA, Walsh PC. Impact of anatomical radical prostatectomy on urinary incontinence. *J Urol* 1991;145:S12–15

75. Hammerer P, Dieringer J, Schuler J, *et al.* Urodynamic parameters to predict continence after radical prostatectomy. *J Urol* 1991;145:292A

76. Barkin M, Dolfin D, Herschorn S, *et al.* Voiding dysfunction in institutionalised elderly men: the influence of previous prostatectomy. *J Urol* 1983;130:258–9

77. Staskin DS, Vardi Y, Siroky MB. Post-prostatectomy continence in the Parkinsonian patient: the significance of poor voluntary sphincter control. *J Urol* 1988;140:117–8

78. Rainwater LM, Zincke H. Radical prostatectomy after radiation therapy for cancer of the prostate: feasibility and prognosis. *J Urol* 1988;140:1455–9

79. Green N, Treible D, Wallack H. Prostate cancer: post irradiation incontinence. *J Urol* 1990;144:307–9

80. Lee WR, Schultheiss TE, Hanlon AL, Hanks GE. Urinary incontinence following external beam radiotherapy for clinically localised prostate cancer. *Urology* 1996;48:95–9

81. Cote RJ, Burke H, Schoenberg HW. Prediction of unusual postoperative results by urodynamic testing in benign prostatic hyperplasia. *J Urol* 1981;125:690–2

82. Thomas AW, Cannon A, Bartlett E, *et al.* The natural history of voiding dysfunction in men: the long term follow up of TURP. *Br J Urol* 1998;81:22

83. Van Kampen M, De Weerdt W, Van Poppel H, *et al.* Effect of pelvic-floor re-education on duration and degree of incontinence after radical prostatectomy: a randomised controlled trial. *Lancet* 2000;355:98–102

84. Burgio KL, Stutzman RE, Engel BT. Behavioural training for post prostatectomy urinary incontinence. *J Urol* 1989;141:303–6

85. Opsomer EJ, Castille Y, Abi Aad AS, van Cangh PJ. Urinary incontinence after radical prostatectomy: is professional pelvic floor training necessary. *Neurourol Urodyn* 1994; 13:382–4

86. Politano VA. Transurethral polytef injection for post prostatectomy incontinence. *Br J Urol* 1992;69:26–8

87. Deane AM, English P, Hehir M, *et al.* Teflon injection in stress incontinence. *Br J Urol* 1985;57:78–80

88. Herschorn S, Radomski S, Fleschner N. Durability of the artificial sphincter in the management of urinary incontinence. *J Urol* 1996;155:456A

89. Webb RJ, Lawson AL, Neal DE. Clean intermittent catheterisation in 172 adults. *Br J Urol* 1990;65:20–3

90. Asplund R, Aberg H. Diurnal variation in the levels of antidiuretic hormone in the elderly. *J Intern Med* 1993;229:131

91. Hilton P, Stanton SL. The use of desmopressin (DDAVP) in nocturnal frequency in the female. *Br J Urol* 1982;54:252–5

92. Reynard J. A novel therapy for nocturnal polyuria: a double-blind randomized trial of furosemide against placebo. *Br J Urol* 1998; 82:215–18

93. O'Donnell PD, Beck C, Walls RC. Serial incontinence assessment in elderly inpatient men. *J Rehab Res Dev* 1990;27:1–9

94. Asplund R, Sundberg B, Bergtsson P. Oral desmopressin for nocturnal polyuria in elderly subjects: a double blind, placebo-controlled randomised exploratory study. *Br J Urol* 1999;83:591–5

95. Norgaard JP, Djurhuus JC, Watanabe H, *et al.* Experience and current status of research into the pathophysiology of nocturnal enuresis. *Br J Urol* 1997;79:825–35

96. Arnell H, Hjalmas K, Jagervall M, *et al.* The genetics of primary nocturnal enuresis: inheritance and suggestion of a second major gene on chromosome 12q. *J Med Genet* 1997;34:360–5

97. Hirasing RA, van Leerdam FJM, Bolk-Benink L, Janknegt RA. Enuresis nocturna in adults. *Scand J Urol Nephrol* 1997;31: 533–6

98. Torrens MJ, Collins CD. The urodynamic assessment of adult enuresis. *Br J Urol* 1975; 47:433–40

99. McGuire EJ, Savastano JA. Urodynamic studies in enuresis and the non-neurogenic, neurogenic bladder. *J Urol* 1984;132: 299–302

100. Fidas A, Galloway NTM, McInnes A, Chisholm GD. Neurophysiological measurements in primary adult enuretics. *Br J Urol* 1985;57:635–40

101. Szonyi G, Collas DM, Ding YY, Malone-Lee JG. Oxybutynin with bladder retraining for detrusor instability in elderly people: a randomized controlled trial. *Age Ageing* 1995; 24:287–91

102. O'Donnell PD. Special considerations in elderly individuals with urinary incontinence. *Urology* 1998;51:20–3

103. Appell RA. Clinical efficacy and safety of tolterodine in the treatment of overactive bladder: a pooled analysis. *Urology* 1997;50: 90–6

104. Engel BT, Burgio LD, McCormick KA, *et al.* Behavioural treatment of incontinence in the long term care setting. *J Am Geriatr Soc* 1990;38:361–3

105. Jilek R. Elderly toiletting: is two hourly too often? *Nursing Standard* 1993;7:25–6

106. Ouslander JG, Schnelle JF, Uman G, *et al.* Predictors of successful prompted voiding among incontinent nursing home residents. *J Am Med Assoc* 1995;273:1366–70

9 Testicular cancer

Axel Heidenreich, MD, and Peter Olbert, MD

Although testicular cancer accounts for only about 1% of all human neoplasms, it represents the most common malignant tumor in young men in the age group of 20–40 years. In 1994, approximately 6800 new cases of testicular cancer were diagnosed[1]. The peak incidence is at age 32; this compares with a median age at diagnosis of 68 years for all other tumors.

EPIDEMIOLOGY

Testicular cancer demonstrates two incidence peaks at the age of under 2 years and among men aged 25–34 years, with rates declining rapidly after the age of 40. There are striking differences in testicular cancer incidences around the world, with the highest incidence of 12–14 per 100 000 person-years in Switzerland and Denmark, and the lowest incidence of less than one per 100 000 person-years among African-Americans and the Chinese populations[2].

Although some risk factors have been identified as being associated with the development of testicular cancer, there are still a number of unknown parameters accounting for the increase in incidence.

ETIOLOGY

Cryptorchidism is the best-known risk factor and, according to case–control studies, the relative risk for testicular cancer is 2.5–8.8[3]. However, an undescended testis accounts for only about 10% of all testicular cancer cases. According to some investigations, there

seems to be an association between the age at correction of cryptorchidism and the risk of developing testicular cancer: patients undergoing orchidopexy prior to age 11 had a three-fold increased risk, compared to a seven-fold increased risk in subjects never having undergone orchidopexy.

Familial and genetic factors have been suggested to be involved in the development of testicular cancer, since first-degree relatives of testicular cancer patients have a six- to ten-fold higher risk of developing this form of cancer[4-6]. Furthermore, family members with testicular cancer have a significantly higher risk of cryptorchidism and bilateral disease and present at a younger age, indicating genetic factors already present at the time of embryological development of the testis. With regard to predisposing genetic events, the Testicular Linkage Consortium[7] has recently identified the locus Xq27 to be predisposing for bilateral testicular cancer and bilateral cryptorchidism. Other studies have reported the loci 1p36, 4p14–13, 5q21–21, 14q13–q24.3 and 18q21.1–21.3 to be highly associated with testicular cancer[8].

Prenatal exposure to estrogens might be associated with the development of testicular cancer, since excessive nausea during the first trimester is attributable to the rapid rise in endogenous estrogens, and the embryological testicular development, highly sensitive to hormonal imbalances, starts at that time[9,10].

No association between vasectomy, testicular trauma and torsion, infertility, inguinal hernia and testicular cancer has been confirmed in case–control studies. Furthermore, there are no consistent occupational exposures predisposing to testicular cancer.

PATHOLOGY OF TESTICULAR GERM-CELL TUMORS

About 90% of all testicular tumors are malignant germ-cell tumors, and the rest comprise benign tumors deriving from Leydig and Sertoli cells and other interstitial components[11–13].

The classification of the World Health Organization (WHO) has become widely accepted in recent years (Table 1). With regard to the classification of a given testicular tumor, it is of major importance to identify each histological pattern present, since the percentages of the various histological subtypes have direct prognostic significance and might be applied for the stratification of further therapy[14,15]. Although the terminology of tumors of a single histological type is straightforward, the classification of tumors consisting of more than one cell type is more controversial. However, mixed germ-cell tumors consist of multiple non-seminomatous elements, whereas combined germ-cell tumors consist of non-seminomatous and seminomatous components.

In many cases it might be possible to identify the major germ-cell tumor component macroscopically from the appearance of the sectioned surface of the tumor (Table 2).

As it is of the utmost importance to identify accurately the various histological subtypes of germ-cell cancer in the primary tumor, a number of immunohistochemical markers have been utilized in the diagnosis of germ-cell cancer. Table 3 summarizes the staining patterns of the most commonly used markers for each of the germ-cell tumor subtypes[13]. Alpha-fetoprotein (AFP) is most commonly associated with yolk-sac tumors, and is consistently negative in seminoma and choriocarcinoma; embryonal carcinoma expresses AFP only focally. Human chorionic gonadotropin (hCG) is specific for syncytiotrophoblasts, and therefore is highly expressed in choriocarcinomas; hCG, however, is also expressed in seminomas and embryonal carcinomas to a lower extent. Placental alkaline phosphatase (PLAP) lacks specificity and is found in basically all types of testicular germ-cell tumors; it is most useful in the detection of testicular intraepithelial neoplasia (TIN) cells and in the differentiation of TIN from normal germinative cells, which do not stain positive. The marker 43-9F has been thought to be specific for embryonal carcinoma; however, follow-up studies demonstrated a common expression of 43-9F in all subtypes of germ-cell tumors and in TIN[16,17].

PATHOGENESIS OF TESTICULAR GERM-CELL TUMORS

Testicular germ-cell tumors originate from totipotent primordial germ cells, which undergo neoplastic transformation as a result of a number of endogenous, exogenous, hormonal and genetic, as well as environmental, events (Figure 1). The neoplastic process results in the development of preinvasive carcinoma in situ (CIS) or TIN representing the common precursor for all testicular germ-cell tumors, except spermatocytic seminoma[18–20].

Some 70% of all patients with TIN will develop an invasive testicular germ-cell tumor within 7 years, based on the data of Skakkebaek and colleagues[20] in cryptorchid testes. Histologically, TIN cells are larger than normal spermatogonia, and have an enlarged and hyperchromatic nucleus, prominent nucleoli and glycogen-rich cytoplasm (Figure 2a). Immunohistochemically, TIN will be detected by the abundant expression of PLAP (Figure 2b). After the initial observation by Skakkebaek[19], a number of groups have demonstrated that approximately 5% of all patients with a unilateral germ-cell tumor will harbor TIN in their remaining testicle[8].

The pathogenetic events resulting in the malignant transformation of atypical spermatogonia to TIN are not well characterized.

Table 1 World Health Organization (WHO) classification of testicular germ-cell tumors (GCTs) and the relative frequency of histological subtypes[11–13]

WHO classification of GCT	Relative frequency (%)	
	Pure histology	More than one histology
Tumors of one histological subtype		
Classical seminoma	43 (35–51)	12 (7–15)
Spermatocytic seminoma	2 (1–4)	0
Embryonal carcinoma	7 (3–11)	36 (28–44)
Yolk-sac tumor	1 (1–2)	25 (10–39)
Polyembryoma	< 1	0
Choriocarcinoma	< 1	17 (7–40)*
Pure teratoma	4 (3–5)	37 (22–44)
mature teratoma	4 (3–5)	37 (22–44)
immature teratoma	0	0
teratoma with malignant transformation	0	0
Tumors of more than one histological subtype		
Teratocarcinoma	11.5	—
Mixed GCT	—	7
Combined GCT	—	10.6

*Includes choriocarcinoma and the presence of syncytiotrophoblasts

Table 2 Clinical characteristics of various histological subtypes of testis cancer

Tumor	Frequency (%)	Macroscopy	Tumor marker	Average age (years)
Seminoma	35–55	homogeneous, white, pale	hCG in 5–15%	35–40
Spermatocytic seminoma	2	yellow–gray, cysts, mucoid or clear fluid	none	55–60
Embryonal carcinoma	3–10	gray–white, soft, necrosis, hemorrhage	AFP, hCG rare	20–35
Yolk-sac tumor	2–5	solid, soft, gray–white, mucoid	AFP	20–35
Choriocarcinoma	< 1	necrosis, hemorrhage	hCG	20–35
Teratoma	< 5	cystic	none	20–35

hCG, human chorionic gonadotropin; AFP, α-fetoprotein

Table 3 Immunohistochemical marker expression by testicular cancer subtypes used for pathohistological differentiation

Marker	Seminoma	Spermatocytic seminoma	Embryonal carcinoma	Yolk-sac tumor	Choriocarcinoma	Teratoma	TIN
AFP	0	0	+	+++	0	0	0
hCG	+	0	+	0	+++	0	0
PLAP	+++	0/+	+++	+++	++	+	++
hPL	0	0	0	0	+++	0	0
EMA	0	0	0/+	0/+	+++	0	0
CEA	0	0	0	+	++	+++	0
NSE	+++	0	+++	++	+	++	0
43-9F	++	+	+++	+++	+	++	0
Vimentin	+	0	++	+/+++	0/+	+/+++	++

AFP, α-fetoprotein; hCG, human chorionic gonadotropin; PLAP, placental alkaline phosphatase; hPL, human placental lactogen; EMA, epithelial membrane antigen; CEA, carcinoembryonic antigen; NSE, non-specific enolase; TIN, testicular intraepithelial neoplasia

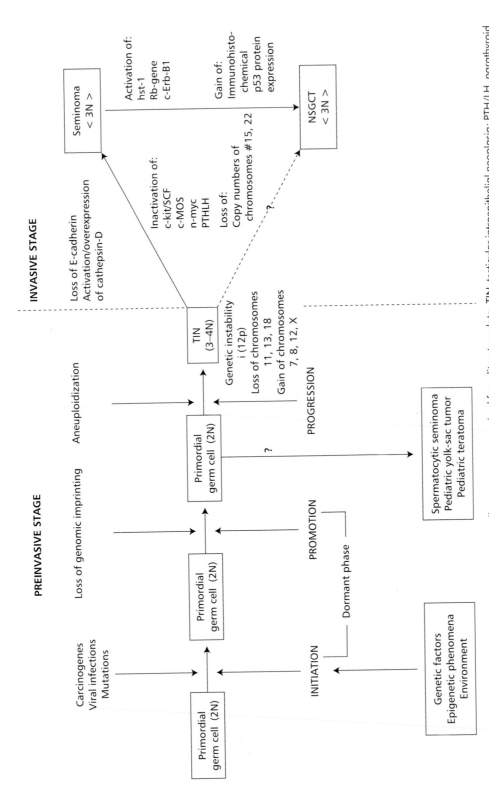

Figure 1 Molecular pathogenesis of testicular germ-cell tumors, as summarized from literature data. TIN, testicular intraepithelial neoplasia; PTH/LH, parathyroid hormone/luteinizing hormone; NSGCT, non-seminomatous germ-cell tumor

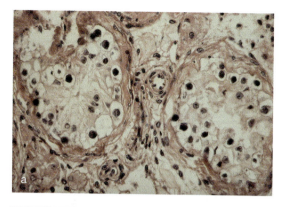

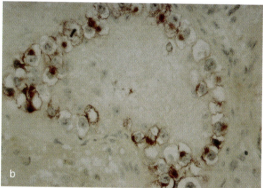

Figure 2 Testicular intraepithelial neoplasia (TIN) exhibiting large cells with enlarged and hyperchromatic nuclei, prominent nucleoli and glycogen-rich cytoplasm (a); TIN and placental alkaline phosphatase (PLAP) staining: TIN cells are depicted by the abundant expression of PLAP at the cell surface (b)

DIAGNOSTIC PROCEDURES AND MANAGEMENT OF TESTICULAR CANCER

Most patients present with a painless, solid testicular mass of varying size and duration; however, about 30% of patients present with scrotal pain. Therefore, any testicular tumor detected in young men 20–40 years of age should be regarded as malignant until proven otherwise.

Whereas the duration of symptoms does not correlate with survival and stage in classical seminoma, Moul[23] demonstrated a direct relationship between the mean symptomatic interval and clinical stage I–IIB, compared to clinical stages IIC and III, with intervals of 8.5–9.7 weeks and 26.4 weeks, respectively. In another study, Oliver[24] reported that delay in diagnosis was only 2 months in patients who were free of disease during follow-up, 4 months in patients who relapsed but were salvaged, and 7 months in patients who died of their disease.

Physical examination should include bimanual palpation of the tumor-bearing and the contralateral testicle, and palpation of the inguinal lymph nodes especially if the patient has had any prior scrotal or inguinal surgery. Scrotal ultrasonography usually reveals a hypoechoic mass within the tunica albuginea as suspicious for malignancy. Differential diagnosis between benign and malignant testicular tumors usually can only be made in the presence of simple testicular cysts and epidermoid cysts presenting either as smooth-lined, hypoechoic masses with a dorsal shadowing, or a well-demarcated cystic mass and an echogenic center caused by multiple acoustical reflections from the keratinous debris[25].

Furthermore, it is still unclear whether differentiation from TIN to embryonal carcinoma might occur directly or whether seminoma always represents the intermediate stage of differentiation. However, based on literature data, an oncogenetic model can be defined, elucidating the pathogenetic events leading to malignant transformation of spermatogonia to TIN and the progression of TIN to invasive germ-cell tumors (Figure 1). According to Damjanov[21] the three stages of initiation, promotion and progression result in the invasive phase of the germ-cell tumor. Pathogenetic events leading to local progression and metastases have been adapted (Figure 1) according to data available in the literature (for a more detailed summary see reference 22).

PRIMARY MANAGEMENT OF THE TESTICULAR MASS

Inguinal exploration and scrotal orchiectomy with early clamping of the spermatic cord is the therapy of choice for testicular cancer, revealing accurate information with regard to

Table 4 Guidelines for tumor enucleation in testicular germ-cell tumors as outlined by the German Testicular Cancer Intergroup based on 72 cases

Tumor diameter less than 20 mm
Tumor must be organ confined
Multiple biopsies from the tumor bed to prove tumor-free resection rims
Normal preoperative testosterone and luteinizing hormone serum levels
Close follow-up, high compliance of patient and physician
Treatment in centers experienced in the management of testicular cancer

histopathology and pathological-stage classification[26]. However, any testicular mass of uncertain ranking must be explored by the inguinal approach to verify or exclude malignancy. Since benign testicular lesions are recognized with increasing frequency, frozen section analysis should be considered intraoperatively, which accurately differentiates malignant from benign testicular lesions[27] with high sensitivity and specificity.

About 5% of all patients with a unilateral testicular germ-cell tumor will harbor TIN in their contralateral testicle, which will be detected by an immunohistochemical evaluation of a randomly taken testis biopsy at the time of orchiectomy. Currently, there exists controversy about the clinical utility of the contralateral biopsy, supposedly unnecessary for 95% of patients. An evidence-based meta-analysis of all studies concerned with the detection of TIN suggests that it is justified to recommend contralateral biopsy for men with a testis volume < 12 ml and age < 30 years at the time of diagnosis, since their risk for contralateral TIN is > 34%[8,26]. It must be emphasized that the biopsy specimen should be fixed in Bouin's or in Stieve's solution to preserve TIN cells for diagnosis.

Only in cases of a second metachronously or synchronously occurring testicular cancer, a testicular tumor developing in a solitary testis or a benign testis tumor might an organ-sparing approach be considered, to maintain endogenous testosterone synthesis, to preserve fertility and to improve quality of life in these long-term survivors. Guidelines identified by the German Testicular Cancer Intergroup based on results from more than 70 patients with a testicular germ-cell tumor and a mean follow-up of 78 months are outlined in Table 4[26,28]. However, it must be emphasized that tumor enucleation for testicular germ-cell tumors should be the exception for the very few patients presenting with bilateral testicular cancer.

PATHOHISTOLOGICAL DIAGNOSIS

Meticulous pathological work-up of the orchiectomy specimen should be performed according to the WHO recommendations, to identify all histological subtypes present and to identify vascular invasion. Especially in clinical stage I non-seminomatous germ-cell tumor (NSGCT), it might also be useful to calculate the percentage of all testicular cancer subtypes present, to obtain prognostic information with regard to the probability of occult metastatic retroperitoneal lymph-node disease[14,15]. As has been shown in previous studies, a high percentage of embryonal carcinoma associated with the presence of vascular invasion identifies patients at high risk of lymph-node metastases in the retroperitoneum, thereby enabling a risk-adapted approach to these patients (Table 5).

RADIOLOGICAL STAGING

Following radical orchiectomy, further staging includes computed tomography (CT) of the abdomen, the chest and the mediastinum, to detect metastatic lymph-node disease or visceral

Table 5 Cut-off for percentage embryonal carcinoma (ECa) and presence or absence of vascular invasion (VI) and their probability to predict final pathological stage in clinical stage I non-seminomatous germ-cell tumor (NSGCT)

| Quantitative pathology | n | Pathological stage (n) | | Stage correct (%) |
		I	II	
≤ 45% ECa	77	68/77	9/77 (11.5%)	88
≤ 45% ECa/VI neg.	71	65/71	6/71 (8.5%)	91.5
45–79% ECa	24	9/24	15/24 (62.5%)	
45–79% ECa/VI neg.	9/24	7/9	2/9 (22.2%)	78
45–79% ECa/VI pos.	15/24	0/15	15/15 (100%)	100
≥ 80% ECa	48	7/48	41/48 (85.4%)	85.4
≥ 80% ECa/VI pos.	42	5/42	37/42 (88.1%)	88
Total	149	86 (57.8%)	63 (42.2%)	87.9

neg., negative; pos., positive

metastases[29]. Unlike other solid neoplasms, the lymphatic spread of testicular cancer follows an anatomically predictable route, with the primary landing zones of the right testis including the interaortocaval region and the primary landing zones of the left side including the para-aortic and preaortic lymph nodes. Micrometastases are present in up to 20% and in approximately 30% of clinical stage I seminomas and non-seminomas, respectively, which will not be detected by classical interpretation of abdominal CT scans owing to the inability of morphological differentiation. Therefore, primary landing zones and the transverse diameter of the largest lymph node might be helpful, as recently demonstrated[30]: using the shortest transaxial lymph-node diameter, the probability of lymph-node metastases increased with increasing diameter. Based on uni- and multivariate logistic regression analysis, an accuracy of 84% was attained at 8 mm to find metastatic disease. Furthermore, the expected primary landing zones of right- and left-sided primaries should be considered in CT interpretation, increasing the predictive ability.

More caudal deposits of metastases usually reflect retrograde spread to the common, external and inguinal lymph nodes; especially in patients having undergone previous scrotal or inguinal surgery or presenting with scrotal tumor infiltration, it advisable to scan the iliac region because of atypical lymphatic spread.

Magnetic resonance imaging (MRI) of the abdomen using currently available techniques does not provide additional clinically useful information, and should be reserved for patients with contraindications to CT[29]. The introduction of new contrast agents for the evaluation of the lymphatic system might improve the diagnostic accuracy of MRI to detect retroperitoneal micrometastases.

In addition, positron emission tomography (PET) scans are not helpful in the detection of retroperitoneal micrometastases in patients with clinical stage I testicular cancer, as has been demonstrated in a variety of studies[31,32].

Although a lateral and posteroanterior chest X-ray will detect pulmonary metastases in approximately 15% of patients, a chest CT should be obtained owing to the higher sensitivity to identify lesions as small as 2 mm in diameter[33]. However, one has to consider that many of these small lesions are benign and do not relate to metastases from testicular cancer[34].

Brain CT and bone scintigraphy are only to be performed in cases of advanced testicular cancer with high-volume metastastic disease (≥ IIC), or in the case of specific symptomatology.

TUMOR MARKERS

Tumor markers are clinically useful for diagnosis, clinical staging, prediction of prognosis (see

Table 6 Clinical staging of testicular germ-cell tumors according to the Lugano classification

Clinical stage	Description
I	no evidence of metastases
IA	tumor limited to testis and epididymis
IB	infiltration of spermatic cord or tumor in cryptorchid testicle
IC	infiltration of the scrotum, trans-scrotal surgery, tumor developing after trans-scrotal or inguinal surgery
IX	extent of primary tumor cannot be evaluated
II	retroperitoneal lymph-node metastases
IIA	all lymph nodes ≤ 2 cm
IIB	more than one lymph node 2–5 cm
IIC	lymph nodes > 5 cm
IID	abdominal tumor palpable, fixed inguinal tumor
III	mediastinal and supraclavicular lymph-node metastases, visceral metastases
IIIA	mediastinal and supraclavicular lymph-node metastases only
IIIB	pulmonary metastases only
IIIC	hematogenous metastases outside the lung
IIID	persistent elevated markers without evidence of metastases

IGCCCG classification below) and monitoring the response of therapy[15,35,36]. The most commonly used markers applied in clinical practice are AFP, the β-subunit of hCG and lactic acid dehydrogenase (LDH); in seminomas, PLAP might be of clinical use. Approximately 40–60% of all testicular cancer patients present with elevated tumor markers at the time of diagnosis.

Serum β-hCG levels might be elevated in 80% of all embryonal carcinomas, in all patients with choriocarcinoma and in 5–20% of patients with classical seminoma. Serum AFP levels might be elevated in patients with yolk-sac tumors and with mixed germ-cell tumors; seminomas are always AFP-negative. LDH reflects primarily tumor burden, and does not represent a specific tumor marker for testicular cancer. There is a correlation with stage and LDH in that 8% of clinical stage I, 32% of clinical stage II and 81% of clinical stage III testicular germ-cell tumors demonstrate elevated serum LDH concentrations.

Following the initiation of therapy, elevated tumor markers should decline according to their half-life, which is 24–36 h for β-hCG and 5–7 days for AFP. Any plateau phase or

any delay in decline is predictive for a poor outcome in terms of response to therapy.

The prognostic significance of tumor markers at the time of diagnosis becomes evident for advanced disease only, adhering to the International Germ Cell Consensus Classification Group (IGCCCG) classification.

CLINICAL STAGING

The Lugano classification[37] represents the most widely used clinical staging system for testicular cancer (Table 6), and describes approximately the extent of metastatic involvement of the lymph nodes and visceral organs. However, in recent years it has been demonstrated that the prognostic relevance of the Lugano classification for clinical stage III patients is too poor to be used for stratification of therapy. Therefore, the IGCCCG has introduced a new staging system[36] defining three prognostic risk groups with regard to therapeutic outcome (Table 7). According to characteristics of the primary testicular tumor, the metastatic involvment of lymph nodes and organs, and the serum tumor marker level, patients are classified to be at good risk (probability of cure

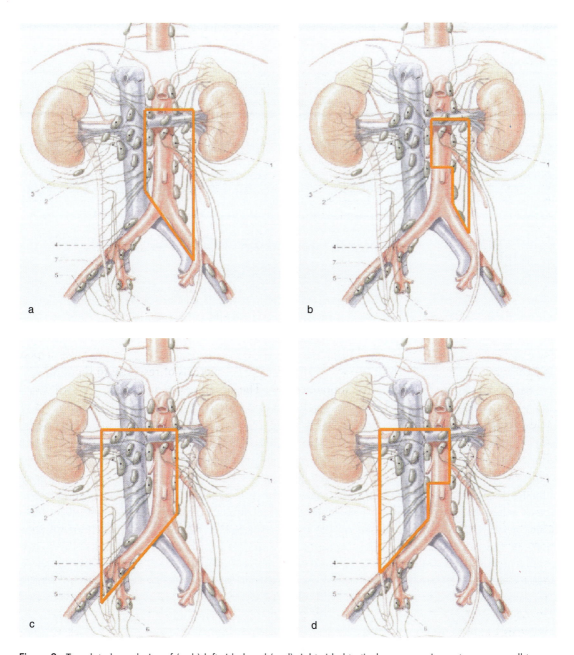

Figure 3 Template boundaries of (a, b) left-sided and (c, d) right-sided testicular non-seminomatous germ-cell tumors as outlined by Donohue and colleagues[38] (a,c) and Weißbach and Boedefeld[39] (b,d)

95%), intermediate risk (probability of cure 70%) or poor risk (probability of cure 50%). The IGCCCG classification gives high prognostic evidence and enables an individualized risk-adapted approach in patients with advanced testicular germ-cell tumor.

MANAGEMENT OF TESTICULAR GERM-CELL TUMORS

Testicular intraepithelial neoplasia

Once TIN is diagnosed, therapeutic intervention is recommended, since 70% of patients will

Table 7 Staging system for advanced testicular germ-cell tumors according to the International Germ Cell Consensus Classification Group (IGCCCG)[36]

Good prognosis	
Non-seminoma	primary testicular cancer or extragonadal retroperitoneal cancer, AFP < 1000 ng/ml, hCG < 5000 IU/ml, LDH < 1.5 × normal
	no extrapulmonary visceral metastases
Seminoma	all primary locations
	all elevated serum markers
	no extrapulmonary visceral metastases
Intermediate prognosis	
Non-seminoma	primary testicular cancer or extragonadal retroperitoneal cancer, AFP 1000 – 10 000 ng/ml, hCG < 5000–50 000 IU/ml, LDH 1.5–10 × normal
	no extrapulmonary visceral metastases
Seminoma	all primary locations
	all elevated serum markers
	extrapulmonary visceral metastases (liver, bones, CNS)
Poor prognosis	
Non-seminoma	extragonadal mediastinal germ-cell tumor
	primary testicular/retroperitoneal germ-cell tumor with extrapulmonary metastases
	AFP > 10 000 ng/ml, hCG > 100 000 IU/ml, LDH > 10 × normal

AFP, α-fetoprotein; hCG, human chorionic gonadotropin; LDH, lactate dehydrogenase; CNS, central nervous system

develop invasive germ-cell tumor within the next 7 years[20].

Local radiation therapy with 18 Gy is the therapy of choice in patients with a contralateral invasive germ-cell tumor, resulting in a 100% cure rate as demonstrated by the eradication of all TIN cells and a Sertoli-cell-only syndrome in follow-up biopsies[18,20]. Only in patients wishing to father a child and having active spermatogenesis does a surveillance strategy with close follow-up seem to be justified. In patients undergoing inductive chemotherapy after orchiectomy, a control biopsy should be performed 6 months after discontinuation of therapy, since about 40% of TIN will be cured by the systemic approach.

In patients with unilateral TIN and a contralateral normal testis, inguinal orchiectomy appears to be the preferred management, since local radiation bears the risk of damaging the healthy testicle.

Non-seminomatous germ-cell tumors

Clinical stage I NSGCT represents a troublesome entity concerning recommendations for optimal management. Approximately 30% of stage I NSGCTs will exhibit microscopic lymph-node disease by means of retroperitoneal lymph-node dissection (RPLND)[26,38,39]; however, for the remaining 70% of patients, RPLND is only a staging procedure without therapeutic benefit. Since quality-of-life issues have assumed great importance for both the patient and the physician, several treatment modalities have been developed for clinical stage I NSGCTs. Primary surveillance protocols were used by Peckham and colleagues[40], with survival rates equal to those with RPLND; however, relapse rates within the first 2 years were almost 30%, necessitating aggressive chemotherapy for advanced disease. Primary chemotherapy represents another treatment modality for clinical stage I NSGCT, with results equal to those for RPLND and adjuvant chemotherapy[26,41–43]. But again, about 70% of patients are unnecessarily treated, underlining the need for non-invasive prognostic risk factors, enabling a more individualized therapy to reduce morbidity without reducing the efficacy of management. Altogether, all three therapeutic options – RPLND, surveillance and primary

Table 8 Chemotherapy and surgery in options for clinical stage I non-seminomatous germ-cell tumor (NSGCT)

Therapy	Surgical intervention (%)	Chemotherapy (%)	Long-term survival (%)
nsRPLND	100	15	> 98
Surveillance	< 10	30–40	> 98
Primary chemotherapy	0	100	> 98

nsRPLND, nerve-sparing retroperitoneal lymph-node dissection

chemotherapy – will result in the same high cure rates of 98%; however, the associated complications and side-effects differ significantly (Table 8). Since the majority of patients are young, classical therapeutic endpoints such as response and survival rates are thrust into the background, and quality of life, protection of fertility and long-term toxicity of the chosen therapy come to the fore[44].

To enable a more individualized therapeutic approach, prognostic risk factors for occult retroperitoneal lymph-node disease can be integrated in the pretherapeutic discussion: vascular invasion has been identified as the most powerful clinical predictor of lymph-node metastasis with 48% of NSGCTs with vascular invasion developing metastases, compared to 14–22% of tumors without vascular invasion[26]. A combination of vascular invasion and percentage of embryonal carcinoma might be even more powerful, but they have not been tested together in prospective clinical trials[14]. Currently, all molecular markers such as p53, Ki-67, bcl-2, cathepsin D and E-cadherin have not been proven to be clinically useful prognosticators[15]; only reverse transcriptase-polymerase chain reaction for AFP, hCG and germ cell alkaline phosphate (GCAP) mRNA for the detection of circulating tumor cells appears to be an interesting approach, with 60% of clinical stage I testicular cancer patients exhibiting positive signals that turn into negative signals following adjuvant chemotherapy[45]. Only patients with clinical stage I pure mature teratoma should undergo primary nerve-sparing RPLND, since up to 20% of all teratomas will harbor occult

retroperitoneal lymph-node metastases at the time of diagnosis[46,47].

Nerve-sparing retroperitoneal lymph node dissection

Nowadays, nerve-sparing RPLND as reported by Jewett[48] and Donohue and colleagues[49] is regarded as the standard approach in clinical stage I NSGCT, using the surgical resection templates described by Donohue and associates[38] and by Weißbach and Boedefeld[39] and depicted in Figure 3. For a right-sided tumor, the paracaval, retrocaval, interaortocaval and preaortic lymphatic tissue superior to the superior mesenteric artery should be dissected. For a left-sided tumor, the para-aortic, interaortocaval and preaortic lymphatic tissue superior to the superior mesenteric artery should be dissected. Up to 10% of patients will suffer from pulmonary relapse within the first 2 years, and will be cured by platinum-based chemotherapy. Even in low-volume lymph-node disease such as pathological stage IIA, the nerve-sparing RPLND can be performed as bilateral radical surgery without compromising the therapeutic outcome. Recurrence and complication rates are low, so that RPLND still has its place in the management of low-volume NSGCT.

Primary chemotherapy or surveillance

In clinical stage I NSGCT, primary chemotherapy consisting of two cycles of cisplatin, etoposide and bleomycin (PEB) results in the same high cure rate of 98% as with primary nerve-sparing RPLND[26,41–43]. In recent years, a

Table 9 Advantages and disadvantages of therapeutic options in management of clinical stage IIA non-seminomatous germ-cell tumor (NSGCT)

nsRPLND + adj. chemotherapy	nsRPLND + surveillance	Primary chemotherapy
Advantages	Advantages	Advantages
Accurate staging	Fewer associated side-effects owing	RPLND necessary in only 10–15%
Risk for relapse 0–7%	to single therapy	Low relapse rate of 4–9%
Primary extraperitoneal recurrences	Accurate staging revealing pathological	
Fewer CT scans for follow-up	stage I in up to 20%	
	Chemotherapy in only 20% of patients	
Disadvantages	Disadvantages	Disadvantages
Potential induction of secondary	Minimum of three cycles in case	Unnecessary chemotherapy in up
malignancies	of relapse	to 20% owing to pathological
Surgical morbidity of 10%	Surgical morbidity of 10%	stage I
Retrograde ejaculation in 5–15%	Retrograde ejaculation in 5–15%	Surgical morbidity due to
operated in centers	operated in centers	secondary RPLND as high as 39%
Higher incidence of associated	Risk for relapse is 20%, compared to	Retrograde ejaculation as high
morbidities	0–7% in first option	as 15–20%
		Higher frequency of follow-up
		CT scans
		Three cycles of chemotherapy,
		compared to two cycles in first option

nsRPLA, nerve-sparing retroperitoneal lymphadenectomy; adj., adjuvant; CT, computed tomography; nsRPLND, nerve-sparing retroperitoneal lymph-node dissection

risk-adapted management of these patients has been proposed, based on the presence of vascular invasion and the percentage of embryonal carcinoma in the primary orchiectomy specimen, which have been identified as significant prognosticators for occult retroperitoneal disease in a number of studies[14,15]. Prospective randomization to two cycles of PEB (presence of vascular invasion) or to surveillance (absence of vascular invasion) results in relapse rates of only 7% and 14%, respectively, compared to the initial observation series describing recurrence rates of 42%[42,43]; all relapsing patients can be salvaged by inductive platinum-based chemotherapy.

Low-stage (IIA/B) NSGCT

Low-stage testicular disease comprises clinical stages IIA and IIB, with the therapeutic options of primary RPLND or primary chemotherapy with 3–4 cycles of PEB[26,50,51]. Both therapeutic options will result in a net cure of about two-thirds of patients with a single therapy; one-third of patients must undergo adjuvant

chemotherapy following nerve-sparing RPLND, or secondary RPLND for residual lymph-node disease following primary chemotherapy. Primary RPLND is a viable approach in clinical stage IIA, since an overstaging is faced in about 20% of patients who would have been subjected to unnecessary chemotherapy otherwise; additional advantages of nerve-sparing RPLND are preservation of sympathetic nerves in 80% of patients and accurate staging in all patients. Furthermore, adjuvant chemotherapy will decrease the risk for relapse to < 3%, facilitating follow-up. Risk of relapse is only about 15% if fewer than three lymph nodes are involved; the maximum lymph node diameter is < 2 cm and there is no extranodal extension, so not all patients must undergo adjuvant chemotherapy and a subgroup of patients might be followed by surveillance. As in clinical stage I disease, both therapeutic options should be intensively discussed with the patient, and parameters such as the wish to father a child, compliance of both patient and physician, and the need for safety must be integrated into the decision (Table 9). The only exceptions are patients with

Table 10 Advantages and disadvantages of therapeutic options in management of clinical stage IIB non-seminomatous germ-cell tumor (NSGCT)

nsRPLA + adj. chemotherapy	nsRPLND + surveillance	Primary chemotherapy
Advantages	Advantages	Advantages
Accurate staging	Fewer associated side-effects owing to single therapy	RPLA necessary in only 30–40%
Risk for relapse 0–7%		Low relapse rate of 11–15%
Primary extraperitoneal recurrences	Accurate staging revealing pathological stage I in up to 20%	
Fewer CT scans for follow-up	Chemotherapy in only 50% of patients	
Disadvantages	Disadvantages	Disadvantages
Potential induction of secondary malignancies	Minimum of three cycles in case of relapse	Unnecessary chemotherapy in up to 20% owing to pathological stage I
Surgical morbidity of 10%	Surgical morbidity of 10%	Surgical morbidity due to secondary RPLA as high as 39%
Retrograde ejaculation in up to 32%	Retrograde ejaculation in 32%	Retrograde ejaculation as high as 15–20%
Higher incidence of associated morbidities due to surgery and chemotherapy	Risk for relapse is 50%, compared to 0–7% in first option	Higher frequency of follow-up CT scans
		Three cycles of chemotherapy, compared to two cycles in first option

nsRPLA, nerve-sparing retroperitoneal lymphadenectomy; adj., adjuvant; CT, computed tomography; nsRPLND, nerve-sparing retroperitoneal lymph-node dissection

elevated markers following radical orchiectomy but no visible metastases on CT scans, who should undergo primary chemotherapy with three cycles of PEB.

Patients with clinical stage IIB testicular cancer, however, will undergo primary chemotherapy with three cycles of PEB followed by secondary RPLND in about 30% of cases[26], although basically the same three therapeutic options are available as for clinical stage IIA (Table 10).

Clinical stages IIC and III

Inductive chemotherapy represents the therapy of choice, with the number of cycles applied depending on the IGCCCG-based prognostic classification[36].

Patients with 'good prognosis' face a long-term survival rate of > 90%, and are best managed by three cycles of PEB, whereas patients with poor prognosis are best treated with four cycles[26,36,52,53]. If there are contraindications for the application of bleomycin, four cycles of platinol and etoposide should be administered.

It appears to be crucial to give all agents without dose reduction at 22-day intervals. Only in the case of neutropenic fever or severe thrombocytopenia is dose reduction or prolongation of the next cycle justified.

Patients with 'intermediate prognosis' face a survival rate of 70–80% and are managed by four cyles of PEB or cisplatin, etoposide and ifosfamide (PEI); however, there are no prospective randomized trials defining a standard therapy[26,54].

Patients with 'poor prognosis' have a survival rate of only about 50%; standard therapy consists of four cycles of PEB or PEI[26,55–58]. A major advantage of primary high-dose chemotherapy has not been demonstrated, but this approach is currently being tested in prospective randomized trials.

Seminomatous germ-cell tumors

Clinical stage I seminoma

Adjuvant retroperitoneal radiation therapy to the para-aortic region with 26 Gy is the standard approach in clinical stage I seminoma,

Table 11 Carboplatinum monotherapy in clinical stage I seminoma: outcome and follow-up

Author	n	Relapse (%)	Survival (%)	Follow-up (months)
Oliver, 1990	25	4	100	16
Kratzik, 1993	39	2.5	100	20
Dieckmann, 1994	16	0	100	16
Oliver, 1994	25	0	100	> 60
Krege, 1997	35	0	100	28
Nöst, 1997	29	0	100	52
Heidenreich, 1999	25	0	100	36
Total	165	2	100	35

resulting in a relapse-free long-term survival of 97%[26,59,60]; these numbers hold true even 21 years after initiation of surveillance strategies in the management of clinical stage I seminoma. Alternative therapeutic options are two cycles of carboplatinum monochemotherapy or surveillance: results of monochemotherapy have been described in 165 patients with relapse rates of 2–4% and a median follow-up of 16–60 months (Table 11). Although the outcome reflects the results obtained with radiation therapy, longer follow-up and results of prospective randomized clinical trials must be awaited before carboplatinum can be recommended as equivalent therapy. Surveillance will result in a 20% relapse rate, and is even more dependent on the patient's compliance (Table 12), as seminomas do not usually produce significant amounts of tumor markers[61]. To provide a more individualized approach to the patient, prognostic risk factors for occult retroperitoneal disease such as tumor size > 4 cm, infiltration of the rete testis, vascular invasion and patient's age (< 34 years) can be integrated into the discussion[26,61].

Low-stage (clinical stage IIA/B) seminoma

Radiation therapy with 30 Gy (IIA) and 36 Gy (IIB), including the ipsilateral iliac and inguinal lymph nodes, is the standard therapeutic approach for low-stage seminomas[26,62]. The radiation field might be enlarged to the iliac and inguinal lymph nodes in the case of prior scrotal surgery. Relapse-free survival is as high as 92.5% in clinical stage IIA/B; relapse rates are about 5% in stage IIA and about 11% in stage IIB seminomas. Primary chemotherapy with two cycles of PEB can be an alternative to radiation in clinical stage IIB seminoma; the clinical utility of three (IIA) and four (IIB) cycles of carboplatinum monotherapy is currently being investigated in a prospective clinical trial, and it cannot be recommended as a viable therapeutic option.

Clinical stage IIC and III

As pointed out for advanced non-seminomatous germ-cell tumors, therapy should be initiated according to the IGCCCG classification[36].

Residual tumor resection following chemotherapy for advanced testicular cancer

Postchemotherapy RPLND in seminomas and non-seminomas following inductive chemotherapy can be omitted only if no residual masses or residual lesions < 1 cm are depicted by CT scans; all other residual tumors should be completely resected, since available standard imaging modalities cannot differentiate between vital tumor masses, mature teratoma and necrosis/fibrosis[26]. PET can depict vital tumor cells; however, it also does not differentiate between mature teratoma and fibrosis/necrosis, with both entities giving negative signals. Steyerberg and colleagues[63] have proposed a risk-adapted model for the prediction of final

Table 12 Advantages and disadvantages of radiation therapy and surveillance in clinical stage I seminomas

Radiation Therapy	Surveillance
Advantages Mild to moderate acute side-effects Relapse rate as low as 3–4% All relapses are outside the radiation field	Advantages No therapy for 80% following orchiectomy
Disadvantages Overtreatment in about 80% of patients Potential risk of radiation-induced secondary malignancies	Disadvantages 20% relapse rate with aggressive salvage therapy Psychological distress owing to close follow-up High intensity of follow-up CT scans

CT, computed tomography

pathology in patients with residual masses, and claim a sensitivity and specificity of close to 90%; this model, however, has to be proven in other institutions before it can be recommended for general use. If secondary RPLND is being performed, it appears to be sufficient to resect the mass only, without repecting the boundaries of modified surgical templates during primary RPLND[26,64]. About 15% of patients will demonstrate vital tumor cells, approximately 30–40% will exhibit mature teratoma and 40% will demonstrate fibrosis/necrosis only. Patients with vital tumor cells should undergo an additional two cycles of conventional polychemotherapy.

Salvage chemotherapy, high-dose chemotherapy

About 50% of relapsing seminomas following conventional chemotherapy can be salvaged with another combination chemotherapy consisting of PEI–etopside, ifosfamide and platinol (VIP) or –vinblastine, ifosfamide and platinol (VeIP). Currently, a 10% benefit of high-dose chemotherapy with regard to survival has been demonstrated; therefore, it seems advisable that all relapsing patients should be treated in a tertiary referral center.

With regard to non-seminomas relapsing following conventional chemotherapy, salvage rates are as low as 15–40% using standard salvage protocols such as PEI–VIP or –VeIP[56,57]. Early consideration of high-dose chemotherapy seems

advisable, according to a number of recently published studies[55,58]. The trials reported from the Memorial Sloan Kettering Cancer Center suggest a benefit for the use of high-dose chemotherapy and autologous bone marrow transfer, with 46% and 50% of the patients being alive and disease-free after a median follow-up of 31 months and 30 months, respectively[58]. In another study including 35 patients, the progression-free survival rate for all patients was 44 months, and the 2-year survival rate was 65%[70]. However, one also has to consider that the results of high-dose chemotherapy combined with autologous bone marrow transfer are not superior to a combination therapy including paclitaxel, ifosfamide and cisplatin as second-line therapy for relapsing germ-cell tumors. In the treatment of 30 patients, a complete response was achieved in 77% and all patients were without evidence of recurrent disease after a median follow-up of 30 months[71]. Therefore, high-dose chemotherapy is an option but not the standard for the management of relapsing testicular germ-cell tumors.

FUTURE DIRECTIONS IN TESTICULAR CANCER

Based on the excellent therapeutic outcome, there appear to be only a few developments possible that will have further impact on the survival or the quality of life of testicular cancer patients. It will be of utmost importance to identify reliable and objective prognostic risk factors in clinical stage I NSGCT, to individualize therapy (surveillance versus active treatment), with reverse transcriptase–polymerase chain reaction (RT-PCR) for GCAP being the most promising approach. Furthermore, the toxicity of adjuvant chemotherapy might be further decreased by applying only one cycle of PEB, as is currently being tested in a prospective randomized trial by the German Testicular Cancer Intergroup. In pathological stage IIA it might be possible to perform nerve-sparing RPLND without the need for adjuvant chemotherapy, by identifiying high-risk and low-risk patients based on the findings of RT-PCR; this is currently under investigation by the German

Testicular Cancer Intergroup. Elucidation of those mechanisms involved in the development of chemo-refractoriness in testicular cancer will be a major issue in the future, to apply effective chemotherapeutic protocols and to save even more lives.

Despite the high cure rates, it will be necessary for testicular cancer to be treated by clinicians and institutions with sufficient experience in diagnosis and management of germ-cell tumors. Specific problems such as extended tumor masses, relapsing tumors or poor prognosis at initial diagnosis must be referred to tertiary centers having the ability of an interdisciplinary approach.

References

1. Boring CC, Squires TS, Tong T, *et al*. Cancer statistics 1994. *Cancer* 1994;44:7–26
2. Coleman MP, Esteve J, Damiecki P, *et al*. *Trends in Cancer Incidence and Mortality*, IARC Science Publication no 121. Lyon, France: International Agency for Research on Cancer, 1993
3. Pottern LM, Brown LM, Hoover RN, *et al*. Testicular cancer risk among young men: the role of cryptorchidism and inguinal hernia. *J Natl Cancer Inst* 1985;74:377–81
4. Forman D, Oliver RTD, Brett AR, *et al*. Familial testicular cancer: a report of the UK family register; estimation of risk and HLA-class I sib-pair analysis. *Br J Cancer* 1992; 65:255–62
5. Heidenreich A, for the German Testicular Cancer Intergroup. Biological and clinical characteristics of familial, bilateral and sporadic germ cell tumors. *J Urol* 2000;163(Suppl 1):145
6. Tollerud DJ, Blattner WA, Fraser MC, *et al*. Familial testicular cancer and urogenital developmental abnormalities. *Cancer* 1985;55:1849–54
7. Rapley E, Crockford GP, Teare D, *et al*. Localization to Xq27 of a susceptibility gene for testicular germ-cell tumors. *Nature Genet* 2000;24:197–200

8. Leahy MG, Tonks S, Moses JH, *et al*. Candidate regions for testicular cancer susceptibility genes. *Hum Mol Genet* 1995;4:1551–5
9. Brown LM, Pottern LM, Hoover RN. Prenatal and perinatal risk factors for testicular cancer. *Cancer Res* 1986;46:4812–16
10. Depue RH, Pike MC, Henderson BE. Estrogen exposure during gestation and risk of testicular cancer. *J Natl Cancer Inst* 1983; 71:1151–5
11. Von Hochstetter AR, Hedinger CE. The differential diagnosis of testicular germ cell tumors in theory and practice. A critical analysis of two major systems of classifications and review of 389 cases. *Virchow's Arch Pathol Anat* 1982;396:247–77
12. Jacobsen GK, Henriksen OB, von der Maase H. Carcinoma *in situ* of testicular tissue adjacent to malignant germ cell tumors: a study of 105 cases. *Cancer* 1981;47:2660–2
13. Mostofi FK, Sesterhenn IA, Davis CJ. Immunopathology of germ cell tumours of the testis. *Semin Diagn Pathol* 1987;4:320–41
14. Heidenreich A, Sesterhenn IA, Mostofi FK, Moul JW. Prognostic risk factors that identify patients with clinical stage I nonseminomatous germ cell tumors at low risk and high risk for metastasis. *Cancer* 1998;83:1002–11

15. Moul JW, Heidenreich A. Prognostic risk factors in low stage nonseminomatous testicular cancer. *Oncology* 1996;10:1359–68

16. Heidenreich A, Sesterhenn IA, Mostofi FK, Moul JW. Immunohistochemical expression of monoclonal antibody 43-9F in testicular germ cell tumors. *Int J Androl* 1998;21:283–8

17. Visfeldt J, Giwercman A, Skakkebaek NE. Monoclonal antibody 43-9F: an immunohistochemical marker of embryonal carcinoma of the testis. *Acta Pathol Microbiol Immunol Scand* 1992;100:63–70

18. Dieckmann KP, Skakkebaek NE. Carcinoma *in situ* of the testis: a review of biological and clinical features. *Int J Cancer* 1999;83:815–22

19. Skakkebaek NE. Abnormal morphology of germ cells in two infertile men. *Acta Pathol Microbiol Immunol Scand* 1972;80:374–8

20. Skakkebaek NE, Bertlesen JG, Giwercman A, *et al.* Carcinoma *in situ* of the testis: possible origin from gonocytes and precursor of all types of germ cell tumours except spermatocytic seminoma. *Int J Androl* 1987;10:19–28

21. Damjano V. Pathogenesis of testicular germ cell tumours. *Eur Urol* 1993;23:2–7

22. Heidenreich A, Srivastava S, Moul JW, Hofmann R. Molecular genetic parameters in pathogenesis and prognosis of testicular germ cell tumors. *Eur Urol* 2000;37:121–35

23. Moul JW. Early and accurate diagnosis of testicular cancer. *Probl Urol* 1994;8:58–66

24. Oliver RTD. Factors contributing to delay in diagnosis of testicular tumours. *Br Med J* 1985;290:356–60

25. Heidenreich A, Engelmann UH, von Vietsch H, *et al.* Organ preserving surgery in testicular epidermoid cysts. *J Urol* 1990;153:1147–50

26. Souchon R, Krege S, Schmoll HJ, *et al.* Interdisciplinary consensus on diagnosis and therapy of testicular germ cell tumors: results of an update conference based on evidence-based medicine. *Strahlenther Onkol* 2000; 176:388–405

27. Tokuc R, Sakr W, Pontes JE, Haas GP. Accuracy of frozen section examination of testicular tumors. *Urology* 1992;40:512–16

28. Schyff van der S, Heidenreich A, Weißbach L, Höltl L, for the German Testicular Cancer Intergroup. Organ preserving surgery in testicular cancer: longterm results. *J Urol* 1990; 163(Suppl 1):145

29. Krug B, Heidenreich A, Dietlein M, Lackner K. Lymph node staging in malignant testicular germ cell tumors. *Fortschr Röntgenstr* 1999;171:87–94

30. Leibovitch I, Foster RS, Kopecky KK, Donohue JP. Improved accuracy of computerized tomography based clinical staging in low stage nonseminomatous germ cell cancer using size criteria of retroperitoneal lymph nodes. *J Urol* 1997;154:1759–63

31. Albers P, Bender H, Ylmaz H, *et al.* Positron emission tomography in the clinical staging of patients with stage I and II germ cell tumors. *Urology* 1999;3:808–11

32. Cremerius U, Wildberger JE, Borchers H, *et al.* Does positron emission tomography using 18-fluoro-2-deoxyglucose improve clinical staging of testicular cancer? Results of a study of 50 patients. *Urology* 1999;54:900–4

33. White PM, Howard GC, Best JJ, *et al.* Imaging of the thorax in the management of germ cell testicular tumors. *Clin Radiol* 1999; 54:207–11

34. Fernandez EB, Moul JW, Foley JP, *et al.* Retroperitoneal imaging with third and fourth generation computed axial tomography in clinical stage I nonseminomatous germ cell tumors. *Urology* 1994;44:548–52

35. Bartlett NL, Freiha NS, Torti FM. Serum markers in germ cell neoplasms. *Hematol Oncol Clin North Am* 1991;5:1245–61

36. International Germ Cell Consensus Classification Group. A prognostic factor-based staging system for metastatic germ cell cancers. *J Clin Oncol* 1997;15:594–603

37. Cavalli F, Manfardini S, Pizzocaro G. Report on the international workshop on staging and treatment of testicular cancer. *Eur J Cancer* 1980;6:1367–72

38. Donohue JP, Zachary JM, Maynard SD. Distribution of nodal metastases in nonseminomatous testicular cancer. *J Urol* 1982;128:315–20

39. Weißbach L, Boedefeld E. Localization of solitary and multiple metastases in stage II non-seminomatous testis tumor as a basis for a

modified staging lymph node dissection in stage I. *J Urol* 1982;128:77

40. Peckham MJ, Barrett A, Husband JE, Hendry WF. Orchiectomy alone in testicular stage I nonseminomatous germ cell tumors. *Lancet* 1982;2:678–80

41. Cullen MH, Stenning SP, Parkinson MC, *et al*. Short course adjuvant chemotherapy in high risk stage 1 nonseminomatous germ cell tumors of the testis: a Medical Research Council report. *J Clin Oncol* 1996;14:1106–13

42. Pont J, Höltl W, Kosak D, *et al*. Risk adapted treatment choice in stage I nonseminomatous testicular germ cell cancer by regarding vascular invasion in the primary tumor: a prospective trial. *J Clin Oncol* 1990;8:16–20

43. Studer UE, Burkhard FC, Sonntag RW. Risk adapted management with adjuvant chemotherapy in patients with high risk clinical stage I nonseminomatus germ cell tumors. *J Urol* 2000;163:1785–7

44. Heidenreich A, Hofmann R. Quality of life issues in the treatment of testicular cancer. *World J Urol* 1999;17:230–8

45. Heidenreich A, Walter B, Hofmann R. RT-PCR for AFP, hCG, GCAP and PDGF-1a to detect circulating tumor cells in testicular germ cell tumors. *Eur Urol* 2000;37 (Suppl 2): 87

46. Heidenreich A, Moul JW, McLeod DG, *et al*. The role of retroperitoneal lymphadenectomy in mature teratoma of the testis. *J Urol* 1997; 157:160–3

47. Leibovitch I, Foster RS, Ulbright TM, Donohue JP. Adult primary pure teratoma of the testis. *Cancer* 1995;75:2244–8

48. Jewett MA. Retroperitoneal lymphadenectomy for testicular tumor with nerve-sparing for ejaculation. *J Urol* 1988;139:1220–4

49. Donohue JP, Foster RS, Rowland RG, *et al*. Nerve sparing retroperitoneal lymphadenectomy with preservation of ejaculation. *J Urol* 1990;144:287–92

50. Pizzocaro G, Monfardini S. No adjuvant chemotherapy in selected patients with pathological stage II nonseminomatous germ cell tumors of the testis. *J Urol* 1994;131: 677–80

51. Weißbach L, Bussar-Maatz R, Flechtner H, *et al*. RPLND or primary chemotherapy in clinical stage IIA/B nonseminomatous germ cell tumors? Results of a prospective multi-center trial including quality of life assessment. *Eur Urol* 2000;37:582–94

52. Horwich A, Sleijfer DT, Fossa SD, *et al*. Randomized trial of bleomycin, etoposide and cisplatin compared with bleomycin, etoposide and carboplatin in good-prognosis metastatic nonseminomatous germ cell cancer: a multiinstitutional Medical Research Council/EORTC trial. *J Clin Oncol* 1997;15:1844–52

53. DeWit R, Stoter G, Kaye SB, *et al*. Importance of bleomycin in combination chemotherapy for good-prognosis testicular nonseminoma: a randomized study of the EORTC Genitourinary Tract Cancer Cooperative Group. *J Clin Oncol* 1997;15:1837–43

54. De Wit R, Stoter G, Sleijfer DT, *et al*. Four cycles of BEP versus four cycles of VIP in patients with intermediate-prognosis metastatic testicular nonseminoma: a randomized study of the EORTC Genitourinary Tract Cancer Cooperative Group. *Br J Cancer* 1998;78:828–32

55. Bokemeyer C, Kollmannsberger C, Meisner C, *et al*. First-line high dose chemotherapy compared with standard-dose PEB/VIP chemotherapy in patients with advanced germ cell tumors: a multivariate and matched-pair analysis. *J Clin Oncol* 1999;17:3450–6

56. Loehrer PJ, Gonin R, Nichols CR, *et al*. Vinblastine plus ifosfamide plus cisplatin as initial salvage therapy in recurrent germ cell tumor. *J Clin Oncol* 1998;16:2500–4

57. Miller KD, Loehrer PJ, Gonin R, *et al*. Salvage chemotherapy with vinblastine, ifosfamide, and cisplatin in recurrent seminoma. *J Clin Oncol* 1997;15:1427–31

58. Motzer RJ, Mazumdar M, Bajorin DF, *et al*. High-dose carboplatin, etoposide and cyclophosphamide with autologous bone marrow transplantation in first-line therapy for patients with poor-risk germ cell tumors. *J Clin Oncol* 1997;15:2546–52

59. Bamberg M, Shmidberger H, Meisner C, *et al*. Radiotherapy for stage I, IIA/B testicular seminoma. *Int J Cancer* 1999;83:823–7

60. Fossa SD, Horwich A, Russel JM, *et al*. Optimal planning target volume for stage I testicular seminoma: a Medical Research

Council randomized trial. *J Clin Oncol* 1999; 17:1146–54

61. Warde P, Gospodarowicz MK, Goodman PJ, *et al*. Stage I testicular seminoma: results of adjuvant irradiation and surveillance. *J Clin Oncol* 1995;13:2255–62

62. Schmidberger H, Bamberg M, Meisner C, *et al*. Radiotherapy in stage IIA and IIB testicular seminoma with reduced portals: a prospective multicenter study. *Int J Radiat Oncol Biol Phys* 1997;39:321–6

63. Steyerberg EW, Keizer HJ, Fossa SD, *et al*. Predicition of residual retroperitoneal mass histology after chemotherapy for metastatic nonseminomatous germ cell tumor: multivariate analysis of individual patient data from six study groups. *J Clin Oncol* 1995;13:1177–87

64. Herr HW. Does necrosis on frozen section analysis of a mass after chemotherapy justify a limited retroperitoneal resection in patients with advanced testis cancer? *Br J Urol* 1997;80:653–7

65. Heidenreich A, Schenkman NS, Sesterhenn IA, *et al*. Immunohistochemical expression of Ki-67 to predict lymph node involvement in clinical stage I nonseminomatous germ cell tumors. *J Urol* 1997;158:620–5

66. International Testis Cancer Linkage Consortium. Candidate regions for testicular cancer susceptibility genes. *Acta Pathol Microbiol Immunol Scnad* 1998;106:64–72

67. Sandberg AA, Meloni AM, Suijkerbuijk RF. Reviews of chromosome studies in urological tumors. III. Cytogenetics and genes in testicular tumors. *J Urol* 1900;155:1531–56

68. Weißbach L. Organ preserving surgery of malignant germ cell tumors. *J Urol* 1995;153: 90–3

69. Williams SD, Stablein DM, Einhorn LH, *et al*. Immediate chemotherapy versus observation with treatment at relapse in pathological stage testicular cancer. *N Engl J Med* 1987;317: 1433–8

70. Dodd PM, Motzer RJ, Bajorin DF. Poor risk germ cell tumors, recent developments. *Urol Clin North AM* 1998;25:485–93

71. Motzer RJ, Mazumdar M, Gulati SC, *et al*. Phase II trial of high-dose carboplatin and etoposide with autologous bone marrow transplantation in first-line therapy for patients with poor-risk germ cell tumors. *J Natl Cancer Inst* 1993;85:1828–35

Section III

Endocrine system

Ronald S. Swerdloff, MD

As men age, there are changes in the functions of many biologic systems of which the endocrine system is no exception. This section reviews the effects of aging on the endocrine system of men. The first chapter sets the tone with an overall introduction to the changes that can be expected with aging, for example, binding protein abnormalities, decreases in the secretion rate of testosterone, adrenal androgen precursors and thyroid hormones, and decreases in hormone action. Subsequent chapters expand on this information, focusing specifically on the issues of androgen deficiency, adrenal androgen deficiency, growth hormone deficiency and impairment of thyroid function.

10 Endocrine system changes in the aging male

Ronald S. Swerdloff, MD, and Christina Wang, MD

ENDOCRINE HYPER- AND HYPOFUNCTION IN AGING

Serum levels of hormones may be higher or lower in older men compared with younger adult men (Table 1). There are decreases in the secretion rate of testosterone, adrenal androgen precursors (e.g. dehydroepiandrosterone and its sulfate, DHEA and DHEAS); thyroid hormones (e.g. triiodothyronine); growth hormone and insulin-like growth factor (IGF); renin and aldosterone; and vitamin D (25-OH and 1,25-(OH)$_2$). There are also alterations in binding proteins (e.g. increased sex hormone-binding globulin (SHBG) and decreased IGF-I) and decreases in hormone action (e.g. insulin resistance).

Hormone binding proteins and age

Binding protein abnormalities caused by aging may in turn differentially influence the bioactive forms of hormones. An example is the increase in SHBG as men age which results in decreased ratios of unbound (bioactive) to bound forms of testosterone and estradiol. Since there are concomitant decreases in testosterone secretion, the net effect of these two abnormalities is an even greater decrease in the biologically active hormone (e.g. testosterone) and greater degrees of androgen deficiency. The binding protein change mandates use of different laboratory tests (i.e. free or bioavailable testosterone instead of total testosterone) in the elderly compared with young males.

Table 1 Circulating levels of hormones in older men relative to younger adults. Data from Cobbs EL, *et al. Geriatric Review Syllabus: A Core Curriculum in Geriatric Medicine*, 4th edn. New York: American Geriatrics Society, 1999

Elevated	Same	Reduced
FSH	ACTH	Growth hormone
LH	Cortisol	IGF-I
Vasopressin	Epinephrine	Testosterone
Atrial natriuretic hormone		Renin
Insulin	TSH*	Aldosterone
PTH	Thyroxine	Triiodothyronine (T$_3$)
Leptin	Glucagon	DHEA and DHEAS
		1,25-(OH)$_2$ Vitamin D
		25-OH Vitamin D

*Increased when primary thyroid disorders co-exist with aging. FSH, follicle-stimulating hormone; ACTH, adrenocorticotropic hormone; LH, luteinizing hormone; IGF-I, insulin-like growth factor type I; TSH, thyroid-stimulating hormone; PTH, parathyroid hormone

Reciprocal changes in hormones associated with endocrine deficiency in older men

In many instances, there are reciprocal increases in hormones that are dysregulated due to the primary endocrine deficiency. These include insulin (increased secretion secondary to target organ resistance), luteinizing and follicle-stimulating hormones (LH and FSH; increased secretion due to decreased negative feedback as a result of decreased Leydig and Sertoli cell function), and parathyroid hormone (PTH; decreased secretion due to increased serum calcium levels). Increases in atrial natriuretic hormone (ANH) in the aged leads to sodium loss and suppression of the renin–angiotensin–aldosterone system[1–5].

Physiologic versus pathologic changes in hormone levels with aging: an enigma

Many of the changes that we see with aging may be considered physiologic changes. Others may be of sufficient severity, and associated with biologic abnormalities, that they can be labeled as hormone deficiencies. Since the endocrine system is one of the key regulators of integrated biologic function, it is not surprising that altered endocrine secretion and actions are important in the development of age-related disorders, such as diabetes mellitus, osteoporosis, frailty, altered libido and erectile function. The endocrine system is also an important regulator of body weight (e.g. obesity) and body composition (e.g. abdominal obesity and male metabolic syndrome), cardiovascular disease, and hypertension. Individual chapters in this section focus on the issues of androgen deficiency, adrenal androgen deficiency, growth hormone deficiency and impairment of thyroid function. Details of the age-associated alterations in erectile function and libido, diabetes mellitus, body weight and composition,

osteoporosis, and frailty are discussed in following sections.

Multifactorial origin of endocrine-associated disease processes in aging

It should be noted that many of the abnormalities that are seen with aging are multifactorial in origin and may be significantly impacted by the frequent multiple drug use in this age group. Polypharmaceutical product use associated with increased age may result in multiple drug interactions, including alterations in binding proteins, resulting in increased or decreased drug metabolism and reduced clearance of hormones. Both age alone and concomitant medicinal use can decrease drug absorption in the gastrointestinal system. Other hormone deficiencies may not represent the extremes of the physiologic deterioration of endocrine function, but rather represent an increase in susceptibility to specific disease states. Examples of the latter include the increased risk of autoimmune thyroid disease (e.g. Hashimoto's thyroiditis) with increase in age. It is presumed that the increased risk is associated with a dysfunctional immune system.

Sleep disorders

Sleep disorders are common in the elderly[6–8]. Melatonin secretion diminishes progressively with age. Aged men with insomnia have lower melatonin levels than non-insomniacs.

Prostate disease and hormones

There are other conditions where enlargement of a hormone-responsive end organ or tissue occurs with age. A classic example of this is the enlargement of the prostate, which is clearly age-dependent. The prostate is an androgen-dependent organ, which is also a major site of conversion of testosterone to dihydrotestosterone (an even more active metabolite). Benign prostatic hyperplasia (BPH) may be present in

10% of men at age 40, but levels can reach 80% by the age of 80 years. Testosterone clearly increases prostate growth and inhibition of testosterone secretion (e.g. GnRH analogs) or action (e.g. antiandrogens or interference with conversion to dihydrotestosterone) will result in decreased prostate size[9–12]. However, despite the above physiologic and pharmacologic observations on testosterone stimulation of the prostate, it is not believed that the process of BPH is caused by testosterone. This apparent enigma can best be understood by hypothesizing that the mechanisms that result in the pathologic disorder of BPH override the prostate growth inhibiting effects of the androgen decline with aging. Nonetheless, there is continuing concern that the clinical manifestations of prostate enlargement could be aggravated by treatment with androgen replacement therapy; this unresolved issue is deserving of much further study. While such data are being generated, there is considerable interest by investigators and pharmaceutical companies in developing prostate-sparing androgen treatments using synthetic androgen receptor modulators (SARMs, e.g. MENT) and the combined use of testosterone preparations and 5α-reductase inhibitors. Not enough data are available to judge the merits of such approaches. Prostate cancer is a common age-related disease. Since prostate cancer is an androgen responsive malignancy, men with existent clinical prostate cancer should not be treated with testosterone. While most investigations have failed to link testosterone treatment as a causal factor in prostate cancer, the use of testosterone preparations for androgen deficiency of aging has raised the question whether such treatment will increase the rate of conversion of preclinical to clinical prostate cancer. Long-term follow-up studies are required to answer this question.

Frailty and aging

Multiple hormone factors have been implicated or considered in the pathogenesis of frailty of aging. These include testosterone, growth hormone, and adrenal androgen precursors. Since there are clear-cut decreases in the concentration of all three of these hormones with increasing age, the prevention or treatment of frailty of aging might involve complex therapeutic regimens.

Osteoporosis

Osteoporosis is another multifactorial disorder where testosterone, estrogen, growth hormone, adrenal androgens and vitamin D deficiencies[13,14] may play a role in its pathogenesis. Vitamin D deficiency, which occurs with increased frequency in older men, is in part dietary, and in part due to limited exposure of skin to UV light and decreased functional capacity of the skin.

Altered endocrine control of salt and water metabolism

Endocrine regulation of salt and water may be affected by the aging process. Depletion and excess of salt and water are pathogenically related to some of the most common and serious metabolic disorders in the elderly. Both extremes of salt and water metabolism result in central nervous system symptoms that are aggravated when associated with concomitant serious illnesses. Age-dependent loosening of homeostatic controls may play a role in the high prevalence and seriousness of these multifactorial disorders. Examples of such dysregulation include impaired thirst in response to hyperosmolality[15–17], impairment at the renal level of the ability to excrete a water load[18–20], as well as a diminished ability to concentrate the urine with increase in age. Vasopressin secretion may also be impaired, with blunting of the sleep-associated rise in plasma vasopressin occurring with increase in age. This change in nocturnal secretion of vasopressin may combine with other factors resulting in nocturnal trips to the bathroom (nocturia)[21,22]. Fluid loss, hypernatremia and dehydration have been reported to occur in 1% of hospitalized patients over the age of 60 years. Half of these patients present with the problem, and half acquire the hypernatremia in the hospital[23]. Endocrine causes of excess fluid loss include: diabetes mellitus, hypercalcemia, partial or severe diabetes insipidus, and aldosterone deficiency[24-29].

References

1. McKnight JA, Roberts G, Sheridan B, Atkinson AB. Relationship between basal and sodium stimulated plasma atrial natriuretic factor, age, sex, and blood pressure in normal men. *J Hum Hypertens* 1989;3:157–63

2. Tajima F, Sagawa S, Iwamoto J, *et al.* Renal and endocrine responses in the elderly during head-out water immersion. *Am J Physiol* 1988;254:R977–83

3. Kario K, Nishikimi T, Yoshihara F, *et al.* Plasma levels of natriuretic peptides and adrenomedullin in elderly hypertensive patients: relationships to 24 h blood pressure. *J Hypertens* 1998;16:1253–9

4. Ohashi M, Fujio N, Nawata H, *et al.* Pharmacokinetics of synthetic alpha-human atrial natriuretic polypeptide in normal men: effect of aging. *Regul Pept* 1987;19:265–71

5. Heim JM, Gottmann K, Weil J, *et al.* Effects of a bolus dose of atrial natriuretic factor in young and elderly volunteers. *Eur J Clin Invest* 1989;19:265–71

6. Gruenewald DA, Matsumoto AM. Aging of the endocrine system. In Hazzard WR, Blass JP, Ettinger WH Jr, *et al.*, eds. *Principles of Geriatric Medicine and Gerontology*, 4th edn. New York: McGraw-Hill, 1999;949–65

7. Brzezinski A. Melatonin in humans. *N Engl J Med* 1997;336:186–95

8. Zeitzer JM, Daniels JE, Duffy JF, *et al.* Do plasma melatonin concentrations decline with age? *Am J Med* 1999;107:432–6

9. Sasagawa I, Nakada T, Kazama T, *et al.* Volume change of the prostate and seminal vesicles in male hypogonadism after androgen replacement therapy. *Int Urol Nephrol* 1990; 22:279–84

10. Behre HM, Bohmeyer J, Nieschlag E. Prostate volume in testosterone-treated and untreated hypogonadal men in comparison to age-matched normal controls. *Clin Endocrinol (Oxford)* 1994;40:341–9

11. Meikle AW, Arver S, Dobs AS, *et al.* Prostate size in hypogonadal men treated with a non-scrotal permeation-enhanced testosterone transdermal system. *Urology* 1977;49:191–6

12. Cooper CS, Perry PJ, Sparks AE, *et al.* Effect of exogenous testosterone on prostate volume, serum and semen prostate specific antigen levels in healthy young men. *J Urol* 1998;159: 44–3

13. Swerdloff RS, Wang CW. Androgens, estrogens and bone in men: the Framington Study. *Ann Intern Med* 2000;133:1002–4

14. Lips P. Vitamin D deficiency and secondary hyperparathyroidism in the elderly: Consequences for bone loss and fracture and therapeutic implications. *Endocr Rev* 2001;22: 477–501

15. Phillips PA, Bretherton M, Johnston CI, Gray L. Reduced osmotic thirst in healthy elderly men. *Am J Physiol* 1991;261:R166–71

16. Phillips PA, Bretherton M, Risvanis J, *et al.* Effects of drinking on thirst and vasopressin in dehydrated elderly men. *Am J Physiol* 1993; 264:R877–81

17. Mack GW, Weseman CA, Langhans GW, *et al.* Body fluid balance in dehydrated healthy older men: Thirst and renal osmoregulation. *J Appl Physiol* 1994;76:1615–23

18. Crow MJ, Forsling ML, Rolls BJ, *et al.* Altered water excretion in healthy elderly men. *Age Ageing* 1987;16:285–93

19. Dontas AS, Karkenos S, Papanayioutou P. Mechanisms of renal tubular defects in old age. *Postgrad Med J* 1972;48:295–303

20. Lye M. Electrolyte disorders in the elderly. *Clin Endocrinol Metab* 1984;13:377–98

21. Kirkland JL, Lye M, Levy DW, Banerjee AK. Patterns of urine flow and electrolyte excretion in healthy elderly people. *Br Med J* 1983;287:1665–7

22. George CP, Messerli FH, Genest J, *et al.* Diurnal variation of plasma vasopressin in man. *J Clin Endocrinol Metab* 1975;41:332–8

23. Snyder NA, Feigal DW, Arieff AI. Hypernatremia in elderly patients: a heterogeneous, morbid, and iatrogenic entity. *Ann Intern Med* 1987;107:309–19

24. Miller M. Water balance in older persons. In Morley JE, van den Berg L, eds. *Endocrinology of Aging*. Totowa, NJ: Humana, 2000;73–92

25. Castrillon JL, Mediavilla A, Mendez MA, *et al.* Syndrome of inappropriate antidiuretic hormone secretion (SIADH) and enalapril. *J Intern Med* 1993;233:89–91

26. Crow M. Hyponatremia due to syndrome of inappropriate antidiuretic hormone secretion in the elderly. *Ir Med J* 1980;73:482–3

27. Goldstein CS, Braunstein S, Goldfarb S. Idiopathic syndrome of inappropriate antidiuretic hormone secretion possibly related to advanced age. *Ann Intern Med* 1983;99:185–8

28. Hirshberg B, Ben-Yehuda A. The syndrome of inappropriate antidiuretic hormone secretion in the elderly. *Am J Med* 1997;10:270–3

29. Davis KM, Minaker KL. Disorders of fluid balance: dehydration and hyponatremia. In Hazzard WR, Blass JP, Ettinger WH Jr, *et al.*, eds. *Principles of Geriatric Medicine and Gerontology*, 4th edn. New York: McGraw-Hill 1999:1429–36

11 Androgens and the aging male

Ronald S. Swerdloff, MD and Christina Wang, MD

INTRODUCTION

Androgen deficiency in older men has become an increasingly important medical consideration. Testosterone has always been considered a sex steroid with major effects on the reproductive axis. Our increasing understanding of the actions of testosterone on multiple tissues that were previously under-appreciated as major testosterone targets (e.g. bone muscle, fat, brain, hematopoietic and immune systems) has broadened our appreciation of the importance of this hormone on body homeostasis.

The decline with age in the serum concentrations of biologically active forms of testosterone in men is an indisputable fact. This decline begins earlier than previously appreciated (approximately age 30) and is progressive and relentless. Eventually, serum testosterone levels fall below the threshold for optimal androgen actions. The question has now turned to whether this decline in testosterone is a physiologic process and should be accepted as 'normal' or as a pathologic process with clinical implications. The pendulum has swung toward a dysfunctional state, as there is increasing recognition that the androgen deficiency with aging has clinical significance and may pose important risk factors for osteoporosis, frailty and cardiovascular disease.

If androgen deficiency of the aging male is a real disorder, this leaves us with the question of whether the manifestations of androgen deficiency of aging are reversible and if so

what will be the adverse effects of replacement therapy. Areas of particular concern for possible negative effects of testosterone are the prostate and cardiovascular system. More information (e.g. long-term safety data) is required to assure physicians, scientists and patients that the net effect of androgen replacement therapy will be positive. If the benefit to risk ratio of testosterone replacement in older men proves to be positive, then we must select an optimal formulation, route of administration, and dosage. Since the biologic actions act on multiple tissues, the optimal therapeutic levels of hormone may differ for different clinical indications. New formations and pharmacologic agents are likely to be designed to enhance benefit and reduce risk. New families of selective androgen receptor modulators (SARMS) are being developed to provide increased biologic and tissue selectivity. These issues will occupy the effects of andrologists and pharmacologists for some time.

SERUM TESTOSTERONE LEVELS AND AGING IN MEN

There is general consensus that the serum levels of testosterone decline with age. This decline begins at about age 30 and decreases progressively as men get older. Cross-sectional studies have shown that serum free testosterone concentrations decrease more than the

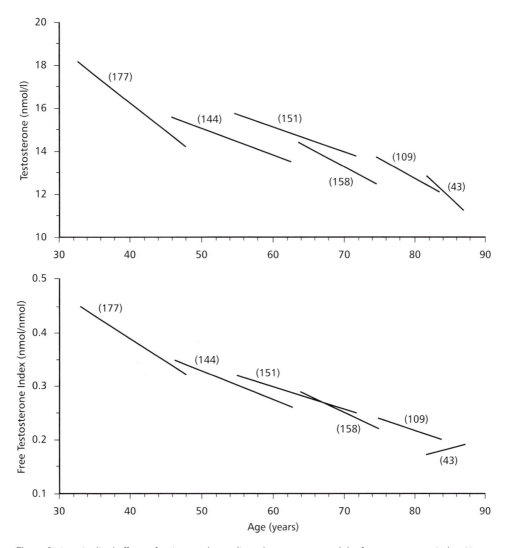

Figure 1 Longitudinal effects of aging on date-adjusted testosterone and the free testosterone index. Linear segment plots for total testosterone and the free testosterone index versus age are shown for men, with testosterone and sex hormone binding globulin values taken on at least two visits. Each linear segment has a slope equal to the mean of the individual longitudinal slopes in each decade, and is centred on the median age, for each cohort of men from the second to the ninth decade. Numbers in parentheses represent the number of men in each cohort. With the exception of the free testosterone index in the ninth decade, segments show significant downward progression at every age, with no significant change in slopes for testosterone or the free testosterone index over the entire age range. Figure reproduced with permission from Harman et al.[4] Longitudinal effects of aging on serum total and free testosterone levels in healthy men. J Clin Endocrinol Metab 2001;86:724–31. © The Endocrine Society

total testosterone because of the increased levels of sex hormone binding globulin (SHBG) in older men[1,2]. Since the circulating non-SHBG-bound testosterone levels (free and albumin-bound) are the biologically available forms for activity at the target organs, measurements of this non-SHBG-bound testosterone better reflect the clinically important state of circulating testosterone than the total testosterone concentrations. A longitudinal study of 77 men showed that total serum testosterone levels decreased over the 15 years

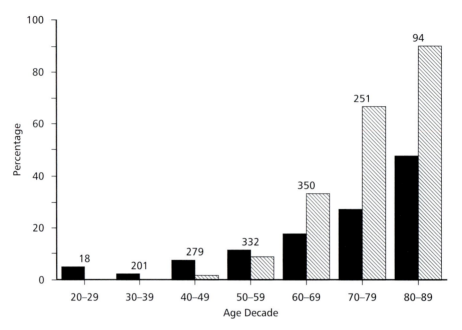

Figure 2 Hypogonadism in aging men. Bar height indicates the percent of men in each 10-year interval, from the third to the ninth decades, with at least one testosterone value in the hypogonadal range, by the criteria of total testosterone (black bars) < 11.3 nmol/l (325 ng/dl) or testosterone/ sex hormone binding globulin (free testosterone index; striped bars) < 0.153 nmol/nmol. Numbers above each pair of bars indicate the number of men studied in the corresponding decade. The fraction of men who are hypogonadal increases progressively after age 50 by either criterion. More men are hypogonadal by free testosterone index than by total testosterone after age 50, and there seems to be a progressively greater difference, with increasing age, between the two criteria. Figure reproduced with permission from Harman et al.[4] Longitudinal effects of aging on serum total and free testosterone levels in healthy men. *J Clin Endocrinol Metab* 2001;86:724–31. © The Endocrine Society

of the study at a rate of 110 ng/dl every decade[3]. The longitudinal effects of aging on serum testosterone and the free testosterone index (serum testosterone/ SHBG) are shown in Figure 1[4]. The percentage of men hypogonadal in each decade by total versus free testosterone criteria is shown in Figure 2. In the Baltimore Longitudinal Study of Aging, 19, 28 and 49% of men over 60, 70 and 80 years had serum total testosterone levels below the normal range for young male adults, and an even higher percentage (34, 68 and 91%, respectively) were below the range for young normal adults when the free testosterone index (total testosterone/SHBG) was used as the criteria for diagnosis (Figure 3)[4]. These studies indicate that chemical hypogonadism is a very common

occurrence in aging men. It should be noted that the decline in serum testosterone in older men is frequently not accompanied by the increase in serum luteinizing hormone (LH) seen in primary hypogonadism of younger men. Furthermore, older men lose the diurnal variation in serum LH and testosterone seen in younger hypogonadal men[5]. This is explained by a dual defect in testosterone secretion at the testicular and hypothalamic/pituitary levels in the elderly[6,7].

What is the clinical significance of the decline in serum testosterone levels in older men? Do the low serum testosterone levels impair healthy aging and increase the risk of frailty in this population? These questions will be addressed in the following discussions.

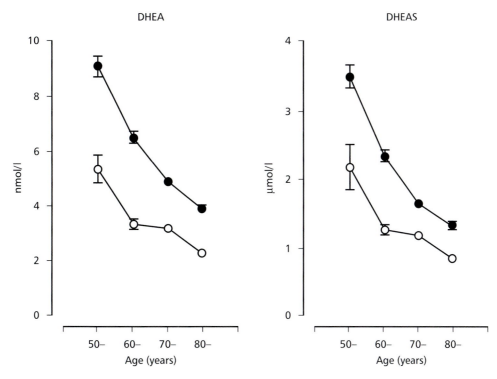

Figure 3 Body mass index-adjusted DHEA and DHEAS levels in men (●) and women (O) stratified by decade of age over 50 years. Modified from reference 43

Sexual activity and erectile function

There is evidence to show that sexual dysfunction including sexual thoughts, enjoyment and performance decreases with age. There is also epidemiological evidence linking serum testosterone levels and bioactive testosterone levels (free and albumin-bound testosterone) with sexual activity[8]. This relationship is consistent with the well-documented evidence that in young hypogonadal men, androgen replacement improves sexual desire and function. Other studies[9,10] have also observed improved libido after androgen replacement in hypogonadal elderly men. Since erectile function declines with age due to multifactorial causes, the most prominent of which is impaired penile nitric oxide (NO) release, erectile dysfunction may not be corrected by testosterone therapy alone unless the local vasodilatory defect is corrected first. It appears from the reported studies that androgen replacement will enhance libido and contribute to improvement of sexual function in older men co-treated with phosphodiesterase-5 inhibitors (e.g. sildenafil). Co-treatment with androgens and phosphodiesterase-5 inhibitors also provides the benefits of androgens on other target sites.

Muscle mass, strength and adipose tissue

Testosterone deficiency results in decreased muscle mass and strength in young hypogonadal men; multiple studies have demonstrated positive effects of androgen replacement on these functions in this age group[11,12]. Muscle mass is also correlated with serum testosterone and free testosterone in older men[13,14], whereas data on muscle strength are not conclusive. In all the reported studies, testosterone replacement in older men increases muscle mass[9,15-18]. Aging is associated with a decrease in lean mass, and an increase in abdominal fat mass is inversely proportional to serum free testosterone levels[19,20]. Therefore testosterone replacement results in decrease abdominal fat[21] and total fat mass[18] in elderly men. There is also evidence to support that muscle strength and power decrease with increasing age[22,23]. The reported studies of testosterone replacement in elderly men do not provide a conclusive answer of whether muscle strength or power is increased by replacement therapy.

Bone mineral density

Hypogonadal young and middle-aged men are often osteopenic and have a higher fracture rate than eugonadal men. Some, but not all, epidemiological studies in older men showed a correlation between bone mineral density (BMD) and serum free or bioavailable testosterone, while most studies demonstrated a stronger correlation with free or bioavailable estradiol (E_2) levels[13,24-26]. Hypogonadism is a recognized cause of osteoporosis in men with fractures. Testosterone replacement is well documented to increase BMD in younger hypogonadal men[11,27], with improvements in bone turnover and bone deposition[27]. Despite the positive effects on bone, it is unclear if the effect is completely or partially through conversion to E_2. The demonstration of an increase in bone formation markers after testosterone treatment of hypogonadal men suggests that a direct androgen effect may complement estrogenic effect on bone[27-29]. Testosterone replacement also results in increases in BMD in all reported studies in androgen-deficient older men but there are no available data on a decrease in fracture risk[30,31].

Brain and psychological function

Hypogonadal young and middle-aged men frequently complain of symptoms of depression and a decreased sense of well being; in contrast, mood is improved after testosterone treatment. Recent studies have also demonstrated that serum testosterone levels correlate with spatial ability[32,33]. Androgen replacement in elderly men also improves spatial ability without changes in memory or verbal fluency[34]. There is also evidence available that depressed mood is inversely related to serum bioavailable testosterone levels[35]. Androgen replacement therapy in aging men has improved general well-being[9]. More detailed studies of androgen replacement on cognition in older testosterone-deficient men are needed as are studies on the benefits on cognitive function in dementia associated with aging.

DIAGNOSIS OF CLINICALLY SIGNIFICANT ANDROGEN DEFICIENCY IN ELDERLY MEN

It is unclear if the diagnosis of testosterone deficiency in the elderly male should be made by hormone testing supported by a symptom complex or vice versa. The Endocrine Society Consensus Committee on this topic decided that the diagnosis should be based on a symptom and sign complex of decreased energy and vitality, libido and erectile function, decreased muscle mass and strength, decreased bone mineral density, increased abdominal fat, lack of a sense of well-being and depression[36]. The presumptive diagnosis, based on one or more of the above symptoms and signs, should be confirmed by a serum testosterone level. A decreased BMD, clinical signs of osteoporosis, or the development of non-traumatic bone fractures should trigger the request for a serum testosterone measurement. Since serum SHBG levels increase with age, non-SHBG-bound testosterone concentrations decrease more profoundly with age than serum testosterone. It is therefore advisable to measure not only serum total testosterone but also either free testosterone (by equilibrium dialysis method), calculated free testosterone (by measuring serum total testosterone and SHBG concentrations) or

Table 1 Testosterone replacement for older men

Preparation	Dose/frequency of administration
Injectable	
T-enanthate/cypionate	100 to 200 mg every 2 weeks
Transdermal	
Scrotal patch	6 mg/day
Non-scrotal patches with enhancers	5 mg/day
Non-scrotal patches without enhancers	5 mg/day
Testosterone gel	5 to 10 mg/day (5–10 g of gel)
Oral	
Testosterone undecanoate (not available in US)	80 mg bid or tid

bioavailable testosterone (non-SHBG-bound)[37] to confirm the diagnosis. It should be noted that measuring free testosterone by the analog displacement assay should be avoided, as this method is poorly reflective of free testosterone and less reliable than total testosterone measurements[38]. Since normal ranges vary significantly between research groups, the results from the patient should be compared with normal ranges established by each laboratory. The most practical approach may be to use the less expensive and more readily available total testosterone level as the first-order test and accept as definitive hormone levels below 200 ng/dl as low, levels above 400 ng/dl as normal and total testosterone concentrations between 200–400 ng/dl as deserving of a more rigorous analysis of either free testosterone by dialysis, bioavailable testosterone or calculated free testosterone.

Exclusion criteria for treatment

Unfortunately there are no long-term data available to fully judge the risk-to-benefit ratio of testosterone replacement therapy in the elderly age group. Until such data are provided symptomatic men with low serum testosterone levels can arguably be treated. Once the diagnosis is confirmed, then androgen replacement can be started, provided that cancer of the prostate, breast and symptomatic benign prostatic hyperplasia have been excluded. A digital rectal exam of the prostate should be performed, and serum prostate-specific antigen

(PSA), hematocrit and liver functions should be checked.

TESTOSTERONE REPLACEMENT THERAPY

At present androgen replacement therapy can be administered as testosterone enanthate or cypionate injections or by transdermal testosterone patches and gels (Table 1). Due to our uncertainty over risk of unmasking prostate cancer, it is not recommended that long-acting testosterone injectables or testosterone pellets be used for androgen replacement therapy in elderly men. These agents, once administered, cannot be removed to lower serum testosterone levels rapidly in cases of serious adverse effects. At the present time in the USA, there are no effective FDA approved oral testosterone preparations other than the 17-alkylated androgens. In general 17-alkylated androgens are not recommended for replacement because of possible hepatic toxicity and marked changes in serum lipoprotein levels associated with these orally administered testosterone preparations. Other androgens under development include testosterone undecanoate (an 8- to 12-week injectable), buccal testosterone (one tablet twice per day), oral testosterone undecanoate (new formulation, one capsule twice per day), other testosterone and DHT gels and selective androgen receptor modulators[39].

Adverse effects of testosterone therapy

The risks of androgen replacement therapy include increases in weight, hematocrit, and sleep apnea. It remains uncertain if there are additional risks of cardiovascular disease and prostate cancer. Weight increase is usually moderate consisting of less than 5 kg. Testosterone replacement may lead to edema and may aggravate symptoms in patients with severe congestive heart failure. Administration of androgens results in increases in hematocrit. Occasionally, clinically significant polycythemia occurs when the hematocrit is over 55%; in this case, testosterone replacement should be stopped or the dose reduced. Sleep apnea and elevated body mass index may increase the risk of developing polycythemia. While the data are sparse, it is believed that testosterone replacement therapy may worsen sleep apnea in hypogonadal men. It is important to inquire about the presence of sleep apnea prior to and during androgen replacement therapy. Administration of testosterone ester injections in supraphysiological or high physiological range results in statistically significant decreases in high-density lipoprotein (HDL) cholesterol. In some studies, the total cholesterol levels are also lowered. It should be noted that although serum HDL cholesterol levels are often decreased, serum lipoprotein (a) levels are also lowered. Moreover, testosterone administration has been reported to have favorable effects in fibrinolysis and coagulation factors. There are also recent studies suggesting a direct action of testosterone on coronary vessel reactivity and dilation[1,40].

The issue of whether androgen replacement therapy will increase the risk of cancer of the prostate (CaP) is not settled. About 30 studies have reported administration of testosterone to middle-aged or elderly men, with most of the studies showing no increase in serum PSA, prostate symptom score, prostate size or urine flow rates[40]. There has not been a reported increase in the incidence of CaP with androgen replacement therapy. In a recent proposed study to examine whether androgen replacement will increase the risk of CaP, it is estimated that 6000 men will have to be enrolled in a 6-year placebo versus testosterone replacement randomized clinical trial to address this question (personal communication: Cunningham G, Bhasin S, Matsumoto A). There is also no evidence that androgen replacement therapy will increase the incidence of benign prostatic hyperplasia. All appropriate screens for prostatic disease should be performed before starting an elderly man on testosterone replacement. The benefits versus risks have to be considered in each individual man.

Summary of benefits of testosterone replacement therapy

It appears that testosterone replacement improves general well-being and sexual function, increases lean body mass and BMD, and decreases body fat in both young and older men with low testosterone levels. The limited data available seem to support similar benefits in older patients.

DHEA AND DHEAS DEFICIENCY IN ELDERLY MEN

It is also known that serum concentrations of adrenal androgens such as dehydroepiandrosterone and its sulfate (DHEA and DHEAS) and androstenedione decrease with increasing age[41–43] (Figure 3). The decline in these adrenally produced androgen precursors are steeper than that for testosterone. Since neither of these steroids binds to the androgen receptor or other known steroid receptors, it is assumed by most investigators that they act either through conversion to androgens and estrogens or by binding to other, ill-defined or unrecognized receptors. Very large amounts of either compound would be required to normalize testosterone levels to the range of normal young male adults. Despite the popularity of these steroids as dietary supplements and their labeling as 'natural steroids', they are not manufactured under FDA guidelines and may have variable purity and consistency. Furthermore, there is no conclusive study that has demonstrated the beneficial effects of DHEA replacement in elderly men compared to that seen in young men[44,45]. Until substantive data to demonstrate beneficial effects on aging in men are available, these authors recommend avoiding the use of either DHEA or androstenedione in androgen-deficient or non-androgen-deficient older men.

References

1. Vermuelen A. Androgen replacement therapy in the aging male – a critical evaluation. *J Clin Endocrinol Metab* 2001;80:2380–9
2. Snyder PJ. Effects of age on testicular function and consequences of testosterone treatment. *J Clin Endocrinol Metab* 2001;86:2369–72
3. Morley JE, Kaiser FE, Perry III HM, *et al*. Longitudinal changes in testosterone, luteinizing hormone, and follicle-stimulating hormone in healthy older men. *Metabolism* 1997;46: 410–13
4. Harman SM, Metter EJ, Tobin JD, *et al*. Longitudinal effects of aging on serum total and free testosterone levels in healthy men. *J Clin Endocrinol Metab* 2001;86:724–31
5. Bremner WJ, Vitiello WV, Prinz PN. Loss of circadian rhythmicity in blood testosterone levels with aging. *J Clin Endocrinol Metab* 1993;51:1278–81
6. Korenman SG, Morley JE, Mooradian AD, *et al*. Secondary hypogonadism in older men: its relation to impotence. *J Clin Endocrinol Metab* 1990;71:963–9
7. Swerdloff RS, Wang C. Androgen deficiency and aging in men. *West J Med* 1993;159: 579–85
8. Nilsson P, Moller L, Solstad K. Adverse effects of psychosocial stress on gonadal function and insulin levels in middle aged males. *J Intern Med* 1995;237:479–86
9. Morley JE, Perry HM, Kaiser FE, *et al*. Effect of testosterone replacement therapy in old hypogonadal males: a preliminary study. *J Am Geriatr Soc* 1993;41:149–52
10. Hajjar RR, Kaiser FE, Morley JE. Outcomes of long-term testosterone replacement therapy in older hypogonadal males: a retrospective study. *J Clin Endocrinol Metab* 1997;82: 3793–6
11. Wang C, Eyre DR, Clark R, *et al*. Sublingual testosterone replacement improves muscle mass and strength, decreases bone resorption, and increases bone formation markers in hypogonadal men. *J Clin Endocrinol Metab* 1996;81:3654–62
12. Wang C, Swerdloff RS, Iranmanesh A, *et al*. Transdermal testosterone gel improves sexual function, mood, muscle strength, and body composition parameters in hypogonadal men. *J Clin Endocrinol Metab* 2000; 85:2839–53
13. Van den Beld AW, de Jong FH, Grobbee DE, *et al*. Measures of bio-available serum testosterone and estradiol and their relationship with muscle strength, bone density and body composition in elderly men. *J Clin Endocrinol Metab* 2000;85:3276–82
14. Baumgartner RN, Waters DL, Gallagher D, *et al*. Predictors of skeletal muscle mass in elderly men and women. *Mech Aging Dev* 1999;107:123–36
15. Tenover JS. Effects of testosterone supplementation in the aging male. *J Clin Endocrinol Metab* 1992;75:1092–8
16. Urban RJ, Bodenburg C, Gilkison C, *et al*. Testosterone administration to elderly men increases skeletal muscle strength and protein synthesis. *Am J Physiol* 1995;269:E820–E826
17. Sih R, Morley JE, Kaiser FE, *et al*. Testosterone replacement in older hypogonadal men: a 12-month randomized controlled study. *J Clin Endocrinol Metab* 1997; 82:1661–7
18. Snyder PJ, Peachy H, Hannoush P, *et al*. Effect of testosterone treatment on body composition and muscle strength in men over 65 years of age. *J Clin Endocrinol Metab* 1999;84:2647–53

19. Vermeulen A, Goemaere S, Kaufman JM. Sex hormones, body composition and aging. *The Aging Male* 1999;2:8–15

20. Tchernof A, Labrie F, Belanger A, *et al.* Relationships between endogenous sex steroid hormones, sex hormone binding globulin and lipoprotein levels in men: contribution of visceral obesity, insulin levels and other metabolic variables. *Atherosclerosis* 1997;133: 235–44

21. Marin P, Holmang S, Gustafson C, *et al.* Androgen treatment of abdominally obese men. *Obesity Res* 1993;1:245–8

22. Frontera WR, Hughes VV, Fiatarone MA, Fielding RA. Aging and skeletal muscle: a 12-year longitudinal study. *J Appl Physiol* 2000;88:1321–6

23. Reed RL, Pearlmutter L, Jochum K, *et al.* The relationship between muscle mass and muscle strength in the elderly. *J Am Geriatr Soc* 1991;39:555–91

24. Greendale G, Edelstein S, Barrett-Connor E. Endogenous sex steroids and bone mineral density in older women and men: The Rancho Bernardo Study. *J Bone Miner Res* 1997;12: 1833–41

25. Khosla S, Melton LJ, Atkinson EJ, *et al.* Relationship of serum sex steroid levels and bone turnover markers with bone mineral density in men: a key role for bio-available estrogen. *J Clin Endocrinol Metab* 1998;83: 2266–75

26. Khosla S, Melton, III LJ, Atkinson, EJ, O'Fallon WM. Relationship of serum sex steroid levels to longitudinal changes in bone density in young versus elderly men. *J Clin Endocrinol Metab* 2001;86:3555–61

27. Wang C, Swerdloff RS, Iranmanesh A, *et al.* Effects of transdermal testosterone gel on bone turnover markers and bone mineral density in hypogonadal men. *Clin Endocrinol* 2001;54:739–50

28. Swerdloff RS, Wang C. Androgens, estrogens and bone in men: The Framington Study. Editorial in *Ann Intern Med* 2000;133: 1002–4

29. Abu EO, Horner A, Kusec V, *et al.* The localization of androgen receptors in human bone. *J Clin Endocrinol Metab* 1997;82:3493

30. Snyder PJ, Peachey H, Hannoush P, *et al.* Effects of testosterone treatment on bone mineral density in men over 65 years old. *J Clin Endocrinol Metab* 1999;84:1966–72

31. Kenny AM, Prestwood KM, Gruman CA, *et al.* Effects of transdermal testosterone on bone and muscle in older men with low bioavailable testosterone levels. *J Gerontol A Med Sci* 2001;56A:M266–M272

32. Christiansen K, Kussmann R. Sex hormones and cognitive functions in men. *Neuropsychobiology* 1987;18:27–36

33. McKeever WF, Deyo A. Testosterone, dihydrotestosterone and spatial task performance of males. *Bull Psychonomic Soc* 1990; 28:305–8

34. Janowski SC, Oviatt SK, Orwoll ES. Testosterone influences spatial cognition in older men. *Behav Neurosci* 1994;108:325–3

35. Barrett-Connor E, von Muhlen DG, Kritz-Silverstein D. Bio-available testosterone and depressive mood in older men. The Rancho-Bernardo Study. *J Clin Endocrinol Metab* 1999;84:573–7

36. Morley JE, Charlton E, Patrick P, *et al.* Validation of a screening questionnaire for androgen deficiency in aging males. *Metabolism* 2000;49:1239–42

37. Vermeulen A, Verdonck L, Kaufman JM. A critical evaluation of simple methods for the estimation of free testosterone in serum. *J Clin Endocrinol Metab* 1999;84:3666–72

38. Rosner W. Errors in the measurement of plasma free testosterone. *J Clin Endocrinol Metab* 1997;82:2014–15

39. Wang C, Swerdloff RS. Androgen replacement therapy, risks and benefits. In: Wang C, ed. *Male Reproductive Function.* Norwell: Kluwer Academic Publishers, 1999:157–72

40. Tenover JL. Risks and benefits of testosterone in older men. In: Robarire B, Chemes H, Morales CR, eds. *Andrology in the 21st Century.* Montreal: Medimond, 2001: 395–405

41. Gray A, Feldman HA, McKinlay JB, Longcope C. Age, disease and changes in sex hormone levels in middle-aged men: results of the Massachusetts Male Aging Study. *J Clin Endocrinol Metab* 1991;73:1016–25

42. Labrie F, Belanger A, Cusan L, *et al.* Marked decline in serum concentrations of androgen C19 sex steroid precursors and conjugated androgen metabolites during aging. *J Clin Endocrinol Metab* 1997;82:2396–402

43. Laughlin GA, Barrett-Connor E. Sexual dimorphism in the influence of advanced aging on adrenal hormone levels: the Rancho Bernardo Study. *J Clin Endocrinol Metab* 2000;85:3561–8

44. Flynn MA, Weaver-Osterholtz D, Sharpe-Timms KL, *et al.* Dehydroepiandrosterone replacement in aging humans. *J Clin Endocrinol Metab* 1999;84:1527–33

45. Baulieu E-E, Thomas G, Legrain S, *et al.* Dehydroepiandrosterone (DHEA) sulfate, and aging: Contribution of the DHEAge study to a sociobiomedical issue. *Proc Natl Acad Sci USA* 2000;1197:4279–84

12 Growth hormone and aging in men

Marc R. Blackman, MD

INTRODUCTION

Aging in man is associated with a progressive loss of function, leading to decreased homeostasic capacity, initially in response to various stressors, and subsequently under baseline conditions. Both aging and growth hormone (GH) deficiency are associated with decreased skeletal muscle and bone mass and strength, increased total and intra-abdominal fat, dyslipidemia, glucose intolerance, reduced cardiac endurance and immunological function, and altered quality of life[1,2]. Recent studies suggest that administration of recombinant GH to non-elderly GH-deficient men ameliorates or attenuates these abnormalities[1,2]. Because normal aging in men is associated with a decline in GH secretion and serum insulin-like growth factor I (IGF-I) levels[1,2], it has been hypothesized that the above-noted alterations in body composition and function in older persons may be due in part to decrements in function of the GH–IGF-I axis. To assess this possibility, the effects of different hormone replacement paradigms are being investigated in selected populations of elderly men. A major goal of this research effort is to assess whether trophic factors such as GH, GH-releasing hormone (GHRH), or other GH-releasing peptides or non-peptide mimetics can be used effectively, safely, ethically and economically to prolong physical and functional independence, and to reduce morbidity and frailty in aged men.

PHYSIOLOGICAL CHANGES IN THE GH–IGF-I AXIS WITH AGING

Age-related changes of spontaneous and stimulated GH release

GH is an important anabolic hormone that exerts stimulatory effects on protein synthesis and on lipolysis[3]. Pituitary GH release is regulated primarily by the interaction of the hypothalamic peptides GHRH, which stimulates[4], and somatostatin, which inhibits[5], GH production.

GH secretion is maximal during puberty, occurring mostly during the night, especially during deep (stages 3–4) slow wave sleep (SWS). Sleep–wake homeostasis is the primary contributor to the temporal organization of GH secretion, whereas the influence of circadian rhythmicity is much less important[6]. In young, healthy men, nearly 60–70% of GH release occurs during delta (stages 3–4) SWS[6]. The usual nocturnal sleep-onset GH secretory pulse results from a burst of hypothalamic GHRH release occurring contemporaneously with a diminished somatostatin tone, although the nocturnal GH surge can occur prior to sleep onset in both sexes. Young adult men given agents that increase SWS, such as γ-hydroxybutyrate, exhibit concomitant increases in nocturnal and 24-h GH secretion[7], suggesting that such drugs may be useful GH secretagogues.

Beginning in early to mid-adulthood, GH production decreases at a rate of about 14% per decade, primarily a result of a decrease in the amplitude of nocturnal GH pulses. By late adulthood, daily spontaneous GH secretion is decreased by 50–70% that exhibited in the third to fourth decades[2]. The acute secretory response of GH to pituitary stimulation with GHRH is reduced in healthy old versus young individuals. This reduced GH secretory response is thought to result from a decrease in the secretion or action of GHRH, and from a rise in somatostatinergic tone[2].

Elderly people and GH-deficient younger adults have decreased delta sleep[8,9]. In a recent cross-sectional survey of 149 healthy men aged 16–83 years, the amount of deep SWS decreased by about 80% from young (16–25 years) to mid- (36–50 years) adulthood, in temporal association with a nearly 75% reduction in spontaneous GH secretion. SWS, independent of age, was a major determinant of 24-h and nocturnal GH release[10].

GH binding proteins

Circulating GH binding protein (GHBP) levels decrease after the fifth to sixth decades in healthy men[11]. Whether the age-related decline in GHBP is a consequence of a decrease in peripheral GH receptors, the putative source of GHBPs, or a reduction in GH secretion with aging and the possible physiological significance of these alterations, remains to be established.

IGF-I

Baseline serum levels of IGF-I are derived primarily from release of hepatic IGF-I, which tends to remain relatively constant throughout the day. IGF-I levels can be augmented directly, by the administration of GH or various GH secretagogues, and indirectly by physical activity and aerobic exercise.

Circulating IGF-I is more than 95% bound to one or more of six specific binding proteins (IGFBPs), of which IGFBP-3 is the predominant circulating binding protein[12]. The major role of the IGFBPs is to prolong the circulating half-life of IGF-I[13] and enhance or restrict the bioavailability of IGF-I to the target tissues[12]. Recent evidence suggests that the IGFBPs may have mitogenic and metabolic properties of their own.

In cross-sectional studies, levels of IGF-I in unextracted serum or plasma decreased with age in men, so that IGF-I levels were 30–50% lower in the seventh than the third decade[14]. A low serum IGF-I concentration (defined arbitrarily as a value below the lowest 2.5th centile of the comparison group) occurred in 85% of healthy elderly compared with young men and in 26% of chronically institutionalized compared with healthy elderly men[15,16]. Co-morbid illness and aging exert independent and additive inhibitory effects on serum IGF-I levels. Using assay methods that reduce or eliminate IGFBPs, such as acid-ethanol extraction, cross-sectional studies have revealed steadily falling IGF-I levels, from a peak of nearly 500 μg/l in young adulthood to values averaging about 100 μg/l by age 80[17].

Baseline serum IGF-I levels are directly related to spontaneous 24-h GH secretion in young, but not older, adults[17]. This may reflect the confounding influences of diminished hepatic synthetic function and reserve, as well as other age-related variables that independently modify IGF-I, including abdominal obesity, hyperinsulinemia, hyperglycemia, aerobic capacity, changing levels of gonadal steroids, the menopause and various disease states. Serum IGF-I is thus a less useful indicator of GH secretion in elderly persons than in younger adults. There is to date no consensus on the optimal clinical method of assessing age-related decrements in GH release.

Changes of IGF-binding proteins with age

Levels of IGFBP-3, the major plasma IGF-I binding protein, decrease with age in men[18]. In elderly persons, plasma levels of IGFBP-3 are positively correlated with levels of IGF-I, but only weakly related to spontaneous GH release[18]. Age-related alterations in the secretory physiology of the other IGFBPs remain to be elucidated.

GH, IGF-I and the gonadal axis

Plasma levels of GH and IGF-I are influenced by endogenous and exogenous gonadal steroids. There is a significant positive relationship between endogenous estradiol levels and spontaneous GH release in healthy elderly men[19]. In older men, some investigators have reported that there are no significant correlations between serum testosterone levels and either GHRH-stimulated or spontaneous GH secretion[19]. More recently, however, significant positive correlations have been observed between serum testosterone levels and spontaneous and GHRH-stimulated GH secretion in old men who had age-related reductions in serum testosterone levels[20-22]. The above observations highlight the importance of considering the influence of the sex steroid milieu in studies of the effects of aging on endogenous GH secretion.

The influence of nutritive status on the somatotropic axis

GH release is suppressed during hyperglycemia[23] and chronic malnutrition, whereas hypoglycemia and acute fasting stimulate GH secretion[24]. The threshold for, and magnitude of, GH release appear to be similar in young and elderly adults[25]. GH release is decreased with obesity[26], particularly with intra-abdominal adiposity[27]. There is a reduction in the frequency of GH secretory bursts and a significant shortening of the circulatory half-life of GH, both of which reduce integrated daily plasma GH concentrations[27]. By comparison with normal weight controls, obese men also have diminished GHRH-stimulated GH secretion[26] which is partly reversible by exogenous administration

of GHRH, arginine and pyridostigmine, perhaps because of increased somatostatinergic tone.

Similarly, plasma IGF-I has been inversely correlated with adiposity and body mass index (BMI)[28] and, especially, with measures of intra-abdominal obesity[29]. This relationship is independent of age[28], is partly reversible with weight loss and may explain the association of low levels of IGF-I with cardiovascular risk factors such as hypertension, hyperlipidemia, hyperglycemia and insulin resistance[30].

Physical activity, exercise and aerobic capacity

The acute GH response to aerobic or resistance exercise is reduced with age[29,31]. Basal and exercise-stimulated plasma IGF-I levels are higher in physically conditioned versus sedentary young men. Because of the general decline in physical activity with advancing age, a decrease in aerobic capacity ($VO_{2\,max}$) may contribute to diminished serum IGF-I levels in elderly persons. Although a positive correlation between $VO_{2\,max}$ and IGF-I levels has been reported in healthy men of various ages, this association may be less robust in elderly men[32]. A sustained program of moderate-intensity resistance exercise training in elderly persons for 1 year failed to increase IGF-I levels[33]. Several current investigations are underway to assess whether chronic aerobic or resistance exercise training elicits an increase in spontaneous GH release and/or IGF-I levels in healthy or frail elderly people.

THE EFFECTS OF AGE-RELATED GH DECLINE ON PHYSIOLOGICAL OUTCOMES

Both aging and GH deficiency in adults are associated with clinically significant decreases in lean body and muscle mass, skeletal muscle strength (sarcopenia)[34] and whole body and skeletal muscle protein synthesis. Aerobic capacity (exercise tolerance) also tends to be reduced. Similarly, bone density is diminished and calcium balance is negative. There are, in addition, increases in total and intra-abdominal fat accompanied by higher levels of total and low-density lipoprotein (LDL) cholesterol. Reduced strength, endurance and lean mass may contribute to falls and frailty. Increased abdominal fat, particularly the visceral as opposed to subcutaneous component, is associated with elevated 'bad' (LDL) cholesterol, increased insulin resistance, and greater cardiovascular disease risk (the so-called 'syndrome X'). Low bone mass (osteopenia) is associated with increased risk of fractures, which are responsible in turn for serious morbidity and mortality in elderly men[35,36]. Administration of GH to GH-deficient non-elderly adults for 6–12 months improved muscle strength[37,38] and lean body mass[39], decreased total and abdominal fat[40], reduced total and LDL cholesterol[41] and serum leptin levels, and resulted in gain of bone mass after 18–24 months of treatment[42] and improved quality of life[43]. In GH-deficient adults, glucose tolerance and insulin sensitivity tend to worsen within the first few months of GH administration, and improve thereafter, concurrent with the reduction in total and intra-abdominal fat.

THE EFFECTS OF GH REPLACEMENT IN GH-DEFICIENT ELDERLY PERSONS

Various metabolic outcomes have been assessed in short-term GH intervention studies conducted in older persons. Treatment of elderly patients with human GH for 2 weeks increased fat oxidation[44], and decreased total and LDL cholesterol, with an early transient rise in very low-density lipoprotein (VLDL) and triglycerides and no change in high-density lipoprotein (HDL)[45]. Both healthy[46,47] and unhealthy[48,49] older adults treated with GH for periods between 2 weeks[44], 4 weeks[50] and 6 months[46] exhibit dose-dependent increases in nitrogen, phosphate and sodium balance, IGF-I, mid-arm

circumference and/or body weight. An increase in *de novo* protein synthesis was demonstrated after GH administration in postsurgical[44,49] but not healthy[51] older individuals.

Administration of GH for periods up to 6 months leads to substantial, predictable changes in body composition. A landmark study[52] demonstrated that administration of recombinant human GH (rhGH) to healthy men > 60 years old could produce highly significant increases in lean body mass and reductions in total body fat over a 6-month period. However, subsequent trials have failed to demonstrate significant improvements in strength or bone mass in men or women treated with rhGH for up to 12 months[46,53,54].

ADMINISTRATION OF RECOMBINANT HUMAN IGF-I

The effects of IGF-I administration have been assessed in healthy non-obese and obese postmenopausal women, but, to date, have not been reported in elderly men. In older women, short-term (e.g. 4 weeks) administration of high doses of IGF-I improved anabolism and body composition, in association with significant side-effects, whereas low-dose IGF-I promoted lesser, but beneficial, changes in body composition with fewer side-effects[50,55,56]. In contrast, long-term (12 months) administration of IGF-I in low doses did not significantly alter body composition, bone density, or indices of psychological function in older women, suggesting that any benefit from monotherapy with IGF-I may be transient in this population group[57]. Whether similar results would be obtained in selected populations of aged men remains to be determined.

GH SECRETAGOGUES

Several GH releasing peptides and related non-peptide GH secretagogues have been synthesized which exert potent stimulatory effects on pulsatile GH release. These novel GH secretagogues exert anti-somatostatinergic functional effects mediated via an endogenous GH secretagogue receptor[58], which, along with a naturally occurring ligand for this GH secretagogue receptor[59], have recently been identified. The physiological role(s) of both synthetic and naturally occurring GH secretagogue(s), and their contribution to the age-related decline in GH production, remain to be elucidated[60–63].

ADVERSE EFFECTS OF GH THERAPY

Several categories of adverse effects are relatively common during treatment of non-elderly adults with GH, whereas others are as yet unproved but of potential concern[64]. The former group includes effects related to salt and water retention (edema, hypertension, headache, papilledema, pseudotumor cerebri), to arthralgias and carpal tunnel syndrome, and to metabolic dysfunction, whereas the latter group relates to possible stimulation of benign or malignant tissue growth. Short-term administration of GH elicited supraphysiological increases in IGF-I in some older individuals, along with hyperinsulinemia, impaired glucose tolerance, decreased daily sodium excretion and edema[47]. However, in other studies in which elderly men were treated for up to 6 months with low doses of GH, either no adverse effects[48] or modest increases in mean systolic blood pressure and fasting plasma glucose concentrations within the normal range[52] were noted. The adverse effects of GH on salt and water retention appear to be dose-dependent, and are more often evident with supraphysiological increases in circulating IGF-I levels[65]. However, even low-dose regimens of GH administration are non-physiological, and serum GH profiles after parenteral administration of GH differ substantially from the normal, diurnal pattern of pulsatile GH secretion. Although there is no definitive evidence that administration of GH enhances risk for *de novo* carcinogenesis in either GH-deficient children

or young adults[1,64], it is uncertain whether GH replacement in elderly persons with age-related decrements in GH secretion enhances the risk for *de novo* mutagenesis, or of promotion or propagation of pre-existent malignant diseases.

CONCLUSIONS

There is a physiological, age-related decline in spontaneous (nocturnal) GH release and IGF-I levels which begins in the third decade and continues into advanced old age, so that GH and IGF-I measurements in the elderly are often indistinguishable from those in younger adults with pathological GH deficiency. This physiological decline in GH and IGF-I, like pathological GH deficiency in non-elderly adults, is associated with adverse changes in body composition such as diminished muscle and bone mass and increased intra-abdominal fat, with their attendant increased risks of muscle weakness, osteoporosis, obesity, diabetes mellitus, dyslipidemia and cardiovascular disease.

Whether the decline of somatotropic function with age represents a treatable hormone deficiency state with associated adverse outcomes (e.g. muscle weakness, osteoporosis, etc.), or an age-appropriate adaptive response protecting frail older persons from increased susceptibility to homeostatic disturbances, is the focus of much current research. Recent studies suggest that administration of GH to elderly people for periods up to 6 months can reverse or attenuate some of these changes in body composition and metabolic function, but whether these effects lead to improvements in physiological and functional status, and the quality and duration of life, remain to be established. Whether the possible clinical improvements after GH administration will be outweighed by undesirable side-effects, and whether they would be sufficient to justify the economic costs, also deserve further inquiry, as does the potential use of the newer, orally active GH-releasing peptides and related non-peptide secretagogues. Finally, the decision to treat otherwise healthy older people with GH or GH secretagogues will inevitably evoke certain ethical considerations, including a re-examination of the distinction between physiological aging and disease, and a redefinition of what constitutes normative and successful aging.

References

1. Corpas E, Harman SM, Blackman MR. Human growth hormone and human aging. *Endocr Rev* 1993;14:20–39
2. O'Connor KO, Stevens TE, Blackman MR. GH and aging. In Juul A, Jorgenson JOL, eds. *Growth Hormone in Adults*. Cambridge, UK: Cambridge University Press, 1996:323–66
3. Rudman D. Growth hormone, body composition and aging. *J Am Geriatr Soc* 1985;33: 800–7
4. Cronin MJ, Thorner MO. Basic studies with growth hormone-releasing factor. In DeGroot LJ, ed. *Endocrinology*, vol. 1. Philadelphia: WB Saunders, 1989:183–91
5. Reichlin S. Somatostatin. *N Engl J Med* 1983; 309:1495–501
6. van Cauter E, Plat L, Copinschi G. Inter-relations between sleep and somatotropic axis. *Sleep* 1998;21:553–66
7. Van Cauter E, Plat L, Scharf MB, *et al.* Simultaneous stimulation of slow-wave sleep and growth hormone secretion by gamma-hydroxybutyrate in normal young men. *J Clin Invest* 1997;100:745–53
8. Prinz PN, Weitzman ED, Cunningham GR, Karacan I. Plasma growth hormone during sleep in young and aged men. *J Gerontol* 1983;38:519–24
9. Astrom C, Lindholm J. Growth hormone deficient young adults have decreased deep sleep. *Neuroendocrinology* 1990;51:82–4
10. van Cauter E, Leproult R, Plat L. Differential rates of aging of slow wave sleep and REM sleep in normal men: impact on growth hormone and cortisol levels. *J Am Med Assoc* 2000;284:861–8
11. Hattori N, Kurahachi H, Ikekubo K, *et al.* Effects of sex and age on serum GH binding protein levels in normal adults. *Clin Endocrinol (Oxf)* 1991;35:295–7
12. Ooi GT. Insulin-like growth factor-binding proteins (IGFBPs): more than just 1,2,3. *Mol Cell Endocrinal* 1990;71:C39–43
13. Guler HP, Zapf J, Schmid C, Froesch ER. Insulin-like growth factors I and II in healthy man. Estimations of half-lives and production rates. *Acta Endocrinol (Copenh)* 1989;121: 753–8
14. Clemmons DR, Van Wyk JJ. Factors controlling blood concentration of somatomedin C. *Clin Endocrinol Metab* 1984;13:113–43
15. Rudman D, Nagraj HS, Mattson D, Erve RR, Rudman IW. Hyposomatomedinemia in the nursing home patient. *J Am Geriatr Soc* 1986; 34:427–30
16. Abbassi AA, Drinka PJ, Mattson DE, Rudman D. Low circulating levels of insulin-like growth factors and testosterone in chronically institutionalized elderly men. *J Am Geriatr Soc* 1993;41:975–82
17. Florini JR, Prinz PN, Vitirello MV, Hintz RL. Somatomedin-C levels in healthy young and old men. Relationships to peak and 24-hour integrated levels of growth hormone. *J Gerontol* 1985;40:2–7
18. Corpas E, Harman SM, Blackman MR. Serum IGF-binding protein-3 is related to IGF-I, but not to spontaneous GH release, in healthy old men. *Horm Metab Res* 1992;24: 543–5
19. Ho KY, Evans WS, Blizzard RM, *et al.* Effects of sex and age on 24-hour profile of growth hormone secretion in men: importance of endogenous estradiol concentrations. *J Clin Endocrinol Metab* 1987;64:51–8
20. Corpas E, Harman SM, Piñeyro MA, *et al.* GHRH 1-29 twice daily reverses the decreased GH and IGF-I levels in old men. *J Clin Endocrinol Metab* 1992;75:530–5

21. Iranmanesh A, Lizarralde G, Veldhuis JD. Age and relative adiposity are specific negative determinants of the frequency and amplitude of growth hormone (GH) secretory bursts and the half-life of endogenous GH in healthy men. *J Clin Endocrinol Metab* 1991;73:1081–8

22. Blackman MR, Christmas C, Münzer T, *et al.* Influence of testosterone on the GH–IGF-I axis in healthy elderly men. In Veldhuis JD, Giustina A, eds. *Sex-Steroid Interactions with Growth Hormone*. New York: Springer-Verlag, 1999:44–53

23. Press M, Tamborlane WV, Thorner MO, *et al.* Pituitary responses to growth hormone releasing factor in diabetes: failure of glucose-mediated suppression. *Diabetes* 1984;33: 804–6

24. Ho KY, Veldhuis J, Johnson ML, *et al.* Fasting enhances growth hormone secretion and amplifies the complex rhythms of growth hormone secretion in man. *J Clin Invest* 1988; 81:968–75

25. Meneilly GS, Cheung E, Tuokko H. Altered responses to hypoglycemia of healthy elderly people. *J Clin Endocrinol Metab* 1994;78: 1341–8

26. Williams T, Berelowitz M, Jaffe SN, *et al.* Impaired growth hormone (GH) responses to GH-releasing factor (GRF) in obesity: a pituitary defect reversed with weight reduction. *N Engl J Med* 1984;311:1403–7

27. Iranmanesh A, Lizarralde G, Veldhuis JD. Age and relative adiposity are specific negative determinants of the frequency and amplitude of growth hormone (GH) secretory bursts and the half-life of endogenous GH in healthy men. *J Clin Endocrinol Metab* 1991;73:1081–8

28. Copeland KC, Colletti RB, Devlin JD, McAuliffe TL. The relationship between insulin-like growth factor-1, adiposity and aging. *Metabolism* 1990;39:584–7

29. Hagberg JM, Seals DR, Yerg JE, *et al.* Metabolic responses to exercise in young and old athletes and sedentary men. *J Appl Physiol* 1988;65:900–8

30. Rasmussen MH, Frystyk J, Andersen T, *et al.* The impact of obesity, fat distribution and energy restriction on insulin-like growth factor-1 (IGF-1), IGF-binding protein-3,

insulin and growth hormone. *Metabolism* 1994;43:315–19

31. Craig BW, Brown R, Everhart J. Effects of progressive resistance training on growth hormone and testosterone levels in young and elderly subjects. *Mech Ageing Dev* 1989;49: 159–69

32. Poehlman ET, Copeland KC. Influence of physical activity on insulin-like growth factor in healthy younger and older men. *J Clin Endocrinol Metab* 1990;71:1468–73

33. Pyka G, Taaffe DR, Marcus R. Effect of a sustained program of resistance training on the acute growth hormone response to resistance exercise in older adults. *Horm Metab Res* 1994;26:330–3

34. Cuneo RC, Salomon F, Wiles CM, Sönksen PH. Skeletal muscle performance in adults with growth hormone deficiency. *Horm Metab Res* 1990;33(Suppl 4):55–60

35. Jackson HA, Kleerkoper M. Osteoporosis in men: diagnosis, pathophysiology, and prevention. *Medicine* 1990;69:137–52

36. Nguyen TV, Eisman JA, Kelly PJ, Sambrook PN. Risk factors for osteoporotic fractures in elderly men. *Am J Epidemiol* 1996;144: 255–63

37. Cuneo R, Salomon F, Wiles CM, *et al.* Growth hormone treatment in growth hormone-deficient adults. II. Effects on exercise performance. *J Appl Physiol* 1991;70: 695–700

38. Johannsson G, Grimby G, Sunnerhagen KS, Bengtsson B-A. Two years of growth hormone (GH) treatment increase isometric and isokinetic muscle strength in GH-deficient adults. *J Clin Endocrinol Metab* 1997;82: 2877–84

39. Amato G, Carella C, Fazio S, *et al.* Body composition, bone metabolism, and heart structure and function in growth hormone (GH) deficient adults before and after GH replacement therapy at low doses. *J Clin Endocrinol Metab* 1993;77:1671–6

40. Gertner JM. Effects of growth hormone on body fat distribution in adults. *Horm Res* 1993;40:10–15

41. Cuneo RC, Salomon F, Watts GF, *et al.* Growth hormone treatment improves serum lipids and lipoproteins in adults with growth

hormone deficiency. *Metabolism* 1993;42: 1519–23

42. Johannsson G, Rosen T, Bosaeus I, *et al.* Two years of growth hormone (GH) treatment increases bone mineral content and density in hypopituitary patients with adult-onset GH deficiency. *J Clin Endocrinol Metab* 1996;81: 2865–73

43. Burman P, Broman JE, Hettat J, *et al.* Quality of life in adults with growth hormone (GH) deficiency: response to treatment with recombinant human GH in a placebo-controlled 21-month trial. *J Clin Endocrinol Metab* 1995;80:3585–90

44. Ponting GA, Halliday D, Teale JD, Sim AJW. Postoperative positive nitrogen balance with intravenous hyponutrition on growth hormone. *Lancet* 1988;2:438–9

45. Oscarsson J, Ottosson M, Wiklund O, *et al.* Low dose continuously infused growth hormone results in increased lipoprotein A and decreased low density lipoprotein cholesterol concentrations in middle aged men. *Clin Endocrinol (Oxf)* 1994;41:109–16

46. Holloway L, Butterfield G, Hintz R, *et al.* Effects of recombinant human growth hormone on metabolic indices, body composition, and bone turnover in healthy elderly women. *J Clin Endocrinol Metab* 1994;79: 470–9

47. Marcus R, Butterfield G, Holloway L, *et al.* Effects of short term administration of recombinant human growth hormone to elderly people. *J Clin Endocrinol Metab* 1990;70:519–27

48. Kaiser FE, Silver AJ, Morley JE. The effect of recombinant human growth hormone on malnourished older individuals. *J Am Geriatr Soc* 1991;39:235–40

49. Binnerts A, Wilson JHP, Lamberts SWJ. The effects of human growth hormone administration in elderly adults with recent weight loss. *J Clin Endocrinol Metab* 1988;67:1312–16

50. Thompson J, Butterfield GE, Marcus R, *et al.* The effects of recombinant human insulin-like growth factor-I and growth hormone on body composition in elderly women. *J Clin Endocrinol Metab* 1995;80:1845–52

51. Zachwieja JJ, Bier DM, Yarasheski KE. Growth hormone administration in older

adults: effects on albumin synthesis. *Am J Physiol* 1994;266:E840–4

52. Rudman D, Feller AG, Nagraj HS, *et al.* Effect of human growth hormone in men over 60 years old. *N Engl J Med* 1990;323:1–6

53. Papadakis M, Grady D, Black D, *et al.* Growth hormone replacement in healthy older men improves body composition but not functional ability. *Ann Intern Med* 1996; 124:708–16

54. Taafe DR, Pruitt L, Reim J, *et al.* Effect of recombinant human growth hormone on the muscle strength response to resistance exercise in elderly men. *J Clin Endocrinol Metab* 1994;79:1361–6

55. Butterfield GE, Thompson J, Rennie MJ, *et al.* Effect of rhGH and rhIGF-I treatment on protein utilization in elderly women. *Am J Physiol* 1997;272:E94–9

56. Thompson J, Butterfield GE, Gylfadottir UK, *et al.* Effects of human growth hormone, insulin-like growth factor-I, and diet and exercise on body composition of obese postmenopausal women. *J Clin Endocrinol Metab* 1998;83:1477–84

57. Friedlander AI, Butterfield GE, Moynihan S, *et al.* One year of insulin-like growth factor-I treatment does not affect bone density, body composition, or psychological measures in postmenopausal women. *J Clin Endocrinol Metab* 2001;86:1496–503

58. Howard AD, Feighner SD, Cully DF, *et al.* A receptor in pituitary and hypothalamus that functions in growth hormone release. *Science* 1996;273:974–7

59. Kojima M, Hosoda H, Date Y, *et al.* Ghrelin is a growth-hormone-releasing acylated peptide from stomach. *Nature (London)* 1999; 402:656–60

60. Copinschi G, Leproult R, Van Onderbergen A, *et al.* Prolonged oral treatment with MK-677, a novel growth hormone secretagogue, improves sleep quality in man. *Neuroendocrinology* 1997;66:278–86

61. Fuh VL, Bach MA. Growth hormone secretagogues: mechanisms of action and use in aging. *Growth Horm IGF Res* 1998;8: 13–20

62. Murphy MG, Bach MA, Plotkin D, *et al.* Oral administration of the growth hormone

secretagogue MK-677, markers of bone turnover in healthy and functionally impaired elderly adults. The MK-677 Study Group. *J Bone Miner Res* 1999;14:1182–8

63. Murphy MG, Weiss S, McClung M, *et al.* Effects of alendronate and MK-677 (a growth hormone secretagogue), individually and in combination, on markers of bone turnover and bone mineral density in postmenopausal osteoporotic women. *J Clin Endocrinol Metab* 2001;86:1116–25

64. Consensus: critical evaluation of the safety of recombinant human growth hormone administration: statement from the Growth Hormone Research Society. *J Clin Endocrinol Metab* 2001;86:1868–70

65. Cohn L, Feller AG, Draper MW, *et al.* Carpal tunnel syndrome and gynecomastia during growth hormone treatment of elderly men with low circulating IGF-1 concentrations. *Clin Endocrinol (Oxf)* 1993;39:417–25

13 The thyroid

Jerome M. Hershman, MD, and Mary H. Samuels, MD

SERUM THYROID HORMONE AND THYROTROPIN CONCENTRATIONS IN THE ELDERLY

Thyroid function has been extensively studied in the elderly. Early studies reported significant alterations in thyroid hormone and thyrotropin (TSH) levels, as well as blunted TSH responses to exogenous thyrotropin-releasing-hormone (TRH) in older subjects. However, more recent studies revealed that most of these alterations are due to the effects of illness and medications on thyroid hormone levels. Acute or chronic nonthyroidal illness decreases serum tri-iodothyronine (T_3) levels, and more severe illness also decreases serum thyroxine (T_4) levels. Serum TSH levels are usually normal, but decrease as the illness becomes more severe, and TSH responses to TRH are blunted. In addition glucocorticoids and dopamine reduce TSH levels and amiodarone and propranolol block conversion of T_4 to T_3, thus elevating serum T_4 and lowering T_3 levels. For these reasons, interpretation of thyroid function tests in the elderly must include an assessment of possible effects of nonthyroidal illness or medications.

In healthy elderly subjects, T_4 production decreases by approximately 25%, but serum T_4 levels are unchanged, due to reductions in T_4 clearance. T_3 production and degradation decrease by approximately 30%, and serum T_3 levels may be slightly lower compared to young subjects while remaining in the normal range[1]. One study reported decreased 24-hour mean serum TSH levels in healthy elderly men, suggesting that 24-hour TSH secretion may be decreased in the elderly[2]. TSH response to TRH are normal or decreased in healthy elderly subjects.

HYPOTHYROIDISM

Prevalence

The prevalence of overt hypothyroidism in the elderly ranges between 0.6 and 3%, depending on the population studied. In most studies, the prevalence is lower among men than among women, because of the increased rate of autoimmune hypothyroidism in women[3]. Subclinical (or mild) hypothyroidism, defined as an elevated serum TSH and normal serum free T_4 concentration, occurs with increasing frequency as subjects age, and is present in approximately 8–15% of the elderly population. Subclinical hypothyroidism is also more common in women (range 7–21% for women vs. 2–15% for men)[4–6]. Elderly subjects with subclinical hypothyroidism have at least a 2–3% annualized rate of progression to overt hypothyroidism. This rate increases to 4–5% per year if antithyroid antibodies are present[7].

Clinical features

It is a common impression that the typical clinical features of hypothyroidism are less pronounced in the elderly. However, one study that addressed this question systematically found that most symptoms and signs of hypothyroidism were present to similar degrees in young and old hypothyroid patients[8]. Specifically, fatigue, weakness, mental status changes, depression, hoarseness, dry skin, decreased heart rate and slowed deep tendon reflexes were equally common in both age groups. However, elderly patients had fewer complaints of weight gain, cold intolerance, paresthesias and muscle cramps. Thus, it appears that the major difficulty in diagnosing hypothyroidism in the elderly is not the lack of symptoms, but rather their non-specific nature. Clinical findings of hypothyroidism in the elderly are often attributed to medical illnesses, medication use, depression or the aging process.

Causes

Most hypothyroidism in the elderly is due to autoimmune (Hashimoto's) thyroiditis, which explains the increased prevalence among elderly women, compared with men[5,9]. There is an age-dependent increase in the prevalence of antithyroid antibodies; 16% of older women and 9% of older men have antithyroid peroxidase antibodies. Between 40 and 70% of older subjects with elevated TSH levels have antithyroid antibodies, although only a minority of older subjects with antithyroid antibodies have elevated TSH levels. Euthyroid subjects with positive antithyroid antibody titers have increased rates of development of subclinical and eventually overt hypothyroidism.

Apart from Hashimoto's thyroiditis, other causes of hypothyroidism in the elderly include thyroid surgery or radiation therapy to the neck, radioiodine treatment of Graves' disease, recovery from subacute or silent thyroiditis, and under-replacement of thyroxine in subjects with known hypothyroidism. In addition, drugs such as lithium, iodine-containing compounds (for example, radiocontrast agents or amiodarone) and cytokines can lead to hypothyroidism.

The issue of hypothyroidism due to iodinated radiocontrast agents or amiodarone is particularly important in the elderly, since older patients are more likely to receive these agents. TSH levels should be monitored routinely in subjects receiving amiodarone, or in subjects with suggestive symptoms within 6 months of radiocontrast administration.

Treatment

Hypothyroidism in an elderly patient should be treated with synthetic levothyroxine, rather than other thyroid hormone preparations such as desiccated thyroid extract or combinations of L-thyroxine and L-tri-iodothyronine. The latter preparations contain unacceptably high levels of tri-iodothyronine, which can precipitate or exacerbate cardiac conditions. The goal of treatment is attainment of a normal serum TSH level. The replacement dose of L-thyroxine is lower than replacement doses used in young subjects, since the elderly have decreased metabolism of thyroxine[9]. It is usually prudent to begin with a low starting does of L-thyroxine (25 μg per day or less), especially in a patient with long-standing hypothyroidism and/or known cardiac disease. The dose is gradually increased every 4–8 weeks until the TSH is normalized. In rare cases, the development of angina precludes the use of full replacement doses of thyroxine. In these cases, it is appropriate to consider surgical therapy or angioplasty while the patient is still hypothyroid[10], followed by attempts to achieve euthyroidism once the angina is well controlled.

It is unclear whether all elderly patients with subclinical hypothyroidism should be treated. Such treatment would prevent progression to overt hypothyroidism and treat the subtle tissue effects of mild hypothyroidism, including neurocognitive symptoms, cardiovascular effects and hyperlipidemia. Patients with suggestive symptoms, abnormal cardiac function or hyperlipidemia may benefit most from therapy for subclinical hypothyroidism, but this has not been rigorously tested.

HYPERTHYROIDISM

Prevalence

Hyperthyroidism occurs in 0.2–2% of the elderly population, with somewhat higher rates in elderly women compared with elderly men[4,5,11]. Subclinical hyperthyroidism, defined as a suppressed serum level of TSH with normal free thyroid hormone concentrations, occurs in about 2% of elderly subjects[1,11], with a variable progression to overt hyperthyroidism[11,12].

Clinical features

It is clear that elderly hyperthyroid subjects do not manifest the same degree of adrenergic symptoms and signs as younger hyperthyroid subjects[13,14]. Older patients have decreased rates of fatigue, weakness, nervousness, sweating, heat intolerance, hyperphagia, diarrhea, tremor, tachycardia and hyperactive reflexes, compared with young patients with hyperthyroidism. Instead, older patients tend to present with confusion, anorexia and atrial fibrillation. This phenomenon has been termed 'apathetic hyperthyroidism' in the elderly. Such patients can be mistakenly diagnosed with cancer, heart disease, dementia or gastrointestinal illness rather than hyperthyroidism, leading to extensive and unnecessary testing.

Causes

The causes of hyperthyroidism in the elderly are similar to the causes of hyperthyroidism in young subjects, and include Graves' disease, toxic multinodular goiter, toxic adenoma, subacute or silent thyroiditis, or over-replacement with thyroid hormone preparations[7,15]. Graves' disease is less common in the elderly, while toxic multinodular goiter is more common. In addition, the development of hyperthyroidism in an elderly patient often occurs after administration of amiodarone or an iodine-containing radiocontrast agent.

Risks

There are two specific risks associated with hyperthyroidism that are particularly important in older patients. First, overt hyperthyroidism has marked effects on the cardiovascular system, including enhanced myocardial contractility, accelerated heart rate, increased cardiac output and peripheral vasodilatation. This may lead to increased myocardial oxygen demand, cardiac hypertrophy or angina in older patients. In addition, the risk of atrial fibrillation is increased by overt or subclinical hyperthyroidism, especially in older subjects[16]. Results from the Framingham Study showed that 28% of subjects with subclinical hyperthyroidism developed atrial fibrillation over 10 years, compared with 11% of age-matched euthyroid subjects[16]. Second, hyperthyroidism leads to excess bone resorption and the development of osteoporosis, especially in women[17]. It may also contribute to osteoporosis in elderly men.

Treatment

The treatment of hyperthyroidism in the elderly depends on the cause of the disease, severity of the hyperthyroidism and condition of the patient. Graves' disease is treated by radioactive iodine-131 or thionamide therapy. Toxic multinodular goiters and toxic adenomas are treated with radioactive iodine (at higher doses than those used to treat Graves' disease) or surgery, with the choice depending on the patient's suitability for surgery and the presence of any worrisome nodules that would warrant excision.

The decision whether to treat subclinical hyperthyroidism is difficult, since treatment options are complicated and carry some risks, and since the overall risk of subclinical hyperthyroidism has not been well quantified. A free

T_3 level should initially be obtained to rule out T_3-toxicosis. One should decide whether to treat subclinical hyperthyroidism based on the presence of symptoms (remembering that hyperthyroidism may be masked in elderly patients), risks for osteoporosis, and risks for atrial fibrillation or other cardiac events. In some cases, it may be prudent to initiate a trial of antithyroid drug therapy. This affords the physician and the patient a chance to see whether symptoms and other parameters improve with treatment of the subclinical hyperthyroidism.

THYROID NODULES

Prevalence

Thyroid nodules, either solitary or multiple, increase in frequency with aging. Studies show that 90% of women over age 60 and 60% of men over age 80 have a nodular thyroid gland. The prevalence of thyroid nodules is much higher in women than in men. Thyroid nodules in asymptomatic individuals ('incidentalomas') have been identified frequently by ultrasonography, which is much more sensitive than palpation. The prevalence of incidentalomas was 67% by high resolution ultrasonography and only 21% by neck palpation[18]. A large autopsy series showed that 50% of the population with no known history of thyroid disease had discrete nodules, and in 35% the nodules were greater than 2 cm in diameter[19].

Clinical evaluation

Evaluation of the thyroid nodule focuses on the detection of malignancy. Although thyroid nodules are more frequent in women, the likelihood of malignancy is somewhat higher in men. Radiation exposure during childhood predisposes to thyroid nodules and thyroid carcinoma, but the latency period probably does not exceed 50 years, so that the chance of radiation-induced thyroid cancer from childhood exposure is low in the elderly. A family history of thyroid cancer suggests familial medullary thyroid cancer as a component of multiple endocrine neoplasia (MEN) type 2 or familial papillary cancer. Multinodular goiter is also prevalent in many families.

Most thyroid nodules are asymptomatic. Hemorrhage into a thyroid nodule or cyst may cause rapid enlargement and pain. Rapid growth of a nodule over a period of several weeks is suspicious of malignancy. Persistent hoarseness may result from recurrent laryngeal paralysis by cancer or a large multinodular goiter.

On physical examination, a firm fixed nodule is more likely to be malignant, but many differentiated carcinomas are soft. Lymphadenopathy suggests malignancy. The distinction between a solitary nodule and multinodular goiter by neck palpation is limited. In approximately 50% of cases of a clinically solitary nodule on palpation, the lesion was subsequently found to be a dominant nodule in a multinodular goiter on histological examination[20]. The relative risk of cancer in solitary versus multinodular thyroid glands is controversial. Many studies have reported lower rates of thyroid carcinoma in palpable multinodular glands (5–13%), compared with the solitary nodules (9–25%), but other studies have found similar incidences of cancer in solitary nodules and in multinodular glands.

Diagnostic tests

A low serum TSH concentration suggests the presence of either an autonomously functioning adenoma, or a toxic multinodular goiter. Elevated antiperoxidase and antithyroglobulin antibody titers indicate lymphocytic thyroiditis, which may present as a nodule. The serum thyroglobulin level is not a useful test to distinguish benign from malignant nodules, because it is increased with any goitrous process.

Thyroid ultrasound scanning is a non-invasive test that discriminates cystic from solid lesions. It has proved useful to differentiate thyroid from non-thyroid neck masses and to localize nodules deep within the gland. In such cases it can be used to guide fine-needle aspiration biopsy. Cystic nodules constitute 15–25% of all thyroid nodules, and a significant fraction may harbor papillary carcinomas[21].

Fine-needle aspiration (FNA) biopsy provides reliable information and is the most effective method of diagnosing the cause of the nodule. Utilization of FNA has dramatically reduced the need for surgery to diagnose benign thyroid nodules. In a large series of patients with FNA biopsy of the thyroid, benign cytology was found in 69% (mainly colloid goiter), malignant cytology in 3.5% and suspicious cytology in 10%[22]. The suspicious category consists of variants of follicular neoplasm, but follicular adenomas are about ten fold more common than follicular carcinomas. Ultrasound-guided FNA is used for sampling of impalpable nodules larger than 1.5 cm and the solid component of cystic nodules. In patients with nodules that are follicular lesions, radioiodine scan should be performed. 'Hot' or functional nodules are rarely malignant.

Management

Treatment of the thyroid nodule depends on the functional state of the nodule and the cytological diagnosis of the FNA biopsy. The hyperfunctioning 'hot' nodule is treated with radioiodine ablation or surgery. The vast majority of thyroid nodules are benign and can be managed medically. Medical management with thyroid hormone suppressive therapy is based on the assumption that growth of the nodule is TSH dependent. Spontaneous regression of thyroid nodules may occur. L-Thyroxine suppressive therapy is useful for nodules that do not decrease in size over several months of initial observation, but is contraindicated in elderly men with cardiac disease. Generally, patients are followed by palpation at intervals of 3–4 months. Ultrasound examination can be performed to assess growth or shrinkage of a nodule if more objective documentation is required.

If the cytological diagnosis indicates malignancy or is strongly suspicious for malignancy, the nodule should be removed surgically.

THYROID CANCER

Thyroid cancer accounts for 0.6–1.6% of all cancers in the USA, and mortality from thyroid cancer is less than 0.5% of all cancer deaths. Thyroid cancer is classified into five major types: papillary, follicular, medullary and anaplastic, and thyroid lymphoma.

Papillary carcinoma is the most common type of thyroid cancer and accounts for 80% of all thyroid cancers. Although its prognosis is generally favorable, it is much more aggressive in the elderly. Surgery, either near-total or total thyroidectomy, is the initial treatment of choice for papillary carcinoma. Radioiodine therapy is used as an adjunct to surgery to treat patients with residual or recurrent papillary cancer in the neck[23]. The prophylactic use of radioactive iodine after surgery reduces the mortality rate and increases survival; it is generally given to any older person with papillary cancer.

Thyroid hormone in a suppressive dose is prescribed after thyroidectomy to reduce recurrence. TSH stimulates growth of thyroid tumors that contain TSH receptors. The does of thyroxine should be adjusted to keep the TSH suppressed without causing clinical thyrotoxicosis.

Follicular thyroid carcinoma accounts for about 5–10% of all thyroid cancers in the USA and occurs more frequently in the elderly. Hurthle-cell carcinoma, a variant of follicular thyroid carcinoma, carries a poorer prognosis. Tumor recurrence in distant sites is more frequently seen with follicular than with papillary carcinoma, and occurs with higher prevalence in highly invasive tumors. Treatment includes total thyroidectomy, and iodine-131 therapy to ablate residual tumor. Radioiodine is the principal treatment of metastatic tumors. If the tumor does not concentrate the isotope, external radiation may be effective. As with papillary carcinoma, thyroxine therapy should be given to suppress serum TSH levels to the subnormal range.

Medullary carcinoma accounts for 2–4% of thyroid cancers and is derived from the calcitonin-secreting cells or parafollicular cells.

Elevated serum calcitonin levels establish the diagnosis and correlate with tumor mass. About 20–30% are familial tumors and are associated with other endocrine neoplasias (MEN 2A or 2B). The recognition of point mutations in RET proto-oncogene on chromosome 10 has enhanced the ability to detect these neoplasms at an early and potentially curable stage in suspected family members. Approximately 70–80% of medullary carcinoma is sporadic and diagnosed later in life, mostly after age 50 years[24]. The preferred treatment consists of total thyroidectomy and a modified radical neck dissection on the side of the tumor.

Anaplastic thyroid carcinoma is the most aggressive and lethal cancer. It accounts for 2% of thyroid cancer. In 28–70% of patients, there is a previous differentiated thyroid carcinoma[25]. The peak occurrence is in the seventh decade; nearly all patients are 60 years or older. It presents with a rapidly growing thyroid mass. Treatment includes surgery followed by external radiation and chemotherapy, but only a small percentage survive more than 1 year.

Thyroid lymphoma accounts for about 1% of thyroid malignancies and is almost always accompanied by chronic lymphocytic thyroiditis. The patients are usually over 60 years of age, and there is a female preponderance. This tumor nearly always arises from B-cell lymphocytes. It presents as a rapidly enlarging thyroid mass in a patient with a long history of a goiter or diagnosis of Hashimoto's disease. FNA may suggest the diagnosis, but definitive diagnosis usually requires an open biopsy. Surgical removal of the lymphoma by total thyroidectomy is unwise. Treatment with external radiation and four to six courses of chemotherapy nearly always produces a permanent remission[26].

References

1. Hershman JM, Pekary AE, Berg L, *et al.* Serum thyrotropin and thyroid hormone levels in elderly and middle-aged euthyroid persons. *J Am Geriatr Soc* 1993;41:823–8
2. Barreca T, Franceschini R, Messina V, *et al.* 24-Hour thyroid-stimulating hormone secretory pattern in elderly men. *Gerontology* 1985;31:119–23
3. Sawin CT, Castelli WP, Hershman JM, *et al.* The aging thyroid. Thyroid deficiency in the Framingham Study. *Arch Intern Med* 1985; 145:1386–8
4. Livingston EH, Hershman JM, Sawin CT, Yoshikawa TT. Prevalence of thyroid disease and abnormal thyroid tests in older hospitalized and ambulatory persons. *J Am Geriatr Soc* 1987;35:109–14
5. Tunbridge WMG, Evered DC, Hall R, *et al.* The spectrum of thyroid disease in a community: the Whickham survey. *Clin Endocrinol* 1977;7:481–93
6. Canaris GJ, Manowitz MR, Mayor G, Ridgway EC. The Colorado thyroid disease prevalence study. *Arch Intern Med* 2000;160: 526–34
7. Vanderpump MPJ, Tunbridge WMG, French JM, *et al.* The incidence of thyroid disorders in the community: a twenty-year follow-up of the Whickham survey. *Clin Endocrinol* 1995;43:55–68
8. Doucet J, Trivalle C, Chassagne PH, *et al.* Does age play a role in the clinical presentation of hypothyroidism? *J Am Geriatr Soc* 1994;42:984–6
9. Sawin CT, Bigos ST, Land S, Bacharach P. The aging thyroid. Relationship between elevated serum thyrotropin level and thyroid antibodies in elderly patients. *Am J Med* 1985;79:591–4
10. Ladenson PW, Levin AA, Ridgway EC, Daniels GH. Complications of surgery in hypothyroid patients. *Am J Med* 1984;77: 261–6

11. Sawin CT, Geller A, Kaplan MM, *et al*. Low serum thyrotropin (thyroid stimulating hormone) in older persons without hyperthyroidism. *Arch Intern Med* 1991;151:165–8

12. Stott DJ, McLellan AR, Finlayson J, *et al*. Elderly patients with suppressed serum TSH but normal free thyroid hormone levels usually have mild thyroid overactivity and are at increased risk of developing overt hyperthyroidism. Q *J Med* 1991;285:77–84

13. Davis PJ, Davis FB. Hyperthyroidism in patients over the age of 60 years. Clinical features in 85 patients. *Medicine* 1974;53: 161–79

14. Tibaldi JM, Barzel US, Albin J, Surks M. Thyrotoxicosis in the very old. *Am J Med* 1986;81:619–22

15. Charkes ND. The many causes of subclinical hyperthyroidism. *Thyroid* 1996;6:391–6

16. Sawin CT, Geller A, Wolf PA, *et al*. Low serum thyrotropin concentrations as a risk factor for atrial fibrillation in older persons. *N Engl J Med* 1994;331:1249–52

17. Lee MS, Kim SY, Lee MC, *et al*. Negative correlation between the change in bone mineral density and serum osteocalcin in patients with hyperthyroidism. *J Clin Endocrinol Metab* 1990;70:766–70

18. Ezzat S, Sarti DA, Cain DR, Braunstein GD. Thyroid incidentalomas. Prevalence by palpation and ultrasonography. *Arch Intern Med* 1994;154:1838–40

19. Mortensen JD, Woolner LB, Bennett WA. Gross and microscopic findings in clinically normal thyroid glands. *J Clin Endocrinol Metab* 1955;15:1270–6

20. Wheeler MH. Investigation of the solitary thyroid nodule. *Clin Endocrinol* 1996;44:245–7

21. Mazzaferri EL. Management of a solitary thyroid nodule. *N Engl J Med* 1993;328: 553–9

22. Gharib H, Goellner JR. Fine needle aspiration biopsy of the thyroid: an appraisal. *Ann Intern Med* 1993;118:282–9

23. Dulgeroff AJ, Hershman JM. Medical therapy for differentiated thyroid carcinoma. *Endocr Rev* 1994;15:500–15

24. Sizemore GW. Medullary carcinoma of the thyroid gland. *Semin Oncol* 1987;14:306–14

25. Ain K. Anaplastic thyroid cancer. *Thyroid* 1998;8:715–26

26. Matsuzuka F, Miyauchi A, Katayama S, *et al*. Clinical aspects of primary thyroid lymphoma: diagnosis and treatment based on our experience of 119 cases. *Thyroid* 1993;3: 93–9

Section IV

Diabetes mellitus

Derek Le Roith, MD, PhD

In the USA, it has been estimated that 5–6% of the population have type 2 diabetes. In certain communities, the percentage increases to almost 20% with aging, and estimates suggest that almost one-third of all cases of type 2 diabetes are undiagnosed. The etiology for this increase in type 2 diabetes with age has not yet been defined, but the aging process is associated with increased levels of insulin resistance as well as deterioration in β-cell function. From a practical point of view, this requires the geriatrician to be even more diligent in correctly diagnosing type 2 diabetes and instituting therapy for this common disorder, which is associated with various ramifications and complications. The diagnostic criteria for this disease have recently been altered to include those individuals who are also prone to microvascular complications secondary to elevated blood glucose levels. Currently, a fasting plasma glucose level of 126 mg/dl or more is considered to be the minimum criterion for the diagnosis of diabetes, whereas a maximal plasma glucose level after a meal or post-glucose challenge remains unchanged at 200 mg/dl. The challenge to the physician, of course, is to provide a balanced treatment. If instituted early, treatment will prevent the micro- and macrovascular complications of diabetes. However, the serious side-effects of these regimens must be carefully monitored, especially in the elderly. Most elderly patients take multiple medications for a number of medical disorders, a fact that clearly complicates management of their disease. Obviously, potential interactions of drugs must be carefully considered. In addition, prescribing multiple drugs must be weighed against the fact that increasing the number of daily tablets the patient requires generally reduces the overall compliance level. Furthermore, many patients today are also using alternative forms of medications including herbs and other 'natural products', many of which can affect the metabolism and efficacy of prescribed medications.

In this section, we present a number of important aspects of diabetes in the aging male. Understanding the pathophysiology of this disorder is an essential prerequisite to appropriate management, as is an understanding of the multiple complications that result from diabetes. Today there are numerous medications available to treat diabetes, but each one needs to be used with caution in the older patient, particularly to avoid the devastating effects of hypoglycemia. Quality of life issues that deal with the patient's feeling of 'well-being' are now being given increased emphasis, in addition to the degree of glucose control. The authors hope that the reader will benefit from these chapters and that our management of the aging diabetic population will afford them continued health and longevity.

14 Pathophysiology of diabetes in the aging male

Nir Barzilai, MD, and Ilan Gabriely, MD

INTRODUCTION

The incidence of type 2 diabetes mellitus is increased approximately three-fold in the elderly population, and is often under-diagnosed[1-4]. The prevalence of the disease is about 3–5% in the 4–5th decade of life and increases to 20–30% in the 6–7th decade in both men and women[2-4]. Thus, it seems that the prevalence of type 2 diabetes increases by 7–10-fold with the transition from the 4th to the 7th decade of life. In addition, many elderly subjects fall into the category of impaired glucose tolerance (IGT; fasting plasma glucose 110–125 mg/dl); hence, the overall prevalence of abnormal glucose metabolism in this population is even greater and probably underestimated[5].

The most characteristic abnormality in glucose metabolism seen in aging is a progressive rise in fasting and postprandial plasma insulin concentrations, which suggests that aging is an insulin-resistance state[1,2,3,6]. The liver maintains normal glucose levels postprandially and during fasting; however, with aging more insulin is required to regulate hepatic glucose production appropriately and avoid hyperglycemia[7-11]. Failure of the β cell adequately to secrete insulin in the face of hepatic and peripheral (muscle and fat) insulin resistance leads to the development of diabetes mellitus[4,7]. Moreover, hyperglycemia itself causes a further

deterioration in muscle and liver sensitivity to insulin and a further impairment in β-cell function (a phenomenon commonly known as 'glucose toxicity'), which leads to a worsening of glucose tolerance in the diabetic patient[12].

Insulin resistance and hyperinsulinemia are associated with increases in total and visceral fat mass, which are typical of aging[13-15]. Insulin resistance *per se* is considered to be an independent risk factor for the development of coronary artery disease[16]. Furthermore, insulin resistance has been associated with hypertension, dyslipidemia and dysfibrinolysis (the insulin resistance syndrome or syndrome X), which is considered to be a major risk factor for atherosclerotic cardiovascular disease, cancer and all-cause mortality in both men and women, and is therefore associated with decreased life expectancy[17-19]. A strong correlation between obesity and insulin resistance has been demonstrated in a variety of epidemiological studies (reviewed in reference 20); the fact that insulin sensitivity improves with weight loss in obese patients suggests a causality relationship between obesity and insulin resistance. Since changes in body composition are observed with aging, it is speculated that the changes in body composition *per se*, i.e. increased fat mass (and not the process of aging), are responsible for the development of insulin resistance and consequently for the increased prevalence of type 2 diabetes with aging[21]. The smaller proportion of type 2 diabetes in men compared to women (approximately 40 : 60%, according to the 1989 National Health Interview Survey) may be explained by the relatively smaller proportion of fat mass in men[22]. However, no clear differences in the pathophysiology of type 2 diabetes have been noted between men and women. Recent advances in the understanding of the pathophysiology of type 2 diabetes in the elderly have led to the development of new therapeutic strategies aimed to affect specific abnormalities (such as peripheral insulin resistance, increased hepatic glucose production and ß-cell failure), as discussed in other chapters in this section.

CHANGES IN BODY COMPOSITION WITH AGING

The process of aging is associated with an increase in the prevalence of obesity. Approximately half of the US population over the age of 50 is obese[23]. An increase in fat mass typically occurs between ages 30 and 70, and the ratio of fat mass to lean body mass (LBM) increases throughout the human life span[14,15]. Increased visceral fat, in particular, is a common and typical change in body composition observed with aging, demonstrated clinically (surgically, and by computed tomography and magnetic resonance imaging) and epidemiologically (increased waist/hip ratio[24,25]). Importantly, the increase in visceral fat associated with aging is independent of body mass index (BMI), which may be normal[25]. Numerous studies in subjects of all ages have demonstrated that increased visceral fat is associated with an increase in fasting and postprandial plasma insulin concentrations and IGT[26,27]. Furthermore, of a cohort of middle-aged men followed for approximately 20 years, those who maintained their waist/hip ratio in the lower decile had no increased risk for developing type 2 diabetes, while subjects in the highest

decile had about 20-fold increased relative risk for developing type 2 diabetes[28]. Additionally, increased visceral fat was an independent risk factor for the development of stroke and coronary artery disease[29,30]. Thus, the visceral fat seems to play an important role in development of the insulin resistance of aging.

INSULIN RESISTANCE WITH AGING

Impaired regulation in glucose homeostasis with aging can be artificially divided into alterations in (peripheral) insulin-stimulated glucose uptake (the muscle being the main site for postmeal glucose disposal) and defects in hepatic glucose production (the liver being the main site for fasting glucose production). Thus, insulin resistance may manifest as a decrease in insulin-stimulated glucose uptake and a decrease in suppression of hepatic glucose production by insulin, both characteristics of IGT and type 2 diabetes in aging men.

Decreases in insulin-mediated glucose uptake with aging

Various studies have demonstrated that fat mass is inversely correlated with insulin-mediated glucose uptake, independent of age[31-34]. The effect of body composition on insulin sensitivity and glucose utilization in lean, older individuals was similar to that in weight-matched young individuals, suggesting that body composition itself rather than age influences insulin sensitivity. A large multicenter study demonstrated that insulin resistance did not increase with aging *per se*, and most of the variation in insulin action could be attributed to increases in body weight and fat mass[31]. The majority of insulin-mediated glucose uptake (IMGU) is accounted for by skeletal muscle. Thus, the typical hyperinsulinemia seen with aging may be attributed to peripheral (muscle) insulin resistance. Consequently, since aging is associated with a progressive increase in fat mass, the latter may have a modulatory effect on skeletal muscle insulin sensitivity. Moreover, various studies have shown a clear association between visceral fat and insulin sensitivity, which suggests that, among the whole body fat mass, visceral fat plays a key role in modulating insulin resistance. To examine whether the effect of fat mass on peripheral insulin sensitivity is 'saturable' and independent of age, a rodent model of aging was examined. This considered that, if the effect of fat mass on peripheral insulin sensitivity is saturable at a relatively young age, then aging *per se* is not further associated with defective peripheral insulin action[35]. Rats were fed *ad libitum* and examined at the age of 2–18 months for body composition and insulin sensitivity using the gold standard tracer methodology. The rate of insulin-stimulated glucose uptake decreased significantly from age 2 months to age 4 months with no further change in the older rats. Analysis of these data demonstrated that reaching a specific body weight was associated with a maximal effect on insulin action; further increases in body weight or further increases in age did not significantly change glucose uptake. To further emphasize the role of decreased fat mass in insulin action with aging, rats were calorie restricted throughout aging and examined for peripheral insulin sensitivity using the hyperinsulinemic clamp. The results demonstrated that chronic calorie restriction, designed to reduce fat mass to below 13% of their body weight, dramatically improved insulin responsiveness[36]. These data suggest that aging *per se* is not associated with a further decrease in peripheral insulin sensitivity. Furthermore, a reduction in fat mass below a certain level dramatically improves the peripheral action of insulin, independent of age. Thus, fat mass accumulation, rather than aging, may be responsible for age-dependent insulin resistance. Of note, it is possible that decreases in muscle mass maybe so severe[31] that the clearance of glucose can be limited by storage capacity. This form of insulin resistance whereby muscle quality is preserved but muscle mass becomes limited is under investigation.

Hepatic insulin resistance in aging

Rates of basal hepatic glucose production (HGP) have been reported to be normal in aging men[10,11,37]. However, suppression of HGP by an oral glucose load or by insulin was significantly impaired with aging, or in subjects with abdominal obesity. As noted above, visceral fat is closely correlated with hepatic insulin sensitivity. Additionally, since hepatic insulin sensitivity is inversely related to increases in fat mass, visceral fat and free fatty acid levels, the age-related changes in body composition, and their biochemical consequences, may lead directly to impairment of the hepatic glucose metabolism. Measuring the rates of hepatic glucose production during hyperinsulinemia has shown an approximate four-fold increase in HGP in the highest versus the lowest tertile of obese subjects with increased visceral fat[31]. Similarly, an approximate three-fold increase in portal insulin levels was needed to suppress HGP in women with upper-body obesity compared with lower-body obesity[38]. As in humans, aging rats develop impairment in the ability of insulin to suppress hepatic glucose production, and a higher insulin concentration is needed to maintain basal HGP[39]. To examine whether a cause–effect relationship exists between visceral fat and hepatic insulin action in aging, rats have been studied after being moderately calorie restricted up to 18 months of age, compared to young and old rats fed *ad libitum*[40]. By changing the ratio of total fat mass to visceral fat by calorie restriction, it was demonstrated that hepatic insulin action is affected by visceral fat and not fat mass. To investigate further a cause–effect relationship between the age-related increase in visceral fat and the impaired action of insulin on HGP, rats were examined after either surgical removal of the epididymal and perinephric fat pads or a sham operation[41]. Total visceral fat was approximately four-fold increased in the sham-operated group. However, whole body fat mass was not significantly different. While plasma glucose, free fatty acids, glycerol and glucagon levels were similar, plasma insulin levels were decreased by half in the rats with surgically removed visceral fat. The rate of insulin infusion needed to maintain plasma glucose levels at baseline during the hepatic–pancreatic clamp was dramatically decreased (about two-fold) following visceral fat removal. These results demonstrate that the hepatic responses to either endogenous (basal) or exogenous (pancreatic clamp) insulin were markedly enhanced by removing the visceral fat. Thus, these data emphasize the pivotal role of visceral fat in the alteration of hepatic carbohydrate metabolism in this model of aging.

ABNORMALITIES IN INSULIN SECRETION WITH AGING

Several studies have shown impaired insulin secretion and lack of ß-cell compensation for insulin resistance in aging, although the mechanism responsible for deficient insulin secretion is still debated[42–44]. Genetic, environmental and behavioral factors are believed to contribute to the impaired ß-cell function in aging; however, none of these mechanisms have been clearly operative in humans[43]. The pancreatic islets in type 2 diabetes are not consistently altered, and normal ß-cell mass appears to be preserved in most patients[45–47]. Pancreatic islet amyloid accumulation characteristically seen in type 2 diabetes does not closely correlate with the pathogenesis of ß-cell failure[48,49]. A large proportion of insulin-resistant subjects develop type 2 diabetes and IGT with aging; this has been hypothesized to be due to a failure by the ß cell to release adequate amounts of insulin[50,51]. In young subjects with peripheral insulin resistance, a proportional increase in insulin secretion maintained euglycemia and normal glucose tolerance; however, in elderly individuals with similar resistance to insulin, less insulin was secreted, suggesting a detrimental effect of aging on ß-cell function.

In obese insulin-resistant subjects, the development of IGT was accompanied by a reduction in ß-cell function and not by a further deterioration in insulin sensitivity, suggesting that the increase in fat mass *per se* may lead to the impaired ß-cell function[52]. Another study of lean, elderly subjects with type 2 diabetes but no apparent insulin resistance showed a decrease in insulin secretion during hyperglycemia, again suggesting an impairment of the ß-cell function with aging[53]. Thus, the development of IGT and type 2 diabetes in the elderly may be artificially divided into two conditions: progressive increases in insulin resistance with a compensatory hyperinsulinemia that eventually fails, and failure of the ß cell in subjects with normal insulin action (in lean individuals). Both may lead to frank diabetes mellitus.

ADDITIONAL FACTORS THAT CONTRIBUTE TO IMPAIRED CARBOHYDRATE METABOLISM IN AGING

Prolonged hyperglycemia *per se* has been shown to have deleterious effects on both insulin sensitivity and insulin secretion (the glucose toxicity phenomenon); thus, a vicious cycle is formed and maintained by primary insulin resistance (peripheral and hepatic) and inadequate insulin secretion, which causes hyperglycemia[12]. The latter causes further impairment in insulin action and secretion; lowering the plasma glucose levels by diet, by exercise or pharmacologically has been shown to improve insulin sensitivity and insulin secretion.

Additionally, it appears that an age-related impairment in non-insulin-mediated glucose uptake (NIMGU) may contribute to the increase in fasting plasma glucose in the elderly[54]. A recent study of elderly patients with type 2 diabetes demonstrated that the effect of NIMGU on glucose uptake was impaired, i.e. during a hypoinsulinemic clamp, the rate of glucose clearance was decreased, compared to controls[55]. This study suggests that fasting hyperglycemia in the elderly may be also due to impaired NIMGU, in addition to frank type 2 diabetes, a notion that may have important implications in the treatment of this population.

SUMMARY

Human aging is associated with a cluster of abnormalities in carbohydrate metabolism leading to a significant increase in the prevalence of type 2 diabetes mellitus and impaired glucose tolerance (IGT). In the past few years, the importance of changes in body-composition, characteristic of human aging, has become a key factor in the pathogenesis of type 2 diabetes in this population. This can easily be missed because the typical elderly man has a normal BMI yet an increased waist/hip ratio. Increased visceral fat with aging seems to be of major importance, not only in modulating muscle insulin sensitivity, hepatic insulin sensitivity and perhaps insulin release, but also in a variety of other physiological functions. Understanding the pathophysiology of aging men has helped researchers to develop newer treatment strategies specifically aimed to combat peripheral insulin resistance (for example, thiazolidinediones), increase hepatic glucose production (metformin) and improve decreased or inadequate insulin secretion (sulfonylureas). Future therapeutic options for diabetes should take into account the central role of changes in body composition seen in the elderly, which currently appear to be an important modulator of insulin secretion and action.

References

1. Reaven GM, Reaven EP. Age, glucose intolerance, and non-insulin-dependent diabetes mellitus. *J Am Geriatr Soc* 1985;33: 286–90

2. Davidson MB. The effect of aging on carbohydrate metabolism: a review of the English literature and a practical approach to the diagnosis of diabetes mellitus in the elderly. *Metabolism* 1979;28:688–705

3. Weingard DL, Sinsheimer P, Barrett-Connor EL, McPhillip JB. Community-based study of prevalence of NIDDM in older adults. *Diabetes Care* 1990;13(Suppl 2):3–8

4. Fernando Samos L, Roos BA. Diabetes mellitus in older persons. *Med Clin North Am* 1998; 82:791–803

5. Harris MI. Impaired glucose tolerance in the US population. *Diabetes Care* 1989;12: 464–74

6. Fraze E, Chiou M, Chen Y, Reaven GM. Age related changes in postprandial plasma glucose, insulin, and FFA concentrations in non-diabetic individuals. *J Am Geriatr Soc* 1987; 35:224–8

7. Meneilly GS, Minaker K, Elahi D, Rowe JW. Insulin action in aging men: evidence for tissue specific differences at low physiological insulin levels. *J Gerontol* 1987;42: 196–201

8. Pagano G, Cassader M, Cavallo-Perin P, et al. Insulin resistance in the aged: a quantitative evaluation of *in vivo* insulin sensitivity and *in vitro* glucose transport. *Metabolism* 1984; 33:976–81

9. Robert JJ, Cummins JC, Wolfe RR, et al. Quantitative aspects of glucose production and metabolism in healthy elderly subjects. *Diabetes* 1982;31:203–11

10. Jackson RA, Hawa MI, Roshania RD, et al. Influence of aging on hepatic and peripheral glucose metabolism in humans. *Diabetes* 1988;37:119–29

11. Barzilai N, Stessman J, Cohen P, et al. Glucoregulatory hormone influence on hepatic glucose production in the elderly. *Age* 1989; 12:13–17

12. Rossetti L, Giaccari A, DeFronzo R. Glucose toxicity. *Diabetes Care* 1990;13:610–30

13. Andres R. In Andres R, Bierman EL, Hazzardeds WR, eds. *Principles of Geriatric Medicine*. New York: McGraw-Hill, 1985: 53–98

14. Norris AH, Lundy T, Shock NW. Trends in indices of body composition in men between ages 30–70 years. *Ann N Y Acad Sci* 1963; 110:623–39

15. Cohn SH, Vartsky D, Yasumura S, *et al.* Compartmental body composition based on total-body nitrogen, potassium and calcium. *Am J Physiol* 1980;239:E524–30

16. Despres JP, Lamarche B, Mauriege P. Hyperinsulinemia as an independent risk factor for ischemic heart disease. *N Engl J Med* 1996;334:952–7

17. Modan M, Halkin H, Almog S, *et al.* Hyperinsulinemia. A link between hypertension, obesity and glucose intolerance. *J Clin Invest* 1985;75:809–17

18. Zavaroni I, Bonora E, Pagliara M, *et al.* Risk factors for coronary artery disease in healthy persons with hyperinsulinemia and normal glucose tolerance. *N Engl J Med* 1989;320: 702–6

19. DeFronzo RA, Ferrannini E. Insulin resistance. A multifaceted syndrome responsible for NIDDM, obesity, hypertension, dyslipidemia, and atherosclerotic cardiovascular disease. *Diabetes Care* 1991;14:173–94

20. Haffner SM. Sex hormones, obesity, fat distribution, type 2 diabetes and insulin resistance: epidemiological and clinical correlation. *Int J Obesity Relat Metab Disord* 2000; 24(Suppl 2):S56–8

21. Cefalu WT, Wang ZQ, Werbel S, *et al.* Contribution of visceral fat mass to the insulin resistance of aging. *Metabolism* 1995;44:954–9

22. Visser M, Harris TB, Langlois J, *et al.* Body fat and skeletal muscle mass in relation to physical disability in very old men and women of the Framingham Heart Study. *J Gerontol A Biol Sci Med Sci* 1998;53:M214–21

23. Kuczmarski RJ, Flegal K, Campbell S, Johnson CL. Increasing prevalence of overweight among US adults. The National Health and Nutrition Examination Survey, 1960 to 1991 (NHANES III). *J Am Med Assoc* 1994;272:238–9

24. Enzi G, Gasparo M, Pinodetti PR. Subcutaneous and visceral fat distribution according to sex, age and overweight, evaluated by computer tomography. *Am J Clin Nutr* 1986; 44:739–46

25. Shimokata H, Tobin JD, Muller DC, *et al.* Studies in the distribution of body fat: I. Effects of age, sex, and obesity. *J Gerontol* 1989;44:M66–73

26. Ferrannini E, Natali A, Capaldo B, *et al.* Insulin resistance, hyperinsulinemia, and blood pressure: role of age and obesity. European Group for the Study of Insulin Resistance (EGIR). *Hypertension* 1997;30: 1144–9

27. Pasquali R, Casimirri F, Cantobelli S, *et al.* Effect of obesity and body fat distribution on sex hormones and insulin in men. *Metabolism* 1991;40:101–4

28. Ferrannini E, Natali A, Bell P, *et al.* Insulin resistance and hypersecretion in obesity. European Group for the Study of Insulin Resistance (EGIR). *J Clin Invest* 1997;100: 1166–73

29. Fujimoto WY, Bergstrom RW, Boyko EJ, *et al.* Visceral adiposity and incident coronary heart disease in Japanese-American men. The 10–year follow-up results of the Seattle Japanese-American Community Diabetes Study. *Diabetes Care* 1999;22:1808–12

30. Lamarche B. Abdominal obesity and its metabolic complications: implications for the risk of ischaemic heart disease. *Coron Artery Dis* 1998;9:473–81

31. Peiris AN, Struve MF, Mueller RA, *et al.* Glucose metabolism in obesity: influence of body fat distribution. *J Clin Endocrinol Metab* 1988;67:760–7

32. Paolisso G, Tagliamonte MR, Rizzo MR, Giugliano D. Advancing age and insulin resistance: new facts about an ancient history. *Eur J Clin Invest* 1999;29:758–69

33. Ferrannini E, Vichi S, Beck-Nielsen H, *et al.* Insulin action and age. European Group for the Study of Insulin Resistance (EGIR). *Diabetes* 1996;45:947–53

34. O'Shaughnessy IM, Kasdorf GM, Hoffmann RG, Kalkhoff RK. Does aging intensify the insulin resistance of human obesity? *J Clin Endocrinol Metab* 1992;74:1075–81

35. Barzilai N, Banerjee S, Hawkins M, *et al.* The effect of age-dependent increase in fat mass on peripheral insulin action is saturable. *J Gerontol A Biol Sci Med Sci* 1998;53: B141–6

36. Gupta G, She L, Ma XH, et al. Aging does not contribute to the decline in insulin action on storage of muscle glycogen in rats. *Am J Physiol Regul Integr Comp Physiol* 2000;278: R111–17

37. Boden G, Chen X, DeSantis RA, Kendrick Z. Effects of age and body fat on insulin resistance in healthy men. *Diabetes Care* 1993;16: 728–33

38. Fink RI, Revers RR, Kolterman OG, Olefsky JM. The metabolic clearance of insulin and the feedback inhibition of insulin secretion are altered with aging. *Diabetes* 1985;34:275–80

39. Barzilai N, Rossetti L. Age-related changes in body composition are associated with hepatic insulin resistance in conscious rats. *Am J Physiol* 1996;270:E930–6

40. Gupta G, Cases JA, She L, et al. Ability of insulin to modulate hepatic glucose production in aging rats is impaired by fat accumulation. *Am J Physiol Endocrinol Metab* 2000; 278:E985–91

41. Barzilai N, She L, Liu BQ, et al. Surgical removal of visceral fat reverses hepatic insulin resistance. *Diabetes* 1999;48:94–8

42. Scheen AJ, Sturis J, Polonsky KS, Van Cauter E. Alterations in the ultradian oscillations of insulin secretion and plasma glucose in aging. *Diabetologia* 1996;39:564–72

43. Coordt MC, Ruhe RC, McDonald RB. Aging and insulin secretion. *Proc Soc Exp Biol Med* 1995;209:213–22

44. Muller DC, Elahi D, Tobin JD, Andres R. The effect of age on insulin resistance and secretion: a review. *Semin Nephrol* 1996;16:289–98

45. Reaven E, Solomon R, Azhar S, Reaven G. Functional homogeneity of pancreatic islets of aging rats. *Metabolism* 1982;31:859–60

46. Borg LA, Dahl N, Swenne I. Age-dependent differences in insulin secretion and intracellular handling of insulin in isolated pancreatic

islets of the rat. *Diabetes Metab* 1995;21: 408–14

47. Aizawa T, Komatsu M, Sato Y, et al. Insulin secretion by the pancreatic beta cell of aged rats. *Pancreas* 1994;9:454–9

48. Mitsukawa T, Takemura J, Nakazato M, et al. Effects of aging on plasma islet amyloid polypeptide basal level and response to oral glucose load. *Diabetes Res Clin Pract* 1992; 15:131–4

49. Clark A, Charge SB, Badman MK, de Koning EJ. Islet amyloid in type 2 (non-insulin-dependent) diabetes. *Acta Pathol Microbiol Immunol Scand* 1996;104:12–18

50. Gray H, O'Rahilly S. Beta cell dysfunction in non-insulin-dependent diabetes mellitus. *Transplant Proc* 1994;26:366–70

51. Polonsky KS, Sturis J, Bell GI. Seminars in Medicine of the Beth Israel Hospital, Boston. Non-insulin-dependent diabetes mellitus – a genetically programmed failure of the beta cell to compensate for insulin resistance. *N Engl J Med* 1996;334:777–83

52. Meneilly GS, Elliott T, Tessier D, et al. NIDDM in the elderly. *Diabetes Care* 1996; 19:1320–5

53. Cavaghan MK, Ehrmann DA, Polonsky KS. Interactions between insulin resistance and insulin secretion in the development of glucose intolerance. *J Clin Invest* 2000;106: 329–33

54. Meneilly GS, Elahi D, Minaker KL, et al. Impairment of noninsulin-mediated glucose disposal in the elderly. *J Clin Endocrinol Metab* 1989;68:566–71

55. Forbes A, Elliott T, Tildesley H, et al. Alterations in non-insulin-mediated glucose uptake in the elderly patient with diabetes. *Diabetes* 1998;47:1915–19

15 Macrovascular complications in the elderly diabetic

Dariush Elahi, PhD, Denis C. Muller, MD, and Grady S. Meneilly, MD

INTRODUCTION

The world-wide epidemic of type II diabetes is the result of two major demographic trends: an increase in the elderly population and an increase in obesity. Improved nutrition and technological advances that lead to a less strenuous life-style have contributed to both trends. Between 1990 and 1998, the prevalence of diabetes in the USA increased by 17.1% in subjects aged 60–69 years and 10.1% in subjects aged 70 years and over[1]. Substantial evidence has been provided to show that increasing age is associated with decreased glucose tolerance[2–6]. The effect of age on fasting and 2–h plasma glucose levels following a glucose tolerance test in healthy men from the Baltimore Longitudinal Study of Aging is shown in Figure 1. There is a progressive decline in glucose tolerance from the third decade to the ninth decade of age. The 2-h plasma glucose level during an oral glucose tolerance test rises on average by 5.3 mg/dl per decade, and the fasting plasma glucose rises on average by 1 mg/dl per decade[4]. This decline is also reflected in the third National Health and Nutrition Examination Survey (NHANES III) on the prevalence of diabetes and impaired fasting glucose and impaired glucose tolerance in US adults[7]. Comparison of the percentages of physician-diagnosed diabetes in middle-aged adults (40–49 years) and elderly adults (≥ 75 years) reveals an increase of 3.9% to

13.2%. Likewise, the percentage of adults with undiagnosed diabetes (defined as a fasting plasma glucose level ≥ 126 mg/dl) rises from 2.5% to 5.7%, and the percentage of adults with impaired fasting glucose (defined as a fasting plasma glucose level of 110–125 mg/dl) rises from 7.1% to 14.1%. Therefore, approximately one-third of elderly adults in the USA have abnormal glucose tolerance as defined by the American Diabetes Association.

In diabetes (types 1 and 2), the most common cause of morbidity and mortality is coronary heart disease. Despite a trend towards a decrease in macrovascular disease following reductions of glycemic levels, as demonstrated in several studies (Diabetes Control and Complications Trial, UK Prevention of Diabetes Study[8–10]), it is still unclear whether hyperglycemia is causally associated with coronary heart disease or if it is just a marker for some other risk factor(s). This issue has been concisely reviewed by Barrett-Connor[11] and is briefly summarized here.

Since there are no animal models to prove or disprove the hypothesis that hyperglycemia causes arteriosclerosis, the evidence is based on epidemiological data. Population studies are not consistent, and the risk ratio of hyperglycemia for the development of coronary heart disease (CHD) ranges from 0.34 to 6.07. A major limitation of studies is the failure to exclude

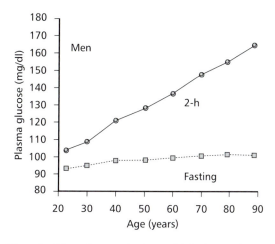

Figure 1 Effect of age on fasting and 2-h plasma glucose levels in men from the Baltimore Longitudinal Study of Aging (BCSA), data unpublished

adults with undiagnosed diabetes. In general, it appears that there is no evidence that, in the absence of diabetes, glycemia is a risk factor for CHD. In diabetes patients, most studies clearly demonstrate a positive relationship between glycemic level and risk of cardiovascular disease. Clinical trials have demonstrated that improved glycemic control reduces the risk of microvascular disease. However, they were usually not designed to examine its effect on macrovascular disease. Furthermore, the volunteers were 'middle-aged', and inferences to elderly diabetic patients may not be accurate. The Diabetes Prevention Program has enrolled elderly patients and its results, expected in 2002, are eagerly awaited. The available data to date suggest that the risk of glycemia for development of CHD is low, and in type 2 diabetes the management of the more important risk factors for heart disease, dyslipidemia and hypertension, in preference to the management of hyperglycemia, is warranted.

EFFECT OF AGE ON GLUCOSE TOLERANCE

Fasting glucose

In the basal state, the decline in carbohydrate metabolism, as assessed by the fasting glucose,

is relatively small. A review of the literature[4] had estimated that fasting glucose levels rise approximately 1 mg/dl per decade. Subsequent studies in populations that cover the adult age span have produced more ambiguous results. In 263 healthy subjects aged 20–69 years, age was positively related to fasting glucose even after adjustment for differences in adiposity[12]. The Baltimore Longitudinal Study of Aging has also shown a positive cross-sectional correlation between age and fasting plasma glucose in both men and women[13,14]. Zavaroni and colleagues[15] demonstrated an age-related increase in fasting glucose levels in Italian factory workers; this increase was significantly reduced in women after adjustments were made for the presence of other age-related variables. Small increases in fasting glucose levels with age were noted in 4170 men and women living in suburban California (0.7 mg/dl per decade in men; 2.0 mg/dl per decade in women)[16]. In a retirement community in California, in subjects aged 47–90 years, Maneatis and co-workers[17] found no significant changes with age in fasting glucose levels in men, but observed a small significant positive correlation in women. However, in several studies, age had little, if any, effect on fasting glucose. Age was not independently related to fasting glucose in a population survey of 740 Danes of The Second Generation Fredericia Study[18]. In a study of 710 healthy individuals, fasting glucose levels increased by only 8% and 6% over seven decades in men and women, respectively[19].

EFFECT OF DIABETES ON MACROVASCULAR DISEASES

Lipoprotein disorders

Type 2 diabetes is associated with high levels of plasma triglycerides[20] and low levels of plasma high-density lipoprotein (HDL) cholesterol, which increase the risk for development of cardiovascular disease. Concentrations of triglycerides and HDL are regulated by a variety of factors including gene regulation of apoproteins, enzymes, lipids and receptors. Hyperlipidemia, which occurs in the majority of type 2 diabetic patients, is due to over-production of apolipoprotein (apo)B-containing lipoproteins[21-23]. ApoB100, synthesized in the liver, is a large hydrophobic protein[24], and is necessary for the secretion of the lipoproteins that transport lipids from the liver to peripheral tissues. Regulation of apoB secretion is not at the transcriptional or mRNA level, and occurs post-translationally. Approximately one-third of newly synthesized apoB100 is secreted from the hepatocytes[25], with the rest degraded intracellularly in the endoplasmic reticulum[26]. The concentration of lipids regulates the post-transitional metabolism of apoB. Plasma triglyceride is the major lipid for the regulation of apoB, and stimulation of triglyceride synthesis stimulates apoB secretion by fatty acids[27]. In type 2 diabetes with increased flow of fatty acids to the liver, more apoB is assembled and secretion of triglyceride-rich lipoproteins is increased.

The risk of development of coronary heart disease is inversely related to the plasma concentration of HDL cholesterol[28]. Low levels of HDL cholesterol are associated with low levels of apoA-I[29], and low levels of apoA-I result from increased catabolic rate and not reduced secretion rate[30]. The mechanics for the accelerated catabolism of apoA-I is due in part to accumulation of HDL apoA-I by the kidney[31], which is filtered by the glomerulus and excreted in the urine. Thus, improved insulin action via reduction of free fatty acid release from fat tissue should result in lower levels of triglyceride and apoB, and increased levels of HDL cholesterol and apoA-I.

Hyperinsulinemia

Multivariate analysis of prospective studies has identified an independent relationship between hyperinsulinemia and cardiovascular disease, which supports the concept of specificity between insulin and atherosclerosis[32]. The Framingham Offspring Study has also identified hyperinsulinemia as being associated with impaired fibrinolysis in subjects with glucose intolerance[33].

Glycation

Advanced glycosylation end-products (AGEs) are produced by rearrangement of early glycation products with a succession of reactive intermediates, which bind to amino aids of diverse proteins (covalent non-enzymatic modification of proteins by glucose, Amadori products). Degradation can also release intermediates that are able to bind again forming new AGEs. Concomitant aging and diabetes is associated with increased accumulation of AGEs[34] and is inversely related to renal function[35]. AGEs elicit cell-mediated responses that result in vascular dysfunction including atherosclerosis and glomerulosclerosis[34], which are mediated by AGE-specific cell surface receptors (RAGEs)[36,37]. RAGEs are expressed on endothelial cells, mononuclear phagocytes and vascular smooth muscle cells[38]. Binding of AGEs to RAGEs induces release of growth factors[39,40] and cytokines[41], resulting in tissue repair. *In vivo* studies in rabbits and rats have shown that administration of AGEs–albumin can produce vascular defects similar to those observed in diabetes[42]. It has also been demonstrated that glomerular hypertrophy basement-membrane thickening, and glomerulosclerosis accompanied by albuminuria/proteinuria occur following prolonged exposure to AGEs[43].

Cerebrovascular disease and mortality

Diabetic subjects have at least twice the risk of stroke, compared with non-diabetics, in addition to higher mortality and slower recovery after stroke. Diabetic patients are 12 times more likely to be hospitalized for cerebrovascular events[44]. Autopsy reports in diabetic patients have demonstrated an increased frequency of cerebral infarction. In a series of 7579 consecutive autopsies, which included 935 diabetic patients aged 23–95 years, the frequency of encephalomalacia was much higher in the diabetic patients and even more if hypertension was present[45]. Very little detailed histopathology is available from autopsy studies in patients with diabetes. In a study where 75 diabetic patients were compared with 77 non-diabetics, endothelial proliferation and hyalinosis of small intraparenchymal vessels were present in 64% of the diabetic patients compared with 23% of the non-diabetics[46]. There are also very few data on cerebral large-vessel atherosclerosis from diabetic patients. The data are not consistent with respect to an association between the disease and large-vessel atherosclerosis. In one series of 16 patients with type 1 diabetes (age < 45), atheromatous changes in large and medium-size arteries were reported[47]. In type 2 diabetes, occlusion of large intracranial arteries is reported to be common[48] or uncommon[45,49]. The difference may be due to hypertension status. Similarly, data regarding a difference between men and women, in relation to cerebral atherosclerosis in diabetic patients, are not consistent. Studies have shown either no difference between men and women in the frequency of atherosclerosis of intracranial large vessels[48] or a greater effect in women in the fifth and sixth decades, compared to men[50].

Many epidemiological studies provide strong evidence for type 2 diabetes as a risk factor for ischemic stroke[51–57]. In the majority of these reports, diabetes is shown to be an independent risk factor for stroke. These studies are rather numerous and, thus, the evidence is compelling. Seven large studies enrolled 1200–16 000 subjects, while one study (the Multiple Risk Factor Intervention Trial, MRFIT) enrolled a total of 340 000 individuals. In studies where both men and women were enrolled, the distribution was generally equal[51,52,54,56,57]. The percentage of individuals with diabetes in these studies ranged from 5 to 19%, with the exception of the MRFIT in which only 1.5% (men) had diabetes. The relative risk for stroke in these studies ranged from 1.3 to 4.9, with men generally having the same average relative risk as women; however, there is a large difference between studies. In some studies, diabetes in men was associated with a lower relative risk for stroke[51,54,57], than in women. An increased relative risk was found in women compared to men in one study[56], while no significant increased risk was found in women with diabetes in another study[52]. The effect of diabetes on increased risk of stroke was generally independent of confounders such as age, systolic blood pressure, antihypertension therapy, cigarette smoking, cardiovascular disease, left-ventricular hypertrophy and atrial fibrillation[47]. Discrepancies in relative risk between studies are in part due to differences in types of stroke (all, ischemic, fatal), the criteria for diabetes, population studies (Framingham; Rochester, MN; Finland; Honolulu; Rancho Bernardo, CA; all sites for the MRFIT) and methods of analysis[51–56]. Another factor that may contribute to the discrepancy is race and ethnicity. Type 2 diabetes is more prevalent in African-Americans, native Americans, Pacific Islander-Americans and Hispanic-Americans than in European-Americans[58]. While African-Americans with type 2 diabetes are more likely to have hypertension, smoke more and have a higher prevalence of microangiopathy than European-Americans, they have a lower prevalence of myocardial infarction.

Type 2 diabetes is associated with a clustering of risk factors for cardiovascular disease[59]. A major disorder is dyslipidemia, with mild to moderate elevation of triglycerides and low-density lipoprotein (LDL) cholesterol and low HDL cholesterol[60]. Elevated triglycerides and low HDL cholesterol are predictors of stroke[61]. The majority of type 2 diabetic patients have hypertension[58], and this may be due in part to obesity, particularly abdominal obesity, and in part to insulin resistance[62-64]. However, these risk factors do not explain the increased risk of vascular disease. Other risk factors that contribute include protein glycation, oxidation and formation of advanced glycation end-products[65,66], platelet aggregation[67,68], endothelial dysfunction[69,70] and hypercoagulability.

Epidemiological studies suggest that glycemic control reduces the risk of macrovascular disease including stroke[71,8]. As yet, there are no data for randomized, controlled trials in elderly patients to determine whether intensive control would reduce the risk of long-term complications. The recently completed UK Prospective Diabetes Study (UKPDS) Control and Complications Trial provided evidence that intensive glycemic control results in a reduction in all macrovascular events, including stroke[8-10]. However, this was not significant, possibly because the cohort was young with a relatively short duration of disease.

The effect reviewed above indicates that type 2 diabetes is a risk factor for stroke. The role of glycemic control in reduction of the risk of stroke is established, but the target level for glucose control has not been defined. The effect of weight loss and increased physical exercise leading to improved or normal glucose homeostasis in patients with impaired glucose tolerance should be re-emphasized[73]. The risk of weight gain and hypoglycemia with oral hypoglycemic agents or insulin should be evaluated in older patients with type 2 diabetes. Other therapies for prevention and treatment of vascular disease in the elderly include antioxidants (vitamins C and E), which reduce endothelium-dependent vascular relaxation[74,75], aminoguanidine, which prevents advanced glycation end-products[76], calcium channel blockers or angiotensin converting enzyme inhibitors for the reduction of urinary protein excretion[77,78], and possibly lipid-lowering agents.

EVIDENCE OF ADDITIVE EFFECT OF AGE AND DIABETES ON MACROVASCULAR DISEASES

Death

At any age, diabetic men exhibit a higher mortality rate than that of non-diabetic men. The preponderance of this excess is due to macrovascular diseases. In the Rancho Bernardo study, the adjusted relative risk for CHD death was 1.9 for diabetic men[79]. Approximately 65% of all deaths in diabetics are secondary to vascular or heart disease[80]. The impact of diabetes on life expectancy in an Iowa population was estimated to be 9.1 fewer years than in non-diabetic men[81]. A Welsh study also showed that diabetic men, on average, lost 7 years of life compared to non-diabetic men[82]. The number of years lost declined in older age-groups. However, since there were a large number of men diagnosed with diabetes in the older age-groups, the total years lost were highest in the elderly. A recent meta-analysis revealed a significant effect of diabetes mellitus on coronary death in men and women after adjustment for other cardiac risk factors; also, women with diabetes were at significantly greater relative (to non-diabetics) risk compared to men with diabetes. Absolute risk of CHD death was still greater in male diabetics than in female diabetics[83].

Myocardial infarction

Myocardial infarction rate is increased in elderly men with diabetes. The increase in heart disease seen in diabetics is a result of the non-atherosclerotic large-vessel abnormalities rather than classical atherosclerosis[84]. Lipoprotein elevation in diabetes mellitus infers increased risk, although the slope of the plot of lipoprotein level versus intimal–medial thickness is the same regardless of diabetes status[85]. Type 2 diabetes was found to be a strong independent predictor of advanced carotid atherosclerosis in 5 years of follow-up[86]. Since elderly diabetics have more coronary atherosclerosis, thrombolytic therapy is less effective. Also, thrombolysis may be contraindicated in the presence of proliferative retinopathy. There are more myocardial lesions and coronary arterial disease in diabetics than in non-diabetics. In addition, diabetes is associated with higher rates of restenosis after angioplasty. Diabetic men experience higher mortality rates after myocardial infarction than do non-diabetic men.

Risk factors for cardiovascular disease

The UKPDS has shown that the incidence of coronary artery disease is significantly associated with baseline levels of hemoglobin (HbA$_{1C}$, systolic blood pressure, triglycerides, LDL cholesterol and HDL cholesterol[9]. However, a subsequent UKPDS analysis revealed that intensive control of glycemia did not decrease the risk of macrovascular complications in subjects with type 2 diabetes[10]. In addition, the non-insulin-dependent diabetes mellitus (NIDDM) Patient Outcomes Research Team found that the prevalence of cardiovascular disease (CVD) did not increase with increasing levels of glycohemoglobin in a cohort of men and women with NIDDM[87]. CVD did increase significantly with age, cigarette smoking and hypertension. Another UKPDS study demonstrated that tight control of blood pressure in patients with hypertension and type 2 diabetes decreased the risk of macrovascular complications[88]. Therefore, CVD seems to be more closely associated with the conventional cardiovascular risk factors than with glycemic control in subjects with type 2 diabetes. Another important factor in the assessment of the effect of diabetes on macrovascular complications in the elderly is the age of onset. In men from the Verona Diabetes Study, the death rate from ischemic heart disease rose with increasing duration of diabetes[89].

SCREENING STRATEGIES AND TREATMENT IN THE ELDERLY MALE

Screening

The American Diabetic Association (ADA) has recommended routine screening for diabetes in adults aged 45 years of age or older by measuring fasting plasma glucose[90]. If levels are normal, the ADA suggests retesting at 3-year intervals. A report on the early detection of undiagnosed diabetes states that screening for diabetes is more advisable in individuals who are know to be at higher risk[91]. The risk can be determined from an individual's demographic (older age, family history of diabetes, ethnic minority) and clinical (obesity, hypertension, dyslipidemia) characteristics and prior evidence of abnormal glucose values.

Although there is a lack of empirical evidence to show that population screening for diabetes will be effective in reducing macrovascular complications, a number of recent reports have examined this issue using statistical models. The Centers for Disease Control (CDC) have recently estimated the cost-effectiveness of early detection and screening for type 2 diabetes using a Monte Carlo computer simulation[92]. Their analysis found that, early detection and treatment of type 2 diabetes (in individuals aged ≥ 25 years) reduced lifetime incidence of many major complications associated with this disease by approximately 25%. The benefit of early detection is postponement of these complications. However, this model gave more weight to the benefit from early treatment in reduction of microvascular complications than of macrovascular complications. Another recent study used decision analysis to compare the relative impacts of screening asymptomatic individuals between 45 and 60 years of age with a fasting glucose test, and not screening[93]. The increase in quality of life from the reduction in cardiovascular complications was weighed against the reduction in quality of life associated with diagnosis and treatment. The authors concluded that, since the prevalence of undiagnosed diabetes increases with increasing age and the elderly are at increased risk of cardiovascular complications, the overall benefit of screening increases with increasing age. They also concluded that the importance of early detection of diabetes lies in the ability to treat other cardiovascular risk factors (hypertension, smoking and dyslipidemia) rather than the raised glucose level. Their finding was that the increase in quality of life from reduction of microvascular risk is minimal in the elderly. A recent review of screening for type 2 diabetes has also concluded that there is little evidence that the incidence of macrovascular complications will be reduced by better glycemic control, but it may be improved by more aggressive treatment of hypertension and hyperlipidemia[94].

Treatment goals

Most clinicians agree that in elderly patients with symptoms of hyperglycemia, glucose levels should be reduced. This can be accomplished by keeping the random glucose level below 12 mmol/l. However, the Diabetes Control and Complications Trial[72] indicated that tight control of diabetes reduces the risk of microvascular complications in young patients with type 1 diabetes.

There are no data from randomized, controlled trials in elderly patients to determine whether intensive control reduces the risk of long-term complications. The optimal level of glycemic control that maximizes benefits, but minimizes the risk of therapy, particularly in relation to hypoglycemia, has not been defined. Results of the UKPDS[10,95] clearly demonstrated that glycemic control in type 2 diabetes worsens as a function of duration of the disease and of pharmacological therapy. Eventually, insulin is required. However, this study also demonstrated that improved glycemic control reduced the risk of microvascular and possibly macrovascular disease in middle-aged patients with diabetes. Unfortunately, many of the patients enrolled in this study were younger than those generally managed by geriatricians, and had minimal comorbidity. As a consequence, the results of the study may not be applicable to the majority of elderly patients, many of whom are frail. The Diabetes Prevention Program (now in its fifth year) is another large study, which enrolls individuals with impaired glucose tolerance. The baseline characteristics of this 27-center randomized clinical trial have recently been reported[96]. The goal of the study is the prevention or delay of type 2 diabetes. This study currently has three arms: an unblinded intensive life-style intervention and two randomized standard life-styles with placebo or metformin. The average follow-up will be 4.5 years, and it is also hoped that the study will demonstrate a reduction of risk factors associated with cardiovascular disease as assessed by carotid artery wall thickness. A major advantage of this study from the gerontological perspective is that 11% of the volunteers currently enrolled are over the age of 65 years.

Although there are no results from randomized trials currently available, epidemiological data suggest that there is a strong correlation between HbA_{1C} and the risk of macrovascular events in elderly patients with diabetes[59,97]. The risk of functional disability and impaired quality of life with complications is of great concern for older diabetics. In older diabetics, the incidence of various diseases associated with disability such as myocardial infarction, stroke and peripheral vascular disease with amputation is increased. The average 80-year-old female in Western society has a life expectancy of approximately 9 years, with a major disability during 60% of this interval[98]. If improved control reduces the risk of complications and associated disability, it will significantly improve the quality of life of older individuals. Although there is no standard treatment recommendation for the elderly, the goal of therapy is a fasting blood glucose level of < 7.0 mmol/l, a 2-h postprandial level of 11 mmol/l, and an HbA_{1C} level < 20% above the upper limit of normal.

The care of elderly patients with diabetes is complicated by a variety of factors including polypharmacy, multiple pathology and alteration of the special senses, as well as numerous social factors including social isolation and poverty. A team approach, consisting of a nurse, dietician, physician and other health professionals is essential[99]. Multidisciplinary programs have been shown to result in better compliance with therapy and improved glycemic control[100–103]. Involvement of family members improves compliance with therapy[104].

Elderly patients with diabetes who have other risk factors for CVD clearly have a much higher risk of complications than those who do not[105–107]. Therefore, risk-factor modification is an essential part of management. Calcium channel blockers are effective antihypertensive agents in older patients with diabetes, and do not worsen glycemic control[108,109]. These agents appear to be equivalent to the angiotensin converting enzyme (ACE) inhibitors in reducing urinary protein excretion[110]. Recently, it has been found that middle-aged patients with type 2 diabetes and hypertension who are taking calcium channel blockers have a greater risk of the occurrence of vascular events than those taking ACE inhibitors[77,78]. There are no data on patients over the age of 70 years to determine whether a similar effect occurs. Until further data are available, prudence is warranted in the use of calcium channel blockers in elderly patients with diabetes. In the Systolic Hypertension in the Elderly Program study, low-dose chlorthalidone was an effective antihypertensive agent, and reduced the risk of major cardiovascular events in older people with diabetes[111].

The Heart Outcomes Prevention Evaluation (HOPE) study showed that the ACE inhibitor, ramipril, reduced the risk of macrovascular complications in older patients with diabetes and one other risk factor, independent of the effects of these drugs on blood pressure[112]. ACE inhibitors have also been found to reduce blood pressure and improve insulin sensitivity in elderly non-diabetic patients with hypertension, and elderly patients with diabetes and congestive heart failure[113,114].

Many elderly patients with diabetes have high lipid values. As yet, there are not data from randomized controlled trials in patients with diabetes over the age of 70 years to determine whether pharmacological treatment of lipid levels improves outcomes in these patients, although such data should be forthcoming in the near future.

CONCLUSION

The current and projected increased prevalence of diabetes in the elderly is epidemic, and warrants a better understanding of the pathogenesis and treatment of this disease. Clinical trials have demonstrated that impaired glycemia results in improvements in microvascular disease and probably macrovascular disease in the populations studied. Control of both hypertension and dyslipidemia should also be undertaken. Despite direct lack of evidence for elderly diabetic patients (> 75 years), the evidence for middle-aged patients strongly suggests that treatment of aggressive hypertension, dyslipidemia and glycemia in the elderly is warranted.

ACKNOWLEDGEMENTS

This work is supported in part by the Canadian Diabetes Association and the Canadian Institutes of Health Research. We are grateful to Brenda I. Vega for her invaluable assistance in the preparation of this manuscript.

References

1. Mokdad AH, Ford ES, Bowman BA, *et al*. Diabetes trends in the US: 1900–1998. *Diabetes Care* 2000;23:1278–83

2. Andres R. Aging and diabetes. *Med Clin North Am* 1971;55:835–45

3. Broughton DL, Taylor R. Deterioration of glucose tolerance with age: the role of insulin resistance. *Age Ageing* 1991;20:221–5

4. Davidson M. The effect of aging on carbohydrate metabolism: a review of the English literature and a practical approach to the diagnosis of diabetes mellitus in the elderly. *Metabolism* 1979;28:688–705

5. DeFronzo R. Glucose intolerance and aging. *Diabetes Care* 1981;4:493–501

6. Reaven GM, Chen N, Hollenbeck C, *et al*. Effect of age on glucose tolerance and glucose uptake in healthy individuals. *J Am Geriatr Soc* 1989;37:735–40

7. Harris MH, Flegal KM, Cowie CC, *et al*. Prevalence of diabetes, impaired fasting glucose, and impaired glucose tolerance in US adults. *Diabetes Care* 1998;21:518–24

8. Diabetes Control and Complications Trial Research Group. The effect of intensive treatment on the development and progression of long-term complications in insulin-dependent diabetes mellitus. *N Engl J Med* 1993;329:977–86

9. UK Prospective Diabetes Group. Risk factors for coronary artery disease in non-insulin dependent diabetes mellitus (UKPDS 23). *Br Med J* 1998;316:823–8

10. UK Prospective Diabetes Group. Intensive blood-glucose control with sulphonylureas or insulin compared with conventional treatment and risk of complications in patients with type 2 diabetes (UKPDS 33). *Lancet* 1998;352:837–53

11. Barrett-Connor E. Does hyperglycemia really cause coronary heat disease? *Diabetes Care* 1997;20:1620–3

12. Berger D, Crowther R, Floyd J, *et al*. Effect of age on fasting plasma levels of pancreatic hormones in man. *J Clin Endocrinol Metab* 1978;47:1183–9

13. Muller D, Elahi D, Tobin J, *et al*. Insulin response during the oral glucose tolerance test: the role of age, sex, body fat and the pattern of fat distribution. *Aging Clin Exp Res* 1996;8:13–21

14. Shimokata H, Muller DC, Fleg JL, *et al*. Age as an independent determinant of glucose tolerance. *Diabetes* 1991;40:44–51

15. Zavaroni I, Dall'Aglio E, Brushi F, *et al*. Effect of age and environmental factors on glucose tolerance and insulin secretion on a worker population. *J Am Geriatr Soc* 1986;34:271–5

16. Barrett-Connor E. Factors associated with the distribution of fasting plasma glucose in an adult community. *Am J Epidemiol* 1980;112:518–23

17. Maneatis T, Condie R, Reaven G. Effect of age on plasma glucose and insulin responses to a test mixed meal. *J Am Geriatr Soc* 1982;30:178–82

18. Vestbo E, Damsgaard EM, Frøland A, *et al*. Clinical features in persons with a family history of diabetes compared to controls (The Second Generation Fredericia Study). *J Intern Med* 1996;240:381–7

19. Colman E, Toth M, Katzel L, *et al*. Body fatness and waist circumference are independent predictors of the age-associated increase in fasting insulin levels in healthy men and women. *Int J Obesity* 1995;19:798–803

20. Ginsberg HN. Lipoprotein physiology in non-diabetic and diabetes states. *Diabetes Care* 1991;14:839–55

21. Kissebah AH. Low density lipoprotein metabolism in non-insulin-dependent diabetes mellitus. *Diabetes Metab Rev* 1987;3:619–51

22. Teng B, Sniderman AD, Soular AK, *et al*. Metabolic basis of hyperapobetalipoproteinemia: turnover of apolipoprotein B in low density lipoprotein and its precursors and subfractions compared with normal and familial hypercholesterolemia. *J Clin Invest* 1986;77:663–72

23. Vega GL, Denke MA, Grundy SM. Metabolic basis of primary hypercholesterolemia. *Circulation* 1991;84:118–28

24. Young SG. Recent progress in understanding apolipoprotein B. *Circulation* 1990;82: 1574–94

25. Borchardt RA, Davis RA. Intrahepatic assembly of very low density lipoproteins: rate of transport out of the endoplasmic reticulum determines rate of secretion. *J Biol Chem* 1987;262:16394–402

26. Furukawa S, Sakata N, Ginsberg HN, *et al.* Studies of the sites of intracellular degradation of apolipoprotein B in Hep G2 cells. *J Biol Chem* 1992;267:22630–8

27. Dixon JL, Furukawa S, Ginsberg HN. Oleate stimulates secretion of apolipoprotein B-containing lipoproteins from Hep G2 cells by inhibiting early intracellular degradation of apolipoprotein B. *J Biol Chem* 1991;266: 5080–6

28. Miller NE, Thelle DS, Forde OH, *et al.* The Tromso heart study: high density lipoprotein and coronary heart disease: a prospective case control study. *Lancet* 1977;8019:965–8

29. Brunzell JD, Sniderman AD, Albers JJ, *et al.* Apoproteins B and A-1 and coronary artery diseases in humans. *Arteriosclerosis* 1984;4: 79–83

30. Nicoll A, Miller NE, Lewis B. High density lipoprotein metabolism. *Adv Lipid Res* 1980;17:53–106

31. Glass C, Pittman RC, Keller GA, *et al.* Tissue sites of degradation of apoprotein A-I in the rat. *J Biol Chem* 1983;258:7161–7

32. Stout RW. Hyperinsulinemia and atherosclerosis. *Diabetes* 1996;46(Suppl 3):S45–6

33. Meigs JB, Middleman MA, Nathan DM, *et al.* Hyperinsulinemia, hyperglycemia, and impaired hemostasis: the Framingham Offspring Study. *J Am Med Assoc* 2000;283:221–8

34. Brownlee M, Cerami A, Vlassara H. Advanced glycosylation endproducts in tissue and the biochemical basis of diabetic complication. *N Engl J Med* 1988;318:1315–21

35. Makita Z, Radoff S, Rayfield EJ, *et al.* Advanced glycosylation endproducts in patients with diabetic nephropathy. *N Engl J Med* 1991;325:836–42

36. Vlassara H, Brownlee M, Cerami A. High-affinity receptor-mediated uptake and degradation of glucose-modified proteins: a potential mechanism for the removal of senescent macromolecules. *Proc Natl Acad Sci USA* 1985;82:5588–92

37. Vlassara H, Brownlee M, Cerami A. Novel macrophage receptor for glucose-modified proteins is distinct from previously described scavenger receptors. *J Exp Med* 1986;164: 1301–9

38. Schmidt AM, Stern D. Atherosclerosis and diabetes: the RAGE connection. *Curr Atheroscler Rep* 2000;2:430–6

39. Kirstein M, Brett J, Radoff S, *et al.* Advanced glycosylation endproducts selectively induce monocyte migration across intact endothelial cell monolayers, and elaboration of growth factors: role in aging and diabetic vasculopathy. *Proc Natl Acad Sci USA* 1990;87: 9010–14

40. Kirstein M, Aston C, Hintz R, *et al.* Receptor-specific induction of insulin-like growth factor I (IGF-I) in human monocytes by advanced glycosylation endproduct-modified proteins. *J Clin Invest* 1992;90:439–46

41. Vlassara H, Brownlee M, Manogue DR, *et al.* Cachectin/TNJ and IL-1 induced by glucose-modified proteins: role in normal tissue remodelling. *Science* 1988;240:1546–8

42. Vlassara H, Fuh H, Makita Z, *et al.* Exogenous advanced glycosylation endproducts induce complex vascular dysfunction in normal animals; a model for diabetic and aging complications. *Proc Natl Acad Sci USA* 1992;89:12043–7

43. Vlassara H, Striker LJ, Teichberg S, *et al.* Advanced glycation endproducts induce glomerular sclerosis and albuminuria in normal rats. *Proc Natl Acad Sci USA* 1994;91: 11704–8

44. Lukovits TG, Mazzone T, Gorelick PB. Diabetes and cerebrovascular disease. *Neuroepidemiology* 1999;18:1–14

45. Kane WC, Aronson SM. Frequency and topographic distribution of intracranial vascular disease in diabetic patients; a necropsy survey. *Am J Pathol* 1968;52:71a–2a

46. Alex M, Baron EK, Goldenberg S, *et al.* An autopsy study of cerebrovascular accident in diabetes mellitus. *Circulation* 1962;25: 663–73

47. Reske-Nielsen E, Lundback K, Rafaelsen OJ. Pathological changes in the central and peripheral nervous system of young long-term diabetics. *Diabetologia* 1965;1:233–41

48. Grunnet ML. Cerebrovascular disease: diabetes and cerebral atherosclerosis. *Neurology* 1963;13:486–91

49. Aronson SM. Intracranial vascular lesions in patients with diabetes mellitus. *J Neuropathol Exp Neurol* 1973;32:183–96

50. Flora GC, Baker AB, Loewenson RB, *et al*. A comparative study of cerebral atherosclerosis in males and females. *Circulation* 1968; 38:859–69

51. D'Agostino RB, Wolf PA, Belanger AJ, *et al*. Stroke risk profile: adjustment for antihypertensive medication. *Stroke* 1994; 25:40–3

52. Davis PH, Dambrosia JM, Schoenberg BS, *et al*. Risk factors for ischemic stroke: a prospective study in Rochester, Minnesota. *Ann Neurol* 1987;22:319–27

53. Stamler J, Vaccaro O, Neaton JD, *et al*. Diabetes, other risk factors, and 12-year cardiovascular mortality for men screened in the Multiple Risk Factor Intervention Trial. *Diabetes Care* 1993;16:434–44

54. Tuomilehto J, Rastenyte D, Jousilahti P, *et al*. Diabetes mellitus as a risk factor for death from stroke. *Stroke* 1996;27:210–15

55. Abbott RD, Donahue RP, MacMahon SW, *et al*. Diabetes and the risk of stroke: The Honolulu Heart Program. *J Am Med Assoc* 1987;257:949–52

56. Barrett-Connor E, Khaw K-T. Diabetes mellitus: an independent risk factor for stroke? *Am J Epidemiol* 1988;128:116–23

57. Kuusisto J, Mykkanen L, Pyorala K, *et al*. Non-insulin-dependent diabetes and its metabolic control are important predictors of stroke in elderly subjects. *Stroke* 1994;25: 1157–64

58. American Diabetes Association. Risk factors for diabetes. *Diabetes 1996: Vital Statistics*. Alexandria, VA: ADA, 1996:21–7

59. Wingard DL, Barrett-Connor E, Criqui MH, *et al*. Clustering of heart disease risk factors in diabetic compared to nondiabetic adults. *Am J Epidemiol* 1983;117:19–26

60. Haffner SM. Management of dyslipidemia in adults with diabetes. *Diabetes Care* 1998; 21:160–78

61. Pujia A, Gnasso A, Irace C, *et al*. Common carotid arterial wall thickness in NIDDM subjects. *Diabetes Care* 1994;17:1330–6

62. Stout RW. Insulin and atheroma: 20-year perspective. *Diabetes Care* 1990;13:631–54

63. DeFronzo RA. The effect of insulin on renal sodium metabolism: a review with clinical implication. *Diabetologia* 1981;21:165–71

64. Rowe JW, Young JB, Minaker KL, *et al*. Effect of insulin and glucose infusions on sympathetic nervous system activity in normal man. *Diabetes* 1981;30:219–25

65. Lyons TJ. Glycation and oxidation: a role in the pathogenesis of atherosclerosis. *Am J Cardiol* 1993;71:26B–31B

66. Vlassara H. Recent progress on the biologic and clinical significance of advanced glycosylation end products. *J Lab Clin Med* 1994; 124:19–30

67. Colwell JA, Winocour PD, Halushka PV. Do platelets have anything to do with diabetic microvascular disease? *Diabetes* 1983; 32(Suppl 2):14–19

68. Davi G, Catalano I, Averna M, *et al*. Thromboxane biosynthesis and platelets in type II diabetes mellitus. *N Engl J Med* 1990;322:1769–74

69. Johnstone MT, Creager SJ, Scales KM, *et al*. Impaired endothelium-dependent vasodilation in patients with insulin-dependent diabetes mellitus. *Circulation* 1993;88:2510–16

70. Cohen RA. Dysfunction of vascular endothelium in diabetes mellitus. *Circulation* 1993;87(Suppl V):V67–76

71. Singer DE, Nathan DM, Anderson KM, *et al*. Association of HbA_{1C} with prevalent cardiovascular disease in the original cohort of the Framingham Heart Study. *Diabetes* 1992;41: 202–8

72. Klein R. Hyperglycemia and microvascular and macrovascular disease in diabetes. *Diabetes Care* 1995;18:258–8

73. Eriksson K-F, Lindgarde F. Prevention of type 2 (non-insulin-dependent) diabetes mellitus by diet and physical exercise. *Diabetologia* 1991;34:891–8

74. Keegan A, Walbank H, Cotter MA, *et al.* Chronic vitamin E treatment prevents defective endothelium-dependent relaxation in diabetic rat aorta. *Diabetologia* 1995;38:1475–8

75. Ting HH, Timimi FK, Boles KS, *et al.* Vitamin C improves endothelium-dependent vasodilation in patients with non-insulin-dependent diabetes mellitus. *J Clin Invest* 1996;97:22–8

76. Brownlee M, Vlassara H, Kooney T, *et al.* Aminoguanidine prevents diabetes-induced arterial wall protein cross-linking. *Science* 1986;232:1629–32

77. Estacio RO, Jeffers BW, Hiatt WR, *et al.* The effect of nisoldipine as compared with enalapril on cardiovascular outcomes in patients with non-insulin-dependent diabetes and hypertension. *N Engl J Med* 1998; 338:645–82

78. Tatti P, Pahor M, Byington RP, *et al.* Outcome results of the fosinopril versus amlodipine cardiovascular events randomized trial (FACET) in patients with hypertension and NIDDM. *Diabetes Care* 1998;21:597–603

79. Barrett-Conner EL, Cohn BA, Wingard DL, Edelstein SL. Why is diabetes mellitus a stronger risk factor for fatal ischemic heart disease in women than in men? *JAMA* 1991; 265:627–32

80. Wilson PWF. Diabetes mellitus and coronary heart disease. *Am J Kidney Dis* 1998;32: S89–100

81. Bale GS, Entmacher PS. Estimated life expectancy of diabetics. *Diabetes* 1977;26: 434–8

82. Morgan CL, Currie CJ, Peters JR. Relationship between diabetes and mortality. *Diabetes Care* 2000;23:1103–7

83. Lee WL, Cheung AM, Cape D, *et al.* Impact of diabetes on coronary artery disease in women and men: a meta-analysis of prospective studies. *Diabetes Care* 2000;23:962–8

84. Andresen JL, Rasmussen LM, Ledet T. Diabetic macroangiopathy and atherosclerosis. *Diabetes* 1996;45(Suppl 3):S91–4

85. Goff DC Jr, D'Agostino RB Jr, Haffner SM, *et al.* Lipoprotein concentrations and carotid atherosclerosis by diabetes status: results from the Insulin Resistance Atherosclerosis Study. *Diabetes Care* 2000;23:1006–11

86. Bonora E, Kiechl S, Oberhollenzer F, *et al.* Impaired glucose tolerance, type II diabetes mellitus and carotid atherosclerosis: prospective results from the Bruneck Study. *Diabetologia* 2000;43:156–64

87. Meigs JB, Singer DE, Sullivan LM, *et al.* Metabolic control and prevalent cardiovascular disease in non-insulin-dependent diabetes mellitus (NIDDM): the NIDDM Patient Outcomes Research Team. *Am J Med* 1997; 102:38–47

88. UK Prospective Diabetes Group. Tight blood pressure control and risk of macrovascular and microvascular complications in type 2 diabetes: UKPDS 38. *Br Med J* 1998; 317:701–13

89. Brun E, Nelson RG, Bennett PH, *et al.* Diabetes duration and cause-specific mortality in the Verona Diabetes Study. *Diabetes Care* 2000;23:1119–23

90. Report of the expert committee on the diagnosis and classification of diabetes mellitus. *Diabetes Care* 1997;20:1183–97

91. Harris MI, Eastman RC. Early detection of undiagnosed diabetes mellitus: a US perspective. *Diabetes/Metab Res Rev* 2000;16:230–6

92. CDC Diabetes Cost-Effectiveness Study Group. The cost-effectiveness of screening for type 2 diabetes. *J Am Med Assoc* 1998; 280:1757–63

93. Goyder EC, Irwig LM. Screening for type 2 diabetes mellitus: a decision analytic approach. *Diabetic Med* 2000;17:469–77

94. Engelgau MM, Venkat Narayan KM, Herman WH. Screening for type 2 diabetes. *Diabetes Care* 2000;23:1563–80

95. UK Prospective Diabetes Group. Efficacy of aterolol and captopril in reducing risk of macrovascular and microvascular complications in type 2 diabetes (UKPDS 39). *Br Med J* 1998;317:713–20

96. The Diabetes Prevention Program Research Group. The diabetes prevention program. *Diabetes Care* 2000;23:1619–29

97. Kuusisto J, Mykkänen, Pyörälä K, *et al.* Non-insulin-dependent diabetes and its metabolic control and important predictors of stroke in elderly subjects. *Stroke* 1994;43: 960–7

98. Manton KG, Stallard E. Cross-sectional estimates of active life expectancy for the US elderly and oldest-old populations. *J Gerontol* 1991;46:S160–82

99. Holvey SM. Psychosocial aspects in the care of elderly diabetic patients. *Am J Med* 1986; 80(Suppl 5A):61–3

100. Funnell MM. Role of diabetes educator for older adults. *Diabetes Care* 1990;13 (Suppl 2):60–5

101. Kronsbein P, Muhlhauser I, Venhaus A, *et al*. Evaluation of structured treatment and teaching program on non-insulin-dependent diabetes mellitus (NIDDM). *Am J Public Health* 1987;77:634–5

102. Wilson W, Pratt C. The impact of diabetes education and peer support upon weight and glycemic control of elderly persons with NIDDM. *Am J Public Health* 1987;77:635–7

103. Gilden JL, Hendryx M, Casia C, *et al*. The effectiveness of diabetes education programs for older patients and their spouses. *J Am Geriatr Soc* 1989;37:1023–30

104. Silliman RA, Bhatta S, Khan A, *et al*. The care of older persons with diabetes mellitus: families and primary care physicians. *J Am Geriatr Soc* 1996;44:1314–21

105. Ford ES, DeStefano F. Risk factors for mortality from all causes and from coronary heart disease among persons with diabetes. *Am J Epidemiol* 1991;133:1200–30

106. Kannel WB, McGee DL. Diabetes and glucose tolerance as risk factors for cardiovascular disease: the Framingham Study. *Diabetes Care* 1979;2:120–6

107. Beks PJ, MacKaay AJC, deNeeling JND, *et al*. Peripheral arterial disease in relation to glycaemic level in an elderly Caucasian population: the Hoorn Study. *Diabetologia* 1995;38:86–96

108. Giugliano D, Saccomanno F, Paolisso G, *et al*. Nicardipine does not cause deterioration of glucose homeostasis in man: a placebo controlled study in elderly hypertensives with and without diabetes mellitus. *Eur J Clin Pharmacol* 1992;43:39–45

109. Antonicelli R, Pagelli P, Paciaroni E. Nicardipine retard in the therapy of elderly diabetic hypertensives: final report of observational study. *J Hypertens* 1992;10(Suppl 2): 569–72

110. Lusardi P, Corradi L, Pasotti P, *et al*. Effects of amlodipine vs fosinopril on microalbuminuria in eldery hypertensive patients with type II diabetes. *J Hypertens* 1996; 14(Suppl):S193.F

111. Curb JD, Pressel SL, Cutler JA, *et al*. Effect of diuretic-based antihypertensive treatment on cardiovascular disease risk in older diabetic patients with isolated systolic hypertension. *J Am Med Assoc* 1996;276: 1886–91

112. The Heart Outcomes Prevention Evaluation study in investigators. Effects of an angiotensin-converting-enzyme inhibitor, ramipril, on cardiovascular events in high-risk patients. *N Engl J Med* 2000;342:145–53

113. Watson N, Sandler M. Effects of captopril on glucose tolerance in elderly patients with congestive cardiac failure. *Curr Med Res Opin* 1991;12:374–8

114. Paolisso G, Gambardella A, Verza M, *et al*. ACE inhibition improves insulin-sensitivity in aged insulin-resistant hypertensive patients. *J Hum Hypertens* 1992;6:175–9

16 Quality of life among older men with diabetes

Ken W. Watkins, PhD, and Cathleen M. Connell, PhD

INTRODUCTION

Health research is increasingly directed towards outcomes measurement, which has been defined as the process of assessing the clinical effectiveness of medical treatment and procedures[1]. Traditionally, outcomes assessment originated from a provider/societal perspective, with a narrow focus on patients' physical status and the economic effectiveness of treatment[2]. Recently, this perspective has been expanded to include patients' evaluation of clinical effectiveness of care and treatment. From the patient's point of view, relevant outcomes include not only objective, physiological measures, but also factors such as satisfaction, social functioning, emotional health and physical functioning[2]. These subjective factors are especially important for people managing chronic illnesses such as diabetes, for whom the treatment regimen involves self-management behaviors that pervade many aspects of their personal lives. Despite this emphasis on the patient's perspective, few studies include subjective measures, such as quality of life, in describing the effects of diabetes or the efficacy of treatment[3], although the number of such studies has increased in recent years[4].

Quality of life is an important outcome measure in this context because diabetes is largely self-managed[5,6]. The individual's subjective interpretation of having diabetes is critical for initiating and regulating the day-to-day regimen of diet, exercise, medication and self-monitoring of blood glucose, as well as maintaining contact with the physician and diabetes treatment team. The patient's subjective evaluations of the effectiveness of the treatment regimen constantly update and modify disease understanding and motivation that drive individual health behaviors. In this respect, quality of life helps to provide researchers and health professionals with a more 'comprehensive assessment of the impact' of diabetes[7-9] in addition to other more traditional measures of diabetes outcomes (for example, glycosylated hemoglobin levels).

The overall objective of this chapter is to describe how diabetes affects quality of life, particularly among older men. Although the prevalence of diabetes increases substantially with age[10], little research has focused on the psychosocial impact of the disease on older men. After a general discussion of diabetes risks among older adults, specific topics addressed include the measurement of quality of life, research findings to date and implications for practitioners.

DIABETES AMONG OLDER ADULTS: UNIQUE RISKS FOR MEN

In some respects, men with diabetes appear to have a health advantage over women with diabetes. Overall, men report fewer chronic illness conditions than women[11], and diagnosed diabetes prevalence and incidence rates are slightly lower in men than in women[10]. In addition, mortality risks associated with diabetes are approximately twice as high for women than for men[10].

Despite this apparent advantage, however, older men with diabetes face several unique health risks. The incidence of peripheral vascular disease is higher among men than among women, and amputation rates are 1.4–2.7 times higher for men than for women[10]. The progression of diabetes-related retinopathy occurs more rapidly for men than for women[10]. Peripheral neuropathy occurs more frequently in men with diabetes than in women: nearly 8% of men with type 2 diabetes experience impotence as a result of neuropathy[10]. Finally, rates of diabetes-related hospitalization are higher for older men than for older women[12]. Together, these health risks suggest that an understanding of the psychosocial context of diabetes as it relates to older men, including quality-of-life concerns, is especially important in terms of research and practice.

MEASURING QUALITY OF LIFE

'Quality of life' is at once an easily identifiable, yet vague concept. Meanings attributed to quality of life are likewise diverse. Quality of life can be categorized as an assessment of functioning[13], a general 'index' of well-being, a multi-attribute health profile, a disease- or population-specific instrument, or a utility measure[14]. This construct has been conceptualized as encompassing physical health and functioning, mental health, cognitive functioning, social functioning, role functioning, satisfaction with treatment, concerns about the future and general well-being[13,15–17], and is often measured in terms of individuals' subjective perceptions[3]. Quality of life is thought to be multidimensional and to cut across different disease categories[3].

The term 'health-related quality of life' shares the broad conceptual domains encompassed by general quality of life measures while maintaining a focus on health status and health care[2,15]. Glasgow and Osteen[5] suggest combining general and disease-specific measures of quality of life to facilitate comparisons of findings across studies and disease treatments, as well as to gain insight into the mechanisms specific to diabetes self-management. However, few published studies have used both general and disease-specific measures (for exceptions, see references 18 and 19).

Among the more popular general measures of quality of life are the Rand Health Insurance/Medical Outcome Study Batteries (for example, SF-36), Sickness Impact Profile (SIP), and the Older Americans Resources and Services (OARS) Multidimensional Functional Assessment Questionnaire (OMFAQ) (see reference 20 for a comprehensive review). The Medical Outcomes Study (MOS) questionnaire comprises eight concepts: physical functioning, role limitations owing to physical problems, social functioning, bodily pain, general mental health, role limitations owing to emotional problems, vitality and general health perceptions[17]. The Sickness Impact Profile (SIP) emphasizes behavioral functioning related to a respondent's perception of illness, and includes items that assess sleep and rest, eating, work, home management, recreation and pastimes, ambulation, mobility, body care and movement, social interaction, alertness behavior, emotional behavior and communication[21]. The OARS Multidimensional Functional Assessment Questionnaire (OMFAQ) was designed specifically for older adults and assesses functional status and service use[20].

While general measures of health status are useful for comparisons across diseases, they may not be sensitive to unique aspects of particular illnesses[3,18]. Several diabetes-specific quality-of-life measures have been developed in recent years (for reviews, see references 22 and 23). For example, the Diabetes Quality of Life Measure (DQOL), developed by the Diabetes Control and Complications Trial (DCCT)

Research Group for use in the landmark DCCT study, measures satisfaction with treatment, impact of treatment, worry about the future effects of diabetes, worry about social/vocational issues, and perceptions of overall well-being[3,19]. The Diabetes Care Profile (DCP) is a comprehensive (234-item) self-administered questionnaire that assesses attitudes, beliefs, self-management behaviors, and quality-of-life concerns (such as social and role functioning, self-care ability) with regard to diabetes[18]. The 22-item self-administered Well-Being Questionnaire[24] assesses depression, anxiety, energy, positive well-being and general well-being among individuals treating diabetes with insulin or oral medication. The Diabetes Quality of Life Clinical Trial Questionnaire – Revised (DQLCTQ–R)[25] assesses physical functioning, energy/fatigue, health distress, mental health, satisfaction, treatment satisfaction, treatment flexibility and frequency of symptoms. Finally, the Diabetes-Specific Quality-of-Life Scale (DSQOLS) measures diabetes treatment goals, satisfaction with treatment success and burden associated with diabetes self-management[26].

RESEARCH FINDINGS TO DATE

Diabetes and quality of life

Although relatively few empirical studies focus exclusively on older adults with diabetes, a growing body of research addresses quality of life among adults with chronic illness, including diabetes. Adults with diabetes report decreased quality of life when compared with healthy adults[9,27,28], but higher levels of quality of life when compared with individuals having other chronic illnesses (such as cardiovascular disease, arthritis, gastrointestinal disorders)[28]. Although improved glycemic control is not consistently related to quality of life[26,29–32], some evidence suggests a positive relationship when diabetes-specific measures of quality of life are used[6]. Decreased quality of life is

also associated with an increased number and severity of complications[4,18,19,33,34]; however, quality of life may be more closely related to the level of disease management required of the individual than to the disease outcomes themselves[3].

Quality of life is also associated with the behavioral regimen required for disease management. Although the physiological benefits (for example, delay or prevention of disease complications) of diabetes self-management are recognized, even among an older adult population[35,36], the psychological impact of maintaining a somewhat demanding treatment regimen over time is less well understood. While some studies show that diabetes-specific health behaviors such as exercise are related to increased quality of life[4,37], other studies conclude that the relationship between quality of life and a wide range of diabetes self-management behaviors is equivocal[29,32,38].

The degree of burden or intrusiveness of diabetes self-management appears to be a primary influence on individuals' perceived quality of life[39–41]. For example, adherence to a dietary regimen is associated with interference with social and personal functioning[41], both of which are related to quality of life. Similarly, taking insulin is associated with decreased quality of life[33], although people who follow a flexible insulin regimen (i.e. pump treatment) report higher levels of quality of life than those who need to take several insulin injections a day[26,42]. In summary, although research suggests that diabetes can impair quality of life, self-management behaviors and regimen characteristics are important factors to consider in this relationship.

Age and gender as moderators of the relationship between diabetes and quality of life

Research evidence suggests that age and gender play a role in the relationship between quality of life and illness outcomes. For example, with age, diabetes becomes increasingly detrimental to physical functioning, social functioning and mental health, all of which impact on qualify of life[4,18,43]. The negative impact of diabetes on quality of life among older adults may be partially explained by their perceptions of control over health[44,45].

As people get older, their perceptions of control over health become particularly relevant to quality-of-life issues. Rodin and Timko[45] suggest that individuals with higher levels of perceived control take greater responsibility for meeting their health needs, and the tendency for individuals with lower perceived control to engage in fewer health-protective behaviors may actually grow stronger with age. This tendency can have serious consequences, as reductions in self-management behavior may be particularly detrimental to the health of older adults. Reductions in perceptions of control and engagement in health behaviors can occur when older adults view physical decline/illness as an inevitable, irreversible consequence of aging[46]. Also, the increased contact of older adults with medical care systems can influence perceived control when this contact is accompanied by restriction of activity, dependency or lack of responsiveness by health professionals.

In addition, older adults' perceptions of and preferences for personal control over health-related issues are more variable than those of younger adults[47]. This variability occurs as a possible result of aging (including loss of roles and physical abilities), cohort differences (older generations may be more accepting of physician authority than younger generations), societal stigmatization (negative stereotypes that older adults cannot adequately self-manage diabetes) or vicarious experiences (observations regarding loss experienced by others).

Related to the concept of personal control, older adults' self-efficacy[48] or confidence regarding their ability to engage in specific physical activities may be lower than that of younger adults. Several factors may help to explain this relationship. First, differences in past and present experiences of performance are more evident with increased age. Second, in observing others' level of physical activity, older adults see an elderly cohort less likely to respond adequately to environmental demands. Third, older adults are at increased risk of physical dependence on others. Finally, lower levels of perceived self-efficacy are common in regard to losses in physical ability associated with some chronic illnesses[47].

Several studies show positive effects on health outcomes of interventions to improve perceived control and self-efficacy for health behaviors among older adults[47,49]. However, an increased desire for control may create problems when health situations do not match an individual's expectations (for example, maintaining normal glycemic levels with the same level of effort as required at a younger age). Such unreasonable expectations regarding control can result in negative psychological and physical outcomes because of the stress they create[45].

In contrast to research that points to decreased quality of life in older adults with diabetes, other studies suggest that, for older adults, diabetes has less of a negative effect on some quality-of-life outcomes than for younger adults. For example, Connell[50] found that older adults with type 2 diabetes perceived less impact of the disease on emotional health (i.e. depression) than did younger adults. Such a difference might exist for several reasons. First, physical health status may become of less subjective importance with increased age and across disease conditions, when considering other factors such as mental and emotional well-being[51]. Likewise, a positive bias in subjective health ratings may be related to three 'rules' regarding health and aging[52]. A first 'rule' suggests that older adults often attribute symptoms of chronic illness to physical aging rather than to illness. This occurs because older adults experience more chronic conditions than younger adults, so there is an increased background of somatic symptoms from which to distinguish. A second 'rule' suggests that when illness symptoms are ambiguous (such as tiredness or lethargy), older adults are more likely than younger adults to attribute them to specific life circumstances (for example, lack of sleep) than to a specific disease condition such as hyperglycemia. Finally, a third 'rule' suggests that older adults tend to compare and discuss illness conditions with peers, and may therefore tend to downplay the seriousness of their condition based upon the number of other older adults who also have similar symptoms and illnesses[53]. In summary, these three 'rules' illustrate how older adults' attribution of diabetes symptoms to factors other than the disease could reduce the perceived negative impact of diabetes on quality of life.

Evidence related to the relationship between gender and quality of life is also mixed. Some research indicates little difference between men and women in terms of the impact of diabetes on their lives[54]. When controlling for other demographic factors (i.e. age, ethnicity, diabetes type and treatment), Watkins and colleagues[41] found that women expressed more positive global quality-of-life ratings than did men. Conversely, other large-scale studies suggest that, compared to men, women with diabetes report poorer overall quality of life[4] and diabetes-specific quality of life[25,31,55]. Rubin and Peyrot[55] found the perceived burden of diabetes self-management to be lower for men than for women (for example, men reported more consistent self-management of diabetes, more confidence in their ability to manage the disease, more satisfaction with spousal support and increased satisfaction with treatment). However, other studies have shown that, while women perceive more barriers to self-management, they also believe more strongly in the efficacy of treatment than do men[56].

Although these studies suggest a possible advantage in the ability to self-manage diabetes among men, little research has investigated gender differences in diabetes quality of life among older adults. An exclusive focus on the main effects of age and gender may result in the failure to detect a possible moderating role for either of these factors. For example, work by Leventhal and associates[57] suggests an age–gender crossover interaction with regard to illness burden (i.e. number of serious illnesses and morbidity). Specifically, they found that younger women reported higher illness burdens than younger men; however, older women reported less illness burden than did older men. This difference was most pronounced among adults 75 years of age and older.

One possible explanation for an age–gender interaction in quality of life associated with diabetes is the differential impact of diabetes-specific social support for older men and women. Social support is associated with better quality of life[26] and an important source of social support for older adults is the spouse. Although widowhood is more common in older women than in older men[12], several factors suggest the experience of widowhood may be more deleterious for older men[58]. First, because older men are more likely to be recently widowed than are older women, they are likely to be experiencing more intense bereavement. Second, older men have 'more to lose' than do their female counterparts. Studies indicate that older men are more likely to be satisfied with spousal support prior to the loss of the spouse[59], and that the loss of diabetes-specific support may have a greater negative impact for older men than for women[60]. Finally, widowhood is perceived as a more normative experience for older women and a more unexpected experience for older men.

Another possible explanation for an age–gender interaction with regard to quality of life might be in the differential impact of diabetes complications for men and women. As mentioned above, older men face increased risks of severe diabetes complications and outcomes (such as end-stage renal disease, neuropathy, amputation) when compared with women. Increased risks for such losses represent a challenge to a traditional masculine identity of autonomy, control and independence[61]; these issues may be especially relevant for older men.

Additional research is needed to untangle the complex relationships among gender, age, and the impact of self-management behaviors on quality of life. These relationships are especially important in an older adult population where diabetes-specific health behaviors and quality of life are necessary, but to some degree conflicting, components of diabetes self-management. While the importance of diabetes-specific health behaviors in preventing or delaying complications of the disease has been conclusively demonstrated[35,62], subjective perceptions of quality of life play an equally critical role in the self-management of diabetes by directly affecting those behaviors. Specifically, people may be less likely to engage in health behaviors that are related to negative assessments of quality of life (such as adopting restrictive dietary changes). The fact that older men view these health behaviors as complicated and difficult to maintain increases the chance that quality of life and successful diabetes management are thought to be competing outcomes[3].

IMPLICATIONS FOR PRACTITIONERS

In working with older male patients with diabetes, it is important to consider individual and contextual factors related to quality of life. Along with comorbid conditions and complications that affect social/physical functioning and emotional well-being, practitioners should be especially aware of individual perceptions of and preferences for control over diabetes. Perceptions of diabetes control are related to personal investment in the disease management process and support from family members, friends and health-care professionals.

An increased sense of personal control over the disease is facilitated by involving the patient in developing a personal diabetes self-management plan. Because of the nature of diabetes and the fact that it is largely self-managed, there has been a growing trend in the medical community towards empowering people to better self-manage their diabetes[63]. In an empowerment model, patients work collaboratively with the physician and diabetes treatment team (nurse, diabetes educator, social worker) to develop an individually tailored regimen plan. The health professional's role in this relationship is neither prescriptive nor 'hands-off' in nature, but instead comprises elements of being an advisor, consultant, motivator and counselor. In this respect, 'successful' self-management of diabetes can positively affect individuals' quality of life by increasing their sense of mastery and control[64] and re-evaluation of the personal meaning of diabetes, issues that have increased relevance for men as they age.

Because having diabetes affects all aspects of physical and social functioning, family members and friends can play an important role in shaping the patient's perceived control of the disease. Therefore, involving family members and friends in diabetes education efforts is recommended for facilitating patient empowerment[65]. For example, interventions that rely on social networks have been found to improve quality of life and knowledge of diabetes[66], assist with behavior change efforts (for example, weight loss)[67,68] and provide protective effects from symptoms of depression for those faced with diabetes-related functional disabilities[69]. Social support from a spouse has been shown to be more strongly related to better blood glucose control for older men than for older women, possibly because women traditionally take on more supportive roles within the home, including food selection and preparation[70]. Some research also suggests that social support facilitates diabetes self-management to a greater extent for certain ethnic groups, such as African-Americans[71].

There are other studies, however, indicating that diabetes-specific social support is not always well received, especially if it is perceived as nagging or is unsolicited. For example, Connell[50] found that older men with diabetes may receive more help than they want with such activities as following a meal plan or taking medications. Wing and colleagues[72] also found that, while women's involvement in a diabetes weight-control program was enhanced by the involvement of the spouse, men preferred to work in the program alone. Ideally, the type and amount of received support need to be congruent with that desired by the patient. Therefore, it is important to take direction from the older male patient regarding how best to involve family members and friends in their self-management efforts.

Finally, practitioners should accept that the older patient's notion of optimal quality of life might not be compatible with the medical community's expectations for ideal diabetes self-management. For example, although older adults can successfully follow an intensive diabetes regimen[73] with clear clinical benefits[36], the level of commitment to such a treatment regimen may be perceived as not worth the cost (e.g., carefully orchestrated blood glucose monitoring, insulin administration, caloric intake). In the case of older men, such a regimen might be viewed as unduly intrusive and in conflict with other priorities, such as maintaining a sense of independence and control in later life. For older men, intensive treatment can also be viewed as a constant reminder of the loss of physical integrity associated with old age. A goal of treatment should therefore involve planning that optimizes outcomes with a minimum of disease burden.

References

1. Greene R, Bondy PK, Maklan CW. The national medical effectiveness research initiative: the search of what really works in treating common clinical conditions. *Diabetes Care* 1994;17(Suppl):45–9
2. Barr JT. The outcomes movement and health status measures. *J Allied Health* 1995;24:13–28
3. Jacobson AM, de Groot M, Samson J. Quality of life research in patients with diabetes mellitus. In Dimsdale JE, Baum A, eds. *Quality of Life in Behavioral Medicine Research.* Hillsdale, NJ: Lawrence Erlbaum Associates, 1995:241–62
4. Glasgow RE, Ruggiero L, Eakin EG, *et al.* Quality of life and associated characteristics in a large national sample of adults with diabetes. *Diabetes Care* 1997;20:562–7
5. Glasgow RE, Osteen VL. Evaluating diabetes education. Are we measuring the most important outcomes? *Diabetes Care* 1992;15:1423–32
6. Rubin RR, Peyrot M. Quality of life and diabetes. *Diabetes Metab Res Rev* 1999;15:205–18

7. Brown I, Renwick R, Nagler M. The centrality of quality of life in health promotion and rehabilitation. In Renwick R, Brown I, Nagler M, eds. *Quality of Life in Health Promotion and Rehabilitation: Conceptual Approaches, Issues, and Applications.* Thousand Oaks, CA: Sage Publications, 1996:13
8. Lau RR. Cognitive representations of health and illness. In Gochman DS, ed. *Handbook of Health Behavior Research.* New York: Plenum Press, 1997:51–69
9. Rodin G. Quality of life in adults with insulin-dependent diabetes mellitus. *Psychother Psychosom* 1990;54:132–9
10. American Diabetes Association. *Diabetes 1996: Vital Statistics.* Alexandria, VA: American Diabetes Association, 1996:13–59
11. Verbrugge LM. Gender and health: an update on hypotheses and evidence. *J Health Soc Behav* 1985;26:156–82
12. Kramarow E, Lentzner H, Rooks R, *et al. Health and Aging Chartbook.* Hyattsville, MD: National Center for Health Statistics, 1999:46–7, 78–9

13. Raphael D. Defining quality of life: eleven debates concerning its measurement. In Renwick R, Brown I, Nagler M, eds. *Quality of Life in Health Promotion and Rehabilitation: Conceptual Approaches, Issues, and Applications*. Thousand Oaks, CA: Sage Publications, 1996:146–65

14. Brooks RG. *Health Status Measurement: A Perspective on Change*. Basingstoke: Macmillan, 1995

15. Shumaker SA, Naughton MJ. The international assessment of health-related quality of life: a theoretical perspective. In Shumaker SA, Berzon RA, eds. *The International Assessment of Health-Related Quality of Life: Theory Translation, Measurement and Analysis*. Oxford: Rapid Communications, 1995:3–10

16. Stewart AL, King AC. Conceptualizing and measuring quality of life in older populations. In Abeles RP, Gift HC, Ory MG, eds. *Aging and Quality of Life*. New York: Springer Publishing, 1994:27–54

17. Ware JE, Sherbourne CD. The MOS 36-item short form health survey (SF-36): I. Conceptual framework and item selection. *Med Care* 1992;30:473–83

18. Anderson RM, Fitzgerald JT, Wisdom K, *et al.* A comparison of global versus disease specific quality-of-life measures in patients with NIDDM. *Diabetes Care* 1997;20:299–305

19. Jacobson AM, The Diabetes Control and Complications Trial Research Group. The Diabetes Quality of Life measure. In Bradley C, ed. *Handbook of Psychology and Diabetes: A Guide to Psychological Measurement in Diabetes Research and Measurement*. Chur, Switzerland: Harwood Academic Publishers, 1994:65–88

20. MacDowell I, Newell C. *Measuring Health: A Guide to Rating Scales and Questionnaires*. New York: Oxford University Press, 1996: 380–472

21. Bergner M, Bobbitt RA, Bergner M, *et al.* Validation of an interval scaling: the Sickness Impact Profile. *Health Serv Res* 1976;11: 516–28

22. Bowling A. *Measuring Health: A Review of Quality of Life Measurement Scales*, 2nd edn. Bristol, PA: Open University Press, 1997

23. Polonsky WH. Understanding and assessing diabetes-specific quality of life. *Diabetes Spectrum* 2000;13:36–41

24. Bradley C. The Well-Being Questionnaire. In Bradley C, ed. *Handbook of Psychology and Diabetes: A Guide to Psychological Measurement in Diabetes Research and Measurement*. Chur, Switzerland: Harwood Academic Publishers, 1994:89–110

25. Shen W, Kotsanos JG, Huster WJ, *et al.* Development and validation of the Diabetes Quality of Life Clinical Trial Questionnaire. *Med Care* 1999;37:AS45–66

26. Bott U, Muhlhauser I, Overmann H, *et al.* Validation of a Diabetes-Specific Quality-of-Life Scale for Patients with type 1 diabetes. *Diabetes Care* 1998;21:757–69

27. Caldwell CM, Baxter J, Mitchell CM, *et al.* The association of non-insulin-dependent diabetes mellitus with perceived quality of life in a biethnic population: the San Luis Valley Diabetes Study. *Am J Public Health* 1998; 88:1225–39

28. Stewart AL, Greenfield S, Hays RD. Functional status and well-being of patients with chronic conditions. *J Am Med Assoc* 1989;262:907–13

29. Aalto AM, Uutela A, Aro AR. Health-related quality of life among insulin dependent diabetics: disease-related and psychosocial correlates. *Patient Educ Couns* 1997;30:215–25

30. Nerenz DR, Repasky DP, Whitehouse FW, *et al.* Ongoing assessment of health status in patients with diabetes mellitus. *Med Care* 1992;30(Suppl 5):MS112–24

31. Petterson T, Lee P, Hollis S, *et al.* Well-being and treatment satisfaction in older people with diabetes. *Diabetes Care* 1998;21:930–5

32. Weinberger M, Kirkman S, Samsa GP, *et al.* The relationship between glycemic control and health-related quality of life in patients with non-insulin-dependent diabetes mellitus. *Med Care* 1994;32:1173–81

33. Bradley C, Todd C, Gorton T, *et al.* The development of an individualized questionnaire measure of perceived impact of diabetes on quality of life: the ADDQoL. *Qual Life Res* 1999;8:79–91

34. Nathan DM, Fogel H, Norman D, *et al.* Long-term metabolic and quality of life results

with pancreatic/renal transplantation in insulin-dependent diabetes mellitus. *Transplantation* 1991;52:85–91

35. American Diabetes Association. Implications of the United Kingdom Prospective Diabetes Study. *Diabetes Care* 1999;22(Suppl 1): S27–31

36. Halter JB. Geriatric patients. In Lebovitz HE. *Therapy for Diabetes Mellitus and Related Disorders*. Alexandria, VA: American Diabetes Association, 1994:164–9

37. Kaplan RM, Hartwell SL, Wilson DK, *et al.* Effect of diet and exercise interventions on control and quality of life in non-insulin-dependent diabetes mellitus. *J Gen Intern Med* 1987;2:220–8

38. Glasgow RE, Toobert DJ, Hampson SE, *et al.* Improving self-care among older patients with Type II diabetes: the 'Sixty Something...' study. *Patient Educ Couns* 1992;19:61–74

39. Connell CM, Davis WK, Gallant MP, *et al.* Impact of social support, social cognitive variables, and perceived threat on depression among adults with diabetes. *Health Psychol* 1994;13:263–73

40. Talbot F, Nouwen A, Gingras J, *et al.* Relations of diabetes intrusiveness and personal control to symptoms of depression among adults with diabetes. *Health Psychol* 1999;18:537–42

41. Watkins KW, Connell CM, Fitzgerald JT, *et al.* Effects of adults' self-regulation of diabetes on quality of life outcomes. *Diabetes Care* 2000;23:1511–15

42. Diabetes Control and Complications Trial Research Group. The effect of intensive treatment of diabetes on the development and progression of long-term complications in insulin-dependent diabetes mellitus. *N Engl J Med* 1993;329:977–86

43. Bourdel-Marchasson I, Dubroca B, Manciet G, *et al.* Prevalence of diabetes and effect on quality of life in older French living in the community: the PAQUID Epidemiological Survey. *J Am Geriatr Soc* 1997;45:295–301

44. Keller ML, Leventhal H, Prohaska TR, *et al.* Beliefs about aging and illness in a community sample. *Res Nurs Health* 1989;12:247–55

45. Rodin J, Timko C. Sense of control, aging, and health. In Ory MG, Abeles RP, Lipman PD,

eds. *Aging, Health, and Behavior*. Newbury Park, CA: SAGE Publications, 1992:174–206

46. Besdine RW. Clinical approach: an overview. In Cassel CK, Cohen HJ, Larson EB, *et al.*, eds. *Geriatric Medicine*. New York: Springer-Verlag, 1997:155–68

47. Deeg DJH, Kardaun JWPF, Fozard JL. Health, behavior, and aging. In Birren JE, Schaie KW, eds. *Handbook of the Psychology of Aging*, 4th edn. New York: Academic Press, 1996:129–49

48. Bandura A. Self-efficacy: toward a unifying theory of behavioral change. *Psychol Rev* 1977;84:191–215

49. Taylor SE, Aspinwall, LG. Psychosocial aspects of chronic illness. In Costa PT, VandenBos GR, eds. *Psychological Aspects of Serious Illness: Chronic Conditions, Fatal Diseases, and Clinical Care*. Washington, DC: American Psychological Association, 1990:3–60

50. Connell CM. Psychosocial contexts of diabetes and older adulthood: reciprocal effects. *Diabetes Educator* 1991;17:364–71

51. Hickey T, Stilwell DL. Health promotion for older people: all is not well. *Gerontologist* 1991;31:822–9

52. Leventhal EA, Crouch M. Are there differences in perceptions of illness across the lifespan? In Petrie KJ, Weinman JA, eds. *Perceptions of Health and Illness: Current Research and Applications*. Amsterdam, The Netherlands: Harwood Academic Publishers, 1997:77–102

53. Croyle RT, Jemmott JB. Psychological reactions to risk factor testing. In Skelton JA, Croyle RT, eds. *Mental Representation in Health and Illness*. New York: Springer-Verlag, 1991:85–107

54. Fitzgerald JT, Anderson RM, Davis WK. Gender differences in diabetes attitudes and adherence. *Diabetes Educator* 1995;21: 523–9

55. Rubin RR, Peyrot M. Men and diabetes: psychosocial and behavioral issues. *Diabetes Spectrum* 1998;11:81–7

56. Glasgow RE, Hampson SE, Strycker LA, *et al.* Personal-model beliefs and social–environmental barriers related to diabetes self-management. *Diabetes Care* 1997;20:556–61

57. Leventhal EA, Leventhal H, Schaefer P, *et al.* Conservation of energy, uncertainty reduction and swift utilization of medical care among the elderly. *J Gerontol Psychol Sci* 1993;48:78–86

58. Lee GR, Willetts MC, Seccombe K. Widowhood and depression: gender differences. *Res Aging* 1998;20:611–30

59. Dean A, Kolody B, Wood P, *et al.* The influence of living alone on depression in elderly persons. *J Aging Health* 1992;4:3–18

60. Connell CM, Fisher EB Jr, Houston CA. Relationships among social support, diabetes outcomes, and morale for older men and women. *J Aging Health* 1992;4:77–100

61. Eckert JK, Rubinstein RL. Older men's health: sociocultural and ecological perspectives. *Med Clin North Am* 1999;83:1151–73

62. American Diabetes Association. Implications of the Diabetes Control and Complications Trial. *Diabetes Care* 1999;22(Suppl 1): S24–26

63. Funnell MM, Anderson RM, Arnold MS, *et al.* Empowerment: an idea whose time has come in diabetes education. *Diabetes Educator* 1991;17:37–41

64. Aldwin CM. *Stress, Coping, and Development.* New York: The Guilford Press, 1994: 258–62

65. Rubin RR. Psychosocial assessment. In Funnell MM, Hunt C, Kulkarni K, *et al.*, eds. *A Core Curriculum for Diabetes Educators.* Chicago, IL: American Association of Diabetes Educators, 1998:87–118

66. Gilden JL, Hendryx MS, Clar S, *et al.* Diabetes support groups improve health care of older diabetic patients. *J Am Geriatr Soc* 1992;40:147–50

67. Glasgow RE, Toobert DJ. Social environment and regimen adherence among type II diabetic patients. *Diabetes Care* 1988;11: 377–86

68. Pratt C, Wilson W, Leklem J, *et al.* Peer support and nutrition education for older adults with diabetes. *J Nutr Elderly* 1987; 6:31–43

69. Littlefield CH, Rodin GM, Murray MA, *et al.* Influence of functional impairment and social support on depressive symptoms in persons with diabetes. *Health Psychol* 1990;9:737–49

70. Eriksson BS, Rosenqvist U. Social support and glycemic control in non-insulin dependent diabetes mellitus patients: gender differences. *Women Health* 1993;20:59–70

71. Ford ME, Tilley BC, McDonald PE. Social support among African-American adults with diabetes, Part 2: a review. *J Natl Med Assoc* 1998;90:425–32

72. Wing RR, Marcus MD, Epstein LH, *et al.* A 'family-based' approach to the treatment of obese type II diabetic patients. *J Consult Clin Psychol* 1991;59:156–62

73. Abraira C, Colwell JA, Nuttall FQ, *et al.* Veterans Affairs Cooperative Study on glycemic control and complications in type II diabetes (VA CSDM). *Diabetes Care* 1995; 18:1113–23

17 Treatment of diabetes in the elderly

Joel Zonszein, MD, FACE, FACP

INTRODUCTION

With advancing age there is a tendency towards worsening of glucose tolerance and increased incidence of diabetes. The prevalence of diagnosed cases is 6% in individuals between the ages of 45 and 64, increasing to 12% in those over the age of 65, and 40% in individuals over the age of 80 years. Medical care is costly, with expenses related to diabetes care of more than $US 100 billion per year, accounting for 50% of all healthcare costs in the USA, and 25% of all Medicare costs[1]. Since diabetes is a treatable condition, there is a tremendous opportunity for early intervention to attenuate the incidence of complications, and their adverse socioeconomic impact.

Treating diabetes in the elderly is complex, and polypharmacy is often necessary owing to comorbidity and other cardiovascular risk factors. This population has age-related organ failure, and higher incidences of cognitive impairment, depression, functional disability and dependency on care-givers. Treatment needs to be carefully prioritized and tailored individually. The goals must be realistic, with treatment of hyperglycemia carefully weighed in the context of the patient's projected life span[2], while avoiding hypoglycemia. There is now an effective armamentarium of medications to combat this disease, and the clinician is confronted with the challenge of how to prescribe wisely to improve disease outcomes, while maintaining an adequate quality of life.

The hyperglycemia of type 2 diabetes is part of a metabolic–cardiovascular syndrome, characterized by a complex interaction of several cardiovascular risk factors. In addition to hyperglycemia and hyperinsulinemia, central obesity, dyslipidemia, hypertension, endothelial dysfunction and a hypercoagulant state are part of this syndrome. The interplay of these factors causes an adverse milieu with a state of accelerated arteriosclerosis[3], with a premature and high morbidity and mortality rate. While this condition has an important genetic component, there are several modifiable or treatable risk factors. Management of diabetes is no longer treatment of hyperglycemia alone; it requires a global and aggressive approach. Improvement of metabolic derangements of carbohydrate metabolism needs to be done in conjunction with amelioration of all other cardiovascular risk factors.

A better understanding of the pathophysiology of diabetes and newer medications have enabled us to treat this condition with a more rational approach. Each patient can have an element of insulin resistance and/or insulin deficiency[4]. Insulin resistance predominates in those with central obesity and hypertriglyceridemia; and insulin deficiency is characteristic of autoimmune type 1 diabetes. As patients with type 2 diabetes live longer, many require insulin replacement as they have 'exhausted' the capacity of their β cells to secrete insulin

Table 1 American Diabetes Association goals for glycemic control

	Normal	Goal	Action suggested
Preprandial plasma glucose (mg/dl)	< 100	90–130	< 90 or > 150
Bedtime blood glucose (mg/dl)	< 120	110–150	< 110 or > 180
HbA$_{1C}$ (%)*	< 6	< 7	> 8

*Normal range 4–6%

Table 2 Other treatment goals for adults with type 2 diabetes

Parameter	Treatment goal*
Blood pressure (mmHg)	< 130/80
Total cholesterol (mg/dl)	< 200
Low-density lipoprotein (LDL) cholesterol (mg/dl)	< 100
High-density lipoprotein (HDL) cholesterol (mg/dl)	> 45
Triglycerides (mg/dl)	< 150–200

*Target should be adjusted based on the presence of additional cardiovascular risk factors

through the duration of their disease[5]. Autoimmune type 1 diabetes in the adult is uncommon in the USA, particularly in individuals of ethnic minorities, but can manifest late in life in Northern European Whites[6]. Since individuals with little or no β-cell function are in a state of insulin deficiency, they need to be treated with insulin. This implies a regimen of multiple insulin injections, similar to that used in the Diabetes Control and Complications Trial (DCCT)[7]. In the elderly, insulin replacement is often done with less intensity to avoid hypoglycemia, and because tight control has less of an impact owing to their life span[2].

Insulin resistance has an irreversible component determined by genetic and phenotypic characteristics, often related to the amount of adipose tissue and its distribution. Medications that improve insulin sensitivity are ideal in these patients. A transient and reversible component of insulin resistance can be caused by 'glucose toxicity', a condition in which hyperglycemia begets more hyperglycemia[8]. The use of insulin or insulin secretagogues can reverse 'glucose toxicity' and can often be discontinued after achieving glycemic control, enhancing the subsequent response to therapy with oral agents[9,10]. When insulin is used chronically in insulin-resistant patients, it is given in small doses as a to overcome the resistant state. One injection of intermediate insulin given at bedtime can be very effective in suppressing the exaggerated rate of hepatic glucose production that plays an important role in the hyperglycemia of type 2 diabetes[11,12].

Treatment of type 2 diabetes needs to be global, including the amelioration of all other cardiovascular risk factors, and not focusing only on 'lowering blood sugar numbers'. There is now a plethora of clinical studies that have been translated into 'evidence based medicine' regarding how best to treat this disorder. Based on this information, the American Diabetes Association (ADA) has made available a consensus of treatment goals for all patients with diabetes[13]; this is given in Tables 1 and 2.

IMPORTANCE OF GLYCEMIC CONTROL

The DCCT[7] established that, in type 1 diabetes mellitus, the risk for microvascular complications can be reduced substantially by maintaining near-normal blood glucose levels with intensive insulin therapy. These findings were immediately applied to type 2 diabetes[14], and similar beneficial effects were found in the largest and longest trial for type 2 diabetes, the UK Prospective Diabetes Study (UKPDS)[15]. Even modest improvement of hemoglobin (Hb)A$_{1C}$ (from 7.9 to 7%) using either sulfonylureas or insulin had a beneficial effect in reducing diabetes-related microvascular complications. A smaller substudy in overweight patients treated with metformin showed a similar reduction in microvascular complications[16]. The incidence of macrovascular complications did not increase in those treated with insulin or sulfonylureas[15], disproving previous concepts of a possible adverse effect of these agents[17,18].

Hyperglycemia is clearly a risk factor for coronary artery disease[19,20], with a direct correlation between duration and severity[19,20]. Patients with type 2 diabetes are at high risk for cardiovascular events and mortality, similar to those with already established arteriosclerotic heart disease (secondary intervention)[21]. In the UKPDS, the incidence of large-vessel disease events was seven times higher than that of microvascular complications[22], and glycemic control had a favorable but not significant impact on decreasing coronary heart disease[15]. On the other hand, blood pressure control was effective in reducing microvascular disease, and had a significant impact on decreasing heart attacks, strokes, congestive heart failure and death[23]. Treatment of dyslipidemia has also been shown to be associated with a major reduction in cardiovascular morbidity and mortality[24–28]. Aspirin therapy has also been found to be beneficial[29–33]. In conclusion, hyperglycemia needs to be addressed as it reduces microvascular complications and is an important marker for coronary heart disease (CHD), but, particularly in the elderly, the concomitant treatment of hypertension[23,34–36], and dyslipidemia[24–28], and antiplatelet therapy[29–33] can be even more important.

MANAGEMENT

A healthy life-style is crucial in the prevention and management of diabetes; unfortunately, those who develop diabetes have already failed in this for most of their life, and significant and protracted changes are difficult in this population. Thus, dietary modifications, while

important[37], often need to be done in parallel with pharmacotherapy. Dietary therapy and calorie restriction in the obese can lead to metabolic improvement within a few days[38], and weight loss can improve insulin sensitivity, glycemic control and other cardiovascular risk factors. Modifications in the elderly need to be realistic, and are difficult because of habitual dietary regimens, ethnic predilections of food and economic constraints. Dietary therapy needs to be individualized, promoting healthy food, and avoiding excessive consumption of simple carbohydrates and saturated fats. It is important to avoid unnecessary restrictions and to recommend weight loss only for the very obese. Vitamin and nutritional supplements may be necessary in some. Exercise enhances insulin sensitivity, improves glucose control and should be encouraged[39,40]. In the elderly, proper evaluation of underlying cardiovascular disease should ideally be performed with a treadmill stress test and simultaneous echocardiographic study, as well as assessment of foot complications, is needed before embarking on a vigorous exercise program. Exercise should be started with low intensity and increased slowly.

Pharmacological antidiabetic treatment

Hypoglycemic agents such as insulin and sulfonylureas used to be the only two agents available. In the past 5 years, a larger armamentarium of antidiabetic medications has become available[41], and there are now five classes of oral agents (Table 3) and several insulin preparations, with more becoming available in the near future. The utility of these various classes of medications is enhanced by their different mechanisms of action, each targeting specific defects in the pathophysiology of type 2 diabetes[41]. Failure of one agent implies adding, but not replacing, another agent, and combinations have additive or synergistic effects. There are no clinical data on which is the best first-line agent; each has its own idiosyncratic advantages and disadvantages. The clinician needs to

Table 3 Commonly used oral antidiabetic agents: mechanism of action and recommended doses

Class	Generic name	Brand name	Effective dose in elderly (mg/day)	Mechanism of action
Sulfonylureas	glipizide	Glucotrol®	2.5–20	⇑ insulin secretion
	glipizide GITS	Glucotrol® XL	2.5–20	
	glyburide	Micronase®, DiaBeta®	2.5–10	
	micronized glyburide	Glynase®	1.5–6	
	glimepiride	Amaryl®	0.5–8	
Biguanide	metformin	Glucophage®	500–2000	⇓ hepatic glucose production
Meglitinide	repaglinide	Prandin®	1.5–6	⇑ insulin secretion
	nateglinide	Starlix	360	
Combination	glyburide + metformin	Glucovance®	glyburide 1.25–10 + metformin 250–2000	⇑ insulin secretion, ⇓ hepatic glucose production
α-Glucosidase Inhibitors	acarbose	Precose®	150–300	⇓ glucose absorption rate
	miglitol	Glynase®		
Thiazolidinediones	rosiglitazone	Avandia®	4–8	⇑ insulin sensitivity in adipose and muscle, ⇓ free fatty acids
	pioglitazone	Actos®	30–45	

GITS, gastrointestinal transport system

choose the one that is effective, has few or no side-effects, and permits an adequate life-style.

Sulfonylureas

Sulfonylureas have been the longest and most commonly used oral hypoglycemic agents. Their primary mechanism of action is enhancement of insulin secretion by binding to a specific sulfonylurea receptor on pancreatic cells[42]; thus, a viable function of pancreatic β cells is needed. The small improvement in insulin-mediated glucose uptake can be explained by improvement in glucose toxicity[8]. As is the case with all antidiabetic agents, the hypoglycemic potency is directly related to the original glucose level[43]: the higher is the fasting plasma glucose level, the greater is the change. In the average patient, the HbA_{1C} value can decrease by 1.5–2.0 percentage points[43], and approximately 25% of patients will achieve the current ADA goal of a fasting plasma glucose level of < 140 mg/dl[13]. A lack of response[44] can be due to poor β-cell function because of very high glucose levels (glucose toxicity), progressive β-cell demise in long-standing diabetes[6], or the rare case of slowly evolving type 1 diabetes presenting in the elderly. The inability of the pancreas to maintain an adequate insulin secretory rate is part of the progression of the disease. The UKPDS results suggest that once the fasting plasma glucose level exceeds a certain value (> 140–160 mg/dl), there is little or no 'rescuing of β-cell function'. Responders may develop secondary failure at a rate of about 5–7% per year[15,16,45] and, after 10 years, most sulfonylurea-treated patients will require other combination therapy[45,46]. Secondary treatment failure can be reversible when caused by stress, acute medical illnesses or concomitant medications that antagonize insulin action or insulin secretion.

Clinical trials have not been able to demonstrate superiority of one sulfonylurea over another[43,47], and glipizide, glyburide and glimepiride exert equipotent glucose-lowering effects[43,47,48]. Glipizide releases insulin more rapidly than does glyburide during a meal, and glyburide has a stronger hepatic glucose suppressive effect[49]. These subtle changes can be significant in the elderly where a more 'gentle insulin secretagogue', such as the long-acting glipizide (glipizide gastrointestinal transport system, GITS) or glymepiride, can result in less hypoglycemia. Sulfonylurea therapy is associated with weight gain[50], which can be less significant with glipizide GITS[43]. The so-called first-generation sulfonylureas are given at higher doses as they have a lower binding affinity to the sulfonylurea receptor[51], and demonstrate more drug-to-drug interaction, therefore are less desirable in the elderly treated with polypharmacy. Responders do so with low doses, and when initiating therapy one should start with the lowest effective dose and titrate upwards. Those who do not respond to lower doses often fail to respond to higher doses[44,51]. Thus, when glycemic goals are not met, combination therapy is indicated.

Adverse effects The major adverse effect is hypoglycemia, which has been reported more commonly with the longer-acting sulfonylureas glyburide and chlorpropamide[15,16,45,50,51]. The risk of hypoglycemia is higher in the elderly, in those with reduced glomerular filtration rate, with congestive heart failure and/or using angiotensin converting enzyme (ACE) inhibitors. Generic sulfonylureas are the least expensive of the oral antidiabetic agents, and the brand-name second-generation sulfonylureas are moderate in price.

In the elderly Sulfonylureas are the longest-used oral agents, and their safety and side-effects are well established. Because older patients are at high risk for hypoglycemia[52], low doses of second-generation agents are preferred with less drug-to-drug interaction[51]. Since there is only a small cost difference, long-acting glucotrol GITS or glimepiride is preferable.

Meglitinides

Repaglinide (Prandin®) is a benzoic acid derivative approved by the Food and Drug Administration (FDA), and nateglinide is a second agent soon to be introduced for the treatment of type 2 diabetes. Repaglinide is a non-sulfonylurea insulin secretagogue that works by closing an adenosine triphosphatase-dependent potassium channel[53], and requires the presence of glucose for its action. When used as monotherapy, the glycemic improvement is similar to that with sulfonylureas[54]. Repaglinide at a dose of 1–4 mg three times daily decreased the HbA_{1C} value by

1.7–1.8 percentage points from baseline[54], and body weight increased by about 3% (5–6 lb)[55]. It is rapidly absorbed (0.5–1 h) and rapidly eliminated (half-life < 1 h). Because of its pharmacokinetic behavior, its administration results in a rapid but brief release of insulin. This medication needs to be given before meals two or three times daily. The starting dose is 0.5 mg three times daily, and can be increased weekly, but a dose of 1 mg three times daily produces 90% of the maximal glucose-lowering effect[54]. Because 90% of repaglinide is recovered in the feces, it is not contraindicated in patients with renal insufficiency. In patients with liver disease, a slower titration schedule is recommended.

Adverse effects As is the case with sulfonylureas, hypoglycemia remains the most serious side-effect. Repaglinide is about 2.5 times more expensive than brand-name sulfonylureas and slightly more expensive than metformin.

In the elderly There are no long-term trials with meglitinides in the elderly, and while they have more physiological pharmacological characteristics than sulfonylureas, the incidence of hypoglycemia is similar, and the multiple daily doses and expense are disadvantages.

Biguanide

Metformin (Glucophage®) is the only biguanide agent available in the USA, and the first combination of antidiabetic agents metformin and glyburide (Glucovance®) has recently been approved by the FDA. Metformin has been in clinical use for 40 years[56], but was only introduced in the USA in 1995[57]. The exact mechanism by which metformin works is unclear, but its major effect is enhancing hepatic insulin sensitivity[58] and inhibiting hepatic gluconeogenesis[59]. By decreasing hepatic glucose production there is improvement in β-cell function, as well as better skeletal muscle glucose uptake. The latter changes however are not directly caused by metformin, and appear to be related to the amelioration of glucose toxicity. Thus by lowering blood glucose level a better glycemic control is achieved with less hyperinsulinemia[58–60]. Metformin therapy improves plasma glucose levels with a decrease in HbA_{1C} value of 1.5–2.0 percentage points, and approximately 25% of patients with metformin monotherapy achieved a HbA_{1C} value of less than 7%[57]. Thus, metformin is equally effective as primary monotherapy when compared with sulfonylureas. An added advantage is its favorable lipid effect, with a decrease in plasma triglycerides and low-density lipoprotein (LDL) cholesterol levels by 10–15%[57,58,61]. Metformin can also decrease the elevated plasminogen activator inhibitor-1 (PAI-1) levels found in diabetes[62]. Weight gain does not occur or is less in individuals treated with metformin alone or in combination[15,16,45,63,64]. The starting metformin dose is 500 mg once daily, given with the largest meals to minimize gastrointestinal side-effects, and needs to be increased gently at weekly or biweekly intervals until achieving 2000 mg daily in divided doses when given as monotherapy[64]. The fasting plasma glucose level begins to decrease within 3–5 days after therapy is started, and reaches a nadir within 1–2 weeks.

Adverse effects Gastrointestinal side-effects, including abdominal discomfort and diarrhea, are common, occurring in 20–30% of patients[57,64]. While these side-effects can be mild and transient, many do not tolerate this medication[57]. Metformin can interfere with vitamin B_{12} absorption, but this is rarely of clinical significance. Because metformin does not increase insulin secretion, biochemically documented hypoglycemia is rare when it is used as monotherapy[15,16,45,57]. Lactic acidosis, the most serious and feared complication, is uncommon at three cases per 100 000 patient-years[56], and no cases were reported in the UKPDS[16]. The possibility of lactic acidosis should be considered in individuals treated with metformin who have concurrent serious medical disorders, including renal insufficiency, severe tissue hypoperfusion, cardiogenic or septic shock, pulmonary insufficiency with

hypoxemia, or severe liver disease[56,57,65]. Impaired renal function is an important contraindication to metformin since the drug is excreted through the kidneys. If the serum creatinine concentration is more than 124 μmol/l (1.4 mg/dl) in women or more than 133 μmol/l (1.5 mg/dl) in men, metformin should not be administered. The cost of metformin is about twice that of a second-generation sulfonylurea, slightly less than that of acarbose and repaglinide, and one-third that of troglitazone.

In the elderly The strong antihyperglycemic effect, the lack of hypoglycemia when used as monotherapy, and the favorable clinical outcomes found in the UKPDS[16] make this drug an excellent choice. However, metformin is not tolerated by all patients, and should be used cautiously or not used at all in the elderly with congestive heart failure, liver disease or decreased renal function. In patients with reduced muscle mass, such as elderly patients, the serum creatinine concentration may underestimate the glomerular filtration rate, and creatinine clearance should be determined. If the creatinine clearance is less than 1.00–1.17 ml/s, metformin should not be given.

α-Glucosidase inhibitors

There are two α-glucosidase inhibitors available in the USA, acarbose (Precose®) and miglitol (Glyset®); both have similar efficacy and side-effects. These drugs competitively inhibit the ability of enzymes (maltase, isomaltase, sucrase and glucoamylase) in the small intestinal brush border to break down oligosaccharides and disaccharides into monosaccharides[66]. By delaying the digestion of carbohydrates, these drugs shift their absorption to more distal parts of the small intestine and colon, and retard glucose entry into the systemic circulation, blunting plasma glucose levels. The hypoglycemic potency of these agents is less than that of sulfonylureas and metformin[66,67]. As monotherapy, they decrease the HbA_{1C} value by 0.7–1.0%[66,67]. They primarily affect the postprandial plasma glucose level[66,67], without increasing the plasma insulin level. The drug is most useful in patients with new-onset type 2 diabetes who have mild fasting hyperglycemia, and in those taking a sulfonylurea or metformin who require additional treatment to reach glycemic goals. Acarbose or miglitol therapy should be ingested with the first bite of food to be effective. It should be initiated with a low dose, 25 mg once or twice daily, to minimize gastrointestinal side-effects, increasing by 25 mg/day every 2–4 weeks. The maximum and more effective dose is 100 mg twice or three times daily. Because these drugs work by interfering with starch digestion and absorption, their effectiveness is diminished in patients with a low carbohydrate intake.

Adverse effects Gastrointestinal side-effects, including bloating, abdominal discomfort, diarrhea and flatulence, occur in up to 30% of diabetic patients treated with α-glucosidase inhibitors, and while transient in some, intolerance to effective doses is common. With very high doses of acarbose, 200–300 mg three times daily, elevated serum aminotransferase levels have been reported, with normalization once therapy is discontinued[66]. Acarbose is contraindicated in patients with inflammatory bowel disease, a plasma creatinine concentration of more than 177 μmol/l ($>$ 2.0 mg/dl) or cirrhosis. Hypoglycemia does not occur when taking α-glucosidase inhibitor as monotherapy, but can be found using combination therapy with sulfonylureas or insulin. Ingestion of pure glucose is advised in diabetic patients who experience hypoglycemia while taking acarbose. The cost for an average daily dose of acarbose is about twice that of a brand-name sulfonylurea and slightly less than that of metformin.

In the elderly These agents are safe and very useful in the elderly when tolerated. Constipation, a common diabetic complication of the elderly, can be helped by the stool-softening effect of these agents. The multiple daily dose and expense are disadvantages.

Thiazolidinediones

Among the class of drugs referred to as the thiazolidinediones[68,69], there used to be three drugs available in the USA: troglitazone (Rezulin®), rosiglitazone (Avandia®) and pioglitazone (Actos®). These compounds were recently reviewed by the FDA, and troglitazone, the first to be introduced, was removed because of the high incidence of hepatotoxicity[70], and similar hypoglycemic potency to that of the two newer compounds[71]. The glucose-lowering effect of the thiazolidinediones is related to the drugs' ability to enhance insulin sensitivity[72,73], but it is not yet clear whether this is a direct effect, or an indirect effect by decreasing fat mobilization and lessening circulating free fatty acid levels[72,74]. Thiazolidinediones bind to a novel receptor called the peroxisome proliferator-activated receptor-γ, leading to increased glucose transporter expression[68]. This effect takes place mainly in fat tissue[74], increasing the number of adipocytes and changing their morphology to smaller, less metabolically active cells, explaining at least in part the weight gain and fat redistribution found with these agents[72]. As monotherapy, the improved glycemic control is less dramatic than that found with metformin or insulin secretagogues[75], with a mean reduction in HbA_{1C} value of 0.6%. This effect is very heterogeneous among patients, with about 25% having primary treatment failure[68,73]. Non-responders can be predicted by a low fasting C-peptide concentration ($<$ 1.5 ng/dl)[68] and low triglyceride levels. Thiazolidinediones consistently reduce plasma triglyceride levels by 10–20%, increase high-density lipoprotein (HDL) cholesterol levels by 5–10%[72], but increase LDL cholesterol levels by 10–15%. Doses of 30–45 mg for pioglitazone and 4–8 mg for rosiglitazone will lower glucose levels within 5–7 days, with a full effect observed at 6–8 weeks.

Adverse effects Liver toxicity was found after troglitazone was approved[70], with some patients having acute hepatic injury and even death from liver failure. Acute liver failure or severe liver dysfunction is less common in either pioglitazone-treated or rosiglitazone-treated patients and the incidence of liver failure remains low. The FDA recommends that the alanine aminotransferase (ALT) level be measured every other month for the first year in rosiglitazone- and pioglitazone-treated patients. If the alanine aminotransferase (ALT) level reaches values that are more than three times the upper limit of normal, therapy should be discontinued. Weight gain is common in those who respond[76], and can be more significant when therapy is combined with a sulfonylurea or insulin[77,78]. A decrease in the plasma hemoglobin level of 3–4% is attributed to a dilutional effect of fluid retention, and expansion of the plasma volume. Edema appears to be more significant with rosiglitazone and pioglitazone, when compared to troglitazone. Congestive heart failure should be monitored and these drugs should not be prescribed to patients with New York Heart Association class III or IV cardiac status. These medications are the most expensive of oral antidiabetic agents, costing three times more than metformin and four times more than brand-name sulfonylureas.

In the elderly Thiazolidinediones are well-tolerated agents, and can be prescribed in patients with impaired renal function. The lack of hypoglycemia when given without sulfonylureas or insulin is another advantage. While these agents can have beneficial non-glycemic-related effects, there is still limited data on their use, particularly in the elderly population. The high cost, fluid retention and need for hepatic failure monitoring have also restricted their use.

Insulin

Insulin replacement and supplementation therapy

Insulin replacement is required for insulinopenic individuals with type 1 diabetes, or those with type 2 who have exhausted the capacity of the β cells to produce insulin. As shown by the DCCT[7], adequate physiological replacement is labor-intensive and far from perfect. Intensive insulin regimens with multiple injections are necessary, since adequate control is rarely achieved with one or two insulin injections a day. Insulin replacement is often associated with periods of hypoinsulinemia resulting in hyperglycemia, and hyperinsulinemia resulting in hypoglycemia. Hypoglycemia, the trade-off of intensive insulin treatment, is undesirable in the elderly. In insulin replacement therapy, a basal insulin regimen is often given by using intermediate or long-acting insulin (NPH®, Lente®, Ultralente®) twice daily. Short-acting insulins, regular or lispro, are used to avoid postprandial glycemic seurges, and need to be given before meals. To be effective, intense therapy with multiple injections requires frequent monitoring and adjustments of insulin doses, and it is therefore recommended in patients who are motivated and proactive. Insulin therapy can also be used as first-line therapy in individuals in a catabolic state with markedly elevated glucose levels, and symptoms of weight loss, impaired vision, confusion, dehydration, urinary incontinence, and/or ketonuria or ketonemia. Some of these patients can be switched to oral agents[9] if the elevated glucose levels were caused by glucose toxicity[8].

Insulin supplements are used in type 2 diabetes to overcome insulin resistance; thus, higher doses are often required. The effectiveness of bedtime insulin therapy is well established; by giving intermediate-acting insulin (such as NPH insulin) at bedtime, the elevated basal rate of hepatic glucose production is effectively reduced[11]. This form of insulin therapy allows good glycemic control using lower doses of insulin, with fewer hypoglycemic events. In clinical settings, insulin treatment has no benefits when compared with sulfonylureas[79]. In the UKPDS there were no advantages or improved outcomes in those treated with insulin, and weight gain and hypoglycemia were common side-effects[10,15]. Specific insulin regimens to treat type 2 diabetes are not discussed here. The reader is referred to several excellent reviews of this topic[80,81].

In the elderly Insulin is highly effective but requires intensive glucose monitoring, affecting cost and quality of life. Patients often need assistance or become dependent on care-givers. Even without changes in insulin regimens, errors in insulin dosing and injection are common, with increased risk of hypoglycemia. When short-acting insulins are used, lispro may be more suitable than regular insulin, but there are very limited data in the elderly. When insulin is used in the elderly, goals of glycemic control need to be balanced with the risk of hypoglycemia. Less aggressive regimens using mainly intermediate or long-acting insulins can improve glycemic control effectively with less effort, and fewer hypoglycemic events.

Combination therapy: oral antidiabetic agents

When monotherapy fails to achieve the desired level of glycemic control, a second oral agent should be added. Triple oral therapy (acarbose or troglitazone plus combined metformin and sulfonylurea therapy) has not been examined formally, and while one might expect additive effects, its role is yet to be defined. Some choose to add bedtime insulin to oral agent monotherapy rather than add a second oral agent. It is important to individualize therapy on the basis of patient and physician preferences, but in the elderly where polypharmacy is common, a simple regimen is preferred. Combination therapy is common since only a portion of individuals taking metformin[57] or sulfonylurea[43,47] can achieve an acceptable level of glycemic control. Moreover, because type 2 diabetes mellitus is a progressive disease[15,16,45], patients will eventually require a second (or third) medication. Substitution of one agent for

another does not improve glycemic control[47,57,64]. The most commonly used combination therapy is metformin plus a sulfonylurea[63,82–84]. Addition of a sulfonylurea to metformin[63,85], or vice versa[63,85], gives an additive glucose-lowering effect. The glucose-lowering effect of repaglinide added to metformin is similarly effective[86]. Addition of acarbose to sulfonylureas or to metformin therapy also provides an additive effect[87,88]. Thiazolidinediones have a more potent blood sugar-lowering effect when used in combination with a sulfonylurea[89], but this combination is associated with weight gain. A similar effective blood glucose-lowering effect can be observed with troglitazone and metformin[90]. As shown in Table 4, when using these combinations improvement of other cardiovascular risk factors needs to be taken into account in addition to glycemic control.

Combination therapy: insulin plus oral antidiabetic agents

Some diabetes experts choose to switch patients from oral antidiabetic failure to a multiple insulin injection regimen, similar to those given to patients with type 1 diabetes. The advantages and disadvantages of this regimen in the elderly are mentioned above. The addition of bedtime intermediate insulin and the continuation of oral agents is preferred by many[91]. This form of therapy effectively reduces elevated plasma glucose levels, requires smaller amounts of insulin and fewer insulin injections, and minimizes weight gain[91–93]. Bedtime insulin and daytime sulfonylureas (BIDS) have been extensively studied[93]. Bedtime insulin added to patients inadequately controlled with metformin alone is more beneficial than switching to a multiple insulin injection regimen[94]. When combination of bedtime insulin with sulfonylureas or metformin is compared, glycemic control is better in the group receiving metformin[92]. Adding oral agents is also useful in patients with type 2 diabetes taking large doses of insulin that result in poor glycemic control.

Table 4 Combination therapy with oral agents: effects on cardiovascular risk factors. Results are expressed as change from baseline

	Metformin + glyburide	Pioglitazone + sulfonylurea
HbA$_{1C}$ (%)	− 1.7	− 1.2
Body weight (lb)	0.9	6.4
LDL cholesterol (% change)	− 6	− 4
HDL cholesterol (% change)	3	10
Triglycerides (% change)	− 9	− 27

LDL, low-density lipoprotein; HDL, high-density lipoprotein

Similar beneficial effects have been found by adding thiazolidinediones[95], and α-glucosidase inhibitors[96].

Treatment of hypertension

The presence of hypertension is more common in type 2 diabetes and is a major hazard for cardiovascular disease. While an adequate diet and increased physical activity are important in the management of these patients, pharmacotherapy is often needed. Previous targets for blood pressure control in the diabetic population have been too high, and the clinician is now challenged to bring the blood pressure control to less than 130/85 mmHg[13]. However, newer recommendations are likely to be < 120/85 mmHg. Perhaps the most important contribution of the UKPDS was to show the impact that modest changes in blood pressure control can have. Small differences in mean blood pressure control between the conventional group (154/87 mmHg) and the tight control group (144/82 mmHg) were associated with a significant reduction of small- and large-vessel complications, with 32% less mortality, 66% less incidence of congestive heart failure and 44% fewer strokes[23]. Furthermore, this was the first study to show that improvement in blood pressure control can decrease microvascular complications by 37%[23]. Long-term prospective studies in the elderly population have also shown that improvement in blood pressure control can reduce cardiovascular events[34,97], as well as decrease the incidence of both hemorrhagic and ischemic (including lacunar) strokes

in the elderly[98]. Antihypertensive medications in the diabetic population not only need to be effective in lowering blood pressure, but also should have favorable metabolic, and cardioprotective and nephroprotective effects. The angiotensin converting enzyme (ACE) inhibitors have been favored as first-line therapy for the diabetic patient[99,100], and angiotensin II receptor antagonists reserved for those who exhibit side-effects to ACE inhibitors. The validity of this concept was reinforced recently with the Heart Outcomes Prevention Evaluation (HOPE) study that showed a low morbidity and mortality effect using ramipril, an ACE inhibitor, in a high-risk non-hypertensive elderly population[36]. While in the UKPDS there was no difference between using an ACE inhibitor or a beta-blocker agent[101], the majority of patients were treated with at least two antihypertensive medications, and nearly 30% needed triple therapy[23,101]. Controversies persist regarding the role of calcium channel blockers in diabetes[102–104]. While these agents are more powerful than ACE inhibitors and have no adverse metabolic effects, they appear to be less effective as monotherapy in decreasing morbidity and mortality when compared to ACE inhibitors[102–104]. In summary, ACE inhibitors or angiotensin II receptor antagonists should be used as first-line therapy, and combination therapy is necessary when goals are not met. Fixed-dose combination pills can reduce the cost of the co-pay and be more effective than single agents[105], and a common logical combination is an ACE inhibitor or angiotensin II receptor blocker combined with a low-dose

Table 5 Clinical trials of lipid-lowering agents in patients with established coronary heart disease (CHD)

Trial	Characteristics	Medication (mg/day)	Reduction in CHD events (%)	Reference
4S	CHD with very high LDL cholesterol	simvastatin 20–40	34	25
LIPID	CHD with moderately elevated LDL cholesterol	pravastatin 40	24	27
CARE	CHD with mildly elevated LDL cholesterol	pravastatin 40	24	26
VA-HIT	CHD with low HDL cholesterol	gemfibrozil 1200	22	28

4S, Scandinavian Simvastatin Survival Study; LIPID, Long-Term Intervention with Pravastatin in Ischaemic Disease; CARE, Cholesterol and Recurrent Events; VA-HIT, Veterans Affairs High-density Lipoprotein Cholesterol Intervention Trial; LDL, low-density lipoprotein; HDL, high-density lipoprotein

diuretic. Also, several tablets with a fixed combination of ACE inhibitors and calcium channel blockers are available.

Treatment of dyslipidemia

The atherogenic effect of hypercholesterolemia is associated with a 2–4-fold increase in CHD in the diabetic population[106]. Individuals with diabetes are at a similar risk of CHD morbidity and mortality than those non-diabetic patients with established CHD (secondary intervention)[21]. This has led both the National Cholesterol Education Program (NCEP)[107] and the ADA[108] to recommend lower target goals for LDL cholesterol, similar to those used for 'secondary intervention'. Thus, individuals with diabetes need to be treated by dietary means, adding pharmacotherapy when necessary, to lower the LDL cholesterol level to < 100 mg/dl, and fasting triglyceride levels to < 150–200 mg/dl. Levels of HDL cholesterol should also be > 35–40 mg/dl; however, there are currently no specific treatment guidelines. Several effective hypolipidemic agents are available, but all can be associated with side-effects, and some are poorly tolerated as in the cases of the bile acid sequestrants and effective doses of nicotinic acid. The latter can also worsen glycemic control, and it is difficult to use particularly in patients treated with oral agents. The hydroxymethyl glutaryl-coenzyme A (HMG-CoA) reductase inhibitors ('statins') are better tolerated, and powerful enough to meet the desirable therapeutic targets. The first step in treating the common dyslipidemia of

diabetes is to use a 'statin' to decrease LDL cholesterol to < 100 mg/dl; if this goal is met and triglyceride levels remain elevated, fish oil or a fibrate should be added. Thus, combination therapy is also being used to meet therapeutic goals, as in the case of treatment of hyperglycemia and hypertension. There are no trials specifically addressing the diabetic population, but substudies from large clinical trials have consistently shown a beneficial effect by improving LDL cholesterol levels with the use of 'statins'[25–27], and increasing HDL cholesterol with the use of gemfibrozil[28] (Table 5). These interventions are as effective in the diabetic population as in the non-diabetic population[109]. The concept that cholesterol-lowering therapy is not as efficacious in the elderly has changed with the outcomes obtained from large clinical trials[25,27,97,98] all showing the benefit of lowering serum cholesterol in this population.

SUMMARY

Type 2 diabetes is common in the elderly, and the association of other cardiovascular risk factors increases the risk of premature morbidity and mortality. There is ample evidence-based medicine to enable the clinician to embark on an early and aggressive intervention. Prevention of type 2 diabetes and its complications should always be the goal. When diabetes is already established, it should be treated aggressively to improve outcomes. Treatment of hyperglycemia is just part of a more comprehensive and global approach to the management of this disease. We now have more effective medications to treat hyperglycemia; thus, we are able to prevent microvascular complications that can lead to blindness and end-stage renal disease. However, improvement of hyperglycemia needs to be done in the context of maintaining a good quality of life and avoiding complications such as hypoglycemia. It has become evident in recent years that the premature morbidity and mortality due to CHD need to be treated early and aggressively. The use of ACE inhibitors, and more important, achieving adequate blood pressure control (< 130/85 mmHg), are paramount for the prevention of vascular events and early mortality. The concomitant treatment of

dyslipidemia in this population by lowering LDL cholesterol levels (< 100 mg/dl) and improving other lipid abnormalities such as elevated triglycerides and low HDL cholesterol levels is also important. Thus, treating the elderly population with diabetes needs to be global in terms of adhering to a healthy life-style, treating all mentioned modifiable cardiovascular risk factors and, in addition, smoking cessation and the prophylactic use of aspirin[13,33]. These approaches should be used in tandem with the treatment of other comorbid conditions, improving the length and quality of life in a non-intrusive and cost-effective manner.

References

1. Roman SH, Harris MI. Management of diabetes mellitus from a public health perspective. *Endocrinol Clin North Am* 1997;26:443–74
2. Vijan S, Hofer TP, Hayward RA. Estimated benefits of glycemic control in microvascular complications in type II diabetes. *Ann Intern Med* 1997;127:788–95
3. Reaven GM, Laws A. Insulin resistance compensatory hyperinsulinemia, and coronary heart disease. *Diabetolgia* 1994;37:948–52
4. DeFronzo RA. Pathogenesis of type II diabetes: metabolic and molecular implications for identifying diabetes genes. *Diabetes Rev* 1997;5:177–269
5. UK Prospective Diabetes Study Group. Intensive blood-glucose control with sulphonylureas or insulin compared with conventional treatment and risk of complications in patients with type II diabetes (UKPDS 33). UK Prospective Diabetes Study Group. *Lancet* 1998;352:837–53
6. Turner R, Stratton I, Horton V, *et al.* UKPDS 25: autoantibodies to islet-cell cytoplasm and glutamic acid decarboxylase for prediction of insulin requirement in type II diabetes. UK Prospective Diabetes Study Group. *Lancet* 1997;350:1288–93
7. The DCCT Research Group. The effect of intensive treatment of diabetes on the development and progression of long-term

complications in insulin-dependent diabetes mellitus. *N Engl J Med* 1993;329:977–86
8. Rossetti L. Glucose toxicity; the implications of hyperglycemia in the pathophysiology of diabetes mellitus. *Clin Invest Med* 1995;18:255–60
9. Ilkova H, Glaser B, Tunckale A, *et al.* Induction of long-term glycemic control in newly diagnosed type II diabetes patients by transient intensive insulin treatment. *Diabetes Care* 1997;20:1353–6
10. Henry RR, Gumbiner B, Ditzler T, *et al.* Intensive conventional insulin therapy for type II diabetes. Metabolic effects during a 6-month outpatient trial. *Diabetes Care* 1993;16:21–31
11. Shank M, Del Prato S, DeFronzo RA. Bedtime insulin/daytime glipizide. Effective therapy for sulfonylurea failures UK Prospective in NIDDM. *Diabetes* 1995;44:165–72
12. Riddle MC. Evening insulin strategy. *Diabetes Care* 1990;13:676–86
13. American Diabetes Association. Clinical Practice Recommendations 2000. Standards of medical care for patients with diabetes mellitus. *Diabetes Care* 2000;23(Suppl 1):S32–42
14. Nathan DM. Inferences and implications. Do results from the Diabetes Control and

Complications Trial apply in NIDDM? Diabetes Study Group. *Lancet* 1998;352: 837–53

15. UK Prospective Diabetes Study (UKPDS) Group. Intensive blood-glucose control with sulphonylureas or insulin compared with conventional treatment and risk of complications in patients with type 2 dia-betes (UKPDS 33). *Lancet* 1998;352:837–53

16. UK Prospective Diabetes Study (UKPDS) Group. Effect of intensive blood-glucose control with metformin on complications in overweight patients with type 2 diabetes (UKPDS 34) *Lancet* 1998;352:854–65

17. Klimt CR, Knatterud GL, Meinert CL, *et al.* A study of the effect of hypoglycemic agents on vascular complications in patients with adult-onset diabetes. I. Design, methods and baseline characteristics. The University Group Diabetes Program. *Diabetes* 1970;19 (Suppl): 747–88

18. Meinert CL, Knatterud GL, Prout TE, *et al.* A study of the effects of hypoglycemic agents on vascular complications in patients with adult-onset diabetes. II. Mortality results. *Diabetes* 1970;19(Suppl):789–830

19. Laakso M. Perspectives in diabetes: hyperglycemia and cardiovascular disease in type 2 diabetes. *Diabetes* 1999;48:937–42

20. Lehto S, Ronnemaa T, Haffner SM, *et al.* Dyslipidemia and hyperglycemia predict coronary heart disease events in middle-aged patients with NIDDM. *Diabetes* 1997; 46:1354–9

21. Haffner SM, Lehto S, Ronnemaa T, *et al.* Mortality from coronary heart disease in subjects with type 2 diabetes and in non-diabetic subjects with and without prior myocardial infarction. *N Engl J Med* 1998; 339:229–34

22. UK Prospective Diabetes Study Group. UK Prospective Diabetes Study UKPDS 17. A 9 year update of a randomized, controlled trial on the effect of improved metabolic control on complications in non-insulin-dependent diabetes mellitus. *Ann Intern Med* 1996;124:136–45

23. UK Prospective Diabetes Study (UKPDS) Group. Tight blood pressure control and risk of macrovascular complications in type 2 diabetes: UKPDS 38 [Published erratum appears in *Br Med J* 1999;318:29]. *Br Med J* 1998;317:703–13

24. Assmann G, Schulte H. The Prospective Cardiovascular Munster (PROCAM) study: prevalence of hyperlipidemia in persons with hypertension and/or diabetes mellitus and the relationship to coronary heart disease. *Am Heart J* 1988;116:1713–24

25. Pyorala K, Pedersen TR, Kjekshus J, *et al.* Cholesterol lowering with simvastatin improves prognosis of diabetic patients with coronary heart disease: a subgroup analysis of the Scandinavian Simvastatin Survival Study (4S) [Published erratum appears in *Diabetes Care* 1997;20:1048]. *Diabetes Care* 1997;20: 614–20

26. Goldberg RB, Mellies MJ, Sacks FM, *et al.* Cardiovascular events and their reduction with pravastatin in diabetic and glucose-intolerant myocardial infarction survivors with average cholesterol levels: sub-group analyses in the Cholesterol and Recurrent Events (CARE) Trial. *Circulation* 1998;98:2513–19

27. The Long-Term Intervention with Pravastatin in Ischaemic Disease (LIPID) Study Group. Prevention of cardiovascular events and death with pravastatin in patients with coronary heart disease and a broad range of initial cholesterol levels. *N Engl J Med* 1998;339:1349–57

28. Rubins HB, Robins SJ, Collins D, *et al.* For the Veterans Affairs High-density Lipoprotein Cholesterol Intervention Trial study group. Gemfibrozil for the secondary prevention of coronary heart disease in men with low levels of high-density lipoprotein cholesterol. *N Engl J Med* 1999;341:410–18

29. Final report on the aspirin component of the ongoing Physician's Health Study. Steering Committee of the Physicians' Health Study Research Group. *N Engl J Med* 1989; 321:129–35

30. ETDRS Investigators. Aspirin effects on mortality and morbidity in patients with diabetes mellitus. Early Treatment Diabetic Retinopathy Study report 14. *J Am Med Assoc* 1992; 268:1292–300

31. Collins R, Baigent C, Sandercock P, *et al.* Antiplatelet therapy for thromboprophylaxis: the need for careful consideration of the

evidence from randomised trials. Antiplatelet Trialists' Collaboration. *Br Med J* 1994;309: 1215–17

32. Colwell JA. Aspirin therapy in diabetes. *Diabetes Care* 1997;20:1767–71

33. American Diabetes Association. Clinical Practice Recommendations 2000. Aspirin therapy in diabetes. *Diabetes Care* 2000;23 (Suppl 1):S61–2

34. Kountz DS. Hypertensive treatment in the elderly diabetic: new answers, new questions. *Clin Geriatr* 2000;8:22–34

35. Perry HM Jr, Davis BR, Price TR, *et al.* Effect of treating isolated systolic hypertension on the risk of developing various types and sub-types of stroke: the Systolic Hypertension in the Elderly Program (SHEP). *J Am Med Assoc* 2000;284:465–71

36. The Heart Outcomes Prevention Evaluation (HOPE) Study Investigators. Effects of an angiotensin-converting-enzyme inhibitor, ramipril, on cardiovascular events in high-risk patients. *N Engl J Med* 2000;342:145–53

37. Kelly DE. Effects of weight loss on glucose homeostasis in NIDDM. *Diabetes Rev* 1995; 3:336–77

38. Henry RR, Schaeffer L, Olefsky JM. Glycemic control and insulin sensitivity during weight loss in obese NIDDM patients. *Diabetes Care* 1994;17:30–6

39. Schneider SH, Khachadurian AK, Amorosa L, *et al.* Ten year experience with exercise-based outpatient life-style modification program in the treatment of diabetes mellitus. *Diabetes Care* 1992;15:1800–10

40. Wing RR, Koeske R, Epstein LH, *et al.* Long-term effects of modest weight loss in type II diabetic patients. *Arch Intern Med* 1987;147: 1749–53

41. DeFronzo RA. Pharmacologic therapy for type 2 diabetes mellitus. *Ann Intern Med* 1999;131:281–303

42. Siconolfi-Baez L, Banerje MA, Lebovitz HE. Characterization and significance of sulfonyl-urea receptors. *Diabetes Care* 1990;13 (Suppl):2–8

43. Simonson DC, Kourides IA, Feinglos M, *et al.* Efficacy, safety, and dose–response character-istics of glipizide gastrointestinal therapeutic system on glycemic control and insulin secre-tion in NIDDM. Results of two multicenter, randomized, placebo-controlled clinical trials. The Glipizide Gastrointestinal Therapeutic System Study Group. *Diabetes Care* 1997; 20:597–606

44. Stenman S, Melander A, Groop P, *et al.* What is the benefit of increasing the sulfonylurea dose? *Ann Intern Med* 1993;118:169–72

45. UK Prospective Diabetes Study Group. United Kingdom Prospective Diabetes Study 24: a 6-year, randomized, controlled trial com-paring sulfonylurea, insulin, and metformin therapy in patients with newly diagnosed type 2 diabetes that could not be controlled with diet therapy. United Kingdom Prospec-tive Diabetes Study Group. *Ann Intern Med* 1998;128:165–75

46. Balodimos MC, Camerini-Davalos R, Marble A. Nine years' experience with tolbu-tamide in the treatment of diabetes. *Meta-bolism* 1966;11:957–70

47. Rosenstock J, Samols E, Muchmore DB, *et al.* Glimepiride, a new once-daily sulfonylurea. A double-blind placebo-controlled study of NIDDM patients. Glimepiride Study Group. *Diabetes Care* 1996;19:1194–9

48. Groop LC, Groop PH, Stenman S, *et al.* Comparison of pharmacokinetics, metabolic effects and mechanisms of action of glyburide and glipizide during long-term treatment. *Diabetes Care* 1987;10:671–8

49. Groop L, Luzi L, Melander A, *et al.* Different effects of glibenclamide and glipizide on insulin secretion and hepatic glucose produc-tion in normal and NIDDM subjects. *Diabetes* 1987;36:1320–8

50. Kelley DE. Effects of weight loss on glucose homeostasis in NIDDM. *Diabetes Rev* 1995; 3:366–77

51. Lebovitz HE, Melander A. Sulfonylureas: basic aspects and clinical uses. In Alberti KG, Zimmet P, DeFronzo RA, eds. *International Textbook of Diabetes Mellitus*, 2nd edn. New York: John Wiley, 1997:817–40

52. Schorr RI, Ray WA, Daughterty JR, *et al.* Individual sulfonylureas and serious hypo-glycemia in older people. *J Am Geriatr Soc* 1996;44:751–5

53. Fuhlendorff J, Rorsman P, Kofod H, *et al.* Stimulation of insulin release by repaglinide

and glibenclamide involves both common and distinct processes. *Diabetes* 1998;47:345–51

54. Schwartz SL, Goldberg RB, Strange P. Repaglinide in type II diabetes: a randomized, double blind, placebo-controlled, dose–response study. Repaglinide Study Group [Abstract]. *Diabetes* 1998;47(Suppl 1):A98

55. Marbury T, Huang WC, Strange P, *et al*. Repaglinide versus glyburide: a one-year comparison trial. *Diabetes Res Clin Pract* 1999; 43:155–66

56. Bailey CJ, Turner RC. Metformin. *N Engl J Med* 1996;334:574–9

57. DeFronzo RA, Goodman AM. Efficacy of metformin in patients with non-insulin-dependent diabetes mellitus. The Multicenter Metformin Study Group. *N Engl J Med* 1995;333:541–9

58. DeFronzo RA, Barzilai N, Simonson DC. Mechanism of metformin action in obese and lean noninsulin-dependent diabetic subjects. *J Clin Endocrinol Metab* 1991;73: 1294–301

59. Stumvoll N, Nurjhan N, Perriello G, *et al*. Metabolic effects of metformin in non-insulin-dependent diabetes mellitus. *N Engl J Med* 1995;333:550–4

60. Rossetti L, DeFronzo RA, Gherzi R, *et al*. Effect of metformin treatment on insulin action in diabetic rats: *in vivo* and *in vitro* correlations. *Metabolism* 1990;39:425–35

61. Reaven GM, Johnston P, Hollenbeck CB, *et al*. Combined metformin–sulfonylurea treatment of patients with noninsulin-dependent diabetes in fair to poor glycemic control. *J Clin Endocrinol Metab* 1992;74:1020–6

62. Vague P, Juhan-Vague I, Alessi MC, *et al*. Metformin decreases the high plasminogen activator inhibition capacity, plasma insulin and triglyceride levels in non-diabetic obese subjects. *Thromb Haemost* 1987;57:326–8

63. Hermann LS, Schersten B, Bitzen PO, *et al*. A therapeutic comparison of metformin and sulfonylurea, alone and in various combinations. A double-blind controlled study. *Diabetes Care* 1994;17:1100–9

64. Garber AJ, Duncan TG, Goodman AM, *et al*. Efficacy of metformin in type II diabetes: results of a double-blind, placebo-controlled, dose–response trial. *Am J Med* 1997;103: 491–7

65. Misbin RI, Green L, Stadel BV, *et al*. Lactic acidosis in patients treated with metformin [Letter]. *N Engl J Med* 1998;338:265–6

66. Lebovitz HE. A new oral therapy for diabetes management: alpha-glucosidase inhibition with acarbose. *Clin Diabetes* 1995;13:99–103

67. Chiasson JL, Josse RG, Hunt JA, *et al*. The efficacy of acarbose in the treatment of patients with non-insulin-dependent diabetes mellitus. A multicenter controlled clinical trial. *Ann Intern Med* 1994;121:928–35

68. Saltiel AR, Olefsky JM. Thiazolidinediones in the treatment of insulin resistance and type II diabetes. *Diabetes* 1996;45:1661–9

69. Spiegelman BM. PPAR-: adipogenic regulator and thiazolidinedione receptor. *Diabetes* 1998;47:507–14

70. Gitlin N, Julie NL, Spurr CL, *et al*. Two cases of severe clinical and histologic hepatotoxicity associated with troglitazone. *Ann Intern Med* 1998;129:36–8

71. Grossman S, Lessem J. Mechanisms and clinical effects of thiazolidinediones. *Exp Opin Invest Drugs* 1997;6:1025–40

72. Maggs DG, Buchanan TA, Burant CF, *et al*. Metabolic effects of troglitazone monotherapy in type II diabetes mellitus. A randomized, double-blind, placebo-controlled trial. *Ann Intern Med* 1998;128:176–85

73. Suter SL, Nolan JJ, Wallace P, *et al*. Metabolic effects of new oral hypoglycemic agent CS-045 in NIDDM subjects. *Diabetes Care* 1992;15:193–203

74. Okuno A, Tamemoto H, Tobe K, *et al*. Troglitazone increases the number of small adipocytes without the change of white adipose tissue mass in obese Zucker rats. *J Clin Invest* 1998;101:1354–61

75. Fonesca VA, Valiquet TR, Huang SM, *et al*. Troglitazone monotherapy improves glycemic control in patients with type 2 diabetes mellitus: a randomized, controlled study. The Troglitazone Study Group. *J Clin Endocrinol Metab* 1998;83:3169–76

76. Iwamoto Y, Kosaka K, Kuzuya T, *et al*. Effects of troglitazone: a new hypoglycemia agent in patients with NIDDM poorly controlled by diet therapy. *Diabetes Care* 1996;19:151–6

77. Horton ES, Whitehouse F, Ghazzi MN, *et al*. Troglitazone in combination with sulfonylurea

restores glycemic control in patients with type 2 diabetes. The Troglitazone Study Group. *Diabetes Care* 1998;21:1462–9

78. Schwartz S, Raskin P, Fonesca V, *et al*. Effect of troglitazone in insulin-treated patients with type II diabetes mellitus. Troglitazone and Exogenous Insulin Study Group. *N Engl J Med* 1998;13:861–6

79. Hayward RA, Manning WG, Kaplan SH, *et al*. Starting insulin therapy in patients with type II diabetes: effectiveness, complications, and resource utilization. *J Am Med Assoc* 1997; 278:1663–9

80. Edelman SV, Henry RR. Insulin therapy for normalizing glycosylated hemoglobin in type II diabetes. Application, benefits, and risks. *Diabetes Rev* 1995;3:308–34

81. Genuth S. Insulin use in NIDDM. *Diabetes Care* 1990;13:1240–64

82. Lebovitz HE. Stepwise and combination drug therapy for the treatment of NIDDM. *Diabetes Care* 1994;17:1542–4

83. UK Prospective Diabetes Study Group. UKPDS 28: a randomized trial of efficacy of early addition of metformin in sulfonylurea-treated type 2 diabetes. UK Prospective Diabetes Study Group. *Diabetes Care* 1998; 21:87–92

84. Bailey CJ. Biguanides and NIDDM. *Diabetes Care* 1992;15:755–72

85. Dunn CJ, Peters DH. Metformin. A review of its pharmacological properties and therapeutic use in non-insulin-dependent diabetes mellitus. *Drugs* 1995;49:721–49

86. Moses R, Slobodniuk R, Boyages S, *et al*. Effect of repaglinide addition to metformin monotherapy on glycemic control in patients with type 2 diabetes. *Diabetes Care* 1999;22: 119–24

87. Coniff RF, Shapiro JA, Seaton TB, *et al*. Multicenter, placebo controlled trial comparing acarbose (BAYg5421) with placebo, tolbutamide, and tolbutamide-plus-acarbose in non-insulin-dependent diabetes mellitus. *Am J Med* 1995;98:443–51

88. Rosenstock J, Brown A, Fischer J, *et al*. Efficacy and safety of acarbose in metformin-treated patients with type 2 diabetes. *Diabetes Care* 1998;21:2050–5

89. Iwamoto Y, Kosaka K, Kuzuya T, *et al*. Effect of combination therapy of troglitazone and sulphonylureas in patients with type 2 diabetes who were poorly controlled by sulphonylurea therapy alone. *Diabetes Med* 1996;13:365–70

90. Inzucchi SE, Maggs DG, Spollett GR, *et al*. Efficacy and metabolic effects of metformin and troglitazone in type II diabetes mellitus. *N Engl J Med* 1998;338:867–72

91. Yki-Järvinen H, Kauppila M, Kujansuu E, *et al*. Comparison of insulin regimens in patients with non-insulin-dependent diabetes mellitus. *N Engl J Med* 1992;327:1426–33

92. Yki-Järvinen H, Ryysy L, Nikkila K, *et al*. Comparison of bedtime insulin regimens in patients with type 2 diabetes mellitus. A randomized, controlled trial. *Ann Intern Med* 1999;130:389–96

93. Johnson JL, Wolf SL, Kabadi UM. Efficacy of insulin and sulfonylurea combination therapy in type II diabetes. A meta-analysis of the randomized placebo-controlled trials. *Arch Intern Med* 1996;156:259–64

94. Chow CC, Tsang LW, Sorenson JP, *et al*. Comparison of insulin with or without continuation of oral hypoglycemic agents in the treatment of secondary failure in NIDDM patients. *Diabetes Care* 1995;18:307–14

95. Buse JB, Gumbiner B, Mathias NP, *et al*. Troglitazone use in insulin-treated type 2 diabetic patients. The Troglitazone Insulin Study Group. *Diabetes Care* 1998;21:1455–61

96. Kelley DE, Bidot P, Freedman Z, *et al*. Efficacy and safety of acarbose in insulin-treated patients with type 2 diabetes. *Diabetes Care* 1998;21:2056–61

97. Curb JD, Pressel SL, Cutler JA, *et al*. Effect of diuretic-based antihypertensive treatment on cardiovascular disease risk in older diabetic patients with isolated systolic hypertension: Systolic Hypertension in the Elderly Program (SHEP). *J Am Med Assoc* 1996;276:1886–92

98. Peny HM Jr, Davis BR, Price TR, *et al*. Effect of treating systolic hypertension in the elderly program (SHEP) Cooperative Research Group. *J Am Med Assoc* 2000;284:465–71

99. Joint National Committee. The Sixth Report of the Joint National Committee on Prevention, Detection, Evaluation, and

Treatment of High Blood Pressure. *Arch Intern Med* 1997;157:2413–46

100. Chalmers J, Zanchetti A. The 1996 report of a World Health Organization expert committee on hypertension control. *J Hypertens* 1996;14:929–33

101. UK Prospective Diabetes Study Group. Tight blood pressure control and risk for macrovascular complications and microvascular complications in type II diabetes: UKPDS 38. *Br Med J* 1998;317:703–13

102. Estacio RO, Jeffers BW, Hiatt WR, *et al*. The effect of nisoldipine as compared with enalapril on cardiovascular outcomes in patients with non-insulin dependant diabetes and hypertension. *N Engl J Med* 1998; 338:645–52

103. Hansson L, Zanchetti A, Carruthers G, *et al*. Effects of intensive blood-pressure lowering and low-dose aspirin in patients with hypertension; principle results of the Hypertension Optimal Treatment (HOT) randomized trial. *Lancet* 1998;351:1755–62

104. Tatti P, Pahor M, Byington RP, *et al*. Outcomes results of the Fosinopril versus Amlodipine Cardiovascular Events Randomized Trial (FACET) in patients with hypertension and NIDDM. *Diabetes Care* 1998;4:597–603

105. Prisant LM, Weir MR, Papademetriou V, *et al*. Low-dose combination therapy: an alternative first-line approach to hypertension treatment. *Am Heart J* 1995;130: 359–66

106. Kannel WB, McGee DN. Diabetes and glucose tolerance as risk factors for cardiovascular disease: the Framingham Study. *Diabetes Care* 1979;2:120–6

107. NCEP Expert panel. Summary of the second report of the National Cholesterol Education Program expert panel on detection, evaluation and treatment of high blood cholesterol. *J Am Med Assoc* 1993;209:3015–23

108. American Diabetes Association: Clinical Practice Recommendations 2000. Management of dyslipidemia in adults with diabetes. *Diabetes Care* 2000;23(Suppl 1):S57–60

109. Haffner SM. Clinical perspective: is all coronary heart disease prevention in type 2 diabetes mellitus secondary prevention? *J Clin Endocrinol Metab* 2000;85:2108–9

Section V

Aging and body composition

Alex Vermeulen, MD

Aging is accompanied by important changes in the body composition in males characterized by a decrease of muscle and bone mass and increase in abdominal fat mass. These changes have important clinical implications: decrease of muscle strength with, as a corollary, decreased statural stability and increased tendency to falls, osteoporosis and increased bone fracture rate, insulin resistance with impaired glucose tolerance, atherogenic lipid profile and atherosclerosis. Aging is also accompanied by important changes in the endocrine system: decrease in gonadal function and growth hormone secretion, decreased adrenal androgen and increased cortisol secretion, and decreased melatonin secretion.

It is tempting to postulate a causal relationship between the altered endocrine functions and the clinical symptomatology of the aging male. This symptomatology is, however, multifactorial in origin, aging being characterized by a decrease of almost all physiological functions. Moreover, changes in life style, in energy balance and physical activity are co-responsible for the decrease in muscle mass, increase in fat mass and osteoporosis. Finally, some of the endocrine changes observed in elderly males may be the consequence rather than the cause of changes in body composition: abdominal obesity, for example, induces a decrease of SHBG and secondarily of testosterone levels; decrease in physical activity is accompanied by decreased growth hormone and androgen secretion, the latter itself influencing growth hormone secretion.

Hence, a complex interplay of different hormonal and non hormonal factors determine the changes in body composition of the elderly men. In this section, we provide an overview of our actual knowledge of the role of the endocrine system in the age-related changes in body composition in males.

Whereas it is evident that the age-associated changes in body composition do play a role in the morbidity and disabilities observed in aging males, the number of well-controlled studies on the effects of the different therapeutic approaches and the ensuing morbidity and invalidity, are disappointingly low and the available data are still too limited to permit a definitive balance between risks and benefits of the different treatment modalities. However, besides eventual pharmacological, hormonal interventions, a healthy lifestyle, including healthy dietary habits and appropriate physical activity remain the corner stones of a healthy aging.

18 Testosterone, aging and body composition

Per Mårin, MD, PhD

INTRODUCTION

It has been well known for many years that normal aging in the male is associated with a decline in lean body mass, muscle mass and strength, as well as an increase in the amount of body fat. The consequences of these changes are significant, and include osteoporosis, diabetes mellitus type 2, cardiovascular disease, stroke and other arteriosclerotic diseases. Although the general opinion has been that decreasing levels of androgens may be an important factor in this process, very few studies have been performed to evaluate the effects of testosterone supplementation on these conditions. Furthermore, a very limited number of studies have explored factors other than the contribution of aging to the decrease in androgen levels, or why a significant population of males do not experience androgen deficiency or the above diseases until very late in life. This chapter deals with possible factors other than pure aging explaining at least in part the development of disease, and also endocrine disturbances other than those related to androgens that may contribute to this process.

CHANGES IN ENDOCRINE STATUS WITH AGE

The decrease in androgen levels with age is a well-known phenomenon. This not only results from impairment of the function of peripheral glands such as the male gonads, but also can be explained by changes in the neuroendocrine centers regulating hormone secretion. In the testis, it is known that there is a morphological change with a decrease both in the numbers of Sertoli and Leydig cells, and in blood perfusion through the testis[1,2]. This probably explains the finding that both follicle stimulating hormone (FSH) and luteinizing hormone (LH) levels increase with age, in an attempt to overcome this impairment[3]. Another explanation for the decrease in androgen levels is that the circadian rhythm of testosterone levels off in elderly men, probably as a result of lower LH amplitudes. Other factors that interact with testosterone secretion at different regulating levels are various somatic diseases occurring throughout life, as well as environmental, psychosocial and socioeconomic factors[4]. This is described in more detail below. Another hormone that declines with age is growth hormone[5]. This seems to result from a decrease in the secretion of growth hormone-releasing hormone (GHRH)[6], as well as a decrease in the stimulating effect of GHRH on the secretion of growth hormone itself[7,8].

An interesting hormone in this context is cortisol, since the secretion of this hormone increases with age[9,10]. This is actually another important factor known to inhibit testosterone secretion[11].

The decline in both testosterone and growth hormone secretion in combination with the increase in cortisol secretion is relevant to the explanation of changed body composition and the various diseases known to occur during aging, and is discussed further below.

CHANGES IN BODY COMPOSITION WITH AGE

It is well recognized that aging in both males and females is associated with significant changes in body composition. Fat-free mass, including organ mass, skeletal muscle, bone mineral content and total body water, decreases[12–14]. The reduction in skeletal muscle mass is a result of a decline in both the number of muscle fibers and the absolute quantity of muscle[15]. It is important to observe that the decline in muscle fiber numbers is most pronounced for the type II fibers[16], since this has implications for both insulin action and glucose transport, as well as physical strength and capacity. The significant decrease in muscle strength with age is a strong predictor for functional problems such as falls, fractures and loss of mobility, leading to impairment in daily life performance and the possible need for institutional care[17]. The clinical correlate to the decline in mineral mass is osteoporosis. This is a major cause of morbidity and mortality in elderly men, owing to the increased risk of fractures. This has been an underestimated problem in men compared to women, and it is of interest that almost one-third of hip fractures occur in men[18], and the incidence of vertebral fractures at age 80 is the same for men as for women[19].

Although it is difficult to calculate exact figures, the most important factors for morbidity and mortality in the aging male are the well-known increase in total adipose tissue mass and the redistribution of fat from peripheral subcutaneous depots to central, intra-abdominal depots that occur with aging[20,21]. Most studies show that abdominal visceral fat increases with age. Several authors[22–24] reported an inverse

correlation with testosterone levels, suggesting that the decline in testosterone levels plays a causal role in the age-associated visceral fat accumulation. As the latter induces decreased SHBG and hence testosterone levels[25] it is, however, not clear whether the decreased testosterone levels induce abdominal fat accumulation or vice versa. Other factors that play a role in this fat accumulation are the age-associated increase in cortisol levels[9,10] as well as decrease in growth hormone levels (see chapter 51). Visceral accumulation of fat, i.e. increased omental and mesenteric adipose tissue depots, represents a special entity that is strongly associated with increased risk for cardiovascular disease and non-insulin-dependent diabetes. The coexistence of visceral obesity, elevated blood lipids, hypertension and impaired glucose tolerance (or manifest diabetes mellitus) defines the 'metabolic syndrome'[26]. A similar complex of symptoms, but without obesity, has been designated 'syndrome X'[27]. The metabolic syndrome is associated with subtle dysfunction of multiple endocrine organ systems[28]. These endocrine abnormalities may be due to the visceral obesity *per se* or to primary central regulatory disturbances that favor central fat accumulation. Because visceral adipose tissue accumulation in the aging male probably represents the most important factor for premature morbidity and mortality from cardiovascular disease and non-insulin-dependent diabetes, this fat depot is discussed in detail separately below.

CHARACTERISTICS OF VISCERAL ADIPOSE TISSUE

Epidemiology and pathophysiology

The critical determinant of the association between obesity and dyslipidemia, hypertension, type 2 diabetes mellitus, and the risk for cardiovascular disease is probably the amount of intra-abdominal fat[29–32]. This is because the visceral fat (omental and mesenteric fat), which constitutes more than 80% of the intra-abdominal fat, has unique metabolic characteristics and anatomical localization. Visceral adipose tissue has a higher turnover rate than that of other adipose tissue depots in both men and women. The visceral fat is drained via the portal vein to the liver, in contrast to peripheral fat depots that are drained by the systemic circulation. The increased lipolytic activity of visceral fat combined with its anatomical location exposes the liver to higher concentrations of free fatty acids (FFAs) than those associated with any other organ. Free fatty acids decrease insulin clearance by the liver, and increase hepatic glucose output and the secretion of very-low-density lipoproteins (VLDLs). These effects of free fatty acids on the liver cause peripheral hyperinsulinemia, hyperglycemia and elevated VLDL. The above three are all known to be important risk factors for type 2 diabetes mellitus and arteriosclerosis. The retroperitoneal fat mass is of minor importance both because of its small size and because its venous drainage bypasses the portal circulation.

Hormonal receptors, circulation and innervation

Several factors account for the increased turnover rate of visceral fat. Compared with fat cells in other regions of the body, the visceral adipocytes have a higher density of β-adrenergic receptors that mediate lipolysis by activation of the sympathoadrenal system[33]. The visceral adipocytes also have a higher density of glucocorticoid, as well as of androgen receptors[34]. Cortisol increases visceral fat mass mainly by increasing the expression of lipoprotein lipase (LPL)[35,36], while testosterone can lead to a decrease in fat accumulation by inhibiting LPL[37–39], and increasing lipolysis[40,41].

In addition, the environment associated with the visceral adipocytes is different from that associated with fat cells in other parts of the body. Blood flow, an important determinant of lipid uptake and mobilization, is higher in visceral fat than in other adipose tissue[42]. The lipolytic process is mainly regulated by catecholamines[43], and visceral adipose tissue contains more catecholamines and catecholaminergic nerves than are found in any other adipose tissue[44]. Therefore, visceral adipose tissue, because of its metabolic properties, higher hormone receptor density, and unique innervation and blood flow, serves as an important metabolic center. The FFAs released by the visceral adipocytes have important effects on the hepatic regulation of glucose and lipoprotein metabolism.

MUSCLE AND BONE TISSUE

As discussed above, aging is associated not only with an increase in the relative and/or absolute amount of adipose tissue mass, but also with a decline in muscle mass and strength as well as osteoporosis. Several studies[45–47] have reported a correlation between testosterone levels and muscle mass in aging men and this independent of age *per se*. The correlation between muscle strength and testosterone levels appears to be more controversial[47,48]. Although clinical studies have demonstrated anabolic effects of testosterone on both muscle and bone tissue, some of these studies are either uncontrolled or small with partly controversial results. Furthermore, the effects of testosterone treatment on these parameters have been investigated in young or middle-aged hypogonadal men with various kinds of underlying disease. It is not clear, therefore, whether these results can be generally transferred to older men. Although the data are limited, studies of testosterone replacement in healthy older men with relative testosterone deficiency have demonstrated some modest improvements in muscle mass and function, the clinical and functional relevance of which is yet to be demonstrated[49–51]. Several large scale studies[45,52,53] showed a weak positive association between free testosterone levels and BMD at several bone sites, but other authors could not confirm this association[54–56].

Recently, a negative correlation between total and bioavailable estradiol (but not bio-T) (which in males originates essentially from peripheral metabolism of androgens) and bone fracture rate in males, independently of age, BMI or exercise has been reported[57]. In another recent study[58] it was suggested that in aging men, estradiol is the dominant sex steroid regulating bone resorption, whereas both estradiol and testosterone maintain bone formation. At least three studies have addressed the issue of bone mineral density in elderly men in more detail. Tenover[59] administered testosterone or placebo for 3 months and found a significant decrease in markers of bone resorption with testosterone. In a similar study, it was shown that 3 months of testosterone replacement increased the level of osteocalcin, a marker of bone formation[60]. In a longer-term study[61], there was no sign of bone formation. Recently in a relatively large scale study[62], an effect of androgen supplementation on BMD was observed in elderly men with clearly decreased testosterone levels but not in the entire elderly population with testosterone levels below 475 ng/dl (16 nMol/l). Therefore, at this stage, it cannot be stated for certain that testosterone improves bone mineral density in older men, as has been shown in younger men. Since the described changes in body composition and aging are very important, especially bearing in mind the rapidly growing population of these men, there is an urgent need and real potential for replacement therapy to increase muscle mass and function and bone mineral density. Such replacement could also have effects on sexual function, mood and other mental functions, and the effects of testosterone replacement on these have not been established at all. In summary, there are strong needs for long-term and controlled clinical studies to determine the benefits and possible drawbacks with testosterone replacement therapy.

THERAPEUTIC CONSIDERATIONS

Choice of patients considered for replacement

There is no internationally accepted definition of what constitutes 'testosterone deficiency' in the aging male. There have been many suggestions for such a definition, including a specific testosterone level $\leq$ 300 ng/dl[63]. Sex hormone-binding globulin (SHBG) and gonadotropin levels have been discussed as other important parameters, but no specific ranges have been yet fully agreed and some elderly men have 'normal' gonadotropin levels.

In the future, it may be reasonble to define a cluster of variables that, taken together, could help physicians to decide which patients should be considered for therapy.

Adverse effects

The main concerns during testosterone replacement therapy relate to the areas of the prostate gland and cardiovascular disease. In the case of the prostate gland, to the author's knowledge there are no published data to suggest that testosterone treatment, given to either hypogonadal or eugonadal men, increases cancer risk compared to healthy men. In severely hypogonadal men, who often have been shown to have a lower incidence of prostatic cancer, the risk can be expected to return to the same as that for normogonadal men when they are treated with testosterone[64,65]. This does not mean that these potentially adverse effects should be neglected; on the contrary, it is of vital importance that the issues concerning both cardiovascular disease and the prostate gland must be carefully followed in future studies for many years to come.

Testosterone replacement strategies

For many years testosterone treatment has most often been given as injections, often in a depot form (testosterone enanthate). For oral use there is a preparation in which testosterone is bound to a fatty acid to assist absorption (by the lymphatic system). During recent years, other ways of administration have been studied, such as sublingual, buccal and transdermal formulations, of which different types of patches or gels are most common today. Injections have the disadvantage of causing fluctuating testosterone levels, and may be painful. There have also been difficulties in

reaching adequate testosterone concentrations with some oral formulations. Some patches can cause local skin irritation. In the future we will see new and improved patches and gels because transdermal administration has several advantages. Patches can mimic the normal diurnal fluctuation of testosterone, and does not cause the same magnitude of the unwanted conversion of testosterone to estradiol and dihydrotestosterone known to occur with injections[66].

References

1. Tenover J, McLachlan R, Dahl K, *et al*. Decreased serum inhibition levels in normal elderly men: evidence for a decline in Sertoli cell function with aging. *J Clin Endocrinol Metab* 1988;67:455–9
2. Vermeulen A. Neuroendocrinological aspects of aging. *Verh K Acad Geeneshd Belg* 1994;56: 267–80
3. Morley J, Kaiser F, Perry H, *et al*. Longitudinal changes in testosterone, luteinizing hormone and follicle-stimulating hormone in healthy older men. *Metabolism* 1997;46:410–13
4. Vermeulen A, Kaufman J. Ageing of the hypothalamo–pituitary–testicular axis in men. *Horm Res* 1995;43:25–8
5. Elahi D, Muller D, Tzankoff S, *et al*. Effect of age and obesity on fasting levels of glucose, insulin, glucagon, and growth hormone in man. *J Gerontol* 1982;37:385–91
6. Russel A, Jaffe C, Demott-Friberg R, Barkan A. *In vivo* semiquantification of hypothalamic growth hormone-releasing hormone (GHRH) output in humans: evidence for relative GHRH deficiency in aging. *J Clin Endocrinol Metab* 1999;84:3490–7
7. Muller E, Cella S, DeGennaro-Colonna V, *et al*. Aspects of the neuroendocrine control of growth hormone secretion in ageing mammals. *J Reprod Fertil* 1993;46(Suppl):99–114
8. Ceda G, Ceresini G, Denti L, *et al*. α-Glycerylphosphorylcholine administration increases the GH response to GHRH of young and

elderly subjects. *Horm Metab Res* 1992;24: 119–21
9. Yen S, Laughlin S. Aging and the adrenal cortex. *Exp Gerontol* 1998;33:897–910
10. Svec F. Ageing and adrenal cortical function. *Baillière's Clin Endocrinol Metab* 1997;11: 271–87
11. Doerr P, Pirke K. Cortisol-induced suppression of plasma testosterone in normal adult males. *J Clin Endocrinol Metab* 1976;43: 622–9
12. Forbes G, Reina J. Adult lean body mass declines with age: some longitudinal observations. *Metabolism* 1970;19:653–63
13. Borkan G, Norris A. Fat redistribution and the changing body dimensions of the adult male. *Hum Biol* 1977;49:495–514
14. Fulop TJ, Worum I, Csongor J, *et al*. Body composition in elderly people. I. Determination of body fat composition by multi-isotope method and the elimination kinetics of these isotopes in healthy elderly subjects. *Gerontology* 1985;31:6–14
15. Tzankoff S, Norris A. ongitudinal changes in basal metabolic rate in man. *J Appl Physiol* 1978;45:536–9
16. Larsson L. Histochemical characteristics of human skeletal muscle during aging. *Acta Physiol Scand* 1983;117:469–71
17. Fiatarone M, Evans W. The etiology and reversibility of muscle dysfunction in the aged. *J Gerontol* 1993;48:77–83

18. Seeman E. The dilemma of osteoporosis in men. *Am J Med* 1995;98:76S–88S

19. Cooper D, Atkinsonn E, O'Fallon W, Melton LD. Incidence of clinically diagnosed vertebral fractures: A population-based study in Rochester, Minnesota. *J Bone Miner Res* 1992;7:221–7

20. Borkan G, Hults D, Gerzof S, *et al.* Age changes in body composition revealed by computed tomography. *J Gerontol* 1983;38:673–7

21. Horber F, Gruber B, Thomi F, *et al.* Effects of sex and age on bone mass, body composition and fuel metabolism in humans. *Nutrition* 1997;13:524–34

22. Vermeulen A, Goemaere S, Kaufman JM. Sex hormones, body composition and aging. *Aging Male* 1999;2:8–15

23. Seidell JC, Björntorp P, Sjöström L, *et al.* Visceral fat accumulation in men is positively associated with insulin, glucose and C-peptide levels but negatively with testosterone levels. *Metabolism* 1990;39:897–901

24. Tchernof A, Labrie F, Belanger A, *et al.* Relationships between endogenous steroid hormones, sex hormone binding globulin and lipoprotein levels in men: contribution to visceral obesity, insulin levels and other metabolic variables. *Artherosclerosis* 1997;133:235–44

25. Vermeulen A, Kaufman JM, Giagulli VA. Influence of some biological indices on the sex hormone binding globulin and androgen levels in aging and obese men. *J Clin Endocrinol Metab* 1996;81:1821–7

26. Herberg L, Bergmann M, Hennigs U, *et al.* Influence of diet on the metabolic syndrome of obesity. *Isr J Med Sci* 1972;8:822–3

27. Reaven GH. Role of insulin resistance in human disease. *Diabetes* 1988;37:1595–607

28. Mårin P, Björntorp P. Endocrine-metabolic pattern and adipose tissue distribution. *Horm Res* 1993;39(Suppl 3):81–5

29. Enzi G, Gasparo M, Biondetti PR, *et al.* Subcutaneous and visceral fat distribution according to sex, age, and overweight, evaluated by computed tomography. *Am J Clin Nutr* 1986;44:739–46

30. Sparrow D, Borkan GA, Gerzof SG, *et al.* Relationship of body fat distribution to glucose tolerance. Results of computed tomography in male participants of the normative ageing study. *Diabetes* 1986;35:411–15

31. Fujioka S, Matsuzawa Y, Tokunaga K, Tarui S. Contribution of intra-abdominal fat accumulation to the impairment of glucose and lipid metabolism in human obesity. *Metabolism* 1987;36:54–9

32. Kissebah AH, Peiris AN, Evans DJ. Mechanisms associating body fat distribution to glucose tolerance and diabetes mellitus: window with a view. *Acta Med Scand* 1988;723:79–89

33. Lönnroth P, Smith U. Intermediary metabolism with an emphasis on lipid metabolism, adipose tissue, and fat cell metabolism – a review. In Björntorp P, Brodoff B, eds. *Obesity*. Philadelphia: Lipincott Press, 1988:3–14

34. Rebuffé-Scrive M, Lundholm K, Björntorp P. Glucocorticoid binding of human adipose tissue. *Eur J Clin Invest* 1985;15:267–72

35. Cigolini M, Smith U. Human adipose tissue in culture. VIII. Studies on the insulin-antagonistic effect of glucocorticoids. *Metabolism* 1979;28:502–10

36. Ottosson M. The effects of cortisol on the regulation of lipoprotein lipase activity in human adipose tissue. *Int J Obesity* 1991;15(Suppl 1):86

37. Rebuffé-Scrive M, Mårin P, Björntorp P. Short communication: effect of testosterone on abdominal adipose tisssue in men. *Int J Obesity* 1991;15:791–5

38. Mårin P, Odén B, Björntorp P. Assimilation and mobilization of triglycerides in subcutaneous abdominal and femoral adipose tissue *in vivo* in men: effects of androgens. *J Clin Endocrinol Metab* 1995;80:239–43

39. Mårin P, Lönn L, Andersson B, *et al.* Assimilation of triglycerides in subcutaneous and intra-abdominal adipose tissues *in vivo* in men. Effects of testosterone. *J Clin Endocrinol Metab* 1996;81:1018–22

40. Xu X, De Pergola G, Björntorp P. The effects of androgens on the regulation of lipolysis in adipose precursor cells. *Endocrinology* 1990;126:1229–34

41. Xu X, De Pergola G, Björntorp P. Testosterone increases lipolysis and the number of

β-adrenoceptors in male rat adipocytes. *Endocrinology* 1991;128:379–82

42. West DB, Prinz WA, Greenwood MRC. Regional changes in adipose tissue, blood flow and metabolism in rats after a meal. *Am J Physiol* 1989;257:R711–16

43. Björntorp P, Östman J. Human adipose tissue dynamics and regulation. *Adv Metab Res* 1971; 6:277–327

44. Rebuffé-Scrive M. Neuroregulation of adipose tissue: molecular and hormonal mechanisms. *Int J Obesity* 1991;15(Suppl 2): 83–6

45. van den Beld AW, de Jong FH, Grobbee DE, *et al.* Measures of bioavailable serum testosterone and estradiol and their relationship with muscle strength, bone density and body composition in elderly men. *J Clin Endocrinol Metab* 2000;85:3276–82

46. Abassi A, Drinka PJ, Mattson DE, Tudman D. Low circulating levels of insulin like growth factors and testosterone in chronically institutionalized elderly men. *J Am Geriatr Soc* 1993;48:975–81

47. Baumgartner RN, Waters DL, Gallagher D, *et al.* Predictors of skeletal muscle mass in elderly men and women. *Mech Aging Dev* 1999;107:123–36

48. Verhaar HJJ, Samson MM, Aleman A, *et al.* The relationship between indices of muscle function and circulating anabolic hormones in healthy elderly men. *Aging Male* 2000; 3:75–80

49. Tenover J. Androgen replacement therapy to reverse and/or prevent age-associated sarcopenia in men. *Baillière's Clin Endocrinol Metab* 1998;12:419–25

50. Vermeulen A. Senile hypogonadism in man and hormone replacement therapy. *Acta Med Austriaca* 2000;27:11–17

51. Snyder P, Peachey H, Hannoush P, *et al.* Effects of testosterone treatment on body composition and muscle strength in men over 65 years of age. *J Clin Endocrinol Metab* 1999;84:2647–53

52. Greendale G, Edelstein S, Barrett-Connor E. Endogenous sex steroids and bone mineral density in men and women. The Rancho Bernardo Study. *J Bone Miner Res* 1997;12: 1833–41

53. Khosla S, Melton LJ, Atkinson EJ, *et al.* Relationships of sex steroid levels and bone turnover markers with bone mineral density in men: a key role for bio-available estrogen. *J Clin Endocrinol Metab* 1998;83: 2266–73

54. Drinka PJ, Olson J, Bauwens S, *et al.* Lack of association between free testosterone and bone density separate from age in elderly males. *Calc Tissue Int* 1993;52:67–9

55. Meier De, Orwoll AS, Keenan EJ, Fagerstrom RM. Marked decline of trabecular bone mineral content in healthy men with age: lack of association with sex steroid levels. *J Am Geriatr Soc* 1987;35:188–97

56. Clarke BL, Ebeling Pr, Jones JD *et al.* Changes in quantitative bone histometry in aging healthy men. *J Clin Endocrinol Metab* 1996; 81:2264–70

57. Barrett-Connor E, Mueller JE, von Mühlen DG, *et al.* Low levels of estradiol are associated with vertebral fractures in older men but not in women. *J Clin Endocrinol Metab* 2000; 85:219–23

58. Falahati-Nini A, Riggs EJ, Atkinson EJ, *et al.* Relative contribution of testosterone and estrogen in regulating bone resorption and formation in normal elderly men. *J Clin Invest* 2000;106:1553–60

59. Tenover J. Effects on testosterone supplementation in the aging male. *J Clin Endocrinol Metab* 1992;75:1092–8

60. Morley J, Perry H, Kaiser F, *et al.* Effects of testosterone replacement therapy in old hypogonadal males; a preliminary study. *J Am Geriatr Soc* 1993;41:149–52

61. Sih R, Morley J, Kaiser F, *et al.* Testosterone replacement in older hypogonadal men. 12-month randomized controlled trial. *J Clin Endocrinol Metab* 1997;82:1661–7

62. Snyder PJ, Peachey H, Hannoush P, *et al.* Effects of testosterone treatment on bone mineral density in men over 65 years old. *J Clin Endocrinol Metab* 1999;84:1966–72

63. Basaria S, Dobs A. Risks versus benefits of testosterone therapy in the elderly man. *Drugs Aging* 1999;15:131–42

64. Gooren L. Endocrine aspects of ageing in the male. *Mol Cell Endocrinol* 1998;145: 153–9

65. Rolf C. Potential adverse effects of long-term testosterone therapy. *Baillère's Clin Endocrinol Metab* 1998;12:521–34
66. Dobs A, Meikle A, Arver S, Sanders S, Caramelli K, Mazer N. Pharmacokinetics, efficacy, and safety of a permeation-enhanced testosterone transdermal system in comparison with bi-weekly injections of testosterone enanthate for the treatment of hypogonadal men. *J Clin Endocrinol Metab* 1999;84:3469–78

19 Somatopause and body composition

Jens O. L. Jørgensen, MD, DMSc, Troels K. Hansen, MD, Flavia L. Conceicao, MD, Jens J. Christiansen, MD, Mikkel T. Kristiansen, MD, Nina Vahl, MD, PhD and Jens S. Christiansen, MD, DMSc

INTRODUCTION

The ability of growth hormone (GH) to mobilize lipids and promote protein anabolism was documented many years ago[1,2], and it is also an old observation that the clinical picture of acromegaly includes alterations in body composition[3].

With the introduction of dependable radioimmunological assays it was recognized that circulating GH was blunted in obese subjects[4], and that normal aging was accompanied by a gradual decline in GH levels[5]. The latter observation led Rudman[6] to the hypothesis that many of the senescent changes in body composition and organ function were causally linked to, or caused by, hyposomatotropinemia. The somatopause can be considered a paraphrase for Rudman's hypothesis, although it remains uncertain who introduced this persuasive term.

Finally, more recent studies have uniformly documented that hypopituitary adults with severe GH deficiency are characterized by increased fat mass, and reduced lean body mass (LBM)[7]. It is also known that normal GH levels can be restored in obese subjects following massive weight loss[8], and that GH substitution in GH-deficient adults normalizes body composition[7].

What remains unknown is the cause–effect relationship between hyposomatotropinemia and senescent changes in body composition. Is the propensity for gaining fat and losing LBM initiated or preceded by a primary age-dependent decline in GH secretion and action? Or is it the other way around: accumulation of fat mass secondary to non-GH-dependent factors (such as life-style, dietary habits) results in a feedback inhibition of GH secretion?

Moreover, little is known about possible age-associated changes in GH pharmacokinetics and action.

The aim of this chapter is to highlight these unresolved issues by reviewing the literature, with a special emphasis on recent studies by the present authors.

INFLUENCE OF BODY COMPOSITION, PHYSICAL FITNESS AND AGE ON STIMULATED AND SPONTANEOUS GROWTH HORMONE LEVELS IN NORMAL ADULTS

Assessment of GH status by means of standardized stimulation tests remains a cornerstone in the diagnosis of GH deficiency in children. The reason for this is that pituitary GH is released in a pulsatile and episodic manner, separated by long intervals with low GH levels. A similar approach is used when evaluating hypopituitary adults, in whom it has been shown that stimulated GH release allows a better distinction between patients and normal subjects, compared to 24-h spontaneous GH release[9]. It is, noteworthy, however, that stimulated GH peak levels are subject to very pronounced inter- and intrasubject variability. A number of physiological variables such as body composition, nutritional status, physical fitness and sex steroids are known to influence GH release, but the degree to which each of these factors contributes to the individual variation is unclarified. In adults it has been reported that the GH response to clonidine declines with age[10], whereas the response to arginine appears to be determined by gender with higher levels in females[11]. However, little is known about the possible association between body composition and stimulated GH release in healthy adults.

We therefore conducted a cross-sectional study in 42 clinically non-obese adults between 27 and 59 years of age (22 females and 20 males) who underwent two stimulation tests (clonidine and arginine) in addition to in-depth investigation of body composition and physical fitness (Vo_2 max.)[12]. 'Older' people (mean age 50 years) had a lower peak GH response to both secretagogues, and females had a higher response to arginine, compared to males. Body mass index and intra-abdominal fat (computed tomography (CT) scan) were higher in 'older' people and in males, compared to 'young' people and females, respectively. Lean body mass was higher in males compared to females, whereas physical fitness was higher in young people compared to older people. Multiple regression analysis, however, revealed that intra-abdominal fat mass was the most important and negative predictor of peak GH levels (Figure 1), whereas age, gender and physical fitness were of minor importance. Lean body mass was not significantly associated with GH status in either males or females.

In the same population, 24-h spontaneous GH levels were also analyzed by means of deconvolution analysis of samples obtained every 20 min. Mean GH levels, GH production rate and GH burst amplitude were higher in young

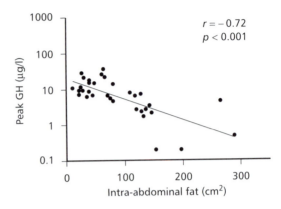

Figure 1 Correlation between peak growth hormone (GH) level following arginine stimulation, and intra-abdominal fat mass, as assessed by computed tomography scan. Data reproduced with permission from reference 12

people and in females, compared to older people and males, respectively[13]. Multiple regression analysis again suggested that intra-abdominal fat mass was the single most important and negative determinant of GH status. Fasting levels of insulin, insulin-like growth factor-I (IGF-I) and free fatty acids did not correlate with either estimate of GH status. Surprisingly, LBM exhibited a weak inverse correlation with mean 24-h GH release, but LBM was not associated with other attributes of GH status and was not an independent determinant by multiple regression analysis.

A detailed analysis of GH secretion in relation to body composition in subjects older than our population has, to the authors' knowledge, not been published. Instead, serum IGF-I has been used as a surrogate or proxy for GH status in several studies of older males[14-16]. These studies comprised large populations of ambulatory, community-dwelling males aged between 50 and 90 years. Not unexpectedly, serum IGF-I declined with age, but IGF-I failed to show any significant association with body composition or functional status[14-16]. As pointed out by some of the authors, however, the validity of IGF-I as an indicator of GH secretion is dubious. It is evident that serum IGF-I levels are low in GH-deficient children and elevated in active acromegaly, but the serum IGF-I level correlates only weakly with GH status in healthy young and mid-life adults, and a large proportion of hypopituitary adults may have IGF-I levels within the normal range[17]. The residual or non-GH-dependent determinants of IGF-I in adults remain elusive and merit future research.

INFLUENCE OF AGE, SEX AND BODY COMPOSITION ON GROWTH HORMONE ACTION AND PHARMACOKINETICS

Considering the great interest in the actions of GH in adults, only a few studies have addressed possible age-associated differences in the responsiveness or sensitivity to GH. In normal adults the senescent decline in GH levels is paralleled by a decline in serum IGF-I, which suggests a downregulation of the GH–IGF-I axis. Administration of GH to older but otherwise healthy adults has generally been associated with predictable, albeit modest, effects on body composition and a high incidence of side-effects[18]. Whether this reflects a different balance between effects and side-effects in older people or that the dosage used was too high is uncertain, but it is evident that older subjects are not resistant to GH. Studies in GH-deficient adults with pituitary disease strongly suggest that the dose requirement declines with age. Short-term dose–response studies clearly demonstrate that older patients required a lower GH dose to obtain a given serum IGF-I level[19,20], and it has been observed that serum IGF-I continues to increase in individual patients during long-term therapy if the GH dosage remains constant. It has also recently been reported that hypopituitary patients above 60 years of age are highly responsive to even a small dose of GH[21]. Interestingly, there appears to be a gender difference in GH-deficient adults, with men being more responsive in terms of IGF-I generation and fat loss during therapy[22]. We have compared the pharmacokinetics and short-term metabolic effects of a near physiological intravenous GH bolus (200 μg) in a group of young (about

30 years) and older (about 50 years) healthy adults[23]. The area under the GH curve was significantly less in older subjects, whereas the elimination half-life was similar in the two groups, which suggests an increase in both metabolic clearance rate and apparent distribution volume of GH in older subjects. Both of these parameters showed a strong positive correlation with fat mass, although multiple regression analysis revealed age to be an independent positive predictor. The short-term lipolytic response to the GH bolus was higher in 'young' than in 'older' subjects. Interestingly, the same study revealed that the GH binding protein (GHBP) correlated strongly and positively with abdominal fat mass[24].

LICENSED INDICATIONS FOR GROWTH HORMONE THERAPY IN ADULTS

Replacement of GH deficiency in adults with hypopituitarism has been studied for nearly 15 years, and the indication was approved by the EU in 1994 and subsequently also in the USA and other countries. According to rather stringent guidelines, therapy should only be considered in patients with documented GH deficiency within an appropriate clinical context, i.e. only patients with evidence of either organic pituitary disease such as a pituitary tumor, or in patients originally diagnosed and treated during childhood[25]. As regards the childhood-onset patients it is noteworthy that approximately 30% of these patients respond normally to GH stimulation upon retesting in adulthood. The insulin tolerance test (ITT) remains the gold standard GH stimulation test, but it is likely that more recent tests such as growth hormone-releasing hormone (GHRH) plus arginine will become viable alternatives. The GH replacement dose declines with age in individual patients, and men are more responsive than women. A suitable dose in adults is 0.2 mg (0.6 IU) per day and the daily dose seldom exceeds 0.8 mg (2.4 IU). The dose should be tailored so that serum IGF-1 levels remain within the normal range. Muscle wasting in association with HIV infection is a licensed indication for GH therapy in the USA, but so far not in other countries. Treatment of muscle wasting or sacropenia with GH remains at the experimental level in other countries.

GROWTH HORMONE ADMINISTRATION IN HEALTHY OLDER MEN

Thanks to the availability of biosynthetic human GH, the original study by Rudman has now been repeated in larger and more adequately controlled trials[26]. Studies with GHRH and GH secretagogues have also been conducted[27]. In general, predictable and potentially favorable changes in body composition are documented with GH treatment for up to 6 months[28]. By contrast, no robust effects have been reported regarding muscle strength, exercise performance or general well-being, whereas side-effects were frequently encountered[28,29].

DISCUSSION

Several lines of evidence suggest a close association between GH status and fat mass in adults. Morbidly obese subjects have severely blunted GH levels, which can be reversed by fat loss[8]. Adult GH deficiency is characterized by excess abdominal adiposity, which becomes normalized after 12 months of GH substitution[7]. The age-associated decline in GH levels appears to be more strongly correlated with fat mass than age *per se*[12,13]. Moreover, it is likely that fat mass – as well as age *per se* – determines the metabolic clearance rate of GH in healthy adults. But the question still remains: is the age-associated decline in GH the cause or the effect of the increased fat mass with aging? We know that the aging pituitary is sensitive to GH secretagogues[30]. It is furthermore documented that the tissues remain responsive to both exogenous and endogenous GH. On the other hand, there is new evidence to suggest that the

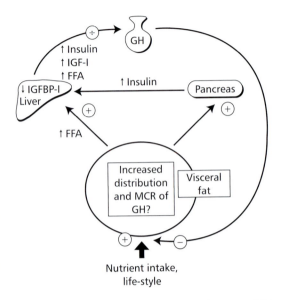

Figure 2 Regulation of pituitary growth hormone (GH) secretion by visceral fat mass. For further details see text. IGF-I, insulin-like growth factor-I; FFA, free fatty acid; IGFBP-1, insulin-like growth factor binding protein-1; MCR, metabolic clearance rate

acute lipolytic response to GH is somewhat reduced in older subjects. It is obvious that the mechanisms underlying the so-called somatopause are more complex than those of the female menopause, which is predominantly caused by gonadal resistance to gonadotropins. A prospective long-term study of normal adults with serial concomitant estimations of GH status and adiposity would provide some answers. Evaluation of GH sensitivity as a function of age, sex and body composition would also be worthwhile. In the mean time, the following hypothesis can be provided (Figure 2):

(1) Changes in life-style and genetic predisposition promote accumulation of body fat with aging.

(2) The increased fat mass increases free fatty acid availability, which stimulates insulin release.

(3) Portal insulin levels suppress insulin-like growth factor binding protein-1 (IGFBP-1), resulting in a relative increase in free IGF-I levels.

(4) Systemic elevations in free fatty acids, insulin and free IGF-I suppress pituitary GH release, which further increases fat mass.

(5) Endogenous GH is cleared more rapidly in subjects with a high amount of fat tissue. The very strong positive correlation between fat mass and GHBP could suggest that GH is cleared in adipose tissue by a receptor-mediated mechanism.

Clearly, future studies are needed to substantiate or refute this simplified model. At present, it is equally premature and unwarranted to recommend GH treatment to reverse the age-associated deterioration in body composition and functional ability.

References

1. Raben MS, Hollenberg CH. Effect of growth hormone on plasma fatty acids. *J Clin Invest* 1959;39:484–8
2. Møller N. In Flyvbjerg A, Ørskov H, Alberti KGMM, eds. *Growth Hormone and Insulin-like Growth Factor I.* New York: John Wiley & Sons, 1993:77–108
3. Bengtsson B-Å, Brummer R-J, Edén S, Bosaeus I. Body composition in acromegaly. *Clin Endocrinol* 1989;30:121–30
4. Copinschi G, Wegienka LC, Hane S, Forsham PH. Effect of arginine on serum levels of insulin and growth hormone in obese subjects. *Metabolism* 1967;16:485–91
5. Rudman D, Kutner MH, Rogers CM, *et al.* Impaired growth hormone secretion in the adult population. Relation to age and adiposity. *J Clin Invest* 1981;67:1361–9
6. Rudman D. Occasional hypothesis: growth hormone, body composition, and aging. *J Am Geriatr Soc* 1985;33:800–7
7. Jørgensen JOL, Vahl N, Hansen TB, *et al.* Growth hormone versus placebo treatment for one year in growth hormone deficient adults: increase in exercise capacity and normalisation of body composition. *Clin Endocrinol* 1996;45:681–8
8. Williams T, Berelowitz M, Joffe SN, *et al.* Impaired growth hormone response to growth hormone-releasing factor in obesity. A pituitary defect reversed with weight reduction. *N Engl J Med* 1984;311:1403–7
9. Hoffman DM, O'Sullivan AJ, Baxter RC, Ho KKY. Diagnosis of growth-hormone deficiency in adults. *Lancet* 1994;343:1064–8
10. Gil-Ad I, Gurewitz R, Marcovici O, *et al.* Effects of aging on human plasma growth hormone response to clonidine. *Mech Age Dev* 1984;27:97–100
11. Parker ML, Hammond JM, Daughaday WH. The arginine provocative test: an aid in the diagnosis of hyposomatotropinism. *J Clin Endocrinol Metab* 1967;27:1129–36
12. Vahl N, Jørgensen JOL, Jurik AG, Christiansen JS. Abdominal adiposity and physical fitness are major determinants of the age associated decline in stimulated GH secretion in healthy adults. *J Clin Endocrinol Metab* 1996;81:2209–15
13. Vahl N, Jørgensen JOL, Skjærbæk C, *et al.* Abdominal adiposity rather than age and sex predicts mass and regularity of GH secretion in healthy adults. *Am J Physiol* 1997;272: E1108–16
14. Papadakis MA, Grady D, Tierny MJ, *et al.* Insulin-like growth factor I and functional status in healthy older men. *J Am Geriatr Soc* 1995;43:1350–5
15. Goodman-Gruen D, Barrett-Connor E. Epidemiology of insulin-like growth factor-I in elderly men and women. *Am J Epidemiol* 1997;145:970–6
16. Kiel DP, Puhl J, Rosen CJ, *et al.* Lack of an association between insulin-like growth factor-I and body composition, muscle strength, physical performance of self-reported mobility among older persons with functional limitations. *J Am Geriatr Soc* 1998;46:822–8
17. Jørgensen JOL, Vahl N, Hansen TB, *et al.* Determinants of serum insulin-like growth

factor I in growth hormone deficient adults as compared to healthy subjects. *Clin Endocrinol* 1998;48:479–86

18. Rudman D, Feller AG, Nagraj HS. Effects of human growth hormone in men over 60 years old. *N Engl J Med* 1990;323:1–6

19. Jørgensen JOL, Flyvbjerg A, Lauritzen T, *et al.* Dose–response studies with biosynthetic human growth hormone in growth hormone deficient patients. *J Clin Endocrinol Metab* 1988;67:36–40

20. Møller J, Jørgensen JOL, Laursen T, *et al.* Growth hormone (GH) dose regimens in GH deficiency: effects on biochemical growth markers and metabolic parameters. *Clin Endocrinol* 1993;39:403–8

21. Toogood AA, Shalet SM. Growth hormone replacement therapy in the elderly with hypothalamic–pituitary disease: a dose-finding study. *J Clin Endocrinol Metab* 1999;84:131–6

22. Burman P, Johansson AG, Siegbahn A, *et al.* Growth hormone (GH)-deficient men are more responsive to GH replacement therapy than women. *J Clin Endocrinol Metab* 1997;82:550–5

23. Vahl N, Møller N, Lauritzen T, *et al.* Metabolic effects and pharmacokinetics of a growth hormone pulse in healthy adults: relation to age, sex and body composition. *J Clin Endocrinol Metab* 1997;82:3612–18

24. Fisker S, Vahl N, Jørgensen JOL, *et al.* Abdominal fat determines growth hormone binding protein levels in healthy non-obese adults. *J Clin Endocrinol Metab* 1997;82: 123–8

25. Consensus guidelines for the diagnosis and treatment of adults with growth hormone deficiency; summary statement of the growth hormone research society workshop on adult growth hormone deficiency. *J Clin Endocrinol Metab* 1998;83:397–401

26. O'Connor K, Blackman MR. Growth hormone and ageing. In Juul A, Jørgensen JOL, eds. *Growth Hormone in Adults*, 2nd edn. Cambridge: Cambridge Univerisity Press, 2000:399–440

27. Chapman IM, Thorner MO. Clinical uses of growth hormone relasing peptides (GHRPs) and GHRP analogues in adults. In Juul A, Jørgensen JOL eds. *Growth Hormone in Adults*, 2nd edn. Cambridge: Cambridge Univerisity Press, 2000:463–83

28. Papadakis MA, Grady D, Black D, *et al.* Growth hormone replacement in healthy older men improves body composition but not functional ability. *Ann Intern Med* 1996; 124:708–16

29. Taaffe DR, Pruitt L, Reim J, *et al.* Effect of recombinant human growth hormone on the muscle strength response to resistance exercise in elderly men. *J Clin Endocrinol Metab* 1994;79:1361–6

30. Chapman IM, Bach MA, Van Cauter E, *et al.* Stimulation of the growth hormone (GH)–insulin-like growth factor I axis by daily oral administration of a GH secretagogue (MK-677) in healthy elderly subjects. *J Clin Endocrinol Metab* 1996;81:4249–57

20 Androgens and lean body mass in the aging male

Melinda Sheffield-Moore, PhD and Randall J. Urban, MD

INTRODUCTION

Considerable public interest and scientific effort has been directed towards the study of the aging male, with particular attention being focused on whether androgens can assist in the maintenance of lean body mass and strength with age. It is well established that with advancing age men undergo a gradual but inevitable decline in gonadal function, often resulting in undiagnosed hypogonadism. A few of the associated symptoms of age-related male hypogonadism or andropause are loss of lean body mass, increased adiposity, and decline in muscle strength and function. It is therefore not surprising that age-related sarcopenia poses a major health concern in old age and is identified world-wide as a significant public-health problem[1,2].

Of primary concern is the progressive reduction in lean muscle mass and strength that occurs with aging. While the mechanisms for the declines in muscle mass and strength with aging remain unclear[3], the resulting loss of contractile tissue and functional capacity contributes to the increased prevalence of lower-extremity weakness and fall-related disability (i.e. bone fracture) in the aging male. Indeed, the ability to counteract progressive losses in skeletal muscle mass and strength in older men has considerable implications. By attenuating or even preventing these losses, older individuals will have an improved quality of life, prolonged independent living and a significantly reduced dependence on structured health-care. Apart from the obvious pitfalls of age-related sarcopenia, there are also metabolic consequences to be considered. These may include a depressed basal metabolic rate, hypothalamic disruption of thermoregulation, glucose intolerance, altered lipid metabolism and enhanced osteoporosis. Thus, as the population of older men grows, the need to develop therapies to counteract losses in skeletal muscle mass and strength with aging takes on added significance.

Recent evidence suggests that, in controlled pharmacological dosing and replacement therapies, androgens are clinically beneficial to various patient populations suffering from muscle wasting[4]. In particular, hypogonadal men benefit from testosterone therapy via enhanced skeletal muscle mass[5-8], increased bone density[7] and increased protein synthesis[6]. Likewise, older men receiving testosterone replacement therapy have increased lean body mass[9], strength[8,10] and protein synthesis[8]. Moreover, changes in body composition, including a loss in lean body mass, are highly correlated with androgen levels in hypogonadal men with acquired immunodeficiency syndrome (AIDS)- related wasting[11]. These findings suggest that androgen therapy, administered in physiological doses to aging males suffering from sarcopenia, is capable of reducing functional losses in lean body mass. This chapter discusses the effects of androgens on skeletal muscle mass, strength, protein synthesis and molecular markers of muscle in aging men.

ANDROGENS AND ANDROPAUSE

The maintenance of skeletal muscle mass and function in the aging male is complicated by the decline in androgens associated with a syndrome termed andropause. In contrast to the menopause in women, the andropause does not occur in all older men, and its presentation and pathophysiology may vary[12,13]. Decreased potency and libido, increased fatiguability and decreased muscle strength are clinical features that define andropause[12–14]. Besides decreased potency and libido and increased fatiguability, other symptoms of andropause include prostatic gland hypertrophy and signs of feminization, for example gynecomastia[14]. Moreover, a significant reduction in serum testosterone concentrations is a core physiological event in those affected by andropause, with the lowest androgen levels seen in men who are aged 70 years or older. While there is no definitive age of onset of andropause, serum testosterone concentrations decrease as men age[15–18], and significant endogenous reductions in testosterone can occur as early as the fifth decade[15]. As a man ages, sex hormone-binding globulin (SHBG) concentration increases[19], and although serum total testosterone concentrations are influenced by SHBG, serum free testosterone concentrations also decrease in healthy aging men[16,17]. Moreover, bioavailable testosterone declines with aging[20] while dihydrotestosterone (DHT) concentrations remain unchanged[21]. Unfortunately, as yet, we do not know the full health impact of these age-related hormonal changes in older men.

It is well accepted that serum testosterone concentrations decline with age; however, the association between lower serum testosterone levels and sarcopenia is less clear. The hypothesized relationship is that age-related reductions in serum testosterone prevent the maintenance of lean muscle mass, which in turn leads to muscle weakness, increased risk for falls and diminished performance of daily living skills. For example, we know that when eugonadal young men are made hypogonadal with a gonadotropin-releasing hormone analog, lean body mass and muscle strength is lost[22]. Considering that 85% of healthy older men (aged 60–98) have serum testosterone concentrations below 480 ng/dl[23], based upon a normal range of 480–1270 ng/dl in healthy 20–30-year-old males, the potential exists for significant numbers of men to be affected by sarcopenia. In fact, chronically institutionalized or rehabilitating older men have been shown to have lower serum testosterone concentrations[24,25], compared to their healthy counterparts[24], indicating that the severity of loss of muscle function correlates with serum testosterone concentration. Furthermore, there is now evidence in older individuals to show that success of strength training is positively correlated with serum testosterone concentration[26]. Thus, a definite link has been established between lower serum testosterone concentrations and reduced skeletal muscle function in older men. However, sarcopenia occurs in both men and women with aging, so testosterone is not the only factor implicated in muscle loss. Nevertheless, androgens are possible therapeutic alternatives to slow age-associated sarcopenia.

ANDROGENS AND MUSCLE PROTEIN SYNTHESIS

There has long existed an unfounded acceptance in the scientific community that exogenous administration of androgens induces myotropic effects in the skeletal muscle of eugonadal males. This unfounded acceptance stems from anecdotal evidence of athletes using anabolic agents. In fact, athletes have long supported the concept that androgens increase lean muscle mass and strength. However, it was only recently that both testosterone and its synthetic analog oxandrolone were proven capable of inducing myotropic effects in the skeletal muscle of post-absorptive young[27–29] and older men[6,8,30,31]. In addition, we recently reported an increase in the rate of protein synthesis (i.e. fractional synthetic rate of muscle protein) in young men after 5 days of androgen administration[29]. Overall, these findings have provided the physiological and molecular evidence that androgens deserve attention in the clinical arena, as a pharmacological intervention against losses in lean body mass associated with age.

While natural androgens such as testosterone clearly stimulate muscle protein synthesis in young and old, they also possess androgenic or virilizing effects in humans. Skeletal muscle, bone and kidneys all show protein-building effects as a result of the androgen-induced positive nitrogen balance. For details on monitoring testosterone replacement therapy, adverse effects and safety considerations see Chapter 27. The clinical use of these androgens is limited to specific patient populations such as hypogonadal men because of these safety considerations. However, efforts have been made to find alternative anabolic agents that can be used in women and children as well as men. If the optimal dose and timing of androgen can be determined in older men or women that gives a maximal anabolic response with minimal side-effects, the expectation is that androgens could be very beneficial in modulating age-related sarcopenia.

been shown between circulating levels of testosterone and strength improvement in older adults involved in a resistance training program[33]. In particular, maximal strength correlates with muscle mass regardless of one's age, but decreases with age to a greater extent than does muscle mass. Thus, the expectation of increasing muscle strength by increasing lean body mass via the administration of therapeutic doses of androgen alone is intriguing.

The primary goal of hormone replacement therapy using androgens in the older male is to maintain strength and function of the appendicular muscles. A few studies have accomplished this by administering therapeutic doses of androgens in hypogonadal men[5,8,31]. However, others have been unable to demonstrate increases in muscle strength with testosterone administration alone[9,30]. In the absence of definitive findings, it is reasonable to consider that a combination of hormone replacement therapy, physical activity (i.e. resistance training) and nutritional intervention will result in optimal increases in muscle strength. However, the equally important variables of power, fatiguability and activities of daily living must not be overlooked when considering intervention programs, whether it be androgen therapy alone or in combination with exercise and nutrition. Clearly, more work is required in the aging male to determine the extent to which androgen replacement therapy positively affects measures of strength, power and fatiguability.

ANDROGENS AND MUSCLE STRENGTH

As men age and lose lean body mass and circulating levels of serum testosterone, physical strength is compromised. Recent evidence from a 12-year longitudinal study of aging skeletal muscle indicates that the quantitative loss in muscle cross-sectional area is a major contributor to the decline in muscle strength seen with aging[32]. In fact, a correlation has

MOLECULAR ASPECTS OF ANDROGEN ACTION

The specific mechanism responsible for the increase in muscle mass and strength during androgen administration is not known. We do know that androgens induce their specific response via the androgen receptor (AR), which in turn regulates the transcription of androgen-responsive target genes. Also, while an accumulation of DNA is therefore essential for muscle growth, we do not know the mechanisms of androgen-induced DNA accretion in skeletal muscle. A study in exercising rats found that skeletal muscle accretion may be dependent on an increased number of ARs[34]. In this study, it was determined that the androgen pathway played a key role in exercise-induced muscle hypertrophy, and found the hypertrophy to be related to an increased number of ARs in the exercised muscle[34]. Moreover, an upregulation of ARs was noted in porcine cells pretreated with testosterone for 24 h without altering the responsiveness of these cells to insulin-like growth factor-I (IGF-I) or other growth factors[35]. Similarly, following 5 days of oxandrolone treatment, we found an increased expression of AR mRNA with no change in intramuscular IGF-I in healthy young men[29]. In a recently completed study, we found that long-term testosterone administration to older men increased AR transcripts at 1 month, but the concentrations returned to baseline values by 6 months[31]. Moreover, IGF-I transcripts were increased at 1 month and continued to be elevated at 6 months, compared with the baseline results. Therefore, the accumulation of DNA required for muscle growth may be directly or indirectly regulated by the AR, and pulsed administration of androgens may have beneficial effects on muscle anabolism when compared with continuous administration.

It has been suggested that prior cellular exposure to androgens may somehow prime muscle cells for the action of secondary agents such as IGF-I. Currently, there is evidence that the increase in muscle protein synthesis that occurs with testosterone administration may be mediated by increasing intramuscular concentrations of IGF-I. We found that in healthy older men, testosterone given for 1 month increased IGF-I mRNA concentrations in muscle while also decreasing mRNA concentrations of the inhibitory IGF binding protein-4[31]. A corollary to this study found that young men who were made hypogonadal for 10 weeks by Lupron® showed a decrease in muscle strength

and a decrease in intramuscular IGF-I mRNA concentration[22].

Myostatin is a recently discovered member of the transforming growth factor-β (TGF-β) superfamily that is a potent regulator of muscle growth. Myostatin is expressed at varying concentrations exclusively in skeletal muscle. A targeted disruption of the myostatin gene in knockout mice resulted in offspring with an approximate 25–30% increase in the musculature of the hip and shoulder regions, compared with their wild-type littermates[36]. Similarly three breeds of cattle (Belgian Blue, Piedmontese, Asturiana do los Valles) show larger muscles ('double-muscled') than those of conventional breeds, and they have a natural homozygous nucleotide deletion, transition, or transversion within the coding region of the myostatin gene[37]. Studies in rats showed that hind-limb atrophy is associated with an increased expression of myostatin in the affected skeletal muscle[38]. However, the function of myostatin is still unclear, because myostatin expression is also increased in regenerating rat skeletal muscle[39]. The only studies in humans measured a myostatin-like protein in the serum of subjects with human immunodeficiency virus (HIV) infection, and found it to be elevated when compared with control subjects without muscle wasting[40]. In a recently completed study, we found no change in the expression of myostatin, using reverse transcriptase–polymerase chain reaction, in skeletal muscle from older men receiving testosterone[31]. However, future studies should investigate myostatin expression at different doses of androgen and at crucial time points of androgen administration.

CONCLUSIONS

While advances in medicine have enabled older persons to live longer, often their quality of life is less than optimal. This is in part due to the alterations in body composition associated with the aging process. Although there is sufficient evidence to believe that androgen therapy is clinically warranted in older men afflicted with symptoms of sarcopenia, we are far from understanding the timing or mechanisms of age-associated sarcopenia. Moreover, we have not yet quieted the debate of the appropriate androgen regimen to be administered to aging males to prevent age-associated sarcopenia. The present review clearly demonstrates the need for additional cross-sectional and longitudinal studies examining the timing, dosing and molecular mechanisms responsible for slowing progressive sarcopenia in the aging male.

References

1. Dutta C, Hadley EC. The significance of sarcopenia in old age. *J Gerontol* 1995; 50A:1–4

2. Schwartz RS. Trophic factor supplementation: effect on the age-associated changes in body composition. *J Gerontol* 1995;50A: 151–6

3. Evans WJ. Functional and metabolic consequences of sarcopenia. *J Nutr* 1997;127: 998S–1003S

4. Sheffield-Moore M. Androgens and the control of skeletal muscle protein synthesis. *Ann Med* 2000;32:181–6

5. Bhasin S, Storer TW, Berman N, *et al.* Testosterone replacement increases fat-free mass and muscle size in hypogonadal men. *J Clin Endocrinol Metab* 1997;82:407–13

6. Brodsky IG, Balagopal P, Nair KS. Effects of testosterone replacement on muscle mass and muscle protein synthesis in hypogonadal men – a clinical research center study. *J Clin Endocrinol Metab* 1996;81:3469–75

7. Katznelson L, Kinkelstein JS, Schoenfeld DA, *et al.* Increase in bone density and lean body mass during testosterone administration in men with acquired hypogonadism. *J Clin Endocrinol Metab* 1996;81:4358–65

8. Urban RJ, Bodenburg C, Gilkison C, *et al.* Testosterone administration to elderly men increases skeletal muscle strength and protein synthesis. *Am J Physiol* 1995;269:E820–6

9. Snyder PJ, Peachey H, Hannoush P, *et al.* Effect of testosterone treatment on body composition and muscle strength in men over 65 years of age. *J Clin Endocrinol Metab* 1999;84:2647–53

10. Morley JE, Perry HM III, Kaiser FE, *et al.* Effects of testosterone replacement therapy in old hypogonadal males: a preliminary study. *J Am Geriatr Soc* 1993;41:149–52

11. Grinspoon S, Corcoran C, Lee K, *et al.* Loss of lean body mass and muscle mass correlates with androgen levels in hypogonadal men with acquired immunodeficiency syndrome and wasting. *J Clin Endocrinol Metab* 1996;81: 4051–8

12. Mastrogiacomo I, Feghali G, Foresta C, Ruzza G. Andropause: incidence and pathogensis. *Arch Androl* 1982;9:293–6

13. Vermeulen A. The male climacterium. *Ann Med* 1993;25:531–4

14. Urban RJ, Veldhuis VJ. Hypothalamo–pituitary concomitants of aging. In Sowers JR, Felicetta JV, eds. *The Endocrinology of Aging.* New York: Raven Press,1988:41–74

15. Moroz EV, Verkhratsky NS. Hypophyseal–gonadal system during male aging. *Arch Gerontol Geriatr* 1985;4:13–19

16. Nankin HR, Caulkins JH. Decreased bioavailable testosterone in aging normal and impotent men. *J Clin Endocrinol Metab* 1986;63: 1418–20

17. Tenover JS, Matsumoto AM, Plymate SR, Bremner WJ. The effects of aging in normal men on bioavailable testosterone and lutenizing hormone secretion: response to clomiphene citrate. *J Clin Endocrinol Metab* 1987;65:1118–25

18. Vermeulen A. Clinical review 24: androgens in the aging male. *J Clin Endocrinol Metab* 1991;73:221–4

19. Purifoy FE, Koopmans LH, Mayes DM. Age differences in serum androgen levels in normal adult males. *Hum Biol* 1981;57:71

20. Morley JE, Kaiser FE, Perry HM III, *et al.* Longitudinal changes in testosterone,

luteinizing hormone, and follicle-stimulating hormone in healthy older men. *Metabolism* 1997;46:410–13

21. Gray A, Feldman HA, McKinley JB, Longcope C. Age, disease and changing sex hormone levels in middle-aged men: results of the Massachusetts Male Aging Study. *J Clin Endocrinol Metab* 1991;73:1016–25

22. Mauras N, Hayes V, Welch S, *et al*. Testosterone deficiency in young men: marked alterations in whole body protein kinetics, strength, and adiposity. *J Clin Endocrinol Metab* 1998;83:1886–92

23. Rudman D, Shetty KR. Unanswered questions concerning the treatment of hyposomatotropism and hypogonadism in elderly men. *J Am Geriatr Soc* 1994;42:522–7

24. Abbasi AA, Drinka PJ, Mattson DE, Rudman D. Low circulating levels of insulin-like growth factors and testosterone in chronically institutionalized elderly men. *J Am Geriatr Soc* 1993;41:975–82

25. Kosasih JB, Abbasi AA, Rudman D. Serum insulin-like growth factor-I and serum testosterone status of elderly men in an inpatient rehabilitation unit. *Am J Med Sci* 1996;311:169–73

26. Hakkinen K, Pakarinen A. Serum hormones and strength development during strength training in middle-aged and elderly males and females. *Acta Physiol Scand* 1994;150:211–19

27. Bhasin S, Storer TW, Berman N, *et al*. The effects of supraphysiologic doses of testosterone on muscle size and strength in normal men. *N Engl J Med* 1996;334:1–7

28. Ferrando AA, Tipton KD, Doyle D, *et al*. Testosterone injection stimulates net protein synthesis but not tissue amino acid transport. *Am J Physiol* 1998;275:E864–71

29. Sheffield-Moore M, Urban RJ, Wolf SE, *et al*. Short term oxandrolone administration stimulates net muscle protein synthesis in young men. *J Clin Endocrinol Metab* 1999;84:2705–11

30. Tenover JS. Effects of testoserone supplementation in the aging male. *J Clin Endocrinol Metab* 1992;75:1092–8

31. Urban R, Gilkison C, Jiang J, *et al*. Testosterone administration to older men for six months increases skeletal muscle strength, net muscle protein balance, and the expression of intramuscular IGF-I transcripts. Presented at *The Endocrine Society*, Toronto, Canada 2000:abstr

32. Frontera WR, Hughes VA, Fielding RA, *et al*. Aging of skeletal muscle: a 12-year longitudinal study. *J Appl Physiol* 2000;88:1321–6

33. Reed RL, Pearlmutter L, Yochum K, *et al*. The relationship between muscle mass and muscle strength in the elderly. *J Am Geriatr Soc* 1991;39:555–61

34. Inoue K, Yamasaki S, Fushiki T, *et al*. Androgen receptor antagonist suppresses exercise-induced hypertrophy of skeletal muscle. *Eur J Appl Physiol* 1994;69:88–91

35. Doumit ME, Cook DR, Merkel RA. Testosterone up-regulates androgen receptors and decreases differentiation of porcine myogenic satellite cells *in vitro*. *Endocrinology* 1996;137:1385–94

36. McPherron AC, Lawler AM, Lee SJ. Regulation of skeletal muscle mass in mice by a new TGF-β superfamily member. *Nature London* 1997;387:83–90

37. McPherron AC, Lawler AM, Lee SJ. Double muscling in cattle due to mutations in the myostatin gene. *Proc Natl Acad Sci USA* 1997;94:12457–61

38. Carlson CJ, Booth FW, Gordon SE. Skeletal muscle myostatin mRNA expression is fiber-type specific and increases during hindlimb unloading. *Am J Physiol* 1999;277:R601–6

39. Yamanouchi K, Soeta C, Naito K, Tojo H. Expression of myostatin gene in regenerating skeletal muscle of the rat and its localization. *Biochem Biophys Res Commun* 2000;270:510–16

40. Gonzales-Cadavid NF, Taylor WE, Yarasheski KE, *et al*. Organization of the human myostatin gene and expression in healthy men and HIV-infected men with muscle wasting. *Proc Natl Acad Sci USA* 1998;95:14938–43

21 Visceral obesity, androgens and the risks of cardiovascular disease and diabetes mellitus

Louis Gooren, MD, PhD

INTRODUCTION

For a long time adipose tissue was considered to be an inactive reserve depot of fat. It is now increasingly recognized that adipose tissue itself is active tissue, directly and actively involved in the control of body weight and energy balance via the secretion of molecules with regulatory potential, such as leptin, a messenger molecule produced by the fat cell. Adipose tissue is metabolically regulated by several genetic, hormonal and nutritional factors[1]. The primary metabolic function of the adipocyte or fat cell, the smallest functional unit of the adipose tissue, is to store fat in the form of triglycerides when the energy intake is in excess, and to release free fatty acids as an energy supply in times of starvation. The amount of triglycerides in adipose tissue is a reflection of the balance between energy intake and energy expenditure over time. Several physiological mechanisms regulate the amount of body fat in order to maintain a more-or-less constant energy store. It is reasonable to believe that the highly efficient and precisely regulated mechanisms to conserve energy in the form of adipose tissue have evolved to ensure an adequate energy supply in times of scarcity of food, necessary for individual survival and for the energy demands that pregnancy and lactation put on women. In modern times this evolutionary adaptive mechanism may overshoot its usefulness and may no longer be favorable for survival in today's Western world. Obesity carries a large number of health risks and shortens life expectancy. The current wide availability of highly palatable, calorically dense foods, and the sedentary life-style promote weight gain. Obesity is a condition that is characterized by an excess storage of triglycerides in adipose tissue. Its development probably involves a very complex interaction between genetic, environmental and developmental factors[2].

SEX DIFFERENCES IN FAT DISTRIBUTION

Adult men and women differ in their fat distribution; the regional distribution of body fat is a sex characteristic. In premenopausal women a larger proportion of fat is stored in peripheral fat depots such as breasts, hips and thighs. Men tend to deposit excess fat in the abdominal regions (both subcutaneous and intra-abdominal or visceral fat depots) and generally have a larger visceral fat depot than (premenopausal) women. As regional localization of body fat is considered a secondary sex characteristic, it is likely that sex steroids are involved in the male and female patterns of fat deposition. This view is strengthened by the observation that variations in sex steroid levels in different phases of (reproductive) life parallel regional differences in fat storage and fat mobilization. Until puberty boys and girls do not differ very much in the amount of body fat and its regional distribution, although girls may have somewhat more body fat than boys. From puberty on differences become manifest. The ovarian production of estrogens and progesterone induces an increase in total body fat as well as selective fat deposition in the breast and gluteo-femoral region. Pubertal boys show a marked increase in fat free mass while the amount of total body fat does not change very much. Adolescent boys lose subcutaneous fat but accumulate fat in the abdominal region, which in most boys is not very apparent at that stage of development but clearly demonstrable with imaging techniques[3].

The sex steroid-induced regional distribution is not an all-or-nothing mechanism; it is a preferential accumulation of excess fat. Obese men and women still show their sex-specific fat accumulation but store their fat also in the 'fat depots of the other sex'. Not only does the distribution of fat differ between the sexes from puberty on, but the dynamics of fat cell size and fat metabolism are different. The amount of fat in a certain depot is dependent on the number and size of the fat cells. Fat cells in the gluteal and femoral region are larger than in the abdominal region. The activity of lipoprotein lipase, the enzyme responsible for the accumulation of triglycerides in the fat cell, is higher in the gluteo-femoral region than in the abdominal area. Conversely, lipolysis is regulated by hormone sensitive lipase, which in turn is regulated by several hormones and by the sympathetic nervous system. Catecholamines stimulate lipolysis via the β-adrenergic receptor while α_2-adrenoreceptors inhibit lipolysis. Hormones affect the number of receptors. Testosterone stimulates the β-adrenergic receptor while estrogens/progesterone favor α_2-adrenoreceptors. Insulin stimulates the accumulation of fat. It is not unreasonable to suppose that the

sex steroid dependent fat distribution serves (or, at least, served!) the different roles of men and women in reproduction. The visceral fat depot has a high metabolic activity with a high turnover of triglycerides which sets rather large amounts of free fatty acids (FFA) free. The visceral fat depot drains via the portal vein which takes blood to the liver, providing FFA as fuel quickly for high degrees of physical activity. So the reserve energy supplies of men can be mobilized rapidly and are readily available to fuel metabolism. Women's fat stores lend themselves less to quick mobilization. Pregnancy and lactation are situations that release energy from female stores at the buttocks and thighs but do so at a slow pace. Again, these sex differences are not absolute but a matter of predominance.

RELATIONSHIPS BETWEEN SEX STEROIDS AND FAT DISTRIBUTION IN ADULTHOOD AND AGING

While there is good evidence that pubertal sex steroids induce a sex-specific fat distribution with preferential abdominal/visceral fat accumulation in males and preferential gluteo-femoral fat accumulation in females, later in life a number of paradoxes occur in the relationship between sex steroids and fat distribution.

Acquired adult onset hypogonadism in men is associated with a higher amount of subcutaneous fat than in eugonadal men but the amount of visceral fat appears to be not less than in a comparable group of eugonadal men[4]. Thus, while androgens apparently induce the accumulation of visceral fat, once fat has been stored in the visceral depot it does not need continued androgen stimulation, as opposed to bone and muscle mass, which were found to be lower in men with adult onset hypogonadism than in eugonadal controls[4]. Correlation studies in large groups of subjects[5,6] have shown that visceral fat increases with aging. There is an inverse correlation between the amount of visceral fat and plasma insulin on the one hand and levels of testosterone and sex hormone-binding globulin (SHBG) on the other. But, with aging, testosterone also shows a decline independently of the amount of visceral fat. Many studies find that an excess of abdominal/visceral fat in men is associated with lowered testosterone levels[5-7], which is paradoxical in view of the effects that testosterone exerts on the accumulation of abdominal/visceral fat in puberty.

The effects of overfeeding and starvation on levels of sex steroid are interesting. In an experiment 12 pairs of identical male twins were overfed for 120 days, resulting in an average weight gain of 8 kg. The excess fat was accumulated both subcutaneously and abdominally/viscerally with a clear preference for the latter localization. Plasma testosterone levels did not decline but SHBG levels did. Even though plasma testosterone did not decline there was a significant negative correlation between changes in the amount of visceral fat and in levels of plasma testosterone. In other words, a gain in visceral fat led to a decrease in plasma testosterone. A further correlation that appeared was between fasting insulin and changes in abdominal fat and in levels of testosterone[8]. The latter is interesting in view of the fact that plasma levels of insulin are negatively correlated with levels of SHBG[7,9]. *In vitro* studies have shown that insulin inhibits hepatic production of SHBG. Lower SHBG levels lead to a fall of total plasma testosterone since this leads to an increase in free testosterone in the first instance and subsequently to a higher metabolic breakdown of testosterone. It could be shown that a higher degree of visceral obesity was correlated with lower SHBG levels and with higher levels of 3α-diol-glucuronide, a metabolite of testosterone, indicating that a lowering of SHBG induces testosterone metabolism. Plasma insulin was positively associated with 3α-diol-glucuronide. Conversely weight loss produced an increase in levels of testosterone[9,10] and/or an increase in levels of SHBG[9,11]. The study of Pritchard and colleagues[10] found that the rise in testosterone levels correlated inversely with loss of abdominal fat and with plasma insulin. Collectively,

these studies suggest that a high degree of visceral adiposity is associated with high insulin levels and low SHBG levels and low total plasma testosterone, and with an increase of metabolites of testosterone, and vice versa.

Correlation studies cannot unravel the cause and effect relationships between the correlates – i.e. whether low testosterone induces visceral fat deposition or whether a large visceral fat depot leads to low testosterone levels. Prospective studies have confirmed that lower endogenous androgens predict central adiposity in men[12] and that these low testosterone levels are significantly inversely associated with levels of blood pressure, fasting plasma glucose and triglyceride, and body mass index and with high density lipoprotein-(HDL) cholesterol[13]. A recent study in Japanese-American men found that low testosterone levels predicted an increase in visceral fat 7.5 years later[14]. Unfortunately, SHBG levels were not measured, but baseline testosterone levels were significantly correlated with fasting C-peptide and fasting insulin levels while adjustment for baseline visceral fat diminished the association between baseline testosterone and plasma insulin, indicating a role for the amount of visceral fat in their inter-relationship. The amount of visceral fat at baseline also predicted an increase in visceral fat over the follow-up period of 7.5 years. The latter is important since in all follow-up studies the hypotestosteronemia associated with visceral obesity may already have been present when the subjects were initially included in the study. Not surprisingly, subjects with a degree of visceral obesity at a younger age show an increase in it later in their lives, as was the case in the study of Tsai and colleagues[14]. Even though low testosterone levels were predictive of future increases in visceral fat accumulation, the already existing excess visceral fat in the men in the study may have been the underlying cause of low testosterone levels in these men.

Women with elevated levels of androgens also tend to have increased amounts of visceral fat, seen most clearly in women with polycystic ovary syndrome (PCOS)[15]. In the medical literature this is often presented as a paradox in the sense that high levels of androgens in women and low levels of androgens in men are associated with visceral obesity. The paradox is partially semantic: high testosterone levels in women (for instance 3–5 nmol/l mean (very) low androgens in men. So the use of the terms high and low testosterone must be related to the individual's sex. A further element is the relation to age. Women with PCOS are relatively young (of reproductive age) when they come to the attention of the medical profession, while the relationship between visceral obesity and low androgen levels in men is typically an epidemiological finding in elderly men. It appears that – similar to the situation in androgen-naïve teenage boys – androgens in women with PCOS are capable of causing accumulations of visceral fat when these women are exposed to androgens postpubertally as their polycystic ovaries start to produce them.

In postmenopausal women there is a larger degree of (male type) upper body fat accumulation in comparison to gluteo-femoral fat storage. Clearly premenopausal estrogen/progesterone levels are required to maintain a premenopausal female type of fat distribution, a finding that is supported by the fact that postmenopausal hormone replacement (partially) restores the premenopausal fat distribution[16].

THE CLINICAL RELEVANCE OF VISCERAL OBESITY

It is now commonly accepted that a preferential accumulation of fat in the abdominal region is associated with an increased risk of non-insulin dependent (type 2) diabetes mellitus and cardiovascular disease, not only in obese subjects but even in non-obese ones[17]. A large number of cross-sectional studies have established a relationship between abdominal obesity and cardiovascular risk factors such as hypertension, dyslipidemia (elevated levels of cholesterol, triglycerides and low-density lipoproteins (LDL), and low levels of HDL impaired glucose tolerance with hyperinsulinemia, a cluster known as the 'insulin resistance syndrome' or 'metabolic syndrome'[18,19]. The explanation of the association between abdominal obesity and the insulin resistance syndrome is still hypothetical. The visceral fat depot has two characteristics that distinguish this depot from the subcutaneous fat stores: the visceral fat depot has a high metabolic activity with a high turnover of triglycerides, producing large amounts of free fatty acids (FFA), and the visceral fat depot drains via the portal vein which leads directly into the liver. The hypothesis states that the liver is unable to handle this high flow of FFA, leading to a disturbance in glucose and lipid metabolism[15]. High levels of FFA may reduce insulin clearance leading to hyperinsulinemia, may further enhance hepatic gluconeogenesis and may reduce glucose uptake by the muscles, resulting in peripheral insulin resistance. While this cluster of risk factors is now well documented, the causal relationships between the components of the cluster is much less certain. Visceral fat may be an epiphenomenon in the cluster of metabolic risk factors, and the contribution of factors such as the amount of subcutaneous fat, muscle tissue characteristics, behavioral aspects and endocrine factors may have been underestimated[18].

As indicated above, a large number of studies have indicated that visceral obesity is associated with low plasma total testosterone levels[19-21]. Part of the explanation for the low total testosterone levels might be the lower plasma levels of SHBG encountered in obese men; these men are often hyperinsulinemic which, in turn, might be part of the explanation for the lowered levels of SHBG[22]. Normally, an increase in SHBG levels is observed in aging men, in all probability due to a decrease of growth hormone and insulin-like growth factor-I (IGF-I) levels with aging[22]. Studies have found that low levels of total and free testosterone are associated with coronary artery disease in men and low levels of total testosterone with cardiovascular risk factors in healthy men[8]. A prospective study found that men with low testosterone and low SHBG levels are more likely to develop insulin resistance and subsequent type 2 diabetes mellitus[23]. It could be established that sleep apnea and daytime sleepiness is much more related to visceral obesity than to general obesity and its occurrence has been related to plasma insulin and leptin levels[24]. Inflammatory cytokines released from adipose tissue produce fatigue and sleepiness in men with visceral obesity.

LEPTIN

The fat cell has traditionally been viewed as a rather passive element in the regulation of reserve energy stores, its main role supposed to be to serve as the site of triglyceride storage in times of caloric excess, and of release of free fatty acids in times of increased energy need. However, several decades ago the theory developed that the fat cell might play a more active role and actually sense excessive energy storage and, in response, provide a signal that leads to a restriction of food intake and induces energy expenditure, thus keeping body weight and fat mass within certain limits. In recent years it has been shown that the fat cell functions as an endocrine cell, producing and secreting molecules with regulatory potential[25]. The discovery of the hormonal signal of the fat cell, termed leptin, was an important step in a better understanding of obesity. The largest proportion of leptin is produced by the fat cells; the subcutaneous fat cells probably produce more leptin than the visceral fat cells. As a result the leptin signal to decrease food intake coming from visceral fat may be weaker than the signal originating from subcutaneous fat. Leptin may be involved in reproductive physiology as well. It is well known that severe weight loss in women is associated with loss of menstrual periods and that puberty in girls develops only when they have attained a certain critical body mass. Leptin is, in all probability, the signal provided

by the adipose tissue to the central nervous system to initiate the release of gonadotropin-releasing hormone, and to discontinue its release when fat mass falls below a critical value as is the case in anorexia nervosa[1] or in women who exercise excessively (athletes).

There are sex differences in levels of leptin. Circulating leptin levels in women are considerably higher than in men. This may be explained partially by the fact that women store their excess fat predominantly subcutaneously in the gluteo-femoral region, and men more in the abdominal/visceral area, the latter producing less leptin[25,26]. Also sex steroids affect leptin levels, with an increase produced by estrogens while androgens have a suppressive effect. Puberty in boys is associated with an initial rise in leptin levels (probably as a result of aromatization of rising levels of testosterone to estradiol) followed by a decline when their androgen levels increase in the further course of puberty. Androgen replacement in hypogonadal men lowers leptin levels, possibly as a result of the decrease of subcutaneous fat, but also as a result of a direct suppressive effect of androgens on its production.

Leptin may be a factor in the association between adiposity and decreased testosterone levels. In men there appears to be a correlation between body mass index and fat mass on the one hand and leptin levels on the other. Leptin receptors are present in the Leydig cell and inhibit the testosterone generated by administration of human chorionic gonadotropin[27]. This may be a model for a less effective stimulation of testosterone production by luteinizing hormone when circulating leptin levels are high as is the case in obesity. Another study found a negative correlation between adiposity, insulin and leptin and testosterone levels[28]. More studies have found that insulin is an important determinant of leptin levels. Feeding and overfeeding increase insulin levels, which leads to an increase in leptin, and vice versa[29].

The main target of leptin is the central nervous system. By modulating neurotransmitters in the hypothalamus it increases energy expenditure and inhibits appetite and weight gain. Leptin influences neuropeptides, affecting appetite and anorexia. The question has arisen whether obesity is an abnormality of leptin physiology. Indeed, both animals and humans with abnormalities of the gene involved in the production of leptin are very obese. In animals this could be partially corrected by the administration of exogenous recombinant leptin. Most obese subjects have high circulating levels of leptin, which is interpreted as a state of leptin insensitivity rather than a state of leptin deficiency. There may be a deficient transport of leptin into the brain[26] or deficient receptor or postreceptor mechanisms of leptin making its action less efficient.

Will the administration of exogenous leptin ever become a tool in the forlorn task of weight reduction? The first studies have been carried out and indeed hold a promise (for review see reference 30). In the studies administering leptin to human subjects visceral fat decreased earlier in the course of weight loss than did subcutaneous fat, which is promising in view of the relation of visceral fat to cardiovascular disease and diabetes mellitus. It is not yet clear which subjects are particularly eligible for leptin administration as the results of leptin administration on adiposity varied strongly between subjects. The long-term efficacy and safety of recombinant leptin have not been studied. In the treatment of diabetes insulin sensitizers are used and, similarly, leptin sensitizers and analogs may be easier to administer and more potent than the subcutaneous administration of recombinant leptin.

INCREASING TESTOSTERONE AND THE EFFECTS ON ADIPOSE TISSUE

It is a widely held belief that androgens have an atherogenic effect and thus lead to cardiovascular disease, but it appears that lower than normal testosterone levels in men are associated with cardiovascular risk factors; visceral obesity, with its association with cardiovascular risk factors, might be the intermediate. Visceral adiposity is associated with low testosterone levels in cross-sectional studies, and their cause and effect relationship are not immediately evident. Does visceral adiposity induce low levels of testosterone, or do low levels of testosterone induce visceral adiposity? Some prospective studies argue that low testosterone levels predict visceral adiposity[12-14]. Three studies have examined the effects of the administration of testosterone on different adipose tissues in men[31-33]; for a review see reference 34. Testosterone inhibits the expression of lipoprotein lipase, the main enzymatic regulator of triglyceride uptake in the fat cell, preferentially in abdominal fat and less so in femoral fat and, maybe, mobilizes lipids from the visceral fat depot. A study of testosterone administration which restored its levels to mid-normal values over a duration of 8–9 months[33] found a decrease in the visceral fat mass, a decrease in fasting glucose and lipid levels and an improvement in insulin sensitivity; in addition, a decrease in diastolic blood pressure was observed[32]. In a recent communication – not yet published – Arver presented the results of the administration of 12 months' transdermal testosterone (5 mg/24 hours) to aging men with type 2 diabetes with plasma testosterone values < 15 nmol/l. There were effects on body composition – a decrease in total adipose tissue and of subcutaneous fat – but no clear effect on abdominal fat or on insulin sensitivity. Many more studies are needed to examine whether raising testosterone levels in viscerally obese men will lead to a reduction of visceral fat and an improvement of the cardiovascular and diabetogenic risk factors associated with it.

THE EPIDEMIC OF OBESITY AND WHAT CAN BE DONE ABOUT IT?

Obesity is a condition that is reaching epidemic proportions not only in the developed world but also in the developing world. Sixty-three per cent of men and 55% of women are overweight in the USA. Twenty-two per cent are grossly overweight, with a body mass index over 30 kg/m^2. The prevalence of obesity has doubled in the past decade with serious consequences (for a review see reference 35). Approximately 80% of obese adults have at least one, and 40% have two or more, associated diseases such as diabetes, hypertension, cardiovascular disease, gallbladder disease, cancers and, last but not least, the morbidity of diseases of the locomotor system such as osteoarthrosis. In the USA 300 000 people die more or less directly from the consequences of obesity and the costs amount to some 10% of the national health care budget, making it not only a personal medical problem but also a public health problem. The frequency of overweight is maximal between the ages of 50 and 60 years and subsequently shows a tendency to decline slowly. Most people over 75 years are not very obese any more. Genetics play a significant role. Studies in identical twins show that 60–70% of overweight can be ascribed to genetic factors and 30–40% to environmental influences. Approximately 80% of children with two obese parents, and 40% of those with one obese parent, will be overweight. If neither parent is obese the probability is less than 10%.

There are several ways of measuring the degree of obesity. The most widely used is the body mass index (BMI), defined as body weight in kilograms divided by the square of the height in meters. Normal BMI is represented by a value between 18 and 25, while values between 25 and 30 indicate overweight and values over 30 obesity. Values over 40 represent extreme obesity. Since the BMI does not provide information on fat distribution, which is relevant for its association with health risks, the waist : hip ratio, or simply the waist circumference, provides additional information. The circumference of the waist is measured midway between the lower rib and the iliac crest and the circumference of the hips over the great trochanters. A ratio of more than 1.0 reveals abdominal obesity or, simply, a waist circumference of

more than 100 cm in men and more than 88 cm in women indicates abdominal/visceral obesity. Still another method is the measurement of skin-fold thickness at various locations. This is less helpful in assessing obesity in the aging population since the sum of skin-fold thickness remains relatively stable with aging, in spite of a larger deposition of fat abdominally/viscerally.

The pathophysiology of obesity is poorly understood. That obesity is a discrepancy between food intake on the one hand and energy expenditure on the other is obvious, but what physiological mechanisms are involved, and how these could be influenced to redress obesity, are much more difficult questions. The central nervous system co-ordinates the checks and balances, with the arcuate and paraventricular nuclei in the hypothalamus as key players. Afferent vagal and sympathetic stimuli and hormonal messengers such as insulin, leptin, cholecystokinin and glucocorticoid modulate in the hypothalamus the neuropeptides involved in appetite and satiety. Efferent signals to the sympathetic and parasympathetic nervous system and to the thyroid regulate food intake and energy expenditure. However this knowledge has not led to the development of powerful tools for intervention. A number of hormonal diseases are associated with increased fat accumulation (hypothyroidism, hypercortisolism) but they are rarely the explanation for overweight. Obesity associated with endocrine disease has characteristic physical features and can relatively easily be recognized by a trained eye. Measurement of the levels of thyroid hormone and cortisol are, therefore, rarely useful in the diagnostic work-up of obesity.

Treatment of obesity is far from simple. Even more difficult is it, after initial success, to maintain reduced weight in the long term. It is evident that the combination of reduced caloric intake and an increase in energy expenditure will lead to a reduction in weight, though the sad thing is that, when on a weight-reducing diet, the body develops counter measures as though the weight loss was undesired and has to be counterbalanced by counter-regulatory mechanisms, slowing the loss of weight. The addition of drugs to a weight-reducing diet has met with some success, though it is difficult, even with drugs, to achieve a weight reduction of more than 6–8% of body weight. With the more modern drugs, sibutramine (with catecholaminergic and serotoninergic agonist action) and orlistat (a pancreatic lipase inhibitor decreasing fat absorption) a certain success in the order of 6–10% can be expected, but their use must be limited over time. Metformin, a drug used in the treatment of type 2 diabetes, may reduce appetite and caloric intake. It has to be admitted that the fight against obesity is largely unsuccessful and probably cannot be won in the setting of clinical therapeutical medicine but must come from health education – starting early

in life – teaching people to eat sensibly and be more physically active. Eating patterns and food preferences seem to become engraved in the mind early in life and are very resistant to change.

A better understanding of the pathophysiology of obesity may lead to better drugs to combat it. The leptin analogs and drugs with β_3-adrenergic properties, stimulating energy expenditure and inhibiting appetite, may become useful additions to the care we have to offer to the obese. Lack of success in the battle against obesity leads to frustrations on the part of patients and physicians who, not having powerful tools, tell the patient that he/she lacks willpower and must take responsibility for his/her own health. This may give rise to an antagonism impairing the doctor–patient relationship.

References

1. Schwartz MW, Seeley RJ. Neuroendocrine responses to starvation and weight loss. N Engl J Med 1997;336:1802–11
2. Rosenbaum M, Leibl RL, Hirsch J. Obesity. N Engl J Med 1997;337:397–407
3. Roemmich JN. Alterations in body composition during adolescence. Curr Opin Endocrinol Diabet 1998;5:11–18
4. Katznelson L, Rosenthal DI, Rosol MS, et al. Using quantitative CT to asses adipose distribution in adult men with acquired hypogonadism. Am J Roentgenol 1998;170: 423–7
5. Vermeulen A, Goemaere S, Kaufman JM. Sex hormones, body composition and aging. The Aging Male 1999;2:8–15
6. Couillard C, Gagnon J, Bergeron J, et al. Contribution of body fatness and adipose tissue distribution to the age variation in plasma steroid hormone concentrations in men: the HERITAGE family study. J Clin Endocrinol Metab 2000;85:1026–31
7. Simon D, Charles MA, Nahoul K, et al. Association between plasma total testosterone and cardiovascular risk factors in healthy adult

men: The Telecom Study. J Clin Endocrinol Metab 1997;82:682–5
8. Pritchard J, Despres JP, Gagnon J, et al. Plasma adrenal, gonadal and conjugated steroids before and after long-term overfeeding in identical twins. J Clin Endocrinol Metab 1998;83:3277–84
9. Vermeulen A, Kaufman JM, Giagulli VA. Influence of some biological indexes on sex hormone binding globulin and androgen levels in aging or obese males. J Clin Endocrinol Metab 1996;81:1821–6
10. Pritchard J, Despres JP, Gagnon J, et al. Plasma adrenal, gonadal and conjugated steroids before and after long-term exercise induced negative energy balance in identical twins. Metabolism 1999:48:1120–7
11. Leenen R, Vander Kooy K, Seidell JC, et al. Visceral fat accumulation in relation to sex hormones in obese men and women undergoing weight loss therapy. J Clin Endocrinol Metab 1994;78:1515–20
12. Khaw KT, Barrett-Connor E. Lower endogenous androgens predict central adiposity in men. Ann Epidemiol 1992;2:675–82

13. Zmuda JM, Cauley JA, Kriska A, *et al*. Longitudinal relation between endogenous testosterone and cardiovascular risk factors in middle-aged men: a 13-year follow-up of former Multiple Risk Factor Intervention Trial participants. *Am J Epidemiol* 1997;146: 609–17

14. Tsai EC, Boyko EJ, Leonetti DL, Fujimoto WY. Low serum testosterone level as a predictor of increased visceral fat in Japanese-American men. *Int J Obesity* 2000;24:485–91

15. Björntorp P. Visceral obesity: a civilization syndrome. *Obesity Res* 1993;1:206–22

16. Tchernof A, Poehlman ET. Effects of the menopause transition on body fatness and body fat distribution. *Obesity Res* 1998;6: 246–54

17. Kannel WB, Cupples LA, Ramaswami R, *et al*. Regional obesity and risk of coronary disease: the Framingham Study. *J Clin Epidemiol* 1991;44:183–190

18. Björntorp P. The android woman – a risky condition. *J Intern Med* 1996;239:105–10

19. Després JP, Marette A. Relation of components of insulin resistance syndrome to coronary disease risk. *Curr Opin Lipidol* 1994;5: 274–89

20. Seidell JC, Björntorp P, Sjöström L, *et al*. Visceral fat accumulation in men is positively associated with insulin, glucose, and C-peptide levels, but negatively with testosterone levels. *Metabolism* 1990;39:897–901

21. Tchernof A, Labrie F, Belanger A, *et al*. Relationships between endogenous sex steroid hormone, sex hormone-binding globulin, and lipoprotein levels in men: contribution of visceral obesity, insulin levels and other metabolic variables. *Atherosclerosis* 1997;133: 235–44

22. Kaufman JM, Vermeulen A. Declining gonadal function in elderly men. *Baillières Clin Endocrinol* 1997;11:189–98

23. Stellato RK, Feldman HA, Hamdy O, *et al*. Testosterone, sex hormone-binding globulin, and the development of type 2 diabetes in middle-aged men: prospective results from the Massachusetts Male Aging Study. *Diabet Care* 2000;23:490–4

24. Vgontzas A, Papanicoaou DA, Bixler EO, *et al*. Sleep apnea and daytime sleepiness and fatigue: relation to visceral obesity, insulin resistance, and hypercytokinemia. *J Clin Endocrinol Metab* 2000;85:1151–8

25. Flier JS. What's in a name? In search of leptin's physiological role. *J Clin Endocrinol Metab* 1998;83:1407–13

26. Mantzoros CS. The role of leptin in human obesity and disease: a review of current evidence. *Ann Intern Med* 1999;130:671–80

27. Isidori AM, Caprio M, Strollo F, *et al*. Leptin and androgens in male obesity: evidence for leptin contribution to reduced androgen levels. *J Clin Endocrinol Metab* 1999;84:3673–80

28. van den Saffele JK, Goemaere S, De Bacquer D, Kaufman JM. Serum leptin levels in healthy aging men: are decreased serum testosterone and increased adiposity the consequence of leptin deficiency? *Clin Endocrinol* 1999;51:81–8

29. Doucet E, St-Pierre S, Almeras N, *et al*. Fasting insulin levels influence plasma leptin levels independently from the contribution of adiposity: evidence from both a cross-sectional and an intervention study. *J Clin Endocrinol Metab* 2000;85:4231–7

30. Mantzoros CS, Flier JS. Leptin as a therapeutic agent – trials and tribulations. *J Clin Endocrinol Metab* 2000;85:4000–2

31. Rebuffe-Scrive CS, Mårin P, Björntorp P. Effect of testosterone on abdominal adipose tissue in men. *Int J Obesity Res* 1991;15:791–5

32. Mårin P, Holmång S, Gustafsson C. Androgen treatment of abdominally obese men. *Int J Obesity Res* 1993;1:245–51

33. Mårin P, Odén B, Björntorp P. Assimilation and mobilization of triglycerides in subcutaneous abdominal and femoral adipose tissue *in vivo* in men. *J Clin Endocrinol Metab* 1995; 80:239–43

34. Mårin P, Arver S. Androgens and abdominal obesity. *Baillière's Clin Endocrinol Metab* 1998;12:441–51

35. Must A, Spadano J, Coakley EH, *et al*. The disease burden associated with overweight and obesity. *J Am Med Assoc* 1999;282: 1523–9

Section VI

Nutrition, digestion and metabolism

John Marks, MA, MD, FRCP

There is a cliché that 'we are what we eat'. While this is indeed a cliché, it is a very true reflection of an important truism in biology and particularly medicine, namely that poor nutrition inevitably leads to poor health, either in the short or more usually the longer term.

However, nutrition is one of the most neglected areas of medical training. In the United Kingdom, for example, the average medical student only receives 1 or 2 hours' formal teaching on nutrition during the whole of the medical and pre-medical curriculum. Moreover, nutrition remains one of the least well practiced of all the medical areas. This despite the fact that type B malnutrition (i.e. inappropriate intake as opposed to the type A – inadequate intake) is now reaching epidemic proportions throughout the First World. Type B malnutrition is causal, to a greater or lesser degree, for a substantial proportion of the disorders covered in this book as a whole.

This section of the book is concerned with a representative sample of the current problems in the area of nutrition and metabolism and aims to provide information on the most recent developments in the field. It examines the management of the epidemic of overweight and obesity, stressing that it is much better to avoid the problem by sensible social behavior than to try to treat it. It explains the importance of equating the energy intake to the energy output of both normal living and exercise; of reducing sloth and gluttony, rather than trying to deal with the problem just by changing food intake patterns.

We also consider the effects of malnutrition of trace elements, both vitamins and minerals, which results from processed foods and from the generation of free radicals and explains how these can be overcome. We consider the requirements of the digestive tract itself, not only in terms of the older concepts of the need for fibre in the diet, but also in relation to the very new concepts of the health benefits of a balance of intestinal health-giving and health-reducing bacteria. Appropriate health giving changes can be effected by the regular ingestion of prebiotics, probiotics and synbiotics. Thus, this section takes note of the new branch of nutrition designated the 'functional foods'. But we are not only interested in the sedentary majority of the population, for we also explain the major new ideas of the special nutritional needs for competitive sports.

Finally, moving away from the nutrition area this section considers the effects that aging exerts on the metabolic processes associated with pharmacodynamics and pharmacokinetics, and ends with an appendix which outlines the concepts of appropriate diets and exercise for the maintenance of health.

22 Hazardous waist: a major problem for men, not just women

John Marks, MA, MD, FRCP

INTRODUCTION

The increasing prevalence of obesity in developed countries must be regarded as a dangerous pandemic. Over the past decade, the incidence of obesity has almost doubled in many countries. One estimate, which cannot be regarded as too much of a doomsday prediction, suggests that within the first half of the 21st century almost 100% of the adult population of the USA will be overweight and some 50% obese. Nor do these dramatic changes apply just to women, for excess weight in men is at least as prevalent as that in women; it is just not so newsworthy. The figures for prevalence of excess weight for men in several European countries are given in Table 1.

The average adult is currently adding about 1 g/day to their weight. Since overweight and obesity are substantial factors in both mortality and morbidity, it is vital that efforts be made not only to prevent any further increase in the problem but also to reduce the weight of those who are already affected.

DEFINITION OF OBESITY

The most common current method of classifying the weight is based upon a proportion of weight for height. Of the formulae, the current preference is for the body mass (BMI or Quetelet) index. This is derived by dividing the weight (in kg) by the height squared (in m)^2.

Whether a weight is normal is based upon actuarial considerations, for above a given range of weight, morbidity and mortality increase. Based on the BMI, the acceptable range in Western populations is defined as between 20 and 25; a BMI between 25 and 30 is regarded as overweight; obesity is taken as starting at 30. Current evidence indicates that the ideal BMI for men is about 20–23, and that an increase in morbidity and mortality starts above this level.

ECONOMIC COSTS OF OBESITY

Although studies in Northern Europe, particularly Finland[1], had identified that there are substantial economic costs from excess weight, these have been quantified only recently. Current estimates are concerned with the more easily quantifiable health-care costs rather than the further community economic costs. These direct costs, i.e. those costs related to the diagnosis and treatment of both obesity and diseases related to obesity, amount to some 2–8% of the total health-care costs. To these should be added those attributable to the diagnosis of overweight, which, with the greater

259

Table 1 Prevalence of overweight and obesity among adult men in representative countries. In several countries there are more than one survey, in different years and in different regions, represented by the range. Note that many of the most recent surveys date back 10 years. There is no evidence that the situation has improved in the mean-time; indeed it is probably worse

Country	Years of survey(s)	Obese (%)	Overweight (%)
Belgium	1990–1993	13–19	47–52
Brazil	1989	10	n/a
Canada	1991	15	n/a
Denmark	1991–1992	13	41
Finland	1992	22–24	46–49
France	1994–1997	13–22	40–51
Germany	1988–1995	13–24	49–56
Hungary	1987–1989	22–23	40–46
Italy	1993–1994	14–17	50–51
Poland	1992–1993	15–22	41–45
Spain	1994–1996	16	53
Sweden	1994–1996	13–14	47–50
Switzerland	1992–1993	13–16	47–53
United Kingdom	1991–1995	14–23	42–49
United States of America	1999	29	33

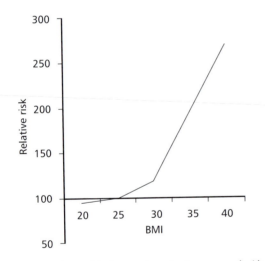

Figure 1 Relative risk of premature death compared with level of obesity/overweight as measured by body mass index (BMI): based upon reference 2

number of patients, would probably amount to at least the same level as those for obesity. Additional, indirect costs to society include not only sick-pay, pensions and so on, but also the loss of productivity from sick-leave, together with the personal costs from higher insurance premiums, job discrimination and adaptations to cope with disability. Hence, the overall economic cost of excess weight is substantial. Against this, the efforts adopted by society to minimize the risk of developing excess weight are derisory.

INFLUENCE OF WEIGHT INCREASE ON MORTALITY AND MORBIDITY

Numerous studies have shown that as the weight increases so does the mortality. Garrow[2] has expressed it very vividly: '[at BMI 40] … the mortality ratio is about 250% of that at [the desired weight] … so this degree of obesity is a greater threat to health than smoking 20 cigarettes a day' (Figure 1). The picture is complicated, because obesity is associated with other disorders that give rise to a reduced life expectancy. Hence, the relationship of weight to mortality is not linear throughout the whole obese group.

The relationship of weight and mortality is also strongly correlated with distribution of the fat. Obesity with a substantial increase of fat around the waist carries the highest risk, both for all-cause mortality and for that associated with cardiovascular disease. The correlation between obesity and reduced life expectancy is

Table 2 Increase in morbidity and mortality associated with obesity (> 30% overweight) in various medical conditions: based on reference 3. The range of figures takes account of age and sex and expresses the risk as a percentage of that in normal-weight people with these conditions

Disorder	Morbidity (%)	Mortality (%)
Diabetes mellitus	110–500	520–790
Cerebrovascular accident	110–440	150–220
Coronary heart disease	130–240	200–210
Cancer	—	130–160
Postoperative wound infection	700	—

greatest among those who are overweight as young adults, although the actual increase in mortality is seen in middle age.

While there is no dispute about the risks associated with obesity, there has been doubt about the health implications of overweight. Some recent studies have demonstrated that overweight *per se* (i.e. a BMI between 25 and 30) carries an increased risk, and that this is greater when the overweight is associated with other disorders. This implies that it is not enough to concentrate on the obese, but that the management of those who are overweight, particularly when young, also requires attention.

Even in the normal group (BMI 20–25), those who are towards the lower limit of normality have a lower mortality than do those who are bordering on being overweight. Although treatment of those in the normal BMI range is not justified, it is now clear that the ideal weight from the point of view of low mortality is about BMI 20–23.

Excess weight carries with it (Table 2) not only an increased risk of death, but also a substantial level of morbidity, embracing a wide range of disorders[3]. These produce ill health in the community and a substantial burden on national health costs. They include cardiovascular problems, diabetes (type II), gall bladder disease, some cancers, excess risk during surgery and a higher incidence of accidents (Table 2). Added to this, excess weight increases the morbidity in various chronic disorders (such as arthritis), and produces several serious social and psychological problems. One area that has not been fully explored is the effect of excess weight on work performance, particularly in manual labor.

CAUSES OF WEIGHT INCREASE

Natural selection in animals for survival has involved the ability to withstand famine. During periods of food abundance, a reasonable store of body fat has been accumulated. In the vast majority of animals in the wild there is competition for the available food, and it is rare for wild animals to accumulate more than a reasonable store of fat, indeed too high a store would result in a reduction in their ability to hunt successfully.

The same concept applied to primitive man. It was only when the human developed the ability to produce food in greater abundance and could harvest it with less effort that body fat stores tended to accumulate to a greater degree. Moreover, since the accumulation of fat demonstrated a lower level of manual labor, society sought to demonstrate status by a more rounded figure. But in previous generations of the so-called 'First World' countries, and even now for those in the Third World, crop failure as a result of disease, weather or wars led to periods of famine. Today these are very rare in developed countries, with the result that not only are reserves not needed, but natural correction does not occur.

At its simplest, obesity that consists of an increase in the number of fat cells, and the quantity of neutral fats they contain, represents an intake of food in excess of the body's energy needs. Fat tissue consists of neutral fats to the

Table 3 Factors leading to excess weight in the individual

Genetic
Reduced energy expenditure
  disability or illness
  aversion to exercise
Excess energy intake
  bad eating habits/food selection – 'junkaholics'
  social eating and drinking
    work-encouraged
    social
Psychological escape mechanism
  comfort foods
  bingeing

extent of some 70–75%, the rest being protein. In consequence, the deposition of 1 g of fat tissue would result from an excess food intake of about 7 kcal. Thus, an increase of, say, 20 kg over a 10-year period will arise with an average excess energy intake of only 40 kcal per day. In food terms this amounts to, say, one plain biscuit or one apple per day above energy needs. An 'apple a day' may not 'keep the doctor away' unless it substitutes for a less healthy energy source.

Although this simple equation still applies, it is clear that the weight increase is multifactorial, involving genetic, environmental and behavioral factors (Table 3). Much has been written recently about the genetic aspects of obesity, probably acting via lectin release. However, it would be false to stress these too much, for if they were of high importance there would not have been the sudden recent explosion in the prevalence of obesity. All the recent evidence points to the major influence of the reduction in exercise of all types – at work and at play. We are now far too sedentary. The current epidemic arises far more from sloth than gluttony[4], although the high proportion of fat in our food is undesirable.

CAUSES OF WEIGHT INCREASE IN THE INDIVIDUAL

As a multifactorial disorder, the influence of the various factors will differ from one person

to another. Without an understanding of the specific factors that lead to an imbalance of energy intake/expenditure in the individual, it is impossible to devise a successful management schedule.

The really important point to appreciate is that excess weight represents a symptom in a chronic, indeed lifelong disease. At present, like the case for so many chronic disorders, we have no means of effecting a cure but merely the means of managing the symptom as well as possible.

WEIGHT REDUCTION AND MAINTENANCE

There is only one really effective method for treating excess weight – avoid it. All other current methods, however effective in the short term, are ineffective in the long term. The vast majority of people are back to their old weight within 5 years.

However, despite this nihilistic long-term view, it behoves the doctor to attempt to try to reduce excess weight in the individual and to try to maintain this lower weight. It is now possible for a substantial proportion of those who are overweight to reduce that weight in the short term.

Non-invasive methods for reducing nutrient intake

Providing that the energy intake is consistently below the energy expenditure, there will be a reduction in weight. Differences will occur in the rate at which the weight will fall, depending only on the margin between the energy intake and the total energy expenditure. This total energy expenditure depends on both the basal energy expenditure (from the fat-free mass) and the energy expenditure of physical activity (Table 4). As the body weight is reduced, by whatever method, there is a reduction in the fat-free mass, since protein and fat are lost together, the accepted proportion being

Table 4 Calculated physical activity levels of men at three levels of occupational and leisure activity. The figures represent the total energy expenditure as a proportion of resting metabolic rate

Leisure activity	Occupational activity		
	Light	Moderate	Heavy
Non-active	1.4	1.6	1.7
Moderately active	1.5	1.7	1.8
Very active	1.6	1.8	1.9

75% fat and 25% protein whatever the starting weight of the individual[5]. To achieve this weight reduction, various non-invasive methods are available, selection depending largely on the individual preferences of doctor and dieter.

Moderation in food intake

For a few overweight people and for the occasional obese person, simple moderation in food consumption will lead to a slow but steady reduction in weight, even down to a normal level. Theoretically, this is the best method, for it should lead on to an easy change in long-term weight management, particularly if the diet stresses reduction in fat intake. In practice, very few tolerate the prolonged dieting.

Conventional food diets

The two types of conventional diets used are 'calorie-counted' or 'fat-restricted'. When the intake is below about 1200 kcal, it is virtually impossible to devise a food-based diet that provides adequate levels of minerals and vitamins, and supplements of these are essential. Self-selected food-based diets usually underestimate the energy content, often by a substantial margin. Food weighing is time consuming and boring, and when this is coupled with the relatively high cost of the low-energy foods it leads to poor compliance.

Formula diets

Formula diets use a very limited number of component food substances (for example, powdered milk) to provide the essential macronutrients, and rely upon artificial fortification with minerals and vitamins to ensure an adequate daily intake of micronutrients. They are often provided in the form of dry powders for reconstitution with water to provide soups or flavored drinks, but are now also available in the form of snack-type bars and prepacked drinks.

They are classified into two categories depending upon whether the daily intake is intended to exceed 800 kcals (low calorie/low-energy diets) or 400–800 kcals (very-low-calorie/low-energy diets). This division by energy content was based upon the mistaken view that those with an energy content below 800 kcals carried greater risks. Many recent studies have demonstrated, however, that the safety depends solely on the levels of the vital macronutrients (particularly the proteins and their constituent essential amino acids) together with the minerals and vitamins. Providing that these requirements are covered and the diet is taken with some sensible precautions, the only difference between the low-calorie and very-low-calorie formula diets is the rate at which weight is lost when there is full compliance (Table 5).

Anorectic drugs

In theory, these should represent a valuable contribution by removing the appetite stimulus. In practice, most anorectic drugs have shown either adverse effects or relatively little benefit.

Food absorption blockers

Theoretically these should be ideal. To date, often as a result of side-effects, these have

Table 5 Average rate of weight loss (over a period of about 8 weeks) in men resulting from total compliance to various weight-losing procedures

Weight loss procedure	Average weight loss (kg/week)
Exercise alone	0.2
1200-kcal formula diet daily	0.5–0.8
800-kcal formula diet daily	0.7–1.1
500-kcal formula diet	1.4–2.2

been poorly tolerated. However, initial results with one recent product appear to be more encouraging.

Methods for increasing energy output

Since body weight depends upon the balance of energy intake and total energy output, physical activity during dieting should help. Unfortunately, there are three fallacies to this argument: those who are overweight find it difficult to exercise, prolonged periods of strenuous exercise would be necessary to produce a significant effect (see Table 5); and compliance with training programs is poor.

Surgical approach to weight reduction

Dental splintage

A few years ago, there was a vogue for the use of dental splintage in those with severe obesity intractable to other procedures. This was based on the concept that it provides a physical barrier to food ingestion. The long-term results were poor.

Jejuno-ileal bypass

A bypass operation produces weight reduction by food malabsorption. The postoperative mortality was unacceptably high, there was substantial later morbidity, and this operation is now rare.

Gastroplasty

The size of the stomach and the passage between the proximal and distal portions is reduced by gastric stapling. Weight loss is good, early mortality and later morbidity are not problems, and the target-weight maintenance is somewhat better than with diets. It is the procedure of choice for those who favor the surgical approach to the management of intractable severe obesity.

As a result of considerable experience, my own preference is for the use of nutritionally complete formula diets below 800 kcals for weight loss programs[6]. Commercially available products intended for use as part of a diet plan are supplied with clear directions on how the daily intake should be constituted, and these directions should be followed to achieve the best results.

Medical role in the use of formula diets

The ideal arrangement for any dieting is for direct or indirect medical supervision. However, while this is vital when other disorders are suspected, there is no evidence that people who have excess weight but who are otherwise healthy are at greater risk using such diets without medical supervision. Nor are the short- or long-term results less good than in those who do consult their practitioners. This is a sad reflection on the medical interest in excess weight as a chronic medical disorder.

There are, however, certain medical contraindications to any form of severe dieting

Table 6 Contraindications to any form of severe dieting

Requires specialist clinic	Use under medical supervision
Children below the age of 12 years	Type II diabetes mellitus
Pregnant and lactating women	Cardiac arrhythmias
Type I diabetes mellitus	Renal disease
Recent myocardial infarction	Gout
Recent stroke	Major psychiatric illness or substance abuse
Recent severe heart failure	Prescription medicines
	diuretics
	antihypertensives
	insulin and oral hypoglycemic agents
	parenteral steroids

(Table 6), and these must be made clear to potential dieters. There is also a further list of disorders for which precautions must be taken, and in this group any form of dieting should be undertaken only under medical supervision (Table 6).

LONG-TERM MAINTENANCE OF WEIGHT LOSS

Losing weight using a modern formula diet is not unduly difficult from either the physical or the psychological point of view, providing that there is an adequate incentive so to do. Until recently, the concept was to define a target weight based upon the recognized weight for height in tables of least mortality. While this is probably still the ideal, it is now recognized that such a target is not attainable unless there is a genuine incentive to achieve it. Of greater importance is the recognition that the major difficulty lies in maintaining the weight loss that has been achieved. The difficulty in weight maintenance has not yet been overcome, but support from family and friends and encouragement to further sustained additional activity certainly help.

Considerable lowering of health risks and improvements in obesity-related disorders can be achieved with only modest weight reductions (of the order of 10%). These smaller, but maintained reductions are more readily achievable, and recent studies have concentrated on these lower expectations.

However, reducing the long-term expectation does not justify taking less interest in the need for a permanent change in life-style (smaller meals of lower energy density, adequate maintained exercise, different approach to stress management, etc.), which is the only process by which good, permanent results will be achieved. Changing the life-style should indeed form an important component of the whole process of dieting, and should not be just brought in at the time when the agreed weight has been achieved.

FUTURE STRATEGIES FOR OVERCOMING THE OBESITY PANDEMIC

In a recent article[7], Egger and Swinburn have proposed a new model for the genesis of excess weight. Their fundamental argument is that we should regard obesity as any other pandemic – not as an abnormal response of the individual to a normal environment, but as the normal response of the individual to an abnormal environment. Most of the information on which their view is based is well established; what differs is their interpretation.

They point out, very cogently, that obesity is a behavioral disorder, a concept with which few would argue. They stress that behavior is modified not only by factors in the individual but more importantly by global factors[8]. The conclusion we should draw is that to overcome the current pandemic requires studies not only by biologists and physicians but, more importantly, by social scientists. A walk down any busy street should convince us that effort spent on this problem is fully justified!

References

1. Rissanen A, Helkiovaara M, Kneckt P, et al. Risk of disability and mortality due to overweight in a Finnish population. *Br Med J* 1990; 301:835–7
2. Garrow JS. Treatment of obesity. *Lancet* 1992;340:409–13
3. Andersen T. Gastroplasty and very-low-calorie diet in the treatment of morbid obesity. *Danish Medical Bulletin* 1990;37:359–70
4. Prentice AM, Jebb SA. Obesity: gluttony or sloth. *Lancet* 1995;346:437–9
5. Kreitzman SR, Howard AN, eds. *The Swansea Trial: Body Composition and Metabolic Studies with a Very Low Calorie Diet (VLCD)*. London: Smith-Gordon, 1993
6. Marks J, Howard AN. *The Cambridge Diet: A Manual for Health Professionals*. Cambridge: Cambridge Export Ltd, 1997
7. Egger G, Swinburn B. An 'ecological' approach to the obesity pandemic. *Br Med J* 1997;315: 477–80
8. World Health Organization. *Obesity: Preventing and Managing the Global Epidemic* (Report of a WHO consultation on obesity). Geneva: WHO, 1997:3–5

23 Nutraceuticals in male health

Paul Clayton, PhD

INTRODUCTION

Throughout history, the leading causes of death have been infection and trauma. Twentieth-century medicine has scored significant victories against these, and the major causes of ill health and death are now the chronic degenerative diseases such as coronary artery disease, arthritis, osteoporosis, Alzheimer's disease, macular degeneration, cataract and cancer.

Five out of six people in their 60s have one or more of these diseases. Drugs may alleviate symptoms, but do little to alter the underlying disease condition, which generally continues to deteriorate. This is because currently available drugs do not address the cause of these diseases. Based on the concept of the 'magic bullet', they are designed to block a single step in the generally multifactorial process leading to the symptoms of illness; this strategy is intrinsically unlikely to cure, and is associated with a high risk of side-effects. Iatrogenic illness is now a leading cause of hospitalization.

An even more fundamental criticism of modern medicine is that it is generally practiced as crisis management: wait until the diagnosis, then start treatment. By the time symptoms of one of these diseases appear, damage has already been done to the body, damage that drugs cannot address.

The chronic degenerative diseases have a long latency period before symptoms appear and a diagnosis is finally made. Coronary artery disease, cancer, Alzheimer's disease and osteoporosis do not occur overnight (although symptoms might do). They are slowly progressing conditions, which develop for years or decades before symptoms finally emerge.

It follows, therefore, that the majority of apparently healthy adults are 'pre-ill'. They contain in their bodies the seeds of the illness that will eventually become overt, and perhaps kill them. An artery is furring, bone is thinning and brain cells are dying, leading eventually, inevitably, to a heart attack, osteoporotic fracture or dementia.

Are these conditions inevitably degenerative? A truly preventive medicine that focuses on the pre-ill, analyzing the metabolic errors that lead to clinical illness, might be able to correct them before the first twinge of angina, or fracture. Will the approach be genomic, or nutraceutical?

Genetic risk factors are known for all the chronic degenerative diseases, and are important to the individuals who possess them. At the population level, however, migration studies confirm that these illnesses are linked for the most part to the life-style factors of exercise, smoking and nutrition. Nutrition is the easiest of these to change, and the most versatile tool for affecting the metabolic changes needed to tilt the balance away from disease.

All biological tissues are dynamic. Their apparent constancy disguises a continual state of flux, with the processes of decay and regeneration running in parallel. Bones are constantly being worn away and rebuilt, as are

Table 1 US Department of Agriculture (USDA) nutrient survey showing percentage of population who do not consume RDA of the essential vitamins, 1994

Vitamin	A	E	C	B_1	B_2	Niacin	B_4	B_6	B_{12}
Percentage(%)	55	68	37	32	31	27	34	54	17

joints. Atheroma is constantly accumulating inside the arteries, and just as constantly being removed. If the anabolic and catabolic processes are in balance, tissue remains intact and good health is sustained. But if the rate of decay is only a little faster than the rate of repair, there is a net loss of healthy tissue, and a pre-illness grows every day until clinical illness finally emerges. This is an important cause of morbidity and mortality because it is obvious that, in middle-aged and older subjects, catabolic processes generally outstrip anabolic capacity. In many cases, this may be due to multiple micronutrient depletion. Depletion is not the near-absolute absence of a nutrient that causes a deficiency disease, like the case of vitamin C and scurvy, but a sub-optimal level of a nutrient or nutrients which slows a restorative process by marginally, but sufficiently, to lead eventually, to clinical illness. Within this definition, chronic degenerative diseases might be regarded as 'depletion diseases'.

It is commonly stated that adequate nutrition is obtained from a well-balanced diet. However, surveys such as that carried out by the US Department of Agriculture (USDA) reveal that malnutrition is common in the developed nations (Table 1). [This is not the calorie and/or micronutrient deficiency associated with developing nations ('type A malnutrition'), but multiple micronutrient depletion, usually combined with calorific balance or excess ('type B malnutrition').]

The above survey measured intakes of classical micronutrients in terms of the recommended daily amount (RDA) values designed to prevent deficiency diseases. Levels of micronutrients needed to sustain prolonged good health appear in many cases to be higher, so the incidence of malnutrition expressed in these terms is obviously greater.

The incidence and severity of type B malnutrition are worsened again if newer micronutrient groups are included, such as the essential polyunsaturated fatty acids, various fiber types, xanthophylls and flavonoids. Commonly ingested levels of all these micronutrients appear to be suboptimal.

The prevalence of multiple micronutrient depletion is due to several structural factors:

(1) *Insufficient calorific throughput* Anthropological studies suggest that we were designed to live active lives, and to consume 3000–4000 kcals per day. No longer hunter–gatherers, we live sedentary lives, and require far fewer calories. Our appetites have shrunk, but not quite enough, which explains why so many people are overweight. When less is eaten, fewer micronutrients are consumed.

(2) *Dietary shift* Many (not all) processed foods are depleted in micronutrients, and more processed foods are being consumed than ever before.

(3) *Depleted soils* Many soils are intrinsically low in key minerals, or have become depleted owing to overintensive farming. Plants or animals raised in these areas are depleted in these minerals also. This is why UK intakes of selenium are so low.

(4) *Life-style* Smoking, sun-bathing, pollution, excessive drinking or exercise, *inter alia*, deplete the body of antioxidants.

(5) *Aging* We become progressively more depleted in many micronutrients as we age. Reduced finances may mean a restricted diet, as does institutionalization. Activity levels are reduced, hence appetite, food

and micronutrient intake fall further. Deteriorating dentition encourages a shift towards softer foods, with fewer of the fruits and vegetables that supply many micronutrients. Finally, older digestive systems may be less efficient at absorbing micronutrients from whatever food is eaten. This is one reason why, with age, we become more likely to sicken and die owing to multiple systems failure, caused in turn by cumulative, multiple micronutrient depletion.

Evidence is growing to support the concept that type B malnutrition is a major cause of the chronic degenerative diseases. Logically, the prevention and treatment of these conditions must be addressed in micronutrient repletion programs.

NEUTRACEUTICAL STRATEGIES

Micronutrients are not medicines, and should not be used as such. The etiology of the degenerative diseases is multifactorial, and intrinsically resistant to monotherapeutic intervention. Furthermore, as most subjects are depleted in most micronutrients, it is not surprising that there is so little evidence of the clinical efficacy of micronutrients, when most studies have used single micronutrients or very limited, low-dose combinations.

Another confounding factor is the variability of local nutritional baselines. A good prospective study[1] demonstrated the anticancer effects of 200 µg/day selenium in the American Midwest, where dietary selenium intakes are as low as 50 µg/day; such an intervention can have no impact in Greenland, where the average daily intake is close to 1.5 mg/day.

A more rational approach to disease management examines the chemical and physiological links in the chain of events that drives the disease process, reviews the micronutrients known to impact on those links, and then combines them in a program designed to impede the overall disease process. One prospective study in particular points the way forward, Salonen and colleagues[2], showed that whereas supplementation with either vitamin C or E had no effect on common carotid atherosclerotic progression, a combined supplementation of C and E vitamins, significantly slowed the disease process. The synergistic impact of the combination was predicted from basic biochemistry. In a textbook of male health, it is appropriate to remain with coronary artery disease as an example of this approach.

NEUTRACEUTICAL PROGRAM FOR CARDIOVASCULAR DISEASE

Retrospective studies[3-5] have suggested that the risk of a heart attack may be reduced by d-α-tocopherol by up to 50%. A similar or greater reduction of risk is associated with a high intake of the xanthophyll lycopene[6], the flavonoid quercitin[7], methyl group donors[8], and omega-3 polyunsaturated fatty acids although intervention studies have been disappointing.

For other micronutrients or food types, only biomarker data are so far available. A 10–15% fall in plasma low-density lipoprotein (LDL) cholesterol, which offers significant cardioprotection, can be obtained by consuming 10–20 g/day of standardized soy protein[9], or 5–10 g/day each of the prebiotic fibers fructo-oligosaccharides (FOS) and inulin[10-12], or 0.3–0.5 l of citrus juice per day[13].

An increase in high-density lipoprotein (HDL) cholesterol is considered to be even more protective[14]. This can be achieved by consuming citrus juice, or monoterpenes such as menthol: 200 mg of menthol per day, combined with pinene (from pine needles), raises HDL cholesterol by up to 40%, which is extremely cardioprotective. The even more potent guggulipids, extracted from the Indian plant *Commiphora mukul*, raise HDL by 60%[15,16].

Of the many potential cardioprotective phytonutrients, three are already being incorporated into a range of functional foods produced by Marks & Spencer plc: soy, FOS and the amino acid trimethyl glycine, also known as betaine, together with vitamins C and E and selenium.

Soy

A meta-analysis of 38 clinical studies[9] found that consumption of soy protein rather than animal protein was associated with significantly reduced levels of total cholesterol, LDL cholesterol and triglycerides. In these studies soy intake varied between 17 and 124 g/day, with an average of 47 g. The average reduction in total cholesterol was 9.3%; LDL cholesterol fell by 12.9%; and triglycerides fell by 10.5%.

The cholesterol-lowering action consists of several components. Studies have shown (in animal models) that soy protein reduces absorption of cholesterol in the intestinal tract, and may also reduce the resorption of bile acids[17], leading to increased fecal excretion of both neutral sterols and bile acids[18]. This would result in increased hepatic cholesterol synthesis of bile acids from cholesterol, leading in turn to hepatic cholesterol depletion. The liver responds by upregulating LDL receptors, resulting in the observed downward shifts in blood cholesterol. This theoretical mechanism is supported by clinical studies which have shown that LDL receptors are upregulated by soy diets[19–21].

Another possible mechanism of action involves the amino-acid composition in soy, specifically the high arginine/lysine ratio, which has been shown in animal models to be hypocholesterolemic[22]. Some authors have suggested that the arginine/lysine ratio may exert its hypocholesterolemic effect via shifts in insulin/glucagon and/or thyroxine levels[23–25]. However, this is not universally agreed[26] and there are as yet no human data.

Other studies indicate that soy protein fractions with higher isoflavone content are more effective in lowering cholesterol in monkeys[27] and in human subjects[28]. However, as purified isoflavones are not hypocholesterolemic, it seems that other components occurring in association with the isoflavones are also involved in the overall cholesterol-lowering effect of soy.

Soy isoflavones are well-known antioxidants, and have been shown to reduce LDL cholesterol oxidation rates in several *ex vivo* studies[29,30]. Unsurprisingly, as cholesterol oxidation products have been shown to disrupt endothelial function, soy isoflavones (and other flavonoid mixtures such as pycnogenol) promote endothelium-modulated vasodilatation. The impact of isoflavones on the endothelium may be augmented by soy protein's content of arginine, which is known to exert vasodilating effects via nitric oxide upregulation; and by the ability of many flavonoids to inhibit angiotensin converting enzyme, which confers additional endothelial and myocardial protection. Protease inhibitors in soy such as the Bowman–Birk lectin may also be involved.

In *in vitro* studies, the soy isoflavone genistein has been shown to impede the activation and accumulation of platelets, to reduce the subsequent production of platelet-derived growth factors, and to inhibit thrombin[31,32]. These effects would tend to reduce the risk of thrombus formation and arterial medial thickening, and would be expected to contribute to an overall reduction of coronary artery disease morbidity and mortality.

Fructo-oligosaccharides

Fructo-oligosaccharides (FOS) are an example of a distinct class of fiber, the non-digestible oligosaccharides.

Non-digestible oligosaccharides are resistant to human digestive enzymes. Instead, they are fermented by bacteria in the large bowel. These fibers, which are stable and well tolerated, form a new therapeutic category of nutrients known as prebiotics. They have a beneficial role in human nutrition, but are seldom listed in food tables because they are not detected by the classical methods of fiber analysis. Their primary effect is the differential stimulation of bacterial growth.

The large bowel contains between 400 and 500 different species of bacteria. Some of these can cause serious illness, while at least two types, the lactobacilli and bifidobacteria, are associated with positive health. Prebiotics encourage the growth of these 'healthy' bacteria, and inhibit other bacteria which can cause disease either by overgrowth or by producing toxic metabolites.

The common prebiotics inulin and oligofructose consist of chains of fructose molecules; the degree of polymerization is higher in inulin. The richest plant sources of inulin and oligofructose are chicory root, which has a long history of medicinal use, and Jerusalem artichoke. Then, in descending order, there are leeks, onions, salsify, wheat, bananas and other fruits, grains and vegetables.

Because prebiotics occur in so many foods everyone consumes them, but dietary intakes vary between 1 and 4 g in the USA, and 3 and 11 g per day in Europe. The highest dose one might encounter would be the 6–18 g of inulin in a bowl of onion soup; scientists have injected themselves with doses of up to 100 g intravenously, without problems[33].

Prebiotics are common plant energy storage compounds, which plants accumulate when solar energy is available, and use as fuel when the skies are dark or overcast. Accordingly, when plants such as onions are stored for long periods, and particularly in cold storage, their prebiotic content declines quite dramatically. Because many of us eat fruit and vegetables that have been in cold storage for some time, their prebiotic content may be very low. This may contribute to many gastrointestinal and other health complaints, because a low intake of prebiotics leads to an increased proportion of potentially disease-causing bacteria in the gut.

When ingested prebiotics cause bifidogenesis, the multiplying bacteria break down the prebiotic polymers to short chain fatty acids. These acids inhibit the growth of potentially disease-causing bacteria. The lactobacilli and bifidobacteria also secrete bacteriocins such as nicin, which have additional inhibitory effects on the 'unhealthy' bacteria, including most of the strains responsible for food poisoning.

As a result of the increase in the 'healthy' bacteria, and the inhibition of the 'unhealthy' bacteria, there is a 1–2 log shift in the flora of the gut in a health-promoting direction. The short-term benefits include improved intestinal 'regularity', and an increased resistance to food poisoning.

As bifidobacteria grow they bind bile acids in the gut, and remove them from the body in the feces. This explains why prebiotics such as FOS lead to a lowering of blood cholesterol. Bile acids are formed in the liver from cholesterol; prebiotics, by increasing bifidobacteria in the gut and bile acid excretion, 'drain' the cholesterol pool.

In this way, prebiotic-induced bifidogenesis leads to a reduction in plasma lipids in animals and in healthy humans. It also lowers LDL and total cholesterol in diabetic, hyperlipidemic and chronic renal failure patients.

In addition, the lactobacilli synthesize B vitamins, including B_1, B_6, B_{12} and folic acid, and are probably the major species of bacteria in the colon that do this. Vitamin B deficiency is surprisingly common in developed countries, and is a major risk factor for coronary artery disease. Logically, prebiotics which increase the population of bifidobacteria in the gut, and stimulate the synthesis of B vitamins, will also be cardioprotective.

Finally, there is some evidence that certain strains of these bacteria synthesize vitamin K analogs. These have been linked to a reduced risk of soft tissue calcification, including inflammatory lesions in the arteries[34]. Taken together, the ability of prebiotics to improve blood cholesterol profiles, vitamin B status and possibly vitamin K status probably constitutes a significant reduction in the risk of coronary artery disease.

Bifidobacteria are particularly important in the new-born, whose immune defenses are not yet fully competent. Breast milk contains bifidogenic substances, which is why bifido-bacteria represent up to 95% of bacteria in the gut of breast-fed infants, but a mere 25% in the bottle-fed infant. This explains the greater resistance of breast-fed babies to stomach upsets and diarrhea, and is strongly supported by studies which show that live yoghurt cultures fed to infants significantly reduce their risk of contracting diarrhea if given preventively, and speed recovery if given as a treatment.

With age, the proportion of bifidobacteria and lactobacilli falls even further. This is one reason why we become more prone to gastro-intestinal upsets, and is probably also linked to the age-related increase in the risk of bowel cancer and other illnesses.

We are reviewing cardioprotection via nutraceutical intervention, but it is probable that the most important health benefits of these fibers may be cancer risk reduction.

There is evidence that prebiotics protect against a number of different cancers, primarily colorectal cancer. One of the anticancer mech-anisms involves the short chain fatty acids pro-duced by bifidobacteria in the gut, which include butyric acid. Butyrate is considered essential for the health and normal growth of colonocytes, the cells that line the colon. Butyrate has various potentially therapeutic effects on colonocytes: studies show that it induces differentiation, slows down abnormal cell growth and accelerates healing after surgery of the gut[35]. It may be no coincidence that the bacteria that produce butyrate concentrate in the ascending colon, which is relatively immune to cancer.

Butyrate production is probably one of the main reasons why prebiotics reduce the risk of colon and other (experimental) cancers, but is unlikely to be the only one.

With longer-term use, prebiotics reduce the numbers of disease-causing bacteria in the gut, and the amount of putrefactive, toxic and carcinogenic compounds they produce. This is

thought to exert an anticancer effect in the colon, and other sites. In one study, prebiotics reduced the incidence of mammary cancer in rats[36].

The risk of colon cancer is increased by a diet high in animal fats. This diet increases the secretion of bile, leading to increased levels of bile acids and cholesterols in the intestine. Many of the gut bacteria (but not the bifidobacteria) convert bile acids into carcino-genic compounds such as aromatic polycyclic hydrocarbons. These bacteria which have been shown in experiments to increase the risk of liver cancer are reduced significantly by prebiotics[37].

Trimethyl glycine

Trimethyl glycine's primary importance in human and animal nutrition is as a methyl group donor.

Because of the strategic role of methyl groups in the nervous, immune, renal and cardiovascular systems, all growing and mature animals including humans require a constant supply of methyl groups in the diet. A deficit of methyl groups is the only dietary deficiency that is intrinsically carcinogenic, via under-methylation of DNA and the activation of oncogenes.

The methyl group cycle is the metabolic point at which methyl groups from the diet are used to transform homocysteine to methionine. Methionine is adenosylated to form S-adenosyl methionine (SAM), which is the ultimate methyl group donor in the body. SAM-provided methyl groups are essential to the formation of a number of physiologically essential com-pounds such as creatine, carnitine, the phos-pholipids, RNA and DNA, polyamines, the stress hormones epinephrine and norepineph-rine, and various monoamine neurotrans-mitters; and to the basic functioning of the immune system.

The body cannot synthesize methyl groups, and therefore a dietary source of methyl groups is essential to maintain the cycle, and to suppress

Table 2 Cardiovascular risk factors showing effects of drugs and a nutraceutical program

Risk factor	Nutrients	Drugs
LDL $\downarrow$	oats, soy, citrus	Statins, cholesterol resins
LDL $\downarrow$ oxidation	vitamins C and E, carotenes, flavonoids	—
ADL $\uparrow$	leuthin, betaine	Statins
HC $\downarrow$	folates, betaine	—
VCAM $\downarrow$	Q3, vitamin E, flavonoids	—
ICAM $\downarrow$	Q3, vitamin E, flavonoids	—
Platelet reactivity	Q3 vitamin E (high dose), flavonoids	aspirin, anti-K agents
BP$\downarrow$	Sodium substitutes	various

plasma and tissue levels of homocysteine. Trimethyl glycine, methionine and choline, along with the coenzymes vitamins B_6, folic acid and B_{12}, are the principal sources of methyl groups in the diet of animals and humans. Trimethyl glycine predominates over folic acid in all species screened.

The main source of methyl groups in the human diet is choline. However, choline is not a methyl donor itself, but must be transformed in the mitochondria to form trimethyl glycine. Trimethyl glycine is the ultimate provider of methyl groups into the methyl group cycle.

Choline is a less effective dietary source of methyl groups than trimethyl glycine, because much dietary choline is used for other purposes. The rate of synthesis of trimethyl glycine from choline is insufficient to meet animals' requirements for methyl groups.

This is why trimethyl glycine has been designated a quasi-vitamin, because many species (fish, chickens, rabbits, etc.) have an obligate dietary need for trimethyl glycine under conditions of stress. This is because methyl groups are required for the formation of stress hormones, for various immune defense mechanisms and for synthesizing polyamines, RNA and DNA, all of which are central to tissue repair and turnover.

Under these conditions, the shortfall of methyl groups leads to an increase in levels of homocysteine, which has been strongly linked to an increased risk of cardiovascular disease[38–40] and, more recently, neurological diseases such as Alzheimer's disease.

In the absence of dietary trimethyl glycine, levels of homocysteine increase if there is a deficiency of certain B vitamins in the diet (vitamins B_6, B_{12} and folic acid). Deficiencies in these B vitamins are very common. One recent study found that people who consumed low levels of folate were 69% more at risk of heart attack death than those whose diet contained high folate levels[8].

A strong B complex preparation reduces levels of homocysteine. For this reason, supplements of folic acid and vitamins B_6 and B_{12} are increasingly being used to reduce homocysteine levels, and the risk of homocysteine-related cardiovascular disease and neurological conditions. However, in as many as 10% of the population, folic acid cannot be metabolized, and the physiological benefits of folic acid are greatly reduced. Trimethyl glycine is a quantitatively more important donor of methyl groups to the cycle, is universally applicable and, in addition, has osmoprotectant and stabilizing functions in tissues such as the kidney and central nevous system.

THE COMBINATION APPROACH

Returning to cardiovascular disease, the major steps in the sequence of events have been identified. No one drug could adequately modify this sequence, but a simple combination of phytonutrients can lower LDL cholesterol, raise HDL, block the oxidation of whatever LDL remains, reduce homocysteine, reduce inflammation in the arterial walls, thereby inhibiting the release of vascular cell adhesion molecule

(VCAM) and intercellular adhesion molecule (ICAM) mediators, and reduce platelet aggregability. The owner of a metabolic system that has been reconfigured in this way is probably largely immune to cardiovascular disease, and has achieved this safely, relatively inexpensively and (in the very near future) as part of a daily diet (Table 2).

References

1. Clark LC, Combs GF Jr, Turnbull BW, *et al*. Effects of selenium supplementation for cancer prevention in patients with carcinoma of the skin. A randomized controlled trial. Nutritional Prevention of Cancer Study Group. *JAMA* 1996;276:1957–63

2. Salonen JT, Nyyssonen K, Salonen R, *et al*. Antioxidant supplementation in atherosclerosis prevention (ASAP) study: a randomized trial of the effect of vitamins E and C on 3-year progression of carotid atherosclerosis. *J Intern Med* 2000;248:377–86

3. Rimms EB, Stampfer MJ, Ascherio A, *et al*. Vitamin E consumption and the risk of coronary disease in men. *N Engl J Med* 1993;328:1450–6

4. Stampfer MJ, Hennekens CH, Manson JE, *et al*. Vitamin E consumption and the risk of coronary disease in women. *N Engl J Med* 1993;328:1444–9

5. Stephens NG, Parsons A, Schofield PM, *et al*. Randomised controlled trial of vitamin E in patients with coronary disease. Coronary Heart Antioxidant Study (CHAOS). *Lancet* 1996;347:781–6

6. Kohlmeier L, Kark JD, Gomez-Gracia E, *et al*. Lycopene and myocardial infarction risk in the EURAMIC Study. *Am J Epidemiol* 1997;146:618–26

7. Hertog MG, Feskens EJ, Hollman PC, *et al*. Dietary antioxidant flavonoids and risk of coronary heart disease. *Lancet* 1993;342:1007–11

8. Morrison HI, Schaubel D, Desmeules M, *et al*. Serum folate and risk of fatal coronary heart disease. *JAMA* 1996;275:1893–6

9. Anderson JW, Johnstone BM, Cook-Newell ME. Meta-analysis of the effects of soy protein intake on serum lipids. *N Engl J Med* 1995;333:276–82

10. Davidson MH, Synecki C, Tryloff MJ, Drennan KB. An inulin-containing dietary supplement for the treatment of hypercholesterolemia in adults. *Presented at the 1st Orafti Research Conference*, Universite Catholique de Louvain, Belgium January 1995:83–94

11. Mitsuoka T, Hidaka H, Eida T. Effects of fructo-oligosaccharides on intestinal microflora. *Die Nabrung* 1987;31:426–36

12. Mitsuoka T. Intestinal flora and human health. *Presented at the 3rd International Symposium on Intestinal flora*. Yakult Bio-science Foundation, Amsterdam 1994:3–21

13. Trovato A, *et al*. *Phytomedicine* 1996;2:221–7

14. Hulley SB, Walsh JM, Newman TB. Health policy on blood cholesterol. Time to change directions. *Circulation* 1992;86:1026–9

15. Nityanand S, Kapoor NK. Cholesterol-lowering activity of the various fractions of guggul'. *Indian J Exp Biol* 1973;11:395–411

16. Satyavati GC. Gum guggul (Comiphora mukul) – the success story of an ancient insight leading to a modern discovery. *Indian J Med Res* 1988;87:327–35

17. Beynen AC. *Dietary Soy Protein and Cholesterol Metabolism*. Department of Laboratory Animal Science, State University of Utrecht, 1989

18. Sugano M, Koba K. Dietary protein and lipid metabolism: a multifunctional effect. *Ann NY Acad Sci* 1993;676:215–22

19. Baum JA, Teng H, Erdman JW Jr, *et al*. Long-term intake of soy protein improves blood lipid profiles and increases mononuclear cell low-density-lipoprotein receptor messenger RNA in hypercholesterolemic, postmenopausal women. *Am J Clin Nutr* 1998;68:545–51

20. Lovati MR, Manzoni A, Canavesi A, *et al*. Soybean protein diet increases low density lipoprotein receptor activity on mononuclear

cells from hypercholerolaemic patients. *J Clin Invest* 1987;80:1498–502

21. Sirtori CR, Lovati MR, Manzoni C, *et al*. Soy and cholesterol reduction: clinical experience. *J Nutr* 1995;125:598S–605S

22. Kirtchevsky D. Dietary protein and experimental atherosclerosis. *Ann NY Acad Sci* 1997;676:180–87

23. Forsythe WA 3rd. Soy protein, thyroid regulation and cholesterol metabolism. *J Nutr* 1995;125:619S–623S

24. Sanchez A, Hubbard RW. Plasma amino acids and the insulin/glucagon ratio as an explanation for the dietary protein modulation of atherosclerosis. *Med Hypoth* 1991;35:324–9

25. Sugano M, Ishiwaki N, Nakashima K. Dietary protein-dependent modification of serum cholesterol level in rats. Significance of the arginine/lysine ratio. *Ann Nutr Metab* 1984;28:192–9

26. Balmir F, Staack R, Jeffrey E, *et al*. An extract of soy flour influences serum cholesterol and thyroid hormones in rats and hamsters. *J Nutr* 1996;126:3046–53

27. Anthony MS, Clarkson TB, Bullock BC, Wagner JD. Soy protein versus soy phytoestrogens in the prevention of diet-induced coronary artery atherosclerosis of male cynomolgus monkeys. *Arterioscler Thromb Vasc Biol* 1997;17:2524–31

28. Crouse JR 3rd, Morgan T, Terry JG, *et al*. A randomized trial comparing the effect of casein with that of soy protein containing varying amounts of isoflavones on plasma concentrations of lipids and lipoproteins. *Arch Intern Med* 1999;159:2070–6

29. Kanzawa T, Osanai T, Zhang XS, *et al*. Protective effects of soy protein on the peroxidisability of lipoproteins in cerebrovascular disease. *J Nutr* 1995;125:639s–46s

30. Tikkanen MJ, Wahala K, Ojala S, *et al*. Effect of soybean phytoestrogen intake on low density lipoprotein oxidisation resistance. *Proc Natl Acad Sci USA* 1998;95:3106–10

31. Raines EW, Ross R. Biology of atherosclerotic plaque formation: possible role of growth factors in lesion development and the potential impact of soy. *J Nutr* 1995;125:624S–630S

32. Wilcox JN, Blumenthal BF. Thrombotic mechanisms in atherosclerosis: potential impact of soy proteins. *J Nutr* 1995;125:631S–638S

33. Shannon JA, Smith HW. Excretion of insulin, xylofructose and urea by normal and phlorizinised men. *J Clin Invest* 1935;14:393–401

34. Hodges SJ. A personal correspondence. 1999

35. Cummings JH. *Presented at the 1st Orafti Research Conference*, Universite Catholique de louvain, Belgium January 1995:95–108

36. Delzenne N. Systemic effect of non-digestible oligosaccharides: their impact on lipid metabolism. *Presented at the 1st Orafti Research Conference*, Universite Catholique de louvain, Belgium January 1995:275–8

37. Mizutani T, Mitsuoka T. Inhibitory effect of some intestinal bacteria on liver tumorigenesis in gnotobiotic C3H/He male mice. *Cancer Lett* 1980;11:89–95

38. Naurath HJ, Joosten E, Riezler R, *et al*. Effects of vitamin B12, folate and vitamin B6 supplements in elderly people. *Lancet* 1995;346:85–9

39. Perry IJ, Refsum H, Morris RW, *et al*. Prospective study of serum total homocysteine concentration and risk of stroke in middle-aged British men. *Lancet* 1995;346:1395–8

40. Jobst KA, Smith AD, Szatmari M, *et al*. Rapidly progressing atrophy of medical temporal lobe in Alzheimer's disease. *Lancet* 1994;343:829–30

24 Current views about dietary fiber

Anthony R. Leeds, FIBiol

INTRODUCTION

Dietary fiber is the non-starch polysaccharide in plants that is not degraded by the enzymes of the small intestine. In the UK the term 'non-starch polysaccharide' is often used instead, and the widespread use of the two terms, which relate to the use of two different analytical methods, introduces scope for confusion in the minds of patients and consumers. The term 'dietary fiber' is that best understood by lay-people world-wide. The term 'soluble dietary fiber' refers to fiber that dissolves in water during laboratory analysis. While lacking a precise definition, the term has come to be used for those types of fiber from oats, beans, barley and rye, fruits and vegetables, which have, in some cases, been shown to lower blood cholesterol levels.

Plants are composed of structural polysaccharides and storage polysaccharides, as well as protein, lipid, vitamin and mineral components. The storage polysaccharide (which provides an energy store for plant growth) is present as starch, which is potentially digestible, or other polysaccharides, which are equally usable by the plant but which are constructed in a manner that is not subject to degradation by mammalian pancreatic α-amylase, and is thus indigestible. Even some of the starch may not be digested in the small intestine (this 'resistant' starch may be inaccessible through encapsulation within intact plant cell walls or as a consequence of starch granule structure), in which case it passes, like dietary fiber, through the small gut to become substrate for fermentation in the large gut. Structural polysaccharides are largely cellulose and pectins, which, along with storage non-starch polysaccharides, make up dietary fiber. Plant composition varies according to the type of tissue and according to the maturity of the plant: for example, tuber composition changes as the tuber grows and matures (the proportions of the types of starch change), and stems become woody with age.

EFFECTS OF FIBER IN THE UPPER GUT

Dietary fiber influences both small- and large-intestinal function. In the upper gut there can be no generalization with respect to gastric emptying. Some purified fiber fractions, when mixed with experimental test meals, have been shown to slow gastric emptying, but under some conditions an increased rate of emptying has been demonstrated. High-fiber foods are generally lower in energy density (fewer calories per gram) than low-fiber foods, and take longer to chew. Thus, gastric filling (measured as intake of food in g/min or cal/min) may be slowed. In the small intestine some types of fiber reduce convective movements and turbulence,

276

thus decreasing mixing and substrate–enzyme interactions. There is clear evidence for a slowing of digestion under some conditions, and a little evidence for impairment of absorption. These effects of some types of fiber result in slower absorption of carbohydrate, which in turn leads to flatter postprandial glucose and insulin curves. Thus, some types of fiber influence the 'glycemic index' of foods (the extent to which a 50-g carbohydrate portion of a food raises the blood glucose level, compared with a glucose control). Glycemic index is, however, also influenced by starch type and structure, the physical structure of food, and the presence of sugar, fat and protein. Thus, while 'high-fiber' carbohydrate foods are important for people with diabetes, the fiber content of food is not the sole determinant of the metabolic response to it.

Some types of fiber appear to have a bile-salt binding effect; this has been shown experimentally but is not as strong as that demonstrated by cholestyramine. This effect probably partly accounts for the blood cholesterol-lowering effect of some types of dietary fiber, for example oat β-glucan.

EFFECTS OF FIBER IN THE LOWER GUT

Polysaccharides (whether fiber or resistant starch) are degraded by colonic bacteria. Starch and pectins are usually totally degraded, while cellulose and isphagula may remain partially intact (the physical structure, solubility and particle size probably determines the extent of degradation). The fermentation process converts carbohydrate to sugars, which are utilized by bacteria for growth and energy supplies; short chain fatty acids (SCFAs; acetate, butyrate and propionate), which stimulate colonic motility and provide substrate for colonic cell metabolism (butyrate being the preferred substrate); and gases (including hydrogen or methane), which are partly absorbed through the colonic mucosa into the blood. Oligosaccharides (intermediate polymers of 3–9 sugar residues) are also fermented in the colon, and enhance the growth of bifidobacteria, which may have health-enhancing effects: scientific support for this is gradually accumulating. The pathways through which energy is recovered following bacterial fermentation result in a contribution of about 1.5 kcal/g of fermented carbohydrate.

In addition to the effects on fermentation, dietary fiber fragments that have not been degraded by bacteria swell and hold water, thus having a stool-bulking effect. This in turn stimulates colonic motility, shortens the transit time through the colon and increases the amount of stool passed each day. Stool weights of less than 100 g/day are associated with complaints of constipation, and population-average stool weights of about 175 g/day are associated with lower rates of colon cancer. In the late 1980s, when the UK Department of Health Committee on Medical Aspects of Food and Nutrition Policy was devising dietary reference values (DRVs) for the UK, the relationships between non-starch polysaccharide (NSP) intake and stool weight, and between stool weight and population colon cancer risk, were used to obtain the current UK non-starch polysaccharide DRV of 18 g/day. Re-examination of the original data shows that 24 g/day is associated with lower risks of colon cancer on a population basis, but the DRV of 18 g/day was a reasonable compromise.

In addition to the stool-bulking effect, which can be beneficial in simple constipation where there is no other physical cause, increasing dietary fiber intake reduces the peak intracolonic pressures that occur in diverticular disease. In the irritable bowel syndrome, individuals who suffer predominantly from constipation may show some improvement of symptoms with increased dietary fiber intakes, but in other cases fiber may exacerbate symptoms, especially if flatulence increases. Increased flatulence is, anyway, a common side-effect of increasing fiber intakes and becomes less troublesome if the patient persists. However, in a small minority of people, flatulence is a major deterrent to eating high-fiber foods.

HEALTH CLAIMS FOR FIBER

In the USA, food claims authorized by the Food and Drug Administration have been allowed since the 1990 Nutrition Labelling and Education Act was passed.

There are two generic claims and two food-specific claims at present.

Cancer risk 'Low-fat diets rich in fiber-containing grain products, fruits, and vegetables may reduce the risk of some types of cancer, a disease associated with many factors.'

Since this claim was allowed, two major reviews of the evidence for dietary factors in influencing the risk of cancer have been published (UK Department of Health and World Cancer Research Fund (WCRF)). The UK report noted that 'Overall there is moderate evidence to conclude that diets rich in NSP (dietary fiber) would reduce the risk of colorectal cancer', while the WCRF report concluded that the evidence was less strong. Prospective trials of fiber with regard to colorectal adenoma growth and dysplasia to date have not demonstrated a convincing beneficial effect of fiber.

Coronary heart disease risk 'Diets low in saturated fat and cholesterol and rich in fruits, vegetables and grain products that contain some types of dietary fiber, particularly soluble fiber, may reduce the risk of heart disease, a disease associated with many factors.'

This general claim, supported (for the soluble fiber part of the claim) by a vast literature on soluble fiber fractions in hyperlipidemic, normolipidemic, diabetic and non-diabetic as well as healthy people, in addition to studies using whole foods especially beans and oats, was followed by a food-specific claim for oats.

Coronary heart disease risk and specific types of fiber 'Diets low in saturated fat and cholesterol that include 3 g of soluble fiber from whole oats per day may reduce the risk of heart disease. One serving of this whole-oats product provides x grams of this soluble fiber.'

This was then followed by a second food-specific claim for soluble fiber in psyllium seed husk, for which there is a convincing body of evidence showing blood cholesterol-lowering effects. Breakfast cereals containing psyllium seed husk are available in the USA and in Australia, and oat-based cereals are available world-wide.

In other countries, legislation and the mechanism for reviewing the scientific evidence to support a claim are not in place (this is so even in Canada where, despite the close trade links with the USA, health claims for food have reached only the discussion stage in the late 1990s).

REQUIREMENTS FOR HEALTH AND DISEASE RISK REDUCTION

Surveys of dietary intakes of large representative samples of populations show that, in most 'Western' countries, population-average dietary fiber intakes are one-half to two-thirds of the levels indicated as being associated (on a population basis) with lower risks of some diseases (such as colon cancer). In the UK, using figures based on the Englyst method of analysis, non-starch polysaccharide intakes are around 12–14 g/day (derived roughly half from cereals and half from fruit and vegetables), whereas the levels associated with the least risk of colon cancer demonstrated in other populations would be about 24 g (the UK DRV, i.e. population recommended daily allowance (RDA), is 18 g/day – a value that represents a compromise recommendation). In populations where analysis is by the American Organisation of Analytical Chemists (AOAC) method (for example the USA), population-average intakes are around 18–20 g and the recommended average intake is 30 g/day.

However, these are recommendations for whole populations, not for individuals or groups within populations. Men generally consume higher-energy diets than do women, especially if following active life-styles; thus, they consume more carbohydrate and more dietary fiber. Yet, among some men, intakes may be low and they may specifically need to achieve an increase as follows:

(1) Based on population-average targets: raise intake to 18 g/day (Englyst) or 30 g/day (AOAC);

(2) To have a reasonable chance of having 'optimal' bowel function: consume about 9 g/day fiber from cereal foods (especially wheat products);

(3) To achieve the maximum likely reduction of blood cholesterol by soluble fiber: consume 3 g/day of soluble fiber.

When judging intake, consumers use food labels; thus, any changes in food labeling legislation are relevant, and any change of what is within the dietary fiber fraction on the label needs to be known. Recently, oligosaccharides (containing 3–9 sugar units and, thus, lying half-way between sugars and polysaccharides), which are known to be a preferred substrate for bifidobacteria growth in the colon, have been included within the AOAC method for dietary fiber, and may be incorporated within the fraction labeled 'dietary fiber' in some countries. While oligosaccharides are an excellent substrate for fermentation, they may not be as potent as polysaccharides in causing the stool-bulking and bowel 'regularizing' effects classically associated with dietary fiber.

HOW TO INCREASE FIBER INTAKE

Dietary guidance should always be given on an individual basis by achieving change within the patient's existing diet and life-style. However, in general terms, there are a few specific points of advice which can be used.

Large-gut function responds to an increase of cereal fiber intake most easily achieved by taking one daily portion of a very high fiber breakfast cereal (such as an All-Bran® type containing about 9.8 g fiber per standard portion of 40 g). Such a simple change is likely to increase stool bulk and defecation frequency in many constipated patients, and will do likewise in people with diverticular disease in whom peak intracolonic pressures should also be reduced. A broader dietary change with more consumption of fruit and vegetables is desirable for other reasons (it increases antioxidant intake, for example), but requires a visit to the dietitian, and may result in more adverse side-effects (such as flatulence from the oligosaccharides in beans, and resistant starch in wholemeal bread) and less long-term compliance. Recommending that a portion of fruit be sliced up and served on top of the All-Bran is a good compromise.

For people with raised blood cholesterol, in whom non-drug diet and life-style changes are to be tried, raising soluble fiber intake can be part of a package of changes (to include spreads containing plant stanols and soluble fiber from oats, beans and rye-bread with the standard low-fat, low-saturated-fat dietary advice) that can achieve a 15–20% reduction of total cholesterol and even larger reductions of low-density lipoprotein (LDL) cholesterol. The literature indicates that at least 3 g soluble fiber per day is needed, and this is obtained from two large bowls of oat porridge, or more realistically one daily portion of an oat product and portions of beans, lentils, rye-bread and barley introduced throughout the day where possible. Advice from the dietitian is essential in achieving these changes.

For diabetic people, the most important dietary variable remains energy (calories), and most dietary guidelines suggest that 55% should come from carbohydrate, choosing high-fiber complex carbohydrate sources. Most guidelines have not quantified the amount of 'soluble' fiber that should be consumed, but high-soluble-fiber foods have low 'glycemic indexes' and thus help to achieve better control of blood glucose.

FUTURE DEVELOPMENTS

The enthusiasm for dietary fiber that began in the early 1970s, following the work of Denis Burkitt who wrote the early 'fiber hypothesis' papers, engendered several decades of scientific investigation, which improved our understanding of both upper- and lower-gut function and established the role for, and limitations of, dietary fiber in clinical practice. In the past 10 years, the accumulation of a body of evidence on metabolic changes following fiber administration has led to the acceptance (in the USA) of health claims for blood cholesterol-lowering effects. The past 10 years has also seen an improved understanding of all fractions of carbohydrate and the importance of the physical structure of carbohydrate foods. Public health in many countries still includes guidance for increased intake of fiber, but there seems to be some resistance to this; this is perhaps due to an intolerance of adverse side-effects. In the coming years, food technological development will result in functional foods (foods that have effects other than the provision of nutrients and energy) that allow effective doses of carbohydrate moieties to be given in acceptable portion sizes (for example, 3 g oat β-glucan in one 40 g portion of a ready-to-eat breakfast cereal). These new food products will allow non-pharmaceutical interventions to contribute effectively towards cholesterol lowering, large-gut 'regularization', blood glucose control and enhancement of beneficial colonic flora, with consequent health benefits and possibly a small reduction of expenditure on drugs.

Further reading

1. Report of a panel on Dietary Reference Values of the Committee on Medical Aspects of Food and Nutrition Policy. *Non Starch Polysaccharides in Dietary Reference Values for Food Energy and Nutrients for the United Kingdom, Report on Health and Social Subjects No. 441*. London: The Stationery Office, 1991:61–71
2. Report of a working group on Diet and Cancer of the Committee on Medical Aspects of Food and Nutrition Policy. *Nutritional Aspects of the Development of Cancer, Report on Health and Social Subjects No. 48*. London: The Stationery Office, 1998:180–2, 205–6
3. *Food, Nutrition and the Prevention of Cancer: a Global Perspective*. Washington: World Cancer Research Fund and American Institute for Cancer Research, 1997
4. US Food and Drug Administration. *Staking a Claim to Good Health*. Science behind health claims on foods. http://vm.csfan.fda.gov/~dms/fdhclm.html reviewed 9 November 2000
5. Report of a joint FAO/WHO Expert Consultation, Rome, April 1997. *Carbohydrates in Human Nutrition*, FAO Food and Nutrition Paper No. 66. Rome: Food and Agriculture Organization, 1998

25 Functional foods: present and future

Colette Shortt, PhD

INTRODUCTION

There is a growing awareness of the link between diet, health and well-being. The concept of the balanced diet has changed from one of providing energy and nutrients to meet the basic needs to one that contributes to optimal health and to the reduction of the risk of disease. Increasingly, consumers are aware that their health can be influenced significantly by personal choices, such as diet, exercise and life-style.

Many consider that the 'Foods for Specific Health Uses' (FOSHU) system established in Japan in 1991 was the start of the functional food concept. Escalating health-care costs and the aging Japanese population were two of the main drives behind this initiative. The FOSHU system stimulated research and development into nutritional products that had clear health impacts. FOSHU foods are evaluated and approved by the Japanese Ministry of Health and Welfare, and are allowed to carry the FOSHU logo and a health claim. Currently, most of the 193 approved products are for the regulation of gastrointestinal conditions, and contain oligosaccharides, probiotic lactic acid bacteria or fiber[1].

The European Union recently supported a Concerted Action on Functional Food Science. A consensus document on the scientific concepts relating to functional foods was developed by this Concerted Action group in 1998, which proposed that 'a food can be regarded as functional if it is satisfactorily demonstrated to affect beneficially one or more target functions in the body, beyond adequate nutritional effects, in a way that is relevant to either improved state of health and well-being and/or reduction of risk of disease'[2,3].

FOODS WITH ADDED HEALTH BENEFITS

Functional foods offer a new dimension to healthy eating, and essentially deliver specific non-nutritive physiological benefits that may enhance health. For exmaple, it is known that oat products influence blood cholesterol and that oligosaccharides stimulate beneficial bacteria in the gastrointestinal tract (GIT)[4]. Foods classed as functional can be natural foods, foods to which a component has been added or removed, foods in which the nature of a component or the bioavailability has been modified, or a combination of these[2,3]. Regular consumption of a functional food is necessary to improve health status and/or reduce the risk of disease.

A functional food must be demonstrated to be effective in amounts that can be expected to be consumed in a normal varied balanced diet. Claims are only justified if there is evidence that a suitable marker relating to an improved state of health and/or reduction of risk of disease is affected. While the level of evidence accepted to demonstrate the functional efficacy of a food is still a matter of intense debate, scientific dossiers should include product-related experimental, *in vitro*, animal, epidemiological and intervention data.

Owing to advances in food technology and nutritional sciences, food products are now reaching the market that are safe, delicious and efficacious[4]. The following section highlights examples of functional ingredients and foods that are relevant to the maintenance of male health in the following areas:

(1) Cardiovascular function;

(2) Gastrointestinal function;

(3) Defense against reactive oxygen species.

FUNCTIONAL FOODS CONTRIBUTING TO A HEALTHY HEART

Coronary heart disease (CHD) is a major cause of morbidity and death among men. Over one in five men die from the disease, accounting for two million deaths in Europe each year. An elevated level of blood cholesterol is one of the established risk factors for CHD. In particular, elevated levels of low-density lipoprotein (LDL) cholesterol are associated with a high risk of CHD[5]. The development of foods with the potential to lower blood cholesterol is one of the most exciting trends in functional foods[6].

Phytosterols

Recently, foods such as margarines, mayonnaise, yoghurts and biscuits have been enriched with phytosterols, a term that includes both plant sterols and stanols. Plant sterols (β-sitosterol, campesterol and stigmasterol) are naturally occurring compounds found in vegetable and sunflower oil, and stanols (sitostanol, campestanol) are saturated plant sterols formed through hydrogenation[7]. To date, several studies

in free-living individuals have demonstrated the benefits of phytosterol consumption[8-11]. Clinical studies have indicated that stanol or sterol intake (1–4 g/day) can significantly reduce serum total and LDL cholesterol, reducing the risk of heart disease[6].

While the mechanism of action of phytosterols is not conclusively understood, many plausible mechanisms have been proposed. Sterols and stanols are structurally very similar to cholesterol, and are thought to compete for absorption in the small intestine. As a consequence, less cholesterol is absorbed, and in turn the liver responds by increasing cholesterol synthesis and increasing LDL receptors, which clear more LDL cholesterol from the blood. In addition to hepatic changes, the intestinal mucosa may produce less cholesterol-rich chylomicrons and LDL precursors, which all contribute to reduce serum LDL cholesterol. It has also been proposed that cholesterol, stanols and sterols may coprecipitate. As the sterol/stanol concentration in the intestinal lumen increases, the solubility of cholesterol is reduced, and it is precipitated in a crystalline form which cannot be absorbed[7].

Intestinal absorption of stanols/sterols is low, and they do not appear to be toxic even at high doses. Fat-soluble vitamins and carotenoids are absorbed in a similar way to cholesterol, and their absorption and transportation may be compromised by phytosterol intake. The long-term effects of this must be considered in further studies.

Sterols are naturally found in seeds, in vegetable and sunflower oils, and in products produced from these. Stanols are derived from natural plant components found in vegetable oils, corn, beans and wood. There are currently several functional foods containing phytosterols on the market, targeted at those who want to reduce their cholesterol levels by dietary means[6]. The benefits observed with these products are midway between the effects seen with dietary and drug treatment in hypercholesterolemic subjects. The dose of phytosterols required is less than 2 g/day, and this amount can be obtained by consuming approximately 20 g/day of a spread supplemented with phytosterols. The phytosterol-containing food needs to be consumed regularly over a 2–3-week period for the effects to be observed, and cholesterol levels return to the baseline within 2–3 weeks after consumption is stopped. It has been estimated that a reduction in the risk of heart disease of about 25% would be expected for the level of reduction in LDL cholesterol found with phytosterols, and this is larger than that expected to be achieved by a reduction in intake of saturated fat[6].

Flavonoids

Flavonoids are a group of substances found in plant matter that are part of the polyphenol family, and consist of over 4000 subgroups including: flavonols, flavanols, flavones, isoflavones and anthocyanidins[12,13]. They have potent antioxidant activity, neutralizing free radicals which can cause oxidative damage to cells[14]. Flavonoids are found naturally in tea, red wine, onions, lettuce, garlic, berries, apples, oranges and grapes. The average intake is in the region of 1 mg/day, and about 80% is obtained from tea in the UK.

Recent epidemiological data suggest that increased levels of flavonoid intake may be associated with reduced CHD risk[13]. Six large-scale cohort studies have investigated the effect of flavonoid intake on CHD risk; half of these identified an inverse association with flavonoid intake and cardiovascular disease, and one found a protective effect for those with a history of CHD[13,15]. These studies identified a stronger relationship with mortality rather than prevention of disease. The proposed modes of action are via an antithrombotic role in reducing platelet aggregation, interfering with atherogenesis, coupled with a potent antioxidant role.

Tea is a rich source of flavonoids, and studies have investigated the role that tea may play in

Table 1 Most common gastrointestinal-related reasons for general practitioner (GP) consultations by men[17].

Rank	Condition
1	intestinal disease presumed infective
2	functional disorders of the stomach
3	irritable bowel syndrome
4	duodenal ulcer
5	inguinal hernia
5	hemorrhoids
6	constipation
7	hiatus hernia
8	other disorders of stomach/small intestine
9	anal fissure/fistula

reducing the risk of CHD. In one study it was observed that men who consumed at least one cup of tea per day had a reduced risk of CHD mortality compared with those who did not drink tea. However, other studies such as the Caerphilly study in Wales have failed to show an association[13,15]. In general, results of studies evaluating the benefits of flavonoids support the dietary recommendation to increase fruit and vegetables in the diet to reduce the risk of CHD. While the flavonoid components may exert beneficial effects, this has not yet been proven, and further clinical and epidemiological trials are required.

FUNCTIONAL FOODS CONTRIBUTING TO GASTROINTESTINAL HEALTH

In general, gastrointestinal health is considered rather a taboo subject among men, leading many to suffer in silence. In a recent study involving 4000 subjects, over one-third of participants considered that the role of the digestive system in general health was not relevant to them, even though they had a high prevalence of gastrointestinal upsets including indigestion, irritable bowel syndrome, diarrhea and constipation[16]. Indeed, we know that diet can play a role in modulating many of the common gastrointestinal conditions for which men regularly seek medical advice (Table 1).

Probiotic foods, optimum gut flora and health

The word probiotic is derived from Greek, meaning 'for life'. Recently, studies have shown that foods containing specific viable bacteria, also known as probiotic foods, can exert beneficial intestinal effects[18]. Our bodies are hosts to 10^{14} bacteria – ten times the number of cells in the body. Most of these bacteria are found in the GIT and are known as the gut flora. Bacterial numbers and composition vary considerably along the GIT, with fewer than 10^3/g in the stomach and more than 10^{10}/g in the intestine. The growth and metabolic activity of the gut flora can have a tremendous influence on our physiological and nutritional well-being.

The gut flora therefore play an important role in the maintenance of health: stimulating the immune system, protecting the host from invading bacteria and viruses, and aiding digestion[18]. An optimum gut flora balance is one in which beneficial bacteria, such as lactobacilli and bifidobacteria, predominate over potentially harmful bacteria[19]. Many factors can influence the balance of the gut flora such as the composition of the diet, antibiotic therapy, infections, food poisoning, stress and aging.

The concept of ingesting live bacteria as a means of modulating the gut flora to maintain health and promote benefical effects is not new. At the beginning of the 20th century, the Nobel laureate Elie Metchnikoff was the first to propose a scientific rationale for the beneficial effects of the bacteria in yoghurt. He postulated that yoghurt consumption played a role in health, and he attributed the long life of Bulgarian peasants to their intake of yoghurt containing *Lactobacillus* species[20]. Gordon and colleagues[21], reporting in the Lancet in 1957, noted that successful *Lactobacillus* therapy depended on certain criteria: it was essential to use a non-pathogenic organism that was a normal inhabitant of the intestine, capable of establishing itself in the gut; and a large number

Table 2 Established health effects of probiotics[18]

Alleviation of symptoms of lactose intolerance
Immune enhancement
Shortening duration of rotavirus diarrhea
Decreasing fecal mutagenicity
Decreasing fecal bacterial enzyme activity
Prevention of recurrence of superficial bladder cancer

of viable cells (10^7–10^9) were required for rapid establishment of a beneficial flora. By the early 1960s, yoghurts were often used to re-establish the balance of the gut flora upset by antibiotics, and to alleviate or prevent conditions such as diarrhea, constipation, dyspepsia, cystitis, mucous colitis, chronic ulcerative colitis and dermatitis.

Recently, a group of European scientists, as part of an EU-supported Concerted Action project, suggested that probiotics for use in human nutrition are best defined as 'live microbial food ingredients that are beneficial to health'[18]. This definition taking into account results from recent research allows for the possibility of non-microflora-mediated probiotic effects, for example probiotic effects on the immune system. Some of the established effects of probiotics are outlined in Table 2.

Probiotic bacteria are generally lactic acid bacteria although not exclusively; for example, *Saccharomyces boulardii* is a probiotic yeast. Other ingredients that influence the gut flora are known as prebiotics. These are non-digestible ingredients that selectively stimulate specific beneficial bacteria in the GIT, and a combination of a prebiotic and a probiotic is known as a synbiotic. There are many studies using classical microbiological techniques and DNA-based techniques confirming that selected probiotic strains remain viable after transit through the GIT[22,23]. For health maintenance, probiotic products with concentrations in the region of 10^8 CFU/ml or greater are generally recommended. Probiotic foods such as fermented dairy products and juices, in addition to providing high stable concentrations of probiotic bacteria, are also good sources of key nutrients and can easily be incorporated into a balanced diet.

Probiotic and/or synbiotic therapy may hold some promise in the future for the amelioration of certain conditions, for example *Helicobacter pylori* infections, inflammatory bowel disease (Crohn's, ulcerative colitis, pouchitis), food allergy, oral rehydration, superficial bladder cancer, urogenital infections and high blood pressure. Research is ongoing in these areas and preliminary results are promising[24–28].

PROTECTION FROM FREE-RADICAL DAMAGE

Recently, much attention has been focused on prostate cancer, as the incidence is rising steadily. It has been suggested that certain food components such as lycopene and selenium may be protective against prostate cancer development.

Lycopene

Lycopene is one of the most effective carotenoids for oxygen radical quenching. It cannot be synthesized within the body, and therefore we rely exclusively on our diet to provide it. Sources of lycopene include tomato, watermelon, guava, papaya, pink grapefruit and apricot. Interestingly, in processed foods such as tomato paste lycopene has a higher bioavailability[29].

There are some preliminary data suggesting an inverse association between lycopene and prostate cancer[30–34]. In particular, 57 of 72 epidemiological studies indicate an inverse association between increased plasma lycopene levels or tomato intake and reduced cancer risk[34]. However, the validity of the results has been questioned, and it has been suggested that the relationship may be due to altered intake or metabolism in the subjects. While plausible mechanisms of action have been hypothesized, the current evidence supporting a relationship between lycopene and prostate cancer risk is inconclusive.

Selenium

Selenium (Se) is an essential trace mineral and a constituent of selenoproteins, which have both structural and enzymatic roles. It is required for immune function, the development of spermatozoa, sperm motility and testosterone biosynthesis[35]. A low intake of Se has been associated with an increased prostate cancer risk, and supplementation of Se has been shown to reduce prostate cancer risk. A high prediagnostic Se level also appears to be associated with an inverse relationship with prostate cancer risk[36]. A Harvard-based health professionals' cohort study found that men with the lowest Se levels were at greater risk of developing advanced prostate cancer than those with increased Se levels[35,36].

The mechanisms resulting in the chemoprotective effect are not understood. However, hypotheses have been put forward including: Se may stimulate and regulate programmed cell death; its antioxidant role may prevent changes in cells which may lead to cancer; the possible production of antitumorigenic metabolites interferes with tumor cell metabolism or inhibits protein and enzyme synthesis. Further studies are required to either refute or confirm recent findings.

Sources of Se include bread, cereals, Brazil nuts, kidney, shellfish and fish. The Reference Nutrient Intake (RNI) for Se is 70–75 µg/day (1 µg/kg body weight). This is the level believed to be required for the functioning of the selenoproteins; however, intake is usually only a half of this value[35]. As Se is a toxic mineral with a relatively small therapeutic threshold, an upper limit of 400–500 µg/day is recommended.

FUTURE TRENDS

A significant driving force in the functional foods arena is consumer demand – the desire of consumers to optimize their health through their dietary intake. Foods are composed of a myriad of biologically active constituents that may contribute to health enhancement, and, given the current advances in food science and nutrition, it is clear that functional foods will contribute to a health-enhancing diet. It is important to note that while some functional foods are for general consumption by the population, others are designed for specific target groups, for example those with high cholesterol levels. In addition, the nutraceutical or supplemental approach may be more appropriate in specific situations, such as where a pharmacological effect is required or where it may be difficult to obtain adequate amounts of a nutrient from dietary sources, for example folate or Se.

With the opportunity provided by functional foods comes the responsibility to ensure that the associated health claims are scientifically substantiated. It is also vital that consumers understand the propositions underpinning functional foods and that they know how to include these foods in a balanced diet, as it is the total dietary balance that is critical to positive nutritional outcomes.

Given that the world population is aging at an accelerated pace, there is a tremendous research interest in the maintenance of health and enhancement of the quality of life. Functional foods are not magic bullets or a universal panacea for poor dietary habits, but the evidence is accumulating that they can play a role in disease risk reduction and health enhancement.

References

1. Japan Health Foods and Nutrition Foods Association. *Foods For Specific Health Uses.* Tokyo: JHFNFA, 2000
2. Diplock A, Aggett P, Ashwell M, *et al.* Scientific concepts of functional foods in Europe: consensus document. *Br J Nutr* 1999; 81:1–27
3. Roberfroid MB. A European consensus of scientific concepts of functional foods. *Nutrition* 2000;16:689–91
4. Mazza G. Introduction. In Mazza G, ed. *Functional Foods, Biochemical and Processing Aspects.* Rowayton, CT USA: Technomic Company, 1998:xi–xiv
5. Willet W. Diet and coronary heart disease. In MacMahon B, ed. *Nutritional Epidemiology.* New York: Oxford University Press, 1990: 341–80
6. Law M. Plant sterol and stanol margarines and health. *Br Med J* 2000;320:861–4
7. Institute of Food Science & Technology. Information statement on phytosterol esters (plant sterols and stanol esters). *Food Sci Technol Today* 2000;14:154–8
8. Weststrate JA, Meijer GW. Plant sterol-enriched margarines and reduction of plasma total- and LDL-cholesterol concentrations in normocholesterolaemic and mildly

hypercholesterolaemic subjects. *Eur J Clin Nutr* 1998;52:334–43
9. Normén L, Dutta P, Lia A, Anderson H. Soy sterol esters and β-sitostanol ester as inhibitors of cholesterol absorption in human small bowel. *Am J Clin Nutr* 2000;71: 908–13
10. Hallikainen MA, Sarkkinen ES, Uusitupa MIJ. Plant stanol esters affect serum cholesterol concentrations of hypercholesterolemic men and women in a dose-dependent manner. *J Nutr* 2000;130:767–76
11. Miettinen TA, Puska P, Gylling H, *et al.* Reduction of serum cholesterol with sitostanol-ester margarine in a mildly hypercholesterolemic population. *N Engl J Med* 1995;333:1308–12
12. Harborne J. Chemistry of the flavonoid pigments. In Rice-Evans C, ed. *Wake Up to Flavonoids.* International Congress and Symposium Series 226. London: The Royal Society of Medicine Press, 2000:3–12
13. Poulter J. Antioxidants in tea. *Br Nutr Found Nutr Bull* 1998;23:203–10
14. Halliwell B. Antioxidant activity and other biological effects of flavonoids. In Rice-Evans C, ed. *Wake Up to Flavonoids.* International Congress and Symposium Series 226.

London: The Royal Society of Medicine Press, 2000:13–24

15. Gaziano M. Epidemiology of flavonoids and coronary heart disease. In Rice-Evans C, ed. *Wake Up to Flavonoids*. International Congress and Symposium Series 226. London: The Royal Society of Medicine Press, 2000:53–61

16. Shortt C. Communicating the benefits of functional foods to the consumer. In Butriss J, Saltmarsh M, eds. *Functional Foods II Claims and Evidence*. London: Royal Society of Chemistry, 2000:70–5

17. Nguyen-van-Tam J, Logan R. Digestive disease. In Charlton J, Murphy M, eds. *Health of Adult Britain 1841–1994*. London: The Stationery Press, 1997:133

18. Salminen S, Bouley C, Boutron-Ruault M-C, *et al*. Functional food science and gastro-intestinal physiology and function. *Br J Nutr* 1998;80:s147–71

19. Gibson GR, Roberfroid MB. Dietary modulation of the human colonic microbiota: introducing the concept of prebiotics. *J Nutr* 1995;125:1401–12

20. Metchnikoff E. *Prolongation of Life*. London: William Heinemann, 1907

21. Gordon D, Macrae J, Wheater D. A *Lactobacillus* preparation for use with antibiotics. *Lancet* 1957;May4:899–901

22. Spanhaak S, Havenaar R, Schaafsma G. The effect of consumption of milk fermented by *Lactobcillus casei* strain shirota on the intestinal microflora and immune parameters in humans. *Eur J Clin Nutr* 1998;52:899–907

23. Yuki N, Koichi W, Mike A, *et al*. Survival of a probiotic, *Lactobacillus casei* strain shirota, in the gastrointestinal tract: selective isolation from faeces and identification using monoclonal antibodies. *Int J Food Microbiol* 1999;48:51–7

24. Naidu AS, Bidlack WR, Clemens RA. Probiotic spectra of lactic acid bacteria (LAB). *Crit Rev Food Sci Nutr* 1999;38:13–126

25. Shortt C. Host–microflora interface in health and disease. *Trends Food Sci Technol* 1999;10:182–5

26. Ohashi Y, Nakai S, Tsukamoto T, *et al*. Habitual intake of lactic acid bacteria and risk reduction of bladder cancer. *Proc Am Cancer Assoc* 2000;abstr.3561

27. Aso Y, Akaza H, the BLP Study Group. Prophylactic effect of a *Lactobacillus casei* preparation on the reoccurrence of superficial bladder cancer. *Urol Int* 1992;49:125–9

28. Michetti P, Dorta G, Wiesel P, *et al*. Effect of a whey-based culture supernatant of *Lactobacillus acidophilus (johnsonii)* La1 on *Helicobacter pylori* infections in humans. *Digestion* 1999;60:203–9

29. Clinton SK. Lycopene: chemistry, biology and implications for human health and disease. *Nutr Rev* 1998;56(2):35–51

30. Gann Ph, Ma J, Giovannucci E, *et al*. Lower prostate cancer risk in men with elevated plasma lycopene levels: results of a prospective analysis. *Cancer Res* 1999;59:1225–30

31. Norrish AE, Jackson RT, Sharpe SJ, Skeaff CM. Prostate cancer and dietary carotenoids. *Am J Epidemiol* 2000;151:119–23

32. Giovannucci E, Clinton SK. Tomatoes, lycopene, and prostate cancer. *Soc Exp Biol Med* 1998;218:129–39

33. Kristal AR, Cohen JH. Invited commentary: tomatoes, lycopene, and prostate cancer. How strong is the evidence? *Am J Epidemiol* 2000;151:124–7

34. Giovannucci E. Tomatoes, tomato-based products, lycopene and cancer: review of the epidemiologic literature. *J Natl Cancer Inst* 1999;91:317–31

35. Rayman MP. The importance of selenium to health. *Lancet* 2000;356:233–41

36. Yoshizawa K, Walter C, Willett WC, *et al*. Study of pre-diagnostic selenium level in toenails and the risk of advanced prostate cancer. *J Natl Cancer Inst* 1998;90:1219–24

26 Sports nutrition

Adrian R. Cassidy, MSc

Many clinical nutritionists wrongly believe that sportsmen in training have no special dietary requirements. Serious training leads to substantial stress, and this can only be avoided and corrected by appropriate food changes. Sports nutrition is therefore an important component in achieving optimum performance in sport of all kinds, but particularly in endurance sports.

Every tissue is in a constant state of flux, and tissue metabolism increases to help the body either perform or recover from training. To maximize training benefit it is important to fuel the body in a way that spares the body as much as possible. The general aim should be to keep the body in an anabolic state, but this is not possible during exercise. Therefore, after exercise, an anabolic state needs to be achieved as soon as possible.

The difference between athletes and sedentary men is not just in the quantity of food required to provide an energy balance, but also in the quality and timing of the dietary intake. This chapter gives a general overview of the principles involved.

HYDRATION

The body is about 75% water, and without adequate hydration athletic performance drops very rapidly. A 3% dehydration of muscle leads to a 10% drop in contractile strength and an 8% drop in the speed of contraction[1]. A further 2% dehydration leads to a 20% drop in performance. During exercise, substantial sweating occurs to maintain a constant body temperature, leading to water loss. As a consequence the blood viscosity increases. To maintain the same level of performance the heart has to work harder and the pulse rises. At the extreme, cell function deteriorates in part owing to raised core temperature. By maintaining hydration the fade in performance can be reduced, but not eliminated.

One of the main problems is the difference between rates of water absorption and water loss, for the athlete can lose water four times more rapidly than he can absorb it. Hence, during performance, athletes are fighting a losing battle, but even during actual performance, hydration should be maintained as far as possible.

To maintain or restore hydration there are three prongs of attack: pre-performance hydration, post-performance hydration and hydration during performance (Table 1).

Hydration is more of a problem for endurance events than for power events. During a marathon, regular hydration is a must. It is also important to drink a lot early in the race. If the athlete waits until he feels thirsty during the race it is too late.

Carbohydrate-loading also helps with pre-competition hydration. As much as 4–5 g of water are stored with every gram of glycogen, and this will be released when the glycogen is metabolized.

Table 1 Principles of maintaining adequate hydration

Pre-performance hydration	drink lots of water, little and often	a dark urine or feeling of thirst implies some dehydration. Water below 10°C is absorbed faster than at room temperature
During performance	drink an 8% solution (m/v) of maltodextrin in water	this is a hypertonic solution aimed at keeping up the blood sugar and body fluid levels
Post-performance hydration	drink water steadily but regularly	adding half a teaspoon of salt after exercise will stimulate the hypothalamus to encourage the athlete to drink

ENERGY NEEDS

Training and competition substantially increase the energy needs, and these must be supplied by the macronutrients of the food: carbohydrate, protein and fat. Both carbohydrates and protein provide about 4 kcal/g while fat provides about 9 kcal/g. If alcohol is imbibed, this provides 7 kcal/g when it is metabolized.

A sedentary man of normal weight would require about 2000–2500 kcal per day on average to maintain an energy balance, but strenuous exercise would raise this figure to around twice this value. The exact daily requirement will depend upon the energy expended, and can be best estimated by regular (say weekly) monitoring of the weight. Minor fluctuations (a kilogram or two) will be frequent and of no importance since they will usually represent changes in the fluid compartment – often the result of modification of the amount of deposited glycogen. A steady change, however, requires appropriate adjustment of total energy intake.

WEIGHT LOSS FOR SPORTSMEN

In those who are directly involved in training, it is rarely necessary to advise any active dieting program. The commitment to the exercise, which not only increases the energy output but also reduces the time available for food intake, is normally sufficient to produce the desired reduction in weight. In those who are not currently in an active training program some form of diet is often desirable before training starts in earnest. Mild exercise alone will reduce the weight by only 0.3 kg or less per week.

On the other hand, although dieting is feasible during training, the best way to achieve the desired weight is slowly over a period of months. The vital aspect, however, is that a competitor should avoid practices such as running with plastic bags under their clothes in the immediate period prior to a competition. They will lose weight, but this will be almost entirely the result of dehydration and counterproductive.

Above all else, the only effective long-term method of managing excess weight is by avoiding it. This implies:

(1) Maintaining low-intensity exercise even when not in training: from the point of view of keeping a level low weight, sloth is a far more dangerous sin than gluttony – although both are bad;

(2) Making sure that the sportsman keeps a regular weight check and avoids weight gain over holiday periods;

(3) Ensuring that the meal size is commensurate with the energy expenditure, that fats, in particular animal fats, are avoided and that there is a substantial fiber and fruit content to the daily food intake.

CARBOHYDRATES

Carbohydrates form the most important energy source for athletes. They can be divided into two main types: simple sugars (glucose, fructose, sucrose) and complex sugars (starches, pasta, rice, potatoes, maltodextrin). Ingested simple sugars are absorbed very quickly into the bloodstream, raising the blood sugar levels and thus providing fuel for the brain, but they also generate a high insulin burst which puts the body in an anabolic state (see section below on 'Anabolic drive'). Complex sugars are less rapidly digested and thus are released more slowly. This in turn leads to a smaller insulin peak and a more sustained energy release. Complex carbohydrates are therefore the preferred source to replenish muscle glycogen.

Carbohydrate-loading for athletes may be effective but only when done properly. Carbohydrate-loading for body-builders differs significantly from that for endurance athletes. For body-builders, the aim is purely cosmetic to increase muscle size and definition by virtue of the water bound to the muscle glycogen. Hence, the loading is undertaken at the last minute, which may disrupt Na^+ and K^+ balance, clearly undesirable in sportsmen.

Carbohydrate-loading in sportsmen should start several days ahead of competition. Thus, the proportion of complex carbohydrate should be elevated to about 55% of the daily calories in the diet some 6 days before competition, at a time when the workload starts to taper. Three days before competition the workload drops to almost nothing, but the carbohydrate intake is increased to 70% of the total calories. This is achieved by tapering the non-carbohydrate energy consumption right down rather than increasing the total calorie intake with carbohydrates. Using this technique, glycogen stores are high, both for the ready provision of glucose and for the release of water.

It is vital that carbohydrate-loading should be practiced ahead of a big training or competition day, to ensure correct procedure and appropriate effect.

PROTEINS

Protein is a reasonable source of energy and is in a constant state of flux. During exercise the rate of protein degradation increases by 3–5 times, and the rate of protein synthesis decreases by 40%[2]. The driving force behind this is to help keep blood sugar at a constant level between 3 and 5 mmol/l. Even when the blood sugar level is stable there is protein flux.

It is essential to keep the blood sugar level stable, because under normal circumstances glucose is necessary for the functioning of the central nervous system. At 2 mmoll glucose, hypoglycemic coma occurs. Fatty acids are not energy substrates for the brain. In humans, acetyl coenzyme A is not gluconeogenic as it is in some animals such as cats. Ketones (hydroxybutyrate, acetoacetate and acetone) become energy sources for the brain only when they are markedly elevated and glucose is depleted. Alternative sources for glucose are the gluconeogenic amino acids, which can be used to maintain blood sugar levels. Branched chain amino acids (leucine, isoleucine and valine) are the major ones involved and their main source is skeletal muscle. They are transaminated in the skeletal muscle into alanine and glutamine. During exercise the alanine and glutamine account for 50% of all free amino acids, far in excess of their relative abundance in proteins[3]. The alanine is then transported to the liver where it is converted into glucose. It is important to reduce the muscle catabolism to a minimum, and therefore high glycogen reserves are desirable.

Since exercise causes muscle catabolism to a greater or lesser extent in all cases, it is important not only to keep it to a minimum but to reverse that state as soon as the exercise is completed (see section 'Anabolic drive').

FATS

Under normal circumstances fats are non-essential nutrients, because in modern Western society fat consumption is usually above healthy levels. However, there are two essential fatty acids (α-linoleic acid and α-linolenic acid), which come mainly from vegetable sources (for example, nuts and extra virgin olive oil), and it is valuable to ensure that some such sources are included in the diet. Fish oils are good, particularly oily cold-water fish (salmon, sardines, mackerel and trout) which are high in omega-3 fats.

Animal fats, on the other hand, should be kept to a minimum, and this can be achieved by advising the use of lean meat such as turkey and chicken, cutting off visible fats, and grilling and baking rather than frying.

A 70-kg athlete at 10% body fat has a fat store of some 50 000 kcal, more than enough for several consecutive marathons. Hence, an athlete will not run out of fat energy if he has a low body fat percentage (for example, 8–10%). However, carrying excess fat is counterproductive. Unsaturated fats are metabolized more readily that saturated fats[4], while fats in the diet encourage greater weight gains than with the equivalent number of calories as protein or carbohydrate. About one-quarter of the calorific value is needed for the interconversion into fat for storage. For this reason all fats, but particularly animal fats, should be avoided by sportsman.

It has been suggested that athletes use medium chain triglycerides (MCTs) as a way of improving endurance performance. A MCT drink is consumed before an endurance performance, and because it contains short chain triglycerides it is rapidly absorbed into the blood and is used as a rapid fuel source. The absorption into the mitochondrion is faster because medium chain fatty acids do not require L-carnitine for transport across the inner mitochondrial membrane. This may have some benefits for endurance performance, but as ingestion of more than 30 g can give stomach cramps and diarrhea, the value is clearly limited since this amount would provide less than 300 kcals. At very high-level competition it might be an option.

VITAMINS AND MINERALS

As a result of modern intensive farming techniques, depletion of minerals from the soil is common. This in turn means that food products from the soil tend to be low in minerals. Processing food, as well as the use of fungicides and pesticides, depletes the food of essential vitamins and some minerals.

The main point that needs to be remembered is that these are essential nutrients and have to be consumed, for the body cannot synthesize minerals, nor can it synthesize all the vitamins that are required even for sedentary men. Moreover, the need for at least several of the vitamins and for some of the minerals is increased by exercise and other stresses. The normally recommended intake for both vitamins and minerals is therefore barely adequate. Exactly how much extra is required is still a matter of dispute. For the vitamins (apart from some of the fat-soluble ones), the therapeutic range (i.e. the ratio between effective and toxic doses) is so substantial that it is not vital to know the ideal intake amount for each level of physical activity. For many minerals there is a low therapeutic ratio, and in consequence greater care must be taken not to overdose as this will be at least counterproductive and at worst frankly dangerous.

If, then, the level of these nutrients in the food is inadequate, particularly for strenuous exercise, it implies that additional supplies must be found elsewhere. To attempt to obtain it from the food is impossible, for this would lead to the conversion of the excess energy that has been consumed into fat. Supplementation in some form is the key. The main difficulty lies in finding a formula that provides the correct balance and in a form that allows ready absorption. There are many vitamin and mineral supplements on the market, but most of these are not ideal for use by sportsmen. The balance may be wrong, or more frequently the compounding is such that the actual substance of the tablet does not dissolve readily when swallowed. This is one of the areas in which economy may not be the best policy. Products from a reliable pharmaceutical company may be more expensive but the extra cost is fully justified. Some mineral supplements are now being produced in a colloidal liquid form, and these are absorbed much better. The key to successful vitamin and mineral supplementation is to find a reliable readily soluble form with the appropriate balance of components. Synergy is the key to proper biochemical function, and this requires a balanced product.

ANABOLIC DRIVE

To maintain the body responding to training, it is essential that sufficient although not always complete recovery is achieved between bouts of exercise. This implies a need to keep the body in an anabolic state as much as possible. There are several factors that influence this.

Good testosterone levels

Testosterone is a strong anabolic hormone which stimulates protein synthesis. Maintaining adequate levels of zinc can help efficient testosterone metabolism.

Making best use of insulin's properties

Insulin stimulates the synthesis of glycogen, protein and fat, while inhibiting gluconeogenesis, and protein degradation. Insulin also increases the ability of skeletal muscles to absorb amino acids. As a crucial anabolic hormone, adequate maintained bloodstream levels of insulin are valuable to aid recovery, rather than large short-lasting peaks. Eating 5–7 smaller meals a day instead of three large meals results in a lower and a more sustained insulin profile. Moreover, eating food with a low glycemic index (see above) is better as it stimulates smaller peaks with a more sustained release (compare Figure 1a and b).

Chromium, in the trivalent form chromium picolinate, may assist in the efficiency of insulin metabolism. The dose will depend on the energy intake and the extent of training. It is best taken with a post-exercise meal, perhaps breakfast if a training session is held before breakfast.

Maintaining a positive nitrogen balance

As discussed previously, nitrogen excretion increases even during gentle exercise (50% of V_{O_2} max.), irrespective of the blood sugar level[3]. So it is critical that sufficient protein is consumed. The required amount varies, depending on the type and volume of training. Weight-lifting and speed athletes should consume 1.2–1.7 g/day of protein per kilogram of body weight; serious endurance athletes need less at 1.2–1.4 g/day/kg body weight[5]. Athletes need more protein than sedentary people, no matter what their volume of training. The quality of protein is also paramount as mentioned above.

Maximizing pulsatile release of growth hormone

Although growth hormone only lasts for 1 h once it has been released from the pituitary, it sets up an anabolic cascade. Human growth hormone (hGH) stimulates the release of insulin-like growth factor-I (IGF-I) by the liver, which lasts for 3–4 h in the bloodstream. IGF-I in turn acts on skeletal muscle to stimulate the absorption of amino acids and lipids, as well as glucose for glycogen synthesis.

Human growth hormone is released in pulses, both at the start of exercise and about 1 h after going to sleep. By eating a post-exercise meal (see below) and then sleeping soon after training, regeneration is encouraged by a rise in hGH and IGF-I in the blood. This enables the most to be made of the available nutrients.

Keeping energy levels high

To keep the metabolic pathways for training, repair and all normal day-to-day function running properly, it is vital that there is enough

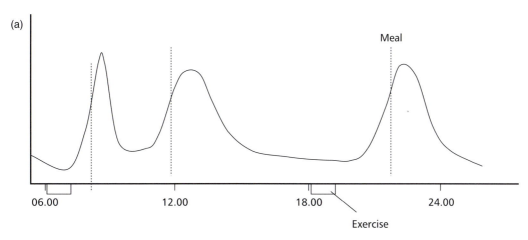

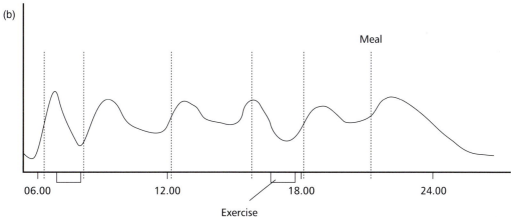

Figure 1 Typical responses to (a) three-meal, two-exercise-period day with exercise before breakfast, and (b) same energy intake but based on six-meal, two-exercise-period day with breakfast before exercise

energy available. Otherwise anabolic processes cannot be achieved.

POST-EXERCISE NUTRITION

When a bout of exercise is completed the body is in a depleted and catabolic state, and to maximize recovery the necessary nutrients are required (see 'Anabolic drive'). The exercise will have depleted muscle and liver glycogen, nitrogen excretion will have risen, and there will have been substantial water loss through sweating. These must all be replenished by the ingestion of appropriate food. To make it easier to obtain enough calorific intake, some sports nutritionists suggest supplementing the regular

meals with a special post-exercise meal which can be readily absorbed. A mixture of the following has been suggested:

(1) Fructose 9 g (replaces liver glycogen);

(2) Glucose 14 g (keeps blood sugar levels up to maintain central nervous system);

(3) Maltodextrin 197 g (complex carbohydrate to replenish the muscle glycogen);

(4) Protein 47 g (as whey protein, to keep a positive nitrogen balance);

(5) 200 mg chromium picolinate.

These would all be blended in 0.5 l of skimmed milk. (Weights are for a 70-kg man, modified according to weight and previous activity level.)

TEXTBOOK OF MEN'S HEALTH

ERGOGENICS

Ergogenics are substances that are reputed to improve maximal performance. All the substances quoted below are legal and currently permitted by the sports authorities at the doses stated. When taken in the proper way they are claimed to enhance an athlete's ability to run, jump and swim faster for longer. None is a substitute for training and good nutrition. When it comes to looking for that little bit extra, some of these might be appropriate. It is still far from clear whether some of these factors rely on a psychological effect to achieve the improvement. Moreover, since they are being used as an artificial energy drive, rather than a true nutrition effect, it could well be held that their use is against the spirit of, if not the wording on, guidelines relating to performance-enhancing substances.

An account of these substances is included to give a complete picture of sports nutrition, and they are not intended as performance-enhancing recommendations.

Inorganic phosphate

Training increases inorganic phosphate (P_i) level but maximal performance lowers it. A study carried out in runners from the Great North Run showed how the weaker performers had low levels of P_i whereas the fast runners had high levels. Those with low P_i also suffered more after their performance[6]. Its effects are to buffer muscle pH and increase 2, 3-diphosphoglycerate, and it is incorporated into glycolytic enzymes.

The appropriate source of P_i is as a sodium (Na^+) or potassium (K^+) salt, for if it is taken as a calcium (Ca^{2+}) salt it is not absorbed. It is recommended that the P_i be taken at a level of 4 g per day for 3 days prior to the performance. In a 40-km bicycle time-trial, the times improved by about 3.5 min, and in a 1-min effort maximum power increased by 17%[7].

Sodium bicarbonate

Oral consumption of sodium bicarbonate (baking powder) enabled oarsmen to row 50 m (2.3%) further in a 6-min test[8]. Cyclists performed five 1-min maximal tests, and were measured on the last test which was continued to exhaustion. Here there was a 42% improvement[9]. Neither calcium bicarbonate nor ammonium bicarbonate produce the desired effect.

The loading of 0.2 mg/kg of body weight is not absorbed by the muscle, but increases the extracellular pH to stimulate a flow of protons out of the intracellular space, to balance the concentration between intracellular and extracellular spaces. This has the effect of reducing the intracellular pH and reducing lactoacidosis.

Creatine monohydrate

Creatine phosphate (PCr) is the instant short-term source of phosphate for the reconversion of adenosine diphosphate (ADP) to adenosine triphosphate (ATP).

$$PCr + ADP + H^+ \longrightarrow ATP + Cr$$

Creatine (Cr) is located mainly in skeletal muscle (about 90% of all creatine), and the supply is depleted within 10–20 s of maximal exercise. It is the first energy source used. After about 1 s glycogen starts to play a role. Then the balance shifts more and more towards glycogen metabolism as the PCr stores run out. The reconversion of Cr back to PCr is linked to oxidative phosphorylation, so aerobic metabolism is required. It takes up to 1 min for 50% of the PCr stores to be replenished, and up to 5 min for full restoration[10]. Loading has mixed results as there is a maximum level of creatine possible in tissue (160 mmol/kg). Depending on diet and genetic make-up, the individual sportsman may already have maximum levels of creatine, and in this case supplementation will not have any effect. Moreover, the nature of the effect is such that, although there may be

294

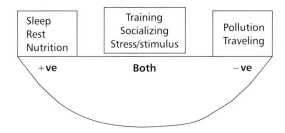

Figure 2 Life-style aspects that affect performance

improvement in those sports that involve short, sharp, repeated bursts (such as for American footballers, sprint runners and power athletes in general), there is considerable debate whether it would help endurance athletes in giving them the ability to change pace. The general feeling has been that it would not help, although there is at least one uncontrolled recent study which seems to show quite substantial and statistically reliable improvement in an endurance sport[11].

There are some worries about the long-term safety of creatine phosphate when taken at marginally high levels, so the risks of this procedure must be kept in mind.

Ginseng

Much has been written about the uses of ginseng. Despite some assertions to the contrary, it seems very unlikely that it has any effect on performance, except psychological. Moreover, there are some unpleasant side-effects with overdosing, including sleeplessness, nausea, nervousness and high blood pressure, and ginseng should be used with great caution, if at all.

LIFE-STYLE DYNAMICS

Good nutrition is not the only aspect of good performance. To maintain optimum sporting performance it is crucial to balance all aspects of an athlete's life. Very few have the luxury of training full-time. Most have to curtail the training they do to keep themselves healthy enough to train. Lack of time also affects nutrition. Most athletes, indeed most people, are too busy

to eat exactly the correct food at the correct time. To perform well requires good nutrition, which in turn requires a balanced life-style.

Figure 2 shows various aspects of life-style that affect performance, either in a positive or a negative way.

Positive aspects of life-style

Sleep

The body starts to recover properly only during sleep, at which time the pulsatile release of growth hormone induces recovery. This occurs about 1 h after going to sleep[12]. With this in mind it is a good idea to get about 1 h sleep after training, as well as a good night's sleep.

Rest

Rest is essential to recovery. Although it does not have the same physiological benefit as sleep, it has more of a psychological effect, for rest (relaxation) helps to balance out the stress. What qualifies as rest varies from person to person, from sitting reading a book to a quiet walk. A run on the other hand is not a rest, although it may be a distraction from worries.

Nutrition

As noted above, this is an underused resource, which helps athletes significantly in balancing their life-style dynamics. Correct nutrition needs to be interwoven with day-to-day life, including not only the amount and nature of each food type eaten, but also the timing of meals and supplements.

Negative aspects of life-style

Pollution

Water, noise, air and food pollution are all damaging. Pollutants gradually reduce energy levels as well as weakening the immune system. Avoiding training in a city center or near a busy road will reduce pollution, as will an ion exchange filter for the drinking water.

Traveling

Traveling to and from training or work always adds to fatigue. It is essential that it is kept to a minimum, and adequate time for traveling allowed to reduce stress.

Either positive or negative depending on circumstances

Training

Although this is the cornerstone of improved performance, it is effective only if recovery is adequate.

Social support

This aspect can be beneficial in that support from family, partners and friends can facilitate training and performance. Social support is particularly important during life's crises.

Socializing

Socializing with fellow performers and friends is a great distraction for sportsmen. On the other hand, taken to extremes with excessive partying, it can have a very detrimental effect. Again, a balance is crucial.

Stress/stimulus

What is stress for one person is stimulus for another. It is vital that each individual realizes what they find stressful and attempts to eliminate it, or learn coping strategies that can turn stress into stimulus.

References

1. Armstrong LE, Costill DL, Fink WJ. Influence of diuretic-induced dehydration on competitive running performance. *Med Sci Sports Exercise* 1985;17:456–61
2. Rennie MJ, Halliday D, Davies CTM, *et al.* Metabolism and clinical implications of branched chain amino and ketoacids. In Walser M, Williamson JR, eds. *Proceedings of the International Symposium on Metabolism and Clinical Implications of Branched Chain Amino and Ketoacids.* 1980:361–6
3. Snell K, Duff DA. Metabolism and clinical implications of branched chain amino and ketoacids. In Walsar M, Williamson JR, eds. *Proceedings of the International Symposium on Metabolism and Clinical Implications of Branched Chain Amino and Ketoacids.* 1980:251–6
4. Jones PJ, Scholler DA. Polyunsaturated : saturated ratio of diet fat influences energy substrate utilisation in the human. *Metabolism* 1988;37:145–51
5. Lemon P. Effects of exercise on protein requirements. *J Sports Sci* 1991;9:53–70
6. Dale G, Fleetwood JA, Weddell A, *et al.* Fitness, unfitness and phosphate. *Br Med J* 1987;11:939
7. Kreider RB. Effects of phosphate loading on oxygen uptake, ventilatory anaerobic threshold and in performance. *Med Sci Sports Exercise* 1990;22:250–5
8. McNaughton LR, Cedaro R. The effect of sodium bicarbonate on rowing ergometer performance in elite rowers. *Aust J Sci Med Sport* 1991;23:66–9
9. Costill DL. Acid-base balance during repeated bouts of exercise. Influence of HCO_3. *Int J Sports Med* 1984;5:225–31
10. Juhn MS, Tarnopolsky M. Oral creatine supplementation and athletic performance: a critical review. *Clin J Sport Med* 1998;8: 286–97
11. Englehart M. Creatine supplementation in edurance sports. *Med Sci Sports Exercise* 1998;30:1123–9
12. Daughaday H. Endocrine control of growth. In William, ed.

27 Pharmacodynamics and pharmacokinetics in aging

Mike A. R. Bosschaert, MD

INTRODUCTION

At the beginning of the 21st century, the elderly constitute a fast growing proportion of the population, responsible for approximately 30–40% of the consumption of all pharmaceutical drugs. However, the elderly present a higher complexity with respect to their medical condition compared with other fractions of the population. During aging, physiological functions tend to decline: for example, renal blood flow, creatinine clearance, glucose tolerance; maximal heart rate and cardiac output, vital capacity of the lungs, and the immune system, to name but a few. This is complicated by a higher chance of the coexistence of chronic diseases, non-specific presentation of disease and a higher sensitivity to drug side-effects. The coexistence of four or more diseases in one elderly individual is not unusual. Commonly found diseases in the elderly are congestive heart failure, angina pectoris, osteoporosis, arthrosis, chronic constipation, urinary incontinence, arterial and venous insufficiency of the lower extremities, diabetes mellitus, depression and sleeplessness. Consequently, the most frequently prescribed drugs belong to the categories of cardio-vascular drugs, diuretics, analgesics, gastrointestinal drugs, antidiabetic drugs and potassium supplements. Of note here is that the reason for requiring potassium supplements is hypokalemia due to diuretics. This illustrates

the dilemma of the medical practitioner. He or she is aware of the problem of polypharmacy in the elderly, and knows that adequate therapy for one disease can contribute to the prevention of other diseases. However, owing to the lack of specificity of symptoms particularly in the elderly, it is not easy to make the correct diagnosis. Conversely, adequate therapy for one disease can cause side-effects. These may be disabling, bringing even more discomfort or risk than with the treated disease, in addition to increased demand for treatment (for example thiazide diuretics and hypokalemia). The medical practitioner should always keep in mind that, with increasing age, improving the quality of life of the patient should prevail over the wish to treat the disease.

The aim of this chapter is to give a general overview of relevant issues in pharmacology and drug treatment in the elderly. For details and justification, the list for 'Further reading' at the end of the chapter is recommended.

GENERAL PRINCIPLES OF PHARMACOLOGY APPLIED TO THE ELDERLY

Absorption

After oral administration, the uptake of drugs across the intestinal wall into the blood circulation can be either a passive process of diffusion following a concentration gradient, or an active process by facilitated transport through the intestinal epithelium. Most lipophilic drugs reach the mesenteric bloodstream by passive diffusion through the intestinal epithelium. Lipophilic drugs then easily pass the cellular barrier of the intestinal wall. The most important limiting factor for these drugs is the mesenteric perfusion rate.

Absorption of hydrophilic drugs is more complicated and influenced by, for example, the transmembrane pH gradient and molecular size. Most hydrophilic drugs are either weak acids or bases. The rate of diffusion of these drugs through the membrane depends heavily on the level of ionization. Most non-ionized drug molecules are lipid soluble, and therefore pass the cellular membrane quite easily. In the elderly, the physiological changes of the intestinal tract have, in general, little effect on the net absorption. Owing to reduced perfusion and increased pH in the intestinal lumen, it could be expected that absorption is less efficient. This is compensated for, however, by the increased exposure of the intestinal wall to the drug as a result of increased intestinal transit time. Nevertheless, if one of these functions becomes less efficient with aging, impaired absorption can occur.

Bioavailability

After the drug is taken up in the portal blood system, the drug first passes the liver, before reaching the systemic circulation. Metabolism and excretion of the drug starts at this initial passage through the liver, even before it has reached its target. Unless there is no hepatic metabolism at first pass a substantial fraction may be lost without having had any therapeutic effect. This is called the first-pass effect. The bioavailability of a drug is defined as the fraction of the biologically active drug that reaches the systemic circulation (or

target site). For drugs that are intended to act on the intestine itself or on the liver, bioavailability calculations are less straightforward. Rectally administered drugs are less subject to the first-pass effect, since approximately 50% of the drug reaches the systemic circulation directly. These drugs usually have a higher bioavailability.

Distribution

As the drug enters the systemic blood flow, an immediate redistribution takes place until a balance between the different 'compartments' is reached. The most important compartments into which drugs diffuse are blood protein (mainly the albumin fraction), adipose tissue and muscle, although drugs can bind to virtually any body tissue. This phenomenon of the redistribution of drugs is responsible for the reduced concentration of drugs in the blood. In particular, highly lipophilic drugs have a high volume of distribution. For these drugs, the serum concentration is much lower than can be expected from the administered dose. As a rule of thumb, one can say that drugs with a large volume of distribution are more dependent on hepatic clearance, whereas drugs with a volume of distribution closer to the actual blood volume are more likely to be excreted in non-metabolized form by the kidneys. In the elderly, various parameters influencing the distribution of drugs are altered. The proportion of adipose tissue is increased, muscle tissue is usually decreased, the plasma albumin concentration is reduced, and the total amount of body water is decreased (Table 1). All these factors lead to a substantial alteration of unbound drug in the systemic circulation. Hydrophilic drugs, with a low volume of distribution, usually yield a higher blood concentration in the elderly, whereas lipophilic drugs, showing a large redistribution into adipose tissue, usually lead to lower serum concentrations.

Table 1 Physiological changes that modify pharmacological behavior in the elderly

Factor	Physiology	Effect	Example
Absorption	gastric pH ⇓ intestinal lumen surface ⇓	probably not relevant	
First-pass effect	hepatic blood flow ⇓ CYP capacity ⇓	increased bioavailability of drugs with high first-pass effect	calcium antagonists, labetalol, metoclopramide, nitrates, opiates
Distribution	adipose tissue ⇑ total body water ⇓ muscle mass ⇓	$t_{1/2}$ ⇑ for lipophilic drugs plasma concentration ⇑ for hydrophilic drugs	diazepam, digoxin, ethanol, flurazepam
Metabolism	first phase of hepatic transformation ⇓	$t_{1/2}$ ⇑ for compounds subject to hepatic first-phase metabolism	carbamazepine, diazepam, flurazepam, sulfonylurea derivatives, tricyclic antidepressants
Elimination	renal perfusion ⇓ glomerular filtration ⇓	$t_{1/2}$ ⇑ for renally excreted drugs	aminoglycosides, digoxin, lithium, morphine metabolites

CYP, cytochrome P450; $t_{1/2}$, half-life

Metabolism

Lipophilic drugs must be metabolized before they can be eliminated from the body. They need to be transformed into hydrophilic substances to be excreted in the urine, or into conjugates to be excreted in the bile. The liver is responsible for these biotransformations. This process takes place in two steps. First the drug is oxidized, reduced/hydrolysed or alkalized, mainly by the cytochrome P450 (CYP) enzyme system. For many drugs this first step is the limiting factor for the rate at which the drug is eliminated. In the second step, the drug is conjugated with, for example, glucuronate, glycine or sulfate, to facilitate excretion in the bile. Owing to reduced hepatic blood flow in the elderly, decreased hepatic weight and, possibly, lower metabolic capacity of the CYP enzyme system, the first step of hepatic transformation is slowed down.

There are indications that the various subsystems for CYP (for example CYP-1A2 and CYP-2D6) show different levels of reduction of capacity with age. A list of the most common drug interactions, with respect to CYP metabolism, is given in Table 2. Although the activity of cytochrome P450 decreases slightly over time, conjugative metabolism is fairly well conserved. Furthermore, drug metabolism can be influenced by clinical conditions that are common in the elderly. For instance drugs that are extensively metabolized in the liver will be less efficiently eliminated from the body in patients with congestive heart failure. In this condition, a reduction of metabolically active hepatic tissue and further reduced hepatic blood flow result in higher steady-state serum levels and increased risk for intoxication, leading to adverse effects.

Excretion

The most important routes of elimination are via the urine and excretion via the bile. After metabolism in the liver, the rate of elimination into the bile is not substantially altered in the elderly. However, for lipophilic drugs, the volume of distribution is increased and the blood concentration is decreased. This slows down elimination. For hydrophilic drugs, the reduced renal clearance is responsible for an increase in half-life. An important difference, however, is that for renally excreted drugs, the plasma concentration is usually increased with age. Renal function gradually declines over time to a level of approximately 50%, compared with that at the age of 30 (Figure 1). The evaluation of renal function, based on calculation of the

Table 2 Drug interactions resulting from interference in first-phase hepatic drug metabolism by cytochrome P450 (CYP) enzyme complex

Inhibitor/ stimulant	Acenocoumarol	Calcium antagonists	Carbamazepine	Cyclosporin	Cisapride	Clonazepine	Diazepam	Ergotamine	Fenprocoumon	Phenytoin	Haloperidol	Metoprolol	Midazolam	Perfenazine	Pimozide	Propranolol	Simvastatin	Terfenadine	Theophylline	Thioridazine	Tolbutamide	Tricyclic antidepressants	Warfarin	Zuclopenthixol	CYP subsets
Amiodarone	I								I	I												I	I		2C9
Carbamazepine			S																S						1A2
Cimetidine	I								I	I									I			I	I		1A2, 2C9, 2C19
Ciprofloxacin										I									I						1A2
Clarithromycin	I	I	I	I			I						I		I		I	I							3A4
Co-trimoxazole							I																		2C19
Diltiazem	I	I	I	I			I						I		I		I	I							3A4
Erythromycin	I	I	I	I			I						I		I		I	I							3A4
Phenobarbital	S	S	S	S	S	S	S	S	S	S			S		S		S	S	S		S		S		1A2, 2C9, 2C19, 3A4
Phenytoin	S	S	S	S	S	S	S	S	S	S			S		S		S	S	S		S		S		1A2, 2C9, 2C19, 3A4
Fluconzaole	I								I	I											I		I		2C9
Fluoxetine							I				I	I		I		I				I		I		I	2C19, 2D6
Fluvoxamine	I					I	I		I	I									I			I		I	1A2, 2C9, 2C19
Grapefruit juice	I	I	I	I			I						I		I		I	I							3A4
Itraconazole	I	I	I	I			I						I		I		I	I							3A4
Ketoconazole	I	I	I	I			I						I		I		I	I							3A4
Kinidine											I	I		I		I				I		I		I	2D6
Miconazole	I	I	I	I	I			I	I	I			I		I		I	I			I		I		2C9, 3A4
Nefazodone	I	I	I	I			I						I		I		I	I							3A4
Paroxetine											I	I		I		I				I		I		I	2D6
Rifampicin	S	S	S	S	S	S	S	S	S	S			S		S		S	S	S		S		S		1A2, 2C9, 2C19, 3A4
Sertraline											I	I		I		I				I		I		I	2D6
Smoking			S																S						1A2
Terbinafine											I	I		I		I				I		I		I	2D6
Verapamil	I	I	I	I			I						I		I		I	I							3A4

I, inhibits CYP and increases plasma concentration; S, stimulates CYP and suppresses plasma concentration

creatinine clearance, may be overestimated in patients with reduced muscle mass.

ADJUSTMENT OF DRUG DOSAGE

The response to drug treatment of the individual can be only partly predicted from a knowledge of the pharmacological properties of the drug and clinical status of the patient. Moreover, it is often difficult to decide whether a modified reaction to a specific drug results from physiological or pathophysiological processes or has an iatrogenic cause. To determine the correct dose, it is often necessary to evaluate the clinical change more regularly than in younger men, and adjust the dose level in a stepwise manner. This is even more important for drugs with a narrow therapeutic range. Small changes in plasma concentration can easily lead to adverse effects. Effective and tolerable therapy with these drugs should be established by starting with a lower dose. This is gradually increased until an effective level is achieved. However, even if a patient shows a

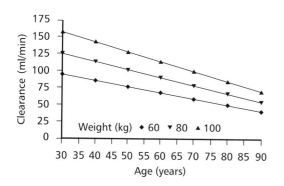

Figure 1 Relationship between creatinine clearance, age and weight in males according to the formula:

$$Cl_{creat} = \frac{(140 - age) \times weight \; ml/min}{70}$$

Table 3 Drugs with small therapeutic range that are likely to be administered to elderly men

Aminoglycosides
Antiepileptic drugs
Anti-Parkinson drugs
Antipsychotic drugs
Coumarin derivatives
Heart glycosides
Tricyclic antidepressants
Opiates

good response to a certain dose level, regular monitoring is required. Small changes in physiology, for example due to progression of cardiac failure or the introduction of another drug, can lead to ineffective therapy or side-effects. Some groups of drugs with a small therapeutic range are given in Table 3. A relatively large variation in plasma concentration can result from, for example, interaction with other drugs as a result of competition with or induction of metabolism (such as CYP induction) or renal excretion.

Even though the dose is adequately adjusted for age, the elderly seem to be more prone to adverse effects, such as hypotension due to psychopharmaceuticals and hemorrhagic diathesis during anticoagulant therapy.

POLYPHARMACY

The elderly tend to take nearly three times as many drugs as younger patients. On average, the older man receives over ten prescribed drugs per year. However, when the number of simultaneously prescribed drugs increases, compliance to the prescribed therapy decreases dramatically. More than 50% of the elderly do not correctly take their drugs, by failing to take the correct dose, by taking the correct dose at the wrong time of day or by failing to take the drugs at all. This contributes to the inefficacy of

medical treatment and consequent modification of therapy or addition of more potent drugs to the previously prescribed drugs.

Many definitions have been used to describe polypharmacy. The common thought behind these definitions is that simultaneous treatment of one individual and/or one disease in an individual with various drugs has a potential risk with respect to interaction and side-effects. The main reasons for prescribing multiple drugs to one patient, however, relate to the fact that the elderly usually have multiple pathologies. For example, in patients with congestive heart failure and chronic obstructive pulmonary disease there is good justification for the prescription of no less than five drugs: a diuretic, an angiotensin converting enzyme inhibitor, digoxin, ipratropium and salbutamol. While polypharmacy often cannot be avoided, it requires more frequent evaluation of the clinical state of the elderly patient than in the young adult, to ensure the aim of the therapy, namely an improvement in the quality of life. The basis for pharmacotherapy in the elderly, perhaps even more than in the young, should be to treat at the lowest effective dose, rather than using a standard dose or maximum tolerable dose. Effective therapy can only be achieved if therapeutic endpoints are defined for each individual drug. These endpoints should be evaluated on a regular basis, and if therapy does not meet the criteria, therapy should be discontinued or modified. Active monitoring of drug therapy in the elderly can reduce polypharmacy and thereby reduce side-effects, interactions and costs.

Further reading

1. Hardman JG, Limbird LE, eds. *Goodman and Gilman's The Pharmacological Basis of Therapeutics,* 9th edn. New York: McGraw-Hill, 1996
2. Melmon KL, Morrelli HF, Hoffman BB, Nierenberg DW, eds. *Melmon and Morrelli's Clinical Pharmacology,* 3rd edn. New York: McGraw-Hill, 1992
3. Rowland M, Tozer TN, eds. *Clinical Pharmaco-kinetics; Concepts and Applications,* 3rd edn. London: Williams & Wilkins, 1995
4. Bressler R, Katz MD, eds. *Geriatric Pharmacology.* New York: McGraw-Hill, 1993

APPENDIX – JOHN MARKS

An appropriate diet

The term 'diet' in the sense used here implies instructions on the quantity of a selection of foods which will provide adequate amounts of both macronutrients and micronutrients for the person for whom the diet is being designed. The construction of diets is a science in its own right and is normally undertaken by dieticians who receive a lengthy period of training. Hence within the framework of a short appendix in a general monograph it is not possible to do other than provide some general principles of the methods applied to the development of suitable diets.

Production of a diet must first be based on making a list of the macronutrients and micronutrients that must be provided per day with a note of the necessary quantities of each. It is usual to define the macronutrients first, namely protein, carbohydrate and fat. Of these, the carbohydrates and fats are concerned with the provision of energy, while proteins provide not only energy but also the amino acids for growth and repair of body tissues.

Energy now should be measured in kilojoules (kJ) but the use of kilocalories (kcal) is so firmly established that calculations are still normally performed in kilocalories. The result is then translated, if necessary, into kilojoules (1 kcal = 4.18 kJ). Very few nutritionists can quote without considerable thought the kJ values for the individual macronutrients while the kcal values are very easy to remember. Thus for practical purposes:

1 g protein provides 4 kcal
1 g carbohydrate provides 4 kcal
1 g fat provides 9 kcal.

It must also be appreciated that any alcohol which is consumed is a potent source of energy with 1 g providing 7 kcals.

Initially it is necessary to define the total amount of energy which must be provided per day. For the vast majority of men this means that the energy provided must equate to the energy expended if the weight is to remain constant. The energy expended per day depends on the resting metabolic rate (or basal metabolic rate (BMR)) together with additional needs for normal or occupational activities and additional needs for recreational or exercise activities.

The resting metabolic rate is determined principally by body mass and composition and it varies also with age. The best estimate for these resting energy needs are based on the equation devised by Schofield and colleagues[1]. For young adult males (age 18–29) the formula is BMR = 0.063W + 2.896; for those aged 30–59 it is 0.048W + 3.653; for those aged 60–74 it is 0.0499W + 2.939, while for those over 75 it is 0.0350W + 3.434. All these values represent W as the weight in kg and the BMR is expressed as MJ/day (where 1 MJ is 1000 kJ. For the purpose of defining food needs it is

Table 1 Total energy needs for adult males as a proportion of basal metabolic needs for three levels of occupational and three independent levels of recreational activity[2]

Recreational activity	Level of occupational activity		
	Light	Moderate	Heavy
Non-active	1.4	1.6	1.7
Moderately active	1.5	1.7	1.8
Very active	1.6	1.8	1.9

preferable to regard 'W' as the ideal body weight read from a chart or table which correlates the ideal weight with the height.

From these calculations it is possible to determine the average BMR per day for an adult male between 20 and 50 years with a weight of about 75 kg (i.e. the average modern man) as about 7.6 MJ/day (1800 kcal/day).

From this basal energy need it is then possible to calculate the additional requirement for various levels of normal and exercise activity based upon the level and time of energy expenditure. For practical purposes the total energy is usually expressed as a multiple of the resting energy figure (e.g 1.2 × BMR for sitting with no physical activity). The total daily energy expenditure can, on this basis, be expressed in terms of three grades of occupational activities and three grades of non-occupational (recreational) activity (Table 1).

The main point to make is that the additional energy which is used between a light occupation with no recreational activity and a heavy occupation with very active recreation is surprisingly little (an additional 35% only).

Having defined the energy needs it is then necessary to convert this into quantities of macronutrients per day. The first substance to establish is protein. Assuming that a high quality protein mixture is selected, the minimum need is about 0.75 g per kg body weight/day. The logical average intake for a man should be about 50–60 g/day which would provide about 220 kcal. If lower quality proteins are included (i.e. those with a lower proportion of essential amino acids, a higher quantity will be required.

Then the fat content per day should be established. The fat level should be kept as low as possible compatible with the provision of an adequate intake of the essential fatty acids (linoleic and α-linolenic acid). Males require at least 3 g and 0.5 g of these, respectively. With a mixed fat intake, these can be provided by a daily intake of around 8 g/day. However there are other factors to be considered. About 10 g fat per day is required to ensure that the gall-bladder contracts adequately to avoid gallstone formation. Indeed there is clear evidence that the fat intake can be maintained at well under 20 g/day with no health problems. Indeed I would suggest that this level has health benefits.

Fat is also necessary to achieve a palatable food pattern. How much is necessary from this point of view is open to substantially different opinions. Taking all these aspects into account, it appears to be agreed in official bodies that a daily intake of about 50 g/day is probably the lowest level that will be tolerated for a long term palatable diet. Although I would prefer an even low recommendation, this figure of 50 g/day is still substantially below the level of 120 g fat per day which represents the current average bad diet of the modern western diet. Quite apart from a substantial reduction in the total quantity of fat, the major component of it should be from vegetable rather than from animal sources.

Assuming that it is possible to persuade the person to substantially reduce their fat intake to at less than 50 g, and for most people this requires a marked change in lifestyle, this

Table 2 Comparison of percentage of each macronutrient in terms of the overall energy intake for A) the composition advised here, B) the levels advised by health authorities (e.g. DHSS)[2] and C) the current average poor Western diet

	A	B	C
Protein	7%	7%	12%
Fat	20%	33%	40%
Carbohydrate	73%	60%	48%

equates to about 450 kcal per day. When added to the energy intake from protein this amounts to a daily intake of around 700 kcal. At this stage it is also necessary to take account of the energy supplied by any alcohol that is consumed. However since alcohol is a food which is empty of any nutritional value other than calories, it will be assumed that none is being drunk.

If we base the calculations on an average energy requirement per day of 300 kcal which is usually about right for an active man in a reasonably active occupation and a deliberate policy of exercising regularly, this means that there are some 2,300 kcal to be supplied by carbohydrate or at 4 kcal/g a daily intake of some 550 g daily.

These quantities can also be presented as percentages of the total energy supplied by each macronutrient and the values suggested here for the average active man compared with the percentages advised by the health authorities and the current poor diets are shown in Table 2. While I accept that the percentage intake concept is widely used I still believe that it is preferable to think in terms of the intake in absolute quantities.

Apart from the calculation of the macronutrients in terms of total daily quantities, it is important to establish the equivalent values for desirable intakes per day of each of the vitamins, minerals and trace nutritional substances. These are defined in many official publications for example by DHSS[2]. Whether they really represent the requirements for full health and avoidance of ill health can be disputed (see, for example Chapter 46). What can be established is that these figures will certainly avoid clinical

evidence of low intakes, for they represent more than adequate levels for the avoidance of clinical deficiency.

Thus we can establish the total composition of the required diet. From this, using one of the numerous sets of tables of the analysis of specific foods, both in their natural form and when cooked, the dietician can suggest a valid and adequately variable menu.

It is important to take account of the following principles in creating this menu:

- Ensure that there is sufficient variability within the food choice to both ensure the availability of a variety of micronutrients, and to increase palatability

- In order to produce a varied diet, use different sources of animal and vegetables, ensuring that not too high a proportion of both protein and fat come from animal sources.

- To avoid wild fluctuations in blood sugar levels, use complex sugar sources for the carbohydrate needs rather than simple sugars. This will also increase the fibre level, which will not only increase satiety but reduce the time spent by food residues in the lower intestine

- Include a high proportion of fruit and vegetables in the diet (to reduce the risk of carcinogenesis)

- Advise an adequate intake of fluid.

- Make sure that any allergens for the individual or items of food intolerance – both physical and psychological are avoided.

While these are the principles which enable any specific diet to be constructed from basics, there are now a substantial number of defined menus available to meet most eventualities. Nowadays most diets are planned by checking and modifying there menus as necessary.

Exercise plans

Exercise can be classified as follows:

(1) Passive movements

(2) Assisted active movements.

(3) Active exercise related to specific muscle groups

(4) Active general exercise.

The first tow of these classes are directly related to remedial exercises during the recovery stage after injury. They should at all times be controlled and organized by a qualified physiotherapist and are well outside the range of topics that should be covered in an appendix of this type.

The third type is primarily concerned with either a later stage of recovery after injury or for specialized training. This may be for either body-building or the development of sporting excellence in specific sports. There are now advisors and coaches that are responsible for such exercises. These exercises are tailored very much for the individual needs and these also are outside the range of topics which can be covered in this appendix. We are indeed concerned here with important topic of general exercise regimes that will assist the development and maintenance of a regular healthy state best exemplified by the latin tag 'mens sano in corpore sano'.

General exercise has three important functions

(1) By imposing an appropriate extra load, it will improve the function of both the cardio-vascular and respiratory systems. This applies not only to the activity of the heart and lungs, but also to improvement in the transport of respiratory gases to the peripheral tissues.

(2) Providing that the exercise is of an appropriate character and does not impose too much strain, it can assist in the establishment and maintenance of normal function in those parts of the skeleto-muscular system that are subjected to the exercise. The important feature is to ensure that too great a strain is avoided, otherwise there may well be long-term damage to the strained areas of the body. Thus, for example, while those who indulge in regular moderate exercise normally remain more supple and less arthritic in old age, those who compete at high levels in sport often damage their tissues badly over the years and suffer badly in old age.

(3) By encouraging a period away from the strains of office work and the un-natural posture imposed by many working activities, general exercise, particularly in clean air can reduce the stresses and strains which are so common in current society.

If these are aims of exercise of this type, as I suggest, then it is important to define some of the characteristics of appropriate exercises.

Probably the most important single feature is to organise the exercise in such a way that it will be undertaken on a very regular basis. Regular, aerobic exercise, i.e that which can be undertaken within the framework of a normal sustainable oxygen load is more valuable from the point of view of general fitness for life, than occasional bursts of activity that impose un-natural strains on the body. We are all familiar with the fact that the gardener who beavers away in his plot at a steady level usually lives to a healthy old age with little tissue damage. On the other hand, when we rush out into the garden on the first fine day in spring, we suffer annoying consequences the following morning when we try to rise from bed. One of the secrets to achieve appropriate levels of exercise for the maintenance of health can be summarised by the phrase 'steady as you go'.

There are those who are prepared to set aside a regular period each day for circuit training in a gymnasium. If they have the time and enthusiasm to maintain this commitment by the year rather than the month, they will achieve substantial benefit providing that they work within their natural capability. On the other hand for every person who takes out an annual subscription for a gymnasium and uses the facilities for the whole year it is possible to find a dozen who go to the gymnasium daily for the first week, but are not to be found there subsequently. The human being is by nature idle. Regular defined exercise over a prolonged period is commitment in time and effort which the vast majority of us are not prepared to make.

I therefore suggest that the best policy on general exercise must be to adopt a general lifestyle which imposes a steady component of exercise as part of living.

- Deliberately reduce the amount of time spent in an armchair watching the television and instead of this undertake some form of physical activity. A pet dog will certainly assist this. The size and energy needs of the dog can be defined depending on the willingness of the owner to exercise both dog and owner.

- As far as possible do not take elevators or escalators. Stairs are much better for ones health.

- Reduce the amount of time spent in cars and increase the amount of time spent either walking or bicycling. With modern city and town congestion, it is often quicker and certainly more beneficial to the health to walk or cycle to work, shops or friends in the neighbourhood. Equally, use public transport for the longer journey when this is available but walk rather than drive to the station or bus-stop.

By adopting the policy of always using the general muscles rather than becoming a couch- or car-potato it is possible to adopt a lifestyle which will improve both health and purse. Regularity is what is important.

References

1. Schofield WN, Schofield C and James WPT. Basal metabolic rate – review and prediction. *Hum Nutr Clin Nutr* 1985;39(Suppl):1–96
2. DHSS. *Dietary reference values for food energy and nutrients for the United Kingdom*. Report (No 41) of the panel on dietary reference values of the Committee on Medical Aspects of Food Policy. London, HMSO, 1991

Section VII

Cardiovascular and respiratory system

David Crook, PhD

As the population ages, arterial diseases such as coronary heart disease (CHD) and stroke become more and more important, not only in the industrialized countries in which they are rampant but increasingly so in developing countries[1]. Despite major advances in the understanding of the causes of these diseases and above all in their treatment once diagnosed, we still are still limited in our success at primary prevention.

Over 40 years ago the classic epidemiological study, the Framingham Heart Study[2], identified male gender as one of the strongest characteristics in predicting which individuals would go on to develop CHD and which do not. When steroid therapies began to be used in large numbers of relatively healthy women requesting oral contraception or postmenopausal hormone replacement therapy (HRT), this issue of the steroid 'androgenicity' began to dominate the discussions of cardiovascular risk. Steroids that were structurally related to testosterone were considered to have the potential to cause CHD in women. Much of the development of both oral contraceptives and postmenopausal HRT over the years has been directed at the neutralization of the androgenic characteristics of progestogens.

Despite extensive epidemiological research, opinion is still split over whether androgenic progestogens – by whatever definition – do increase CHD risk. Data from animal studies and, more recently, human vascular research suggests that androgens may have beneficial effects on cardiovascular function. What was once a simple concern – that androgens had an unwanted influence on plasma lipoprotein metabolism – is now more complex as androgens reduce plasma levels of triglycerides and lipoprotein (a), changes that in both cases would be expected to reduce, not increase, the risk of CHD.

Given this background, the evaluation of the cardiovascular potential of androgens in the aging male needs to proceed in as cautious a manner as possible. Current attitudes range from fear of androgen-induced arterial disease through to excitement that androgen therapies will play a major role in reducing the risk of these diseases. Similarly, concerns have been expressed over the ability of androgen therapy to exacerbate sleep apnea (a risk marker for arterial disease), but others argue that androgens may strengthen the muscles of the respiratory system, especially in aging men with chronic airways disease.

Ultimately there is no substitute for placebo-controlled prospective trials of androgens on the clinical endpoints of cardiovascular and respiratory diseases, but the experience with steroid therapies in women's healthcare is that the success of such a venture will be dictated by the choice of androgen type, dose and route of administration, as well as by the baseline health of the volunteers. The contributions to this section provide biochemical, physiological and clinical evidence that is likely to help formulate such a protocol.

References

1. Lopez AD, Murray CCJL. The global burden of disease: 1990–2020. *Nature Med* 1998;4:1241–3
2. Kannel WB, Dawber TB, Kagan A, *et al*. Factors of risk in the development of coronary heart disease – six-year follow-up experience: the Framingham Study. *Ann Intern Med* 1962;55:33–50

28 Atherosclerotic risk assessment of androgen therapy in aging men

David Crook, PhD

INTRODUCTION

Testosterone has traditionally been regarded as a hormone that is harmful to the heart, in the same way that estrogen is perceived as a hormone that is good for the heart[1]. The development of androgen therapies for men has often struggled against the perception that any benefit in terms of improved sexual function or protection from osteoporosis, for example, will be at a cost of myocardial infarction and strokes, in addition to concern over prostatic disease. In fact this has never been a unanimous concern: a vocal minority, increasingly evident on the World Wide Web[2], extols the virtue of androgens as *treatments* for these very same diseases.

Risk–benefit analysis of androgen supplementation in the aging male is essential but cannot proceed until this fundamental uncertainty is resolved. Even minor effects of androgens on coronary heart disease (CHD) risk may have major implications when expressed in large populations of aging men. In the context of clinically-hypogonadal men an increased risk of CHD might well be considered acceptable, but if androgens are to be used as a more general supplementation therapy in aging men then such an increased risk may prove to be a major obstacle. Conversely, if the claims that androgen therapies can protect some men from CHD

are true, then this benefit could be used to 'fast-track' the wider acceptance of androgen therapies in aging men.

ATHEROSCLEROSIS: A CRITICAL ISSUE IN WORLD HEALTH

Arterial diseases have come to be regarded as an inevitable consequence of a 'western' lifestyle – addiction to tobacco, abhorrence of physical activity and possession of a hunger that can only be sated by processed foods rich in salt and animal fats. Arterial diseases are now the major cause of morbidity and mortality in the USA and much of Europe, with 'hot spots' being seen in Scotland, Northern Ireland and parts of Scandinavia.

There is an old adage that arterial disease is the leading cause of death in all countries who have achieved such a level of economic progress that they can afford to perform epidemiological studies. In an unwanted deviation to this pattern, the fallout from the dismantling of the former Soviet Union in the 1980s saw the beginning of an epidemic of arterial disease in Eastern bloc countries. On a more global scale, arterial diseases are likely to become major causes of morbidity and mortality[3] (Figure 1). As life expectancy in

**THE GLOBAL BURDEN OF DISEASE
PROJECTIONS FOR THE YEAR 2020**

'Disability-Adjusted Life Years'

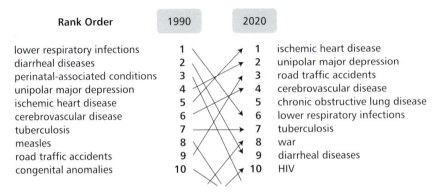

Rank Order	1990		2020	
lower respiratory infections	1		1	ischemic heart disease
diarrheal diseases	2		2	unipolar major depression
perinatal-associated conditions	3		3	road traffic accidents
unipolar major depression	4		4	cerebrovascular disease
ischemic heart disease	5		5	chronic obstructive lung disease
cerebrovascular disease	6		6	lower respiratory infections
tuberculosis	7		7	tuberculosis
measles	8		8	war
road traffic accidents	9		9	diarrheal diseases
congenital anomalies	10		10	HIV

Figure 1 Arterial diseases are predicted to become the major global cause of mortality and morbidity by 2020. Data from reference 3

under-developed countries is extended by public health policies, their people survive long enough to enter the age groups in which arterial disease will be prevalent, a trend now exacerbated by the drive to promote tobacco products to these countries.

The underlying pathology of atherosclerosis is believed to represent a preventable process. Understanding of the pathogenesis of arterial disease is a surprisingly recent development, originating with the post-World War II investment in medical research in the USA[4]. The discovery of risk factors such as hypertension, cigarette smoking and dyslipidemia held out the dual possibility of prevention and treatment. More recently, molecular biology has led to major advances in our understanding of that most complex organ, the vascular endothelium. This research supports the proposal by the late Russell Ross[5] that atherosclerosis involves an inappropriate and overenthusiastic inflammatory response by the body to endothelial damage caused by free radicals or other noxious agents. These interlaced phenomena are slowly being unravelled and the list of factors thought to be involved (positively or negatively) in the arterial disease now runs to many

hundreds. Steroid hormones are very much a part of this complex scheme.

STEROID HORMONES AND ARTERIAL DISEASE

Both estrogens and androgens have been linked to the pathogenesis of arterial disease, originating with the observation that clinically-evident CHD is rare in young women compared to young men[1]. The evidence that this gender difference is due to a protective action of estrogen is strong, although final proof – protection of postmenopausal women from CHD in placebo-controlled trials of hormone replacement therapy (HRT) – is still lacking.

The widespread use of estrogens in oral contraception and HRT has meant that the anti-atherogenic potential of estrogen has been studied in depth, while interest in the cardiovascular effects of androgens remains something of a niche area of research. Review articles on androgens and CHD were hard to find until the last decade, but when they did appear they were unusually consistent in their conclusion that treatment of relatively healthy men with modest doses of 'natural' androgens is as likely to reduce CHD risk as it is to increase it[6–9].

ANDROGENS AND ARTERIAL DISEASE

The current predictions of the effects of androgen therapies on CHD in men are based on measurement of 'surrogates' such as blood chemistries, animal models of atherosclerosis and non-invasive evaluations of vascular function. There are no formal randomized controlled trials in which the incidence of myocardial infarction or stroke in men treated with androgens has been compared to that in men given placebo. Such studies are planned but it is unlikely that their results will be available within this current decade.

The prevalence of androgen supplementation in the male population, though increasing in many countries, is unlikely to reach the levels whereby observational epidemiology can be used. This contrasts with the situation in women, in which epidemiologists were able to track the occurrence of diseases such as CHD in large communities of aging women, many of whom were HRT users. It is possible to envisage a time in which androgen replacement therapy in men has become so commonplace in certain countries that such groups of users are easily identifiable but then a new problem is likely to emerge: the use of different therapies and routes of administration. An interim approach is to break the current published literature into a set of themes relating to androgens and CHD in men.

'Maleness' as a risk factor for CHD

Attempts to discuss androgen therapy in men often flounder at an early stage due to the ingrained popular belief that 'maleness' causes CHD. This is partly due to the heavy promotion of cardiovascular risk assessment strategies that score 'maleness' as a risk factor of similar weight to diabetes or hypertension. What is rarely acknowledged is that the scoring of male gender as a positive factor is essentially an administrative convenience. The term 'femaleness' could just as well be used but there is a convention that such protective factors should be kept out of the equation. Overall it has proved simpler to score male gender as a positive risk factor than to introduce the negative risk factor of female gender.

If the plasma androgen levels associated with being male are responsible for the gender difference in CHD, then castration in men should reduce their CHD risk. The evidence for this is inconclusive[9].

Arterial disease in men abusing androgenic anabolic steroids

Another widely-held view is that androgen therapies in aging men will increase CHD risk because androgenic anabolic steroids (AAS) induce the disease. The evidence for this involves a dozen or so case-reports that describe premature CHD, often of atypical pathology, in young male athletes abusing AAS[10]. However, the toxicity problem highlighted in these case-reports has yet to be validated in formal epidemiological studies, leading Rockhold[11] to contend that the frequency of such reports is actually lower than would be expected, given the widespread abuse of AAS and the awareness within the medical community of a potential problem.

Parsinnen and colleagues[12] investigated the health of 62 male elite powerlifters who had competed in the Finnish championships in 1977–1982. AAS abuse was commonplace at that time because doping controls had yet to be introduced in Finland. By 1993 eight of these men had died, giving a relative risk of death of 4.6 compared to 1094 population controls (95% confidence interval (CI) 2.0–10.5). Three of these eight deaths were suicides. The authors consider the prevalence of cardiovascular deaths in the two groups to be similar. Even if it is shown that CHD risk is increased in AAS users, could such findings be extrapolated to

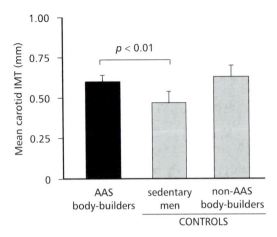

Figure 2 Carotid intima-media thickness (IMT), a surrogate for atherosclerosis, in body-builders who used androgenic anabolic steroids (AAS). Note that these men showed evidence of increased atherosclerosis, but not when compared to body-builders who did not use AAS. Data from reference 14

healthy men taking low doses of androgens under medical supervision? In most studies the AAS abusers were using combinations of oral and injectable steroids, often involving multiple drugs and supplemented with many other agents of unknown arterial safety, such as amphetamines and cocaine. A further complication is the role of strenuous physical exercise in 'triggering' plaque rupture in individuals who may otherwise have peacefully co-existed with their atherosclerotic plaques. Strenuous exertion, as distinct from regular moderate exercise, is strongly linked to acute myocardial infarction events[13].

The validity of the control subjects used in these studies is also under question. In one recent study, researchers at the University of Sydney performed a panel of cardiovascular tests in 20 elite body-builders whose self-reporting of AAS abuse was confirmed by urine screening[14]. These men had impaired vascular reactivity and increased carotid intima-media thickness (CIMT) compared with non-bodybuilding sedentary controls, but, critically, such differences were lost when body-builders

who denied AAS abuse were used as controls (Figure 2). The claim that this latter group was 'clean' must be taken seriously as they belonged to an athletic society in which continued membership relied on repeated negative urine drug screens. However this does not exclude the possibility that these men were previously exposed to AAS and so had some residual arterial damage.

Thus, studies of CHD in AAS abusers pivot on the choice of control group. This uncertainty could be resolved in the setting of a randomized controlled trial but such a study is unlikely to be commissioned. These studies should alert us to the possibility of an adverse effect of androgen therapy in aging men, but do not in themselves prove that such intervention would be dangerous. Their strength may lie in identifying potential atherogenic mechanisms, such as hypertension, plasma lipoprotein levels, platelet aggregation, myocyte toxicity or coronary spasm, that can then be investigated in a more clinically-relevant population.

Arterial disease in experimental animals treated with androgens

Laboratory animals such as mice, rats, rabbits and monkeys have been used as a shortcut to understanding drug effects on atherosclerosis. With few exceptions these species do not develop atherosclerosis and must be fed highly artificial diets rich in saturated fats and crystalline cholesterol in order to induce a gross and atherogenic dyslipidemia. These models are gradually being replaced by genetically-engineered animals such as the apoE knock-out mouse.

Many such studies find that androgens protect rabbits from diet-induced atherosclerosis in rabbits (see Chapter 30), with a possible link to induction of androgen receptors in arterial tissue[15]. In contrast, two reports in the cynomolgus monkey have contributed to the fears that androgen administration will induce atherosclerosis[16,17]. Both studies should be regarded with caution as the adverse effects were seen in female animals. There is increasing evidence that androgens may not have the same cardiovascular effects in women as in men. Cynomolgus monkeys have been extensively used for the safety evaluation of HRT and oral contraceptive steroids but their relevance to human vascular disease is increasingly under question.

ANDROGENS AND CARDIOVASCULAR RISK FACTORS

Androgens, like estrogens, affect many aspects of cardiovascular risk (see review by von Eckardstein[18]). The interpretation of these changes is becoming increasingly difficult. Androgens often reduce plasma levels of high density lipoproteins (HDL) and this change has historically been used to categorize such steroids as 'harmful' to vascular health[1]. But these changes are often seen in parallel with reductions in plasma levels of triglycerides and lipoprotein (a), a pattern that would be considered to reduce CHD risk[18,19]. The effects of androgens on plasma levels of low density lipoproteins (LDL), the classic metabolic risk factor in men, are difficult to interpret. Some AAS regimens grossly elevate plasma LDL levels, suggestive of an increase in CHD risk[18], but these levels are often unchanged when considering the doses of androgens being considered for male contraception or androgen replacement[18] and in one recent study in AAS users LDL levels were reduced[19].

The increased hemoglobin levels seen with some androgens could be considered to increase CHD risk but in the context of older men may be beneficial. Studies in AAS abusers suggest an increase in platelet aggregation[20], especially in older men, and activation of hemostasis as monitored by plasma levels of F1+2 and D-dimer[21].

There is still no agreement as to which risk factor is the most important in terms of cardiovascular disease and thus there is no way that the complex metabolic data now being generated can be synthesized to produce an estimate of the net effect of a specific androgen therapy on CHD risk. The position is further complicated by emerging evidence from studies in women that steroid-induced changes in plasma levels of CHD risk factors may not reflect changes in underlying pathological processes[22,23].

A striking finding from many clinical studies of androgens is the change in body mass, in particular the reduction in fat mass. The status of obesity itself as a CHD risk factor is still controversial: in many studies the relationship disappears once corrections are made for lack of exercise, diet and diabetes. Obesity, in particular central or 'android' obesity, is linked to insulin resistance and many other CHD risk factors. Without doubt (1) plasma testosterone levels correlate negatively with abdominal fat content, and (2) aging in men is associated with a shift towards central adiposity, but this is likely to reflect a complex interplay between sex hormones, insulin, leptin, growth hormone, changes in physical activity and so on. Where hypogonadal men have been studied an androgen-induced reduction in android fat mass is quite convincing but the evidence that moderate doses of androgens will have this effect in healthier men is dubious[24]. This issue needs resolution in placebo-controlled clinical trials. In the USA and many western countries the existence of a 'six-pack' culture makes it likely that any claims that androgens will reduce abdominal fat (and perhaps increase muscle mass) will attract considerable popular interest.

Cardiological studies of arterial health in androgen users

If androgens are indeed atherogenic (due to changes in plasma lipoproteins or other factors) then men with coronary artery disease would be expected to have higher plasma androgen levels

313

compared to those free of the disease. The epidemiological evidence fails to support such a contention[7] but it is the unexpected inverse relationship with angiographically-assessed coronary artery disease that has intrigued many cardiologists. The association of low plasma testosterone levels with coronary atherosclerosis first described by Phillips[25] has been confirmed by other researchers[26] and has also been shown to exist with plasma DHEA levels[27]. Of particular interest is the subsequent observation by Phillips of a positive relationship between plasma testosterone and angiographically assessed coronary disease in women[28], reinforcing the theme of a gender difference in the way androgens influence arterial disease.

Testosterone appears to be a vasorelaxant, though one that operates through different and more complex mechanisms than are seen with estradiol[29]. This is an attractive attribute of the steroid, but other aspects of the vascular influence of androgens remain a concern, such as the demonstration of increased monocyte adherence to endothelial cells in culture, at least in part due to overexpression of vascular adhesion molecules[30].

The true test of the hypothesis that androgens reduce the severity or incidence of arterial diseases will come from placebo-controlled studies using clinical endpoints. The evidence so far – reviewed in Chapter 33 – is encouraging

although it is largely based on the study of men with pre-existing arterial disease.

One issue yet to be addressed is that of androgen resistance in aging men: when testosterone was used to vasodilate rat coronary arteries, it appeared that vessels from older rats were less sensitive to testosterone than were those from young animals[31].

CONCLUSIONS

Over recent years the exciting evidence that androgens might reduce CHD risk has been balanced by some concerns: we simply do not know what any specific androgen supplementation therapy will do in a specific population of men. The experience so far should lead to a wider acknowledgement of the potential of androgens to protect at least some men from arterial disease. The animal data are confusing: androgens appear to be beneficial in some species but harmful in others. The risk factor data are especially difficult to interpret and are overshadowed by the possibility that steroid-induced changes in blood chemistries do not reflect underlying changes in pathological processes. The present enthusiasm on the part of cardiologists for the beneficial effects of androgen therapy relates to men with established CHD; information on clinical endpoints in men without symptomatic arterial disease is still lacking.

References

1. Godsland IF, Wynn V, Crook D, Miller NE. Sex, plasma lipoproteins and atherosclerosis: prevailing assumptions and outstanding questions. *Am Heart J* 1987;114:1467–503
2. Kennedy R. http://www.medical-library.net/sites/framer.html?/sites/testerone therapy.html
3. Lopez AD, Murray CCJL. The global burden of disease: 1990–2020. *Nature Med* 1998;4:1241–3
4. Braunwald E. Shattuck Lecture – cardiovascular medicine at the turn of the millennium:

triumphs, concerns and opportunities. *New Engl J Med* 1997;337:1360–9
5. Ross R. Atherosclerosis – an inflammatory disease. *New Engl J Med* 1999;340:115–25
6. Barrett Connor EL. Testosterone and risk factors for cardiovascular disease in men. *Diabetes Metabol* (Paris) 1995;21:156–61
7. Alexandersen P, Haarbo J, Christiansen C. The relationship of natural androgens to coronary heart disease in males: a review. *Atherosclerosis* 1996;125:1–13

8. English KM, Steeds R, Jones TH, Channer KS. Testosterone and coronary heart disease: is there a link? *Q J Med* 1997;90: 787–91

9. Crook D. Androgen therapy in the aging male: assessing the effect on heart disease. *Aging Male* 1999;2:1–6

10. Sullivan ML, Martinez CM, Gennis P, Gallagher EJ. The cardiac toxicity of anabolic steroids. *Prog Cardiovasc Dis* 1998;41: 1–15

11. Rockhold RW. Cardiovascular toxicity of anabolic steroids. *Ann Rev Pharmacol Toxicol* 1993;33:497–520

12. Parssinen M, Kujala U, Vartiainen E, *et al.* Increased premature mortality of competitive powerlifters suspected to have used anabolic agents. *Int J Sports Med* 2000;21: 225–7

13. Mittleman MA, Maclure M, Tofler GH, *et al.* Triggering of acute myocardial infarction by heavy physical exertion. Protection against triggering by regular exertion. Determinants of Myocardial Infarction Onset Study Investigators. *New Engl J Med* 1993;329: 1677–83

14. Sader MA, Griffiths KA, McCredie RJ, *et al.* Androgenic anabolic steroids and arterial structure and function in male bodybuilders. *JACC* 2001;37:224–30

15. Hanke H, Lenz C, Hess B, *et al.* Effect of testosterone on plaque development and androgen receptor expression in the arterial vessel wall. *Circulation* 2001;103: 1382–5

16. Adams MR, Williams JK, Kaplan JR. Effects of androgens on coronary artery atherosclerosis and atherosclerosis-related impairment of vascular responsiveness. *Arterioscler Thromb Vasc Biol* 1995;15:562–70

17. Obasanjo IO, Clarkson TB, Weaver DS. Effects of the anabolic steroid nandrolone decanoate on plasma lipids and coronary arteries of female cynomolgus macaques. *Metabolism* 1996;45:463–8

18. Von Eckardstein A. Androgens, cardiovascular risk factors and atherosclerosis. *In:* Nieschlag E, Behre HM, eds. *Testosterone.* Berlin: Springer, 1998;229–58

19. Dickerman RD, McConathy WJ, Zachariah NY. Testosterone, sex hormone binding globulin, lipoproteins and vascular disease risk. *J Cardiovasc Risk* 1997;4:363–6

20. Ferenchick G, Schwartz D, Ball M, Schwartz K. Androgenic-anabolic steroid abuse and platelet aggregation: a pilot study in weight lifters. *Am J Med Sci* 1992;303:78–82

21. Ferenchick GS, Hirowaka S, Mammen EF, Schwartz KA. Anabolic-androgenic steroid abuse in weight lifters: evidence for activation of the hemostatic system. *Am J Hematol* 1995;49:282–8

22. Crook D, Von Eckardstein A, Dieplinger H, *et al.* Tibolone lowers HDL concentrations but does not impair cholesterol efflux from cells. *Maturitas* 2000;35:7–8

23. Van Kesteren PJ, Kooistra T, Lansink M, *et al.* The effects of sex steroids on plasma levels of marker proteins of endothelial cell functioning. *Thromb Haemostasis* 1998;79: 1029–33

24. Vermeulen A, Goemaere S, Kaufman JM. Testosterone, body composition and aging. *J Endocrinol Invest* 1999;22(5 Suppl): 110–6

25. Phillips GB, Pinkernell BH, Jing T-Y. The association of hypotestosteronemia with coronary artery disease in men. *Arterioscler Thromb* 1994;14:701–6

26. English KM, Mandour O, Steeds RP, *et al.* Men with coronary heart disease have lower levels of androgens than men with normal coronary androgens. *Eur Heart J* 2000;21: 890–4

27. Adamkiewicz M, Zgliczynski S, Slowinska-Srzednicka J, *et al.* Androgens (testosterone and dehydroepiandrosterone-sulfate) and coronary arteriosclerosis in men. Presented at III Internationales Grazer Andrologie-Symposion, Graz, 31 August–2 September 2000

28. Phillips GB, Pinkernell BH, Jing T-Y. Relationship between serum sex hormones and coronary artery disease in postmenopausal women. *Arterioscler Thromb Vasc Biol* 1997; 17:695–701

29. Crews JK, Kahil RA. Antagonistic effects of 17 β-estradiol, progesterone and testosterone

on calcium entry mechanisms of coronary vasoconstriction. *Atheroscler Thromb Vasc Biol* 1999;19:1034–40

30. McCrohon JA, Jessup W, Handelsman DJ, Celermajer DS. Androgen exposure increases human monocyte adhesion to vascular endothelium and endothelial cell expression of vascular cell adhesion molecule-1. *Circulation* 1999;99:2317–22

31. English KM, Jones RD, Jones TH, *et al*. Aging reduces the responsiveness of coronary arteries from male Wister rats to the vasodilatory action of testosterone. *Clin Sci* 2000;99:77–82

29 Changes in metabolic, inflammatory and endothelial indices of cardiovascular risk

Ian F. Godsland, PhD

INTRODUCTION

The development of cardiovascular disease may be understood in terms of exposure to risk factors. These damage the vasculature and, if exposure is chronic, may overwhelm natural repair mechanisms and set in motion processes which ultimately lead to the catastrophic consequences of arterial occlusion, including stroke and heart attack. Evaluation of cardiovascular risk is generally considered separately in men and women for, although there is uncertainty over whether a given risk factor is equally damaging to both sexes, exposure to risk can differ considerably. There are two aspects to risk factor exposure, one relating to cultural, life-style and environmental influences and the other to inherent differences in physiology dictated by differences in sex hormone levels. These two arenas of risk factor relationship embody a broad range of interactions and are themselves interrelated. In men, these interactions and interrelationships are exemplified by the changes in risk factor status that accompany aging.

To fully appreciate the complexities of risk factor interactions in the aging male, it is essential to recognize the extraordinary interconnectedness of the biochemical and physiological systems involved, and the ways in which disturbances in any one of them can disturb other systems, and thus augment the risk of vascular damage. Therefore, before describing the shifting patterns of cardiovascular risk in the aging male, this chapter will begin with a detailed consideration of cardiovascular risk factors themselves.

CARDIOVASCULAR RISK FACTORS

A core trinity of risk factors underlies cardiovascular disease: cigarette smoking, hypertension and hypercholesterolemia. In the prediction of coronary heart disease (CHD) epidemiological studies have shown each of these to be of comparable importance, albeit depending on the degree of exposure. With regard to stroke, however, elevated blood pressure emerges as an especially strong indicator of risk, whereas both low and high cholesterol levels have been implicated in the risk of stroke. The shared common factor for this trinity is damage to the arterial endothelium. Hypertension exposes vessels to increased mechanical stress; cigarette smoking

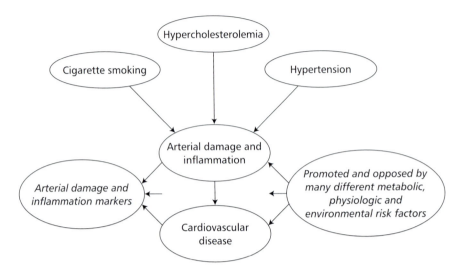

Figure 1 Risk factors and cardiovascular disease

causes a transient but intense release of oxidative free radicals into the arterial system; and oxidized cholesterol can act as an endothelial toxin. How this damage then progresses depends on local conditions and the intensity of the exposure to these insults.

The effects of one such insult may be seen when cholesterol is deposited in the subendothelial space to form atherosclerotic plaque. This can ultimately rupture to expose thrombotic tissue surfaces and release into the vessel lumen the highly oxidized lipid hitherto contained under the cap of the plaque. When this occurs in the coronary arteries the consequence is angina or myocardial infarction. When the blood supply to the brain is affected, transient ischemic attack or ischemic stroke results. On the other hand endothelial damage may sufficiently disrupt the fine vessels of the tissues surrounding the brain, perhaps already weakened as a consequence of low cholesterol levels, to cause catastrophic hemorrhagic stroke.

Such an outline, however, provides only the broadest depiction of some of the main features of arterial disease. Beyond the three factors described above, a host of variables may be distinguished, each of which is in some way linked with the development of the disease, either as a possible cause or as a marker of progressing damage (Figure 1). Many of these variables may be measured in serum, in contrast to variables that relate directly to endothelial or arterial structure or function. What follows will exclusively concern such serum-based measures, their relationships to atherosclerosis, and changes in these measures as men age.

Risk factors versus risk markers

A frequently-made distinction is to separate measures that relate to substances (or processes) directly involved in the development of cardiovascular disease, so-called 'risk factors', and those providing a secondary index of such factors, but which are not themselves directly involved in the disease process, 'risk markers'. Hitherto, epidemiology has identified probable risk factors on the basis of their ability to predict cardiovascular disease. However, an increasing appreciation of the manifold intercorrelations between different risk factors or markers and the basic physiology underlying such interrelationships suggests that many so-called 'independent risk factors' may be no more than the most prominent and precisely measurable indices of entire constellations of physiological disturbance. The emergence of clinical arterial disease can be viewed as a consequence of sustained, co-ordinated disturbances at many levels, which ultimately swamp the numerous processes that work to maintain arterial health.

Beyond the recognition that no index of risk exists or works in isolation, a number of novel measures have been explored which relate not to the causal development of arterial disease, but to the presence or progression of sub-clinical disease. All of these measures may provide potentially important signals for intervention, although it may yet take many years of intensive research for their usefulness to be established.

MEASURES OF CARDIOVASCULAR RISK

Cholesterol metabolism

The paradigm for a metabolic risk factor for cardiovascular disease is found in the role of cholesterol in the development of CHD. Atherosclerotic plaques often contain large amounts of cholesterol; serum cholesterol concentrations are high in those with CHD and in those who are subsequently diagnosed with CHD. Furthermore, conditions have been identified in which specific defects in cholesterol metabolism were inherited along with a predisposition to CHD, and mechanisms identified whereby cholesterol could enter and be deposited in the subendothelial space. Conclusive evidence comes from the fact that specific pharmacological interventions have been designed which substantially lower both cholesterol concentrations and rates of CHD. However, most people with high serum cholesterol concentrations do not develop CHD. Neither do all people with CHD have high cholesterol concentrations. There is merely a greater proportion of people with high cholesterol among those who will develop CHD than among those who will not, and this is generally true of other disturbances that have been linked to CHD. Exceptions to this may be found among those with homozygous inherited conditions that cause, for example, familial hypercholesterolemia. In such cases heart disease invariably develops early in life. But such exceptions are very rare, emphasizing how, in the great majority of cases of CHD, no single factor can fully account for the condition.

Variation in serum cholesterol concentration is itself the net expression of a complex underlying metabolic system, different elements of which can independently affect the development of atherosclerosis (Figure 2). Being insoluble in water, cholesterol must be carried within particles made water soluble by a hydrophilic coating. These particles comprise the lipoproteins, which provide the means by which not only cholesterol but other lipids, primarily triglycerides, are transported around the body.

Three principal systems of lipoprotein metabolism may be distinguished. The central system, or endogenous pathway, of lipoprotein metabolism involves the assembly in the liver of very-low-density lipoprotein (VLDL) particles, which have a core of triglycerides and cholesterol esters and a surface comprising a single molecule of apolipoprotein (apo) B_{100}, and molecules of apolipoprotein AI and AII, phospholipids and cholesterol esters. Once released into the circulation, VLDL particles acquire further surface apolipoproteins, E, CI and CIII, from high-density lipoproteins (HDL), and are acted on by endothelial lipoprotein lipase, which hydrolyses the core triglycerides. Non-esterified fatty acids thus released are then available for oxidation, incorporation into adipose tissue fat depots, or reincorporation into VLDL triglyceride in the liver. Progressive delipidation of the VLDL particles leads to their increasing cholesterol enrichment and the emergence of intermediate-density lipoprotein (IDL), which may be acted on by a further lipolytic enzyme, hepatic lipase, and, finally, low-density lipoprotein (LDL). LDL is the principal medium through which cholesterol is made available throughout the body, entering tissues via the LDL (or B_{100}/E) receptor. LDL also interacts with HDL to deliver excess cholesterol to the liver for excretion into the bile.

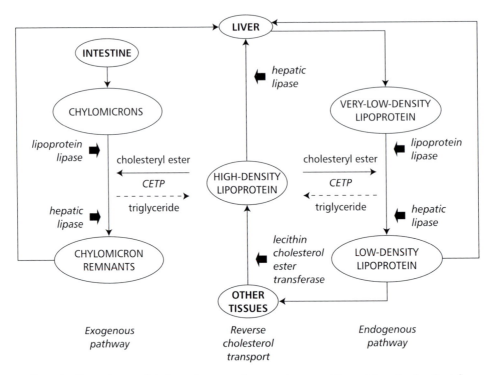

Figure 2 The pathways of cholesterol transport between tissues and lipoproteins, showing the influences of the principal enzymes of lipoprotein metabolism and of cholesterol ester transfer protein (CETP)

The endogenous pathway of lipoprotein metabolism has further interconnections. As triglyceride is removed from the VLDL particle, surface apolipoproteins are released and are reincorporated into HDL. Via cholesterol ester transfer protein (CETP), triglyceride from intermediates in the delipidation pathway may be exchanged for cholesterol esters in cholesterol-rich HDL or LDL particles. Triglyceride enrichment of LDL makes it a preferred substrate for the action of hepatic lipase, resulting in the production of a smaller, denser, cholesterol-rich LDL particle. Conversely, cholesterol enrichment of intermediates in the delipidation pathway leads to the production of cholesterol-rich VLDL remnants. Beyond the consequences of lipid exchange between different lipoprotein particles, cellular uptake of LDL via the LDL receptor downregulates the activity of the principal enzyme of cholesterol synthesis, hydroxymethyl glutaryl coenzyme A (HMG CoA) reductase.

In parallel with the endogenous pathway, the exogenous pathway of lipoprotein metabolism performs a similar function, using freshly absorbed triglycerides and fatty acids from the intestine rather than the liver. Instead of VLDL, the particles produced are the larger triglyceride-rich chylomicrons. These have around their surface, in additon to phospholipids, cholesterol esters and molecules of apolipoprotein AI and AII, and a smaller variant of apoB, apolipoprotein B-48. Like VLDL, the chylomicrons acquire apolipoproteins E, CI and CIII from HDL and are acted on by lipoprotein lipase. Intermediates in the delipidation of chylomicrons can provide triglyceride for exchange with cholesterol esters from cholesterol-rich lipoproteins, and surface components for reintegration into HDL. The cholesterol ester-rich chylomicron remnants that are the end product of the exogenous pathway of lipoprotein metabolism are finally removed from the circulation via the hepatic chylomicron remnant receptor.

The third lipoprotein system is reverse cholesterol transport, which mediates removal of excess cholesterol from the body via HDL. Nascent HDL particles are secreted by the liver and intestine and progressively mature with the acquisition of apolipoproteins AI, AII, CI and CIII, free cholesterol and phospholipid released during delipidation of VLDL and chylomicrons. HDL-free cholesterol is esterified by the action of lecithin cholesterol acyl transferase (LCAT), which also esterifies tissue free cholesterol for transfer to HDL. HDL thus becomes progressively more laden with cholesterol esters and progresses from the HDL_3 particle to the cholesterol ester-rich HDL_2 particle. The remaining free cholesterol in HDL_2 may then be exchanged via CETP for triglycerides from intermediates in VLDL delipidation. This cholesterol is then ultimately removed along with LDL by the liver. The triglyceride in HDL_2 may then be hydrolyzed by the lipolytic enzyme hepatic lipase. Apolipoprotein AI is released for reincorporation into nascent HDL particles and a smaller, denser HDL_3 particle emerges ready to receive further loads of cholesterol ester. In this way, cholesterol can be removed from the tissues and excreted via LDL and the liver. Other transfer processes centered on HDL are being elucidated. For example, there is at present intensive research into the roles of the hepatic SRB-1 receptor, which can accept cholesterol ester for excretion from HDL, and the ABC-1 protein, which facilitates HDL-mediated efflux of cellular lipid[1].

Variation in plasma cholesterol concentrations is, therefore, the net result of an extremely complex transport system that, between cholesterol synthesis and excretion, mediates the distribution of cholesterol throughout the body. Disturbances in any one of the elements of this system may, theoretically – and in many cases demonstrably – result in elevated cholesterol concentrations. The question then arises, what

is the relationship between total cholesterol measured as a predictor of risk in epidemiological studies and arterial cholesterol deposition itself?

A critical factor in the accumulation of cholesterol in the subendothelial space appears to be oxidation of LDL that has passed through the endothelium. Cell-induced peroxidation of LDL polyunsaturated fatty acids initiates oxidation of phospholipids and cholesterol esters and results in modification of LDL apoB. Oxidized lipid in the subendothelium acts as an endothelial toxin and initiates recruitment of monocytes into the subendothelium by chemotaxis, as well as their differentiation into macrophages. Moreover, oxidative modification of apoB renders the LDL particle less likely to be taken up by the LDL receptor and more likely to be taken up by macrophages. Given sufficient internalization of oxidized lipoprotein, macrophages develop into lipid-laden foam cells which undergo necrosis and release their lipid into the subendothelial space to form the lipid core of the developing atherosclerotic plaque.

The principal medium through which cholesterol promotes atherosclerosis therefore appears to be the LDL particle which, in excess and, possibly, in the absence of sufficient antioxidant activity, provides the vehicle for cholesterol accumulation in the atherosclerotic plaque. VLDL and chylomicron remnants may also provide a similar vehicle. Since the greatest proportion of cholesterol in the circulation is carried on LDL, measurement of total serum cholesterol provides an index of potentially atherogenic LDL levels, with some contribution from VLDL and chylomicron remnants, and it is as an index of these species that serum total cholesterol concentration is an effective index of CHD risk.

Variations in total cholesterol levels may result from changes in the structure or activity of LDL receptors, the various apolipoproteins, CETP, hepatic lipase, lipoprotein lipase, etc. Variations may also depend on dietary intake of saturated fatty acids, which can downregulate the LDL receptor. Measures of each of these species could provide an index of risk, but the net atherogenic effect is effectively quantified by a straightforward measurement of total cholesterol. Measurement of LDL cholesterol has hitherto been more difficult, although, with the availability of direct assays, LDL cholesterol may yet provide a better index of risk. Measurement of remnant cholesterol is more difficult still, but, again, relatively straightforward assays are becoming available[2], so this measure may also prove useful. It should be noted, however, that some proportion of total cholesterol represents cholesterol in the HDL fraction and, as might be expected from the role of HDL in reverse cholesterol transport, high levels of HDL cholesterol are associated with a decreased risk of CHD. In other words, HDL is a negative predictor. HDL also has other antiatherogenic effects on account of its various protein components. Principal among these are apolipoprotein AI, which can act as a prostacyclin stabilizer, prostacyclin having antithrombotic, anti-inflammatory and vasodilatory actions. HDL also carries antioxidant enzymes, such as paraoxonase. Ideally, therefore, cardiovascular risk assessment as it relates to cholesterol metabolism should include the measurement of LDL cholesterol and either HDL cholesterol or apolipoprotein AI concentrations.

The metabolic syndrome

Clearly, a central element in cholesterol metabolism is the synthesis and output of VLDL by the liver and its progressive delipidation. This, in turn, provides an area of interaction with another metabolic system that has ramifications entirely beyond cholesterol metabolism, a system with insulin as its central element. Several key control points in lipoprotein metabolism are powerfully affected by insulin. The most sensitive of these is lipolysis of fat stores in adipose tissue, which is acutely suppressed by insulin. Adipose tissue lipolysis provides non-esterified fatty acids (NEFAs) for synthesis of triglycerides by the liver, and the supply of such

substrates largely determines the rate of synthesis of VLDL by the liver. Suppression of this supply then suppresses hepatic VLDL synthesis. Insulin also appears able to suppress VLDL release from the liver[3], and it has a third control point in its stimulation of lipoprotein lipase activity. Insulin, therefore, blocks release of VLDL from the liver, and promotes the elimination of such VLDL as is released.

There are two linked states in which insulin action is deficient. One is insulin resistance, associated with a subnormal tissue response to insulin, and the other is impaired glucose tolerance and diabetes, themselves associated with insulin resistance, but with the predominant contribution to deficient insulin action being an impaired pancreatic insulin response to glucose. Each of these conditions – insulin resistance, impaired glucose tolerance and diabetes – is associated with increased NEFA supply to the liver, increased output of VLDL and decreased elimination of VLDL and chylomicrons. This has several consequences. Primarily there is a net increase in circulating triglycerides and VLDL concentrations and a greater tendency to postprandial lipemia. But possibly the most atherogenic consequence of these changes relates to the enhanced exchange of triglycerides and cholesterol esters via CETP. HDL and LDL become enriched in triglycerides and are more readily acted on by hepatic lipase. With regard to LDL, small dense particles result, which are less readily taken up by the LDL receptor, tend to penetrate into the subendothelium more readily and are more susceptible to oxidation. With regard to HDL, there are fewer HDL particles available for reverse cholesterol transport and the accompanying cholesterol enrichment of VLDL and chylomicrons results in greater cholesterol enrichment of remnant particles. This, in turn, leads to greater arterial cholesterol deposition as a result of their uptake into macrophages in the subendothelium.

There is, therefore a typical dyslipidemia of impaired insulin action that includes increased triglyceride levels, decreased HDL levels, a greater proportion of LDL in the small dense form and more cholesterol-rich intermediates of VLDL and chylomicron metabolism. The importance of elevated triglycerides as a cardiovascular risk factor has been controversial, but several influential studies, including the Framingham and PROCAM studies, have found the serum triglyceride concentration to be an independent predictor[4].

Beyond these changes in lipid metabolism, deficient insulin action may result in a number of further disturbances, depending on whether the principal cause of deficient insulin action is insulin resistance or insulin deficiency, the former being characterized by hyperinsulinemia and the latter by hyperglycemia. Although controversial, insulin resistance and its accompanying hyperinsulinemia have been linked with increased blood pressure, increased catecholamine levels, increased concentrations of the antifibrinolytic factor, plasminogen activator inhibitor-1 (PAI-1, levels of which can also be increased by increased triglyceride concentrations), increased fibrinogen and increased uric acid concentrations. Each of these changes can independently predict the development of CHD and some may independently promote the atherosclerotic process. It has therefore been proposed that the so-called 'insulin resistance syndrome', which encompasses these manifold changes, may be as critical a factor in cardiovascular risk as hypercholesterolemia. Evidence for this is equivocal, however, possibly owing to a lack of agreement over exactly what constitutes such a syndrome and to uncertainties over how to quantify it. This has, nevertheless, been attempted in one of the first studies to demonstrate insulin as a risk factor for cardiovascular disease, the Helsinki Policemen Study[5]. A syndrome score derived using factor analysis was found to predict CHD mortality during the course of 20 years of follow-up.

One uncertainty regarding the syndrome of disturbances centered on insulin resistance is whether it can exist independently of increased body fat accumulation, particularly in the visceral (omental or central) region. This body fat depot appears to have a relatively high lipolytic rate and is therefore a particularly rich source of NEFAs. As described below, it is also a source of inflammatory cytokines, one of which, tumor necrosis factor-α, can induce insulin resistance and promote triglyceride release. A reduction in central fat, including its removal surgically, results in a significant improvement in insulin sensitivity and its accompanying metabolic disturbances. It is therefore possible that visceral fat deposition rather than insulin resistance is the primary disturbance. The contributions of insulin resistance and visceral fat to a range of intercorrelated metabolic disturbances linked with cardiovascular disease are illustrated in Figure 3.

In addition to being a well-characterized risk factor for CHD, obesity is a key risk factor for the development of insulin deficiency. The resulting fasting hyperglycemia, impaired glucose tolerance or diabetes have each been linked with the development of cardiovascular disease. Weight loss may considerably reduce the degree of hyperglycemia and it is possible that in predisposed individuals a complex of insulin resistance and mildly elevated glucose levels can adversely affect pancreatic insulin output itself. Improved insulin sensitivity can then restore normal pancreatic function. In others, however, deficient pancreatic insulin secretion is irreversible, leading to the typical profile of type 2 diabetes.

Several mechanisms have been proposed for vascular disease associated with hyperglycemia, including increased release of oxidative free radicals, mitochondrial DNA damage and protein glycation. With regard to protein glycation, the formation of advanced glycation end-products is now a well-characterized feature of diabetes, and such changes extend to LDL. Glycation of LDL renders it less able to be taken up by the LDL receptor and more likely to accumulate in oxidized form in the subendothelium.

Deficient insulin action is therefore accompanied by a core of adverse metabolic changes, particularly in lipid metabolism, and these alone

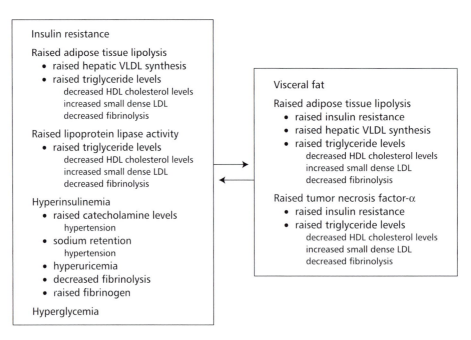

Figure 3 Interrelated disturbances of the metabolic syndrome. First-level effects are a direct consequence of insulin resistance or visceral fat. Second-level effects resulting from these first-level effects are bulletted. Third-level effects resulting from the second-level effects are shown in smaller type

could justify the delineation of a distinct metabolic syndrome. The extensive additional consequences of these changes, albeit varying somewhat according to the causes of deficient insulin action, add to this co-ordinated series of atherogenic changes. Central fat deposition may have an independent role to an extent which has yet to be determined. Measurements of triglyceride, HDL, insulin and glucose concentrations and adiposity can nevertheless delineate a complex of disturbances that could account for a considerable number of cases of CHD not explained by the classic three risk factors: smoking, hypertension and hypercholesterolemia.

While the metabolic syndrome has been an influential concept in our developing understanding of risk factor disturbances and their interrelationships, it remains to be established whether simultaneous evaluation of all its various manifestations can provide a better index of cardiovascular risk than any single measure. There is still no agreed quantitative definition

of the syndrome, and disagreement over the features that constitute it remains. These uncertainties will only be resolved by large prospective epidemiological studies in which the full range of putative components of the syndrome is measured in each individual.

Markers of inflammation and vascular damage

Cigarette smoking, hypertension, hypercholesterolemia and the metabolic syndrome, in its various manifestations, either cause vascular damage or exacerbate its consequences. Reducing their impact either by life-style modification or pharmacological intervention offers the possibility of reducing cardiovascular disease risk. However, it may also be useful to have measures which provide indices of actual vascular damage rather than indices of risk of developing atherosclerosis. Clinical manifestations of atherosclerotic vascular disease are the consequence of a slowly developing subclinical process and if it were known that this was occurring in an individual, more intensive intervention might be considered beyond that suggested by evaluation of other risk factors.

An important feature of atherosclerosis is inflammation, one aspect of the normal healing response to injury, but which may become chronic, causing further damage beyond the original lesion that initiated the inflammatory process. Leukocyte count, globulin concentrations and erythrocyte sedimentation rate are amongst the traditional indices of inflammation, although they have been evaluated generally in relation to acute infection or chronic inflammatory diseases, in which their levels are substantially increased. More recently, however, it has come to be recognized that relatively minor elevations in these measures may also be indicative of underlying inflammation, particularly as it relates to cardiovascular disease[6]. Furthermore, other, so-called 'acute phase markers', in particular C-reactive protein (CRP) and fibrinogen, have recently been the subject of intensive investigation in relation to cardiovascular disease, and others, including serum amyloid-A[7] and lipoprotein-associated phospholipase-A2[8] are being actively investigated. There is now substantial information from prospective studies confirming that subclinical elevations in each of these measures can predict subsequent cardiovascular disease[6,9], thus providing strong evidence for the importance of chronic, low-grade inflammation in the underlying development of vascular disease.

Several of these measures are undoubtedly simply markers of pre-existing subclinical inflammation. However, there is increasing evidence that CRP may be an active agent in promoting cardiovascular disease[10–12]. Adipose tissue is a source of inflammatory cytokines and obesity may be accompanied by a chronic low grade inflammatory response that includes stimulation of CRP production and release of tumor necrosis factor-α. As described above, this latter agent can induce insulin resistance

and hypertriglyceridemia. These disturbances and the metabolic effects of obesity itself provide a link between low-grade inflammation and a broad range of other disturbances. This argues in favor of a metabolic syndrome that includes inflammation as one of its accompanying features[13].

A further dimension to the complex of relationships surrounding inflammatory risk markers is the possibility that they may reflect an infection of the vascular wall, which itself may be atherogenic[14]. Cytomegalovirus, *Helicobacter* and *Chlamydia* have each been nominated as potential causative agents. However, prospective studies investigating the possible presence of these agents by measurement of specific immunoglobulin titers prior to diagnosis of CHD have not provided strong evidence overall for an association[15].

Endothelial damage markers provide another potential index of subclinical vascular disease, although existing studies provide only equivocal evidence for their usefulness. Normally, the selectin and adhesion molecules that are involved in the process of anchoring leukocytes to the vascular wall appear to be tightly bound to the endothelium. However in the presence of vascular inflammation and atherosclerosis, these molecules are released into the circulation and the moderate elevations that ensue can provide an index of existing damage. E-selectin, vascular cell adhesion molecule-1 (VCAM-1), and intercellular adhesion molecule-1 (ICAM-1) have been the most studied of these species. Their measurement does, however, require expensive assays and there is currently relatively little prospective information on their ability to predict the emergence of clinical vascular disease.

A surrogate measure of more advanced stages of endothelial damage is provided by microalbuminuria, measured as the albumin/creatinine ratio (upper limit in men 2.5 nmol/mg) in an early morning urine sample, which primarily reflects damage to the renal tubule. Hypertension and diabetes are its most common clinical correlates although, interestingly, there is an association between microalbuminuria, hyperinsulinemia and CHD in non-diabetic individuals[16]. Also associated with microalbuminuria in diabetes are elevated homocysteine levels and it has been suggested that homocysteine may itself be a correlate of insulin resistance. However, this does not appear to be the case[17], and the status of homocysteine as an indicator of cardiovascular risk is, in any case, somewhat uncertain at present[18]. Despite consistent evidence for elevated homocysteine levels in cases of cardiovascular disease compared with controls, in prospective studies homocysteine has generally failed to predict the subsequent diagnosis, suggesting that it may be a marker of existing vascular disease rather than an active causative agent. Nevertheless, as with hypercholesterolemia, there is a precedent for the importance of homocysteine, which is the cardiovascular disease that develops in association with the grossly elevated homocysteine levels seen in the inherited condition of homocysteinuria. Moreover, experimental studies have shown that homocysteine is capable of acting as an endothelial toxin.

A complication in distinguishing whether homocysteine is important in vascular disease is the role of vitamin status in modulating its concentration. Vitamins B_6 and B_{12} and folate are each important cofactors in homocysteine metabolism, so there is an underlying association between elevated homocysteine levels and poor nutrition. Given the possible importance of low vitamin B_6 and low antioxidant vitamin levels in the development of cardiovascular disease, it is possible that elevated homocysteine levels provide a marker for deficiencies in these agents, which, despite being subclinical, nevertheless predispose to the development of cardiovascular disease.

Lipoprotein (a) (Lp(a)) bears a structural resemblance to LDL, but the extent to which it is involved in lipid transport is unclear. Lp(a) also resembles tissue plasminogen activator (tPA) and may act as a competitive inhibitor of tPA action, thus inhibiting fibrinolysis. It has been proposed that this may be the principal influence underlying the association between high Lp(a) levels and CHD, seen both in prospective studies in humans and in transgenic animals in which the apolipoprotein (a) gene has been inserted. Synthesis of Lp(a) can, however, be influenced by inflammatory cytokines, and Lp(a) is present in high concentrations at sites of vascular inflammation. Its role in this respect is uncertain, although one possibility is that it provides cholesterol for membrane synthesis at sites of vascular damage.

METABOLIC AND INFLAMMATORY RISK FACTORS IN MEN

The epidemic of coronary heart disease that developed during the first part of the 20th century had, as its most dramatic manifestation, sudden death from myocardial infarction in men aged between 45 and 65 years, who would otherwise have been expected to enjoy several more decades of active life. It is now recognized that women are equally affected, but later in life. Nevertheless, the focus of research into cardiovascular disease risk factors has until very recently been mainly on men, and the associations described above have all been confirmed, albeit to varying degrees, in men.

Whether a particular risk factor is especially damaging in men relative to women is not clear, since risk factors do not work in isolation and there may be different modulating factors in men and women. One such factor could be the lower HDL cholesterol levels seen in men, which may account for the observation that mortality is greater in men for a given degree of cigarette smoking, hypertension or hypercholesterolemia[19]. However, a given ratio of total to HDL cholesterol level may itself be associated with higher CHD incidence in men than in women[20]. In women, on the other hand, diabetes appears to have particularly deleterious consequences, since women developing diabetes lose their relative protection from CHD compared with men. Diabetes is characterized by high triglyceride and low HDL cholesterol levels, and evidence from the influential Lipid Research Clinics Prevalance Study suggests that these are more closely related to CHD risk in women than in men[21]. However, triglyceride metabolism and cholesterol metabolism are so closely linked that considering either in isolation is questionable. Moreover, triglyceride levels vary from day to day in an individual to a greater extent than do cholesterol levels so cholesterol will inevitably tend to emerge from multivariate statistical analysis as a stronger predictor of CHD because there is less variance associated with it as a risk measure.

CHANGES IN RISK-FACTOR STATUS WITH AGE IN MEN

Puberty and adolescence

Puberty in boys is accompanied by a rise in testosterone levels and a fall in HDL cholesterol concentrations, possibly as a result of the induction of the sex-hormone sensitive enzyme of lipoprotein metabolism, hepatic lipase[22]. This fall in HDL levels thus establishes one of the principal risk factor differences that may underlie the higher age-standardized CHD rates in men than in women. Puberty is also accompanied by a transient increase in insulin resistance on account of the increase in growth hormone levels taking place at the time[23]. However, the increases in both androgen and growth hormone levels combine to induce a substantial increase in lean body mass. Since muscle is one of the principal sites of action of insulin, this net increase in insulin-sensitive metabolic tissue as boys pass from puberty to adulthood restores whole body insulin sensitivity to levels which are probably somewhat higher than those seen in women.

Adulthood

Although the rise in testosterone in boys at puberty is associated with a decrease in HDL levels, in men there is a positive correlation between testosterone and HDL levels. This may

reflect the predominance of a further effect of testosterone on HDL metabolism, beyond induction of hepatic lipase, namely stimulation of hepatic synthesis of apolipoprotein AI[24]. HDL does not appear to change appreciably in adult males in passing from youth to middle-age, but most other risk indices deteriorate. To what extent this is due to life-style and environmental influences or to factors intrinsic to the aging process is unclear, but both are likely to be operating. Excessive calorie intake and an increasingly sedentary life-style in men can combine to promote the deposition of visceral fat, a process which becomes increasingly noticeable as middle-age approaches. As described above, visceral fat has manifold adverse metabolic effects, and it is possible that these contribute to the tendency for cardiovascular disease to manifest in mid-life in men. The chronic insulin resistance associated with central fat deposition may be a precursor of maturity onset, or type 2, diabetes, thus further compounding the impairment of insulin action associated with insulin resistance.

Diet in men may be suboptimal not only in relation to total caloric intake but to the quality of food as well. Prospective epidemiological studies of cardiovascular disease have included increasingly accurate evaluations of dietary composition, particularly in terms of vitamin and fruit and vegetable intake, and there is increasing evidence for these as significant modulators of cardiovascular risk[25-27]. Total cholesterol levels, too, increase steadily with age. Again life-style influences may contribute, but there is also a progressive impairment of cholesterol elimination[28]. Protein turnover decreases with increasing age, and proteins involved in lipoprotein metabolism, such as $apoB_{100}$ and the LDL receptor, are therefore more likely to undergo glycation or oxidative modification.

Late life

Risk factor status worsens with increasing age, although different rates of change may be detected for some factors in men and women. For example, the age-related increase in procoagulatory factor VII may be significantly less in men[29]. Beyond maturity, the rates of adverse change in risk factor profiles appear to diminish. Much of the information relating to risk factor changes later in life comes from cross-sectional studies. It could, therefore, be argued that those susceptible to adverse risk factor changes may have already died, leaving a population with somewhat healthier intrinsic risk factor characteristics. Nevertheless, although risk factor changes may diminish, the clinical consequences of earlier disturbances do not. By this time, irrevocable damage may already have been done in terms of the onset of diabetes and vascular disease and there may be additional factors, in particular declining testosterone concentrations, which exacerbate the effects of such damage. In men testosterone levels start to decline after 20 years of age[30] and this leads to an appreciable deficit in testosterone concentrations beyond about 50 years of age[30-32]. There could be an intrinsic, physiological reduction in testosterone levels associated with aging[33-36], but there is also evidence for a contribution from psychosocial and life-style factors.

Type A personality classification could contribute to the age-related decline in testosterone levels[37-39], as might be expected since the increased cortisol levels in type A individuals could suppress testosterone levels in men[39]. Life-style influences apparent in associations between low testosterone levels and cigarette smoking, alcohol intake and obesity may also be important. Two longitudinal studies[39,40] and several cross-sectional studies[41-43] have found evidence for lower testosterone levels, or a more rapid decline in testosterone levels with age in cigarette smokers. Not all cross-sectional studies support these findings, however[30,44-48]. Nevertheless, reductions in testosterone levels would be expected on the basis of animal experimental data showing a dose-dependent reduction in testosterone levels in response to cigarette smoking[49,50] or to the components of cigarette smoke[51].

Evidence regarding the effects of alcohol intake on testosterone levels is also inconsistent. Chronic alcoholism[52] and acute intake[53] have been linked to reduced gonadal function. However, with regard to moderate alcohol intake, no association has been observed with testosterone levels[39,47,54,55].

Evidence relating obesity to low testosterone levels is more consistent, the association being apparent over a broad range of degrees of overweight[56,57] and in the increases in testosterone levels accompanying weight loss[46]. Moreover, there is evidence, both from cross-sectional and prospective studies, that the association may be particularly strong with abdominal obesity[58-61].

In adult men low testosterone levels have been linked with low HDL cholesterol, both cross-sectionally[62] and longitudinally[39]. An association between low testosterone and high blood pressure has also been reported[61,63,64], although the majority of reports have been negative[39,65,66]. Other associations with a low testosterone level have included elevated plasma insulin concentrations[67,68], suggesting an association between low testosterone concentrations and insulin resistance, and this is supported by the observation that low testosterone levels can predict the development of type 2 diabetes[69]. Potentially adverse changes in factors of the hemostatic system have also been linked to low testosterone levels. These include elevated fibrinogen and factor VII antigen[65,70] and PAI-1[71].

The strongest risk factor correlates of a low testosterone level therefore appear to be central obesity, low HDL cholesterol and increased insulin concentration. The resemblance of these changes to the classic metabolic syndrome is striking, and it is noteworthy that low testosterone concentrations are linked with elevated leptin levels[72,73], another potential feature of the metabolic syndrome[74]. Metabolically, these associations are likely to synergize. Moreover, they could be augmented by the decreasing muscle mass associated with increasing age and decreasing testosterone levels, which diminishes available metabolizing tissue. Risk factor correlates of

Table 1 Risk factor correlates of a low testosterone level in adult men

Central obesity
Low HDL cholesterol concentrations
Increased insulin concentrations
Type 2 diabetes
Increased leptin concentrations
Increased fibrinogen and factor VII concentrations

a low testosterone level are listed in Table 1. Such associations could account for the observation that, although testosterone levels correlate negatively with severity of coronary disease measured angiographically[75–77], low testosterone levels do not independently predict CHD[64,78–80]. This would be expected if low testosterone was either an initiating or exacerbating factor in a syndrome of changes each of which independently promoted the development of CHD; statistically it will be these changes that emerge as significant in multivariate analysis rather than testosterone itself.

INTERVENTION IN CARDIOVASCULAR RISK-FACTOR DISTURBANCES

In the continuum of risk factor disturbances, prescribed interventions only exist for the most extreme manifestations: hypertension, hyperlipidemia and diabetes. A range of pharmacological strategies, which generally act by inhibiting a key step in the processes involved, are available for dealing with these, for example the angiotensin converting enzyme inhibitors in the case of hypertension, or the HMG CoA reductase inhibitors in the case of hypercholesterolemia. Treatment strategies for diabetes generally involve stimulation either of insulin sensitivity or of insulin secretion, but this may be combined with therapies for any accompanying hypertension or dyslipidemia.

Although, in deteriorating beyond diagnostic limits, risk factor disturbances become disease entities around which systems of clinical practice develop, the relationship between risk factor disturbances and the development of cardiovascular disease is, if not always linear, then at least continuous. In other words there is no such thing as a completely safe level of risk. Many of the consequences of subclinical disturbances in risk factor levels in men have hitherto been regarded simply as the inevitable accompaniments of aging, as has the progressive rise in rates of cardiovascular disease and diabetes with age. But if risk-factor impact could be minimized throughout the male life span, such apparent inevitabilities might be effectively prevented.

While avoiding obesity by limiting calorie intake has been recognized for many years as necessary for general good health, a better understanding of risk-factor relationships has identified a number of specific components of foods that are to be avoided or encouraged. The role of saturated fatty acids in increasing cholesterol levels is well known, but other types of fats may have equally adverse consequences. Trans fatty acids are formed by partial hydrogenation of unsaturated vegetable oils and have been the subject of several epidemiological and experimental studies, which show that some of these fats may be associated with similar increases in risk to those seen with saturated fats[81]. Conversely, fish oils, the omega-3 and omega-6 polyunsaturated fatty acids, may improve the antiatherogenic properties of the tissues into which they are incorporated, as well as improving insulin sensitivity and having antithrombotic properties.

More generally, the effects of increased fruit and vegetable intake have recently been the subject of several large epidemiological investigations, which have consistently found reduced CHD rates in those with the highest intakes[25–27]. This has been ascribed to the accompanying enhancement in the intake of antioxidant vitamins, in particular vitamins E and C, but trials of vitamin E supplementation in the prevention of CHD have generally been negative, so uncertainty remains about the role of specific components of a diet rich in fruit and vegetables.

For men, there are several specific areas in which risk factor modification may be expected

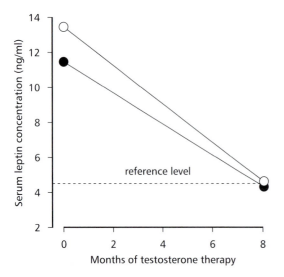

Figure 4 Normalization of serum leptin levels by testosterone therapy in 22 hypogonadal men (serum testosterone < 3.6 nmol/l). Men were randomized to treatment with depot testosterone (open circles: mean level on therapy 14.3 nmol/l) or subcutaneous testosterone pellets (closed circles: mean level on therapy 25.0 nmol/l). The leptin reference level of 4.28 nmol/ml (SD ± /0.52 nmol/ml) was derived from 393 healthy adult men. Data from reference 86

to have particular benefits. In addition to the independent effects of cigarette smoking, the complex of smoking, poor living conditions and respiratory infection has the potential for increasing cardiovascular risk as it relates to infection and inflammation, and there is evidence to support the importance of such a complex[82]. A further complex may be found in decreasing physical activity, increased central body fat and the decreasing testosterone levels seen in the aging male. As described above, this complex could have particularly damaging consequences, with the features of the metabolic syndrome, including dyslipidemia and proinflammatory cytokine release, emerging in force. However, in contrast to the analogous changes in postmenopausal women, endogenous testosterone levels are highly variable and there is considerable overlap in the range between older and younger men[31]. Therefore, it remains to be established whether, in aging men, the combination of low testosterone level

and central obesity, or even low testosterone in itself, could constitute a distinct clinical entity. However, this complex of changes that could particularly affect the aging male does offer points of intervention at all levels. Increased physical activity is clearly the most straightforward of these, and this, in itself, can diminish fat deposition and increase testosterone levels. Physical activity can also increase growth hormone levels. Given the strong association observed between increased adiposity and reduced testosterone levels, reducing fat stores might be expected to increase testosterone levels. Given that the age-related fall in testosterone levels may be an intrinsic physiological change, analogous to the menopause in women, replacement administration of testosterone itself could be of value. Testosterone replacement would be expected to reduce central fat and increase muscle mass, and there is some evidence from both healthy and clinically hypogonadal men that this is indeed the case[83,84]. Beneficial effects of testosterone administration in healthy men have also been demonstrated with regard to fibrinogen and PAI-1[85], and the raised leptin levels seen in hypogonadal men have been shown to fall in response to testosterone (Figure 4)[86]. There is only equivocal evidence at present that these changes extend to insulin resistance or HDL[87-90]. It is possible, however, that beneficial changes in these areas might be primarily a consequence of improvements in body composition and that it would therefore be some time before they become apparent.

This is an area where considerable research will be needed to establish when, or even if, such intervention is appropriate. Administration of androgens, except in a few clearly-defined clinical conditions, has traditionally been viewed as unwarranted and potentially dangerous since, in healthy adults, synthetic androgens cause adverse changes in both HDL levels and insulin sensitivity. However, given the associations between low testosterone levels and an adverse risk-factor profile, it is possible that there is an optimum level in men and that it would be appropriate to correct states of moderate deficiency. Studies evaluating the relative merits of interventions at the life-style or hormonal level will be needed to establish the most effective approach to diminishing the impact of the age-related metabolic syndrome of low levels of testosterone and increased visceral fat in men.

CONCLUSIONS

The broad outline given here of measurements made primarily in the serum and plasma to evaluate cardiovascular risk identifies several key areas in which our knowledge is now sufficiently advanced to justify and provide effective interventions in the aging male. The use of

pharmacological agents, in addition to diet, to alleviate the risk factor disturbances in hypercholesterolemia and diabetes is now a well-established strategy. Dietary strategies long believed to be of benefit, particularly increased fruit and vegetable consumption, are now receiving increasing support from epidemiological studies. The causes and consequences of obesity are increasingly well-understood and emphasize the adverse cardiovascular consequences of excessive calorie intake and physical inactivity. Finally, new areas in which intervention may be of value are being identified, particularly subclinical insulin resistance and the various manifestations of the metabolic syndrome, chronic low-grade inflammation and, in men, the correlated changes that accompany aging and declining testicular function.

References

1. Brousseau ME, Eberhart GP, Dupuis J, *et al.* Cellular cholesterol efflux in heterozygotes for Tangier disease is markedly reduced and correlates with high density lipoprotein cholesterol concentration and particle size. *J Lipid Res* 2000;41:1125–35

2. Nakajima K, Okazaki M, Tanaka A, *et al.* Separation and determination of remnant-like particles in human serum using monoclonal antibodies ro apo B-100 and apo A-1. *J Clin Ligand Assay* 1996;19:177–83

3. Lewis GF, Uffelman KD, Szeto LW, *et al.* Interaction between free fatty acids and insulin in the acute control of very low density lipoprotein production in humans. *J Clin Invest* 1995;95:158–66

4. Austin MA, Hokanson JE, Edwards KL. Hypertriglyceridemia as a cardiovascular risk factor. *Am J Cardiol* 1998;81(4A):7B–12B

5. Pyörälä M, Miettinen H, Halonen P, *et al.* Insulin resistance syndrome predicts the risk of coronary heart disease and stroke in healthy middle-aged men – the 22-year follow-up of the Helsinki Policemen Study. *Arterioscler Thromb Vasc Biol* 2000;20:538–44

6. Danesh J, Collins R, Appleby P, Peto R. Association of fibrinogen, C-reactive protein, albumin, or leukocyte count with coronary heart disease. *J Am Med Assoc* 1998;279: 1477–82

7. Danesh J, Whincup P, Walker M, *et al.* Low grade inflammation and coronary heart disease: prospective study and updated meta-analysis. *Br Med J* 2000;321:199–204

8. Packard CJ, O'Reilly DS, Caslake MJ, *et al.* Lipoprotein-associated phospholipase A2 as an independent predictor of coronary heart disease. West of Scotland Coronary Prevention Study Group. *N Engl J Med* 2000; 343:1148–55

9. Danesh J, Collins R, Peto R, Lowe G. Haematocrit, viscosity, erythrocyte sedimentation rate: meta-analysis of prospective studies of coronary heart disease. *Eur Heart J* 2000;21:515–20

10. Griselli M, Herbert J, Hutchinson WL, *et al.* C-reactive protein and complement are important mediators of tissue damage in acute myocardial infarction. *J Exp Med* 1999; 190:1722–39

11. Lagrand WK, Visser CA, Hermens WT, *et al*. C-Reactive protein as a cardiovascular risk factor: more than an epiphenomenon? *Circulation* 1999;100:96–102

12. Pasceri V, Willerson JT, Yeh ETH. Direct proinflammatory effect of C-reactive protein on human endothelial cells. *Circulation* 2000; 102:2165–8

13. Yudkin JS, Kumari M, Humphries SE, Mohamed-Ali V. Inflammation, obesity, stress and coronary heart disease: is interleukin-6 the link? *Atherosclerosis* 2000;148:209–14

14. Brull D, Humphries S, Montgomery H. Infection, inflammation and coronary artery disease: more than just an association? *Br J Cardiol* 2000;7:681–91

15. Danesh J, Whincup P, Walker M, *et al*. *Chlamydia pneumoniae* IgG titres and coronary heart disease: prospective study and meta-analysis. *Br Med J* 2000;321:208–13

16. Kuusisto J, Mykkänen L, Pyorälä K, Laakso M. Hyperinsulinemic microalbuminuria: a new risk indicator for coronary heart disease. *Circulation* 1995;91:831–7

17. Godsland IF, Rosankiewicz JR, Proudler AJ, Johnston DG. Plasma total homocysteine concentrations are unrelated to insulin sensitivity and components of the metabolic syndrome in healthy men. *J Clin Endocrinol Metab* 2001;86:719–23

18. Christen WG, Ajani UA, Glynn RJ, Hennekens CH. Blood levels of homocysteine and increased risks of cardiovascular disease: causal or casual? *Arch Intern Med* 2000; 160:422–34

19. Wingard DL, Suarez L, Barrett-Connor E. The sex differential in mortality from all causes and ischemic heart disease. *Am J Epidemiol* 1983;117:165–72

20. Kannel W. Metabolic risk factors for coronary heart disease in women: perspective from the Framingham Study. *Am Heart J* 1987;114: 413–19

21. Miller Bass K, Newschaffer CJ, Klag MJ, Bush TL. Plasma lipoprotein levels as predictors of cardiovascular death in women. *Arch Intern Med* 1993;153:2209–16

22. Tan KCB, Shiu SWM, Kung AWC. Alterations in hepatic lipase and lipoprotein subfractions with transdermal testosterone replacement therapy. *Clin Endocrinol* 1999;51:765–9

23. Amiel SA, Sherwin RS, Simonson DC, *et al*. Impaired insulin action in puberty. *N Engl J Med* 1986;315:215–19

24. Tang J, Srivastava RAK, Krul ES, *et al. In vivo* regulation of apolipoprotein A-I gene expression by estradiol and testosterone occurs by different mechanisms in inbred strains of mice. *J Lipid Res* 1991;32:1571–85

25. Liu S, Manson JE, Lee IM, *et al*. Fruit and vegetable intake and risk of cardiovascular disease: the Women's Health Study. *Am J Clin Nutr* 2000;72:922–8

26. Kant AK. Consumption of energy-dense, nutrient-poor foods by adult Americans: nutritional and health implications. The third National Health and Nutrition Examination Survey 1988–1994. *Am J Clin Nutr* 2000; 72:929–36

27. Hu FB, Rimm EB, Stampfer MJ, *et al*. Prospective study of major dietary patterns and risk of coronary heart disease in men. *Am J Clin Nutr* 2000;72:912–21

28. Ericsson S, Eriksson M, Vitols S, *et al*. Influence of age on the metabolism of plasma low density lipoproteins in healthy males. *J Clin Invest* 1991;87:591–6

29. Ariens RA, Coppola R, Potenza I, Mannucci PM. The increase with age of the components of the tissue factor coagulation pathway is gender-dependent. *Blood Coagul Fibrinolysis* 1995;6:433–7

30. Simon D, Preziosi P, Barrett-Connor E, *et al*. The influence of aging on plasma sex hormones in men: the Telecom Study. *Am J Epidemiol* 1992;135:783–91

31. Vermeulen A, Rubens R, Verdonck L. Testosterone secretion and metabolism in male senescence. *J Clin Endocrinol Metab* 1972; 34:730–5

32. Gray A, Feldman HA, McKinlay JB, Longcope C. Age, disease, and changing sex hormone levels in middle-aged men: results of the Massachusetts Male Aging Study. *J Clin Endocrinol Metab* 1991;73:1016–25

33. Rubens R, Dhont M, Vermeulen A. Further studies on Leydig cell function in old age. *J Clin Endocrinol Metab* 1974;39:40–5

34. Takahashi J, Higashi Y, LaNasa JA, et al. Studies of the human testis XVIII. Simultaneous measurement of nine intratesticular steroids: evidence for reduced mitochondrial function in testis of elderly men. *J Clin Endocrinol Metab* 1983;56:1178–87

35. Harman SM, Tsitouras PD, Costa PT, Blackman MR. Reproductive hormones in aging men. II. Basal pituitary gonadotropins and gonadotropin responses to luteinizing hormone-releasing hormone. *J Clin Endocrinol Metab* 1982;54:547–51

36. Harman SM, Metter EJ, Tobin JD, et al. Longitudinal effects of aging on serum total and free testosterone levels in healthy men. *J Clin Endocrinol Metab* 2001;86:724–31

37. Zumoff B, Rosenfeld RS, Friedman M, et al. Elevated daytime urinary excretion of testosterone glucuronide in men with the type A behavior pattern. *Psychosom Med* 1984;46:223–5

38. Nilsson PM, Moller L, Solstad K. Adverse effects of psychosocial stress on gonadal function and insulin levels in middle-aged males. *J Intern Med* 1995;237:479–86

39. Zmuda JM, Cauley JA, Kriska A, et al. Longitudinal relation between endogenous testosterone and cardiovascular disease risk factors in middle-aged men: a 13-year follow-up of former multiple risk factor intervention trial participants. *Am J Epidemiol* 1997;147:609–27

40. Pearson JD, Blackman MR, Metter EJ, et al. Effects of age and cigarette smoking on longitudinal changes in androgens and SHBG in healthy men. Presented at the *77th Annual Meeting of the Endocrine Society*. Washington DC, 1995;abstr.323

41. Briggs MH. Cigarette smoking and infertility in men. *Med J Aust* 1973;1:616–17

42. Sofikitis N, Miyagawa I, Dimitriadis D, et al. Effects of smoking on testicular function, semen quality, and sperm fertilising capacity. *J Urol* 1995;154:1030–4

43. Shaarawy M, Mahmoud KZ. Endocrine profile and semen characteristics in male smokers. *Fertil Steril* 1982;38:255–7

44. Deslypere JP, Vermeulen A. Leydig cell function in normal men: effect of age, life-style, residence, diet and activity. *J Clin Endocrinol Metab* 1984;59:955–62

45. Vogt HJ, Heller WD, Borelli S. Sperm quality of healthy smokers, ex-smokers, and never-smokers. *Fertil Steril* 1986;45:106–10

46. Dai WS, Gutai JP, Kuller LH, Cauley JA. Cigarette smoking and serum sex hormones in men. *Am J Epidemiol* 1988;128:796–805

47. Field AE, Colditz GA, Willett WC, et al. The relation of smoking, age, relative weight, and dietary intake to serum adrenal steroids, sex hormones, and sex-hormone-binding globulin in middle-aged men. *J Clin Endocrinol Metab* 1994;79:1310–16

48. Barrett-Connor E, Khaw K-T. Cigarette smoking and increased endogenous estrogen levels in men. *Am J Epidemiol* 1987;126:187–92

49. Mittler JC, Pogach L, Ertel NH. Effects of chronic smoking on testosterone metabolism in dogs. *J Steroid Biochem* 1983;18:759–63

50. Yardimci S, Atan A, Delibasi T, et al. Long-term effects of cigarette smoke exposure on plasma testosterone, luteinizing hormone and follicle stimulating hormone levels in male rats. *Br J Urol* 1997;79:66–9

51. Yeh J, Barbieri RL, Friedman AJ. Nicotine and cotinine inhibit rat testis androgen biosynthesis *in vitro*. *J Steroid Biochem* 1989;33:627–30

52. Irwin M, Dreyfus E, Baird S, et al. Testosterone in chronic alcoholic men. *Br J Addict* 1988;83:949–53

53. Gordon CG, Altman K, Southren AL, et al. Effect of alcohol (ethanol) administration on sex-hormone metabolism in normal men. *N Engl J Med* 1976;295:793–7

54. Sparrow D, Bosse R, Rowe JW. The influence of age, alcohol consumption, and body build on gonadal function in men. *J Clin Endocrinol Metab* 1980;51:508–12

55. Dai WS, Kuller LH, LaPorte RE, et al. The epidemiology of plasma testosterone levels in middle aged men. *Am J Epidemiol* 1981;114:804–16

56. Glass AR, Swerdloff RS, Bray GA, et al. Low serum testosterone and sex-hormone-binding-globulin in massively obese men. *J Clin Endocrinol Metab* 1977;45:1211–19

57. Zumoff B, Strain GW, Miller LK, *et al.* Plasma free and non-sex-hormone-binding-globulin-bound testosterone are decreased in obese men in proportion to their degree of obesity. *J Clin Endocrinol Metab* 1990;71: 929–31

58. Seidell JC, Bjorntorp P, Sjostrom L, *et al.* Visceral fat accumulation in men is positively associated with insulin, glucose, and C-peptide levels, but negatively with testosterone levels. *Metabolism* 1990;39:897–901

59. Khaw K-T, Barrett-Connor E. Lower endogenous androgens predict central adiposity in men. *Ann Epidemiol* 1992;2:675–82

60. Haffner SM, Karhapaa P, Mykkanen L, Laakso M. Insulin resistance, body fat distribution and sex hormones in men. *Diabetes* 1994;43:212–19

61. Simon D, Charles MA, Nahoul K, *et al.* Association between plasma total testosterone and cardiovascular risk factors in healthy adult men: The Telecom Study. *J Clin Endocrinol Metab* 1997;82:682–5

62. Barrett-Connor EL. Testosterone and risk factors for cardiovascular disease in men. *Diabetes Metab* 1995;21:156–61

63. Khaw KT, Barrett-Connor E. Blood pressure and endogenous testosterone in men: an inverse relationship. *J Hypertens* 1988;6: 329–32

64. Barrett-Connor E, Khaw KT. Endogenous sex hormones and cardiovascular disease in men. A prospective population-based study. *Circulation* 1988;78:539–45

65. Bonithon-Kopp C, Scarabin PY, Bara L, *et al.* Relationship between sex hormones and hemostatic factors in healthy middle-aged men. *Atherosclerosis* 1988;71:71–6

66. Dai WS, Gutai JP, Kuller LH, *et al.* Relation between plasma high-density lipoprotein cholesterol and sex hormone concentrations in men. *Am J Cardiol* 1984;53:1259–63

67. Simon D, Preziosi P, Barrett-Connor E, *et al.* Interrelation between plasma testosterone and plasma insulin in healthy adult men: the Telecom Study. *Diabetologia* 1992;35:173–7

68. Haffner SM, Valdez RA, Mykkanen L, *et al.* Decreased testosterone and dehydroepiandrosterone sulfate concentrations are associated with increased insulin and glucose concentrations in nondiabetic men. *Metabolism* 1994;43:599–603

69. Stellato RK, Feldman HA, Hamdy O, *et al.* Testosterone, sex hormone binding globulin, and the development of type 2 diabetes in middle-aged men: prospective results from the Massachusetts Male Aging Study. *Diabetes Care* 2000;23:490–4

70. Glueck CJ, Glueck HI, Stroop D, *et al.* Endogenous testosterone, fibrinolysis, and coronary heart disease risk in hyperlipidaemic men. *J Lab Clin Med* 1993;122:412–20

71. Caron P, Benet A, Camare R, Louvet JP. Plasminogen activator inhibitor in plasma is related to testosterone in men. *Metabolism* 1988;38:1010–15

72. Vettor R, De Pergola G, Pagano C, *et al.* Gender differences in serum leptin in obese people: relationships with testosterone, body fat distribution and insulin sensitivity. *Eur J Clin Invest* 1997;27:1016–24

73. Baumgartner RN, Waters DL, Morley JE, *et al.* Age-related changes in sex hormones affect the sex difference in serum leptin independently of changes in body fat. *Metabolism* 1999;48:378–84

74. Leyva F, Godsland IF, Ghatei M, *et al.* Hyperleptinemia as a component of a metabolic syndrome of cardiovascular risk. *Arterioscler Thromb Vasc Biol* 1998;18: 928–33

75. Barth JD, Jansen H, Hugenholtz PG, Birkenhager JC. Post-heparin lipases, lipids and related hormones in men undergoing arteriography to assess atherosclerosis. *Atherosclerosis* 1983;48:235–41

76. Chute CG, Baron JA, Plymate SR, *et al.* Sex hormones and coronary artery disease. *Am J Med* 1987;83:853–9

77. Phillips GB, Pinkernell BH, Jing TY. The association of hypotestosterinaemia with coronary artery disease in men. *Arterioscler Thromb* 1994;14:701–6

78. Cauley JA, Gutai JP, Kuller LH, Dai WS. Usefulness of sex steroid hormone levels in predicting coronary artery disease in men. *Am J Cardiol* 1987;60:771–7

79. Phillips GB, Yano K, Stemmermann GN. Serum sex hormone levels and myocardial infarction in the Honolulu Heart Program.

Pitfalls in prospective studies on sex hormones. *J Clin Epidemiol* 1988;41:1151–6

80. Yarnell JW, Beswick AD, Sweetnam PM, Riad-Fahmy D. Endogenous sex hormones and ischaemic heart disease in men. The Caerphilly prospective study. *Arterioscler Thromb* 1993;13:517–20

81. Oomen CM, Ocké MC, Feskens JM, *et al.* Association between trans fatty acid intake and 10-year risk of coronary heart disease in the Zutphen Elderly Study: a prospective population-based study. *Lancet* 2001;357: 746–51

82. Grimes DS, Hindle E, Dyer T. Respiratory infection and coronary heart disease: progression of a paradigm. *Q J Med* 2000;93:375–83

83. Marin P, Holmang S, Jonsson L, *et al.* The effects of testosterone on body composition and metabolism in middle aged men. *Int J Obes Relat Metab Disord* 1992;16:991–7

84. Bhasin S, Storer TW, Berman N, *et al.* Testosterone replacement increases fat-free mass and muscle size in hypogonadal men. *J Clin Endocrinol Metab* 1997;82:407–13

85. Anderson RA, Ludlam CA, Wu FC. Hemostatic effects of supraphysiological levels of testosterone in normal men. *Haemost* 1995;74:693–7

86. Jockenhovel F, Blum WF, Vogel E, *et al.* Testosterone substitution normalizes elevated serum leptin levels in hypogonadal men. *J Clin Endocrinol Metab* 1997;82:2510–13

87. Ebeling P, Stenman UH, Seppala M, Koivisto VA. Acute hyperinsulinemia, androgen homeostasis and insulin sensitivity in healthy men. *J Endocrinol* 1995;146:63–9

88. Arslanian S, Suprasongsin C. Testosterone treatment in adolescents with delayed puberty: changes in body composition, protein, fat, and glucose metabolism. *J Clin Endocrinol Metab* 1997;82:3213–20

89. Pasquali R, Macor C, Vicennati V, *et al.* Effects of acute hyperinsulinemia on testosterone concentrations in adult obese and normal-weight men. *Metabolism* 1997;46: 526–9

90. Zgliczynski S, Ossowski M, Slowinska-Srzednicka J, *et al.* Effect of testosterone replacement therapy on lipids and lipoproteins in hypogonadal and elderly men. *Atherosclerosis* 1996;121:35–43

rogens and nary heart disease: evidence from animal models of atherosclerosis

Peter Alexandersen, MD

INTRODUCTION

The effects of steroids and other drugs on human coronary heart disease (CHD) and stroke are difficult to evaluate, not least because of the confounding effect of life-style factors such as diet, smoking and exercise as well as the emerging area of responses specific to certain genetic polymorphisms. Animals have been extensively used as experimental models of human atherosclerosis for over 80 years, ever since Anitschkow[1] induced atheromatous lesions in rabbits by feeding a cholesterol-rich diet. This experimental approach, now extended to rodents, dogs and monkeys, offers the added benefit of allowing us to investigate the underlying mechanisms of drug effects on atherosclerosis, for instance by culturing and studying arterial cells from hormone-treated animals and by using invasive techniques such as quantitative coronary angiography to look at arterial function. Animal studies may provide hints as to the likely effects of steroid hormones on human metabolism and ultimately on the risk of cardiovascular disease.

In the area of steroid hormones, female fat-fed cynomolgus monkeys have been extensively studied as a model of human atherosclerosis, as they have a 28-day menstrual cycle and show menopausal and steroid-induced changes in plasma lipoprotein levels. Despite these attractions there are now serious concerns over whether the endpoints used in these monkey studies, such as changes in the size of atherosclerotic plaques in response to estrogen, accurately reflect the clinical effects of such hormones in humans.

Accumulating evidence suggests that steroid treatment of monkeys and rabbits produces rather similar results in terms of atherosclerosis. As primates are in increasingly short supply, owing to national bans on their export, rabbits provide an attractive alternative. There are drawbacks: the plasma lipoprotein responses to diet and steroid hormones show some dissimilarities to those seen in humans. There is also a problem with the heterogeneity in plaque size resulting from cholesterol feeding, necessitating rather larger numbers of animals in the treatment groups. Nevertheless, the relatively low cost, easy availability and affordable housing requirements of rabbits have led to the common use of this species in atherosclerosis research. A role in the safety evaluation of androgens and other therapies for the aging male is now firmly established.

EXPERIMENTAL STUDIES OF EXOGENOUS ANDROGENS IN FAT-FED ANIMALS

Published studies investigating the influence of androgens on atherogenesis in fat-fed animals are summarized in Table 1[2-16]. The most commonly used steroids are natural androgens such as testosterone and dehydroepiandrosterone (DHEA); synthetic androgens such as stanozolol and nandrolone have also been used. There are differences in the diets used in these studies, confounded by the use of female animals in many studies. The endpoints in these studies range from the direct determination of the cholesterol content of the arterial wall to the presence or extent of atherosclerotic plaques. Others have looked at the arterial content of collagen as a marker of atherosclerosis.

Overall, these data indicate that androgens are perhaps more likely to protect males from atherosclerosis than to cause it. In a well-conducted study, Gordon and colleagues[6] studied the effect of oral DHEA administration on atherogenesis in 34 cholesterol-fed male rabbits. In order to accelerate the atherogenic process the authors used 'balloon' catheterization to strip the intimal layer of arteries in two of the groups. Twelve weeks of therapy resulted in supraphysiological plasma DHEA levels and a 50% reduction in plaque size compared with the findings in control animals ($p = 0.006$). Although the reduction in plaque size was found to correlate inversely with plasma DHEA levels, no such correlations were seen with changes in plasma lipoprotein levels, suggesting other pathogenic mechanisms. In a study of cardiac transplantation in rabbits[10] DHEA was given to cholesterol-fed male rabbits, some of which had received donor-heart implants

anastomosed to the abdominal aorta, a procedure known to accelerate atherosclerosis. Transsectional cuts of coronary arteries from both unmodified and transplanted rabbits treated with DHEA showed a marked and significant reduction in atherogenic plaque formation compared with the findings in controls (62 and 45%, respectively; $p < 0.05$), and the number of stenosed vessels was reduced by 50% compared with the number in controls ($p < 0.05$). Although the number of animals dying during surgery is a cause for concern, these results strongly support the ability of DHEA to retard atherosclerosis, at least in this model system.

In another study, castrated male rabbits were treated with testosterone enanthate (twice weekly for 17 weeks); plasma cholesterol levels were then 'clamped', i.e. maintained at constantly elevated levels by adjusting the fat content of their diet[11]. The authors found no statistically significant difference in aortic accumulation of cholesterol between the testosterone- and placebo-treated animals at necropsy, concluding that testosterone had no effect on atherogenesis. However, methodological problems in terms of absorption and/or metabolism of testosterone may have influenced these results, since half of the animals showed only modest increases in serum total cholesterol concentrations compared with the remaining half, despite individual feeding. In an interesting study[14], castrated cholesterol-fed male and female rabbits were treated with testosterone (given intramuscularly as enanthate), estradiol, or a combination of both for 12 weeks. An untreated group served as controls. Morphometric analysis of the intimal thickening of the proximal aorta showed a significant ($p < 0.05$) reduction in plaque size in male rabbits treated with testosterone and in female rabbits treated with estrogen. In rabbits treated with both steroids, plaque size was significantly smaller than in control animals ($p < 0.05$), effects independent of plasma lipid

Table 1 Published studies on cholesterol-fed animals to investigate the effect of exogenous androgens on atherogenesis

Species	Authors	Year	No. of animals	Duration of study	Androgen(s)	Influence of androgen(s)
Female dogs	Sirek et al.[2]	1977	22	11 weeks	T	↔
Cockerels	Copeman et al.[3]	1984	36	87 days	T	→
Male chicks	Toda et al.[4]	1984	24	7 weeks	T	←
Female rabbits	Fischer et al.[5]	1985	54*	10 weeks	T	←
Male rabbits	Gordon et al.[6]	1988	34	12 weeks	DHEA	→
Male rabbits	Wojcicki et al.[7]	1989	20	12 weeks	T	→
Male and female rabbits	Arad et al.[8]	1989	15 (2m + 13f)	8 weeks	DHEA	→
Male rabbits	Fogelberg et al.[9]	1990	17	12 weeks	STAN	↔
Male rabbits	Eich et al.[10]	1993	48	5 weeks	DHEA	→
Male rabbits	Larsen et al.[11]	1993	36	17 weeks	TE	↔/↓
Female cynomolgus monkeys	Adams et al.[12]	1995	64	32 months	T	↑
Female cynomolgus monkeys	Obasanjo et al.[13]	1996	59	2 years	NAN	↑
Male and female rabbits	Bruck et al.[14]	1997	64 (32m + 32f)	12 weeks	T	→
Male rabbits	Alexandersen et al.[15]	1999	100	30 weeks	TE, TU, DHEA	→
Female rabbits	Hayashi et al.[16]	2000	48	10 weeks	DHEA	→

DHEA, dehydroepiandrosterone; NAN, nandrolone decanoate; STAN, stanozolol; T, testosterone; TE, testosterone enanthate; TU, testosterone undecanoate; m, males; f, females. ↑, ↓ and ↔ indicate an increase, decrease or no change, respectively, in atherogenesis vs. contol animals. *The number is estimated, as the exact number is not given by the authors ($52 \leq n \leq 56$)

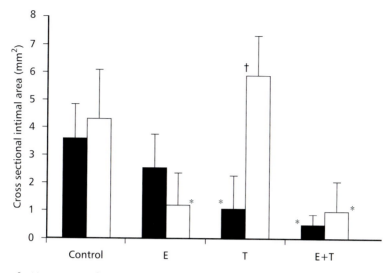

Figure 1 Mean extent of neointimal thickening (from three serial cross sections of the aortic arch in male (■) and female (□) cholesterol-fed rabbits (0.5%). Controls were fed cholesterol without hormones. E, estradiol valerate (1 mg/kg body weight, once a week); T, testosterone enanthate (25 mg/kg body weight intramuscularly once a week). Treatment lasted for 12 weeks. In females, plaque development was inhibited by E or E + T compared with controls ($p < 0.05$). In males, plaque development was inhibited by T or E + T compared with controls ($p < 0.05$).*Between hormone-treated groups and control group for each gender. †Between corresponding male and female rabbits with regard to their respective control groups. Data from reference 14

and lipoprotein levels. However, plaque size was significantly increased in female animals treated with testosterone compared with males ($p < 0.05$) (Figure 1), in line with two studies of female monkeys treated with testosterone[12,13]. There was also a trend towards an increased plaque size in male animals treated with estrogen compared with females. These data are important in that they suggest that both testosterone and estradiol may possess gender-specific effects in terms of atherogenesis.

A protective effect of both DHEA and testosterone (both oral and parenteral) was found in a larger study of castrated, cholesterol-fed male rabbits[15]. This was linked to changes in plasma lipoprotein levels. Castration also resulted in a significant ($p < 0.01$) reduction in the aortic accumulation of cholesterol. New studies using transgenic animals such as apoE knockout mice may help towards further investigation of the impact of exogenous androgens on atherogenesis.

ANDROGENIC MECHANISM OF ACTION

Studies using male and/or female animals to investigate the mechanisms behind the changes in atherosclerosis are summarized in Table 2. In sharp contrast to the whole animal studies detailed in Table 1, 15 out of 23 studies in Table 2 suggested that natural androgens in general (and testosterone in particular) have a deleterious influence on arteries, which suggests that androgens may increase the risk of CHD. However, in many of the 'mechanistic' studies, no discrimination was made as to the sex (male or female) of cells used in the cell/tissue cultures or of the vascular rings studied. Often a mixture of males and females was used which may be crucial as to genomic effects of androgens[14]. For DHEA, the mechanistic studies consistently indicated a favorable effect of this androgen on cardiovascular risk factors. There appears to be a distinct trend whereby

Table 2 In vitro studies of androgen effects on isolated cell cultures or vascular rings and experimental in vivo studies on vascular resistance or serum lipoproteins.

Species	Authors	Year	Type of study or cell culture used	Androgen(s)	Influence of androgen(s)	Consideration of effect
Male and female cats	Bhargava et al.[17]	1967	in vivo	T	blood pressure ↑	unfavorable
Male rats	Fischer and Swain[18]	1977	in vivo	T	vascular connective tissue ↑	unfavorable
Male rats	Wolinsky[19]	1972	in vivo	T	vascular connective tissue ↑	unfavorable
Male and female dogs	Greensberg et al.[20]	1974	in vivo	T	vasoconstriction	unfavorable
Male and female rats	Baker et al.[21]	1978	in vivo	T	blood pressure ↑	unfavorable
Male rats	Nakao et al.[22]	1981	aortic VSMCs	T	prostacyclin synthesis ↓	unfavorable
Male and female rats and rabbits	Karanian et al.[23]	1982	aortic rings	T	vasoconstriction	unfavorable
Male (?) calves	Bronson et al.[24]	1987	aortic VSMCs	T	lysyl oxidase activity ↑	unfavorable
Male and female rats and rabbits	Wakasugi et al.[25]	1989	rat aortic rings, rabbit aortic VSMCs	T	prostacyclin synthesis ↔ in males but ↓ in females	
Male rats	Masuda et al.[26]	1991	aortic VSMCs	T	TxA_2 receptors ↑	unfavorable
Male rats	Hölmang and Björntorp[27]	1992	in vivo	T	insulin resistance ↑	unfavorable
Male cynomolgus monkeys	Weyrich et al.[28]	1992	in vivo	T	TxB_2 ↑, HDL-C ↓	unfavorable
Female rats	Mohan and Jacobson[29]	1993	peritoneal Mφ	DHEA, T	superoxide generation ↓*	favorable
Male rats	Fujimoto et al.[30]	1994	aortic VSMCs	T, DHT	androgen receptor expression ↑, proliferation of VSMCs ↑	unfavorable
Male guinea pigs	Schror et al.[31]	1994	coronary artery VSMCs	T	vasoconstriction	unfavorable
Male and female rabbits	Yue et al.[32]	1995	vascular rings	T	vasodilatation	favorable
Male and female pigs	Farhat et al.[33]	1995	coronary artery rings	T	vasoconstriction	unfavorable
Male dogs	Chou et al.[34]	1996	in vivo	T	vasodilatation	favorable
Male (?) mice[†]	Taniguchi et al.[35]	1996	Mφ	DHEA	cholesteryl ester accumulation ↓	favorable
?	Mohan and Benghuzzi[36]	1997	endothelial cells	DHEA	proliferation ↓	favorable
Male rabbits	Hutchison et al.[37]	1997	aortic rings	T	endothelium-dependent relaxation ↓	unfavorable
Male (?) rabbits[†]	Furutama et al.[38]	1998	VSMCs	DHEA	proliferation ↓ and migration ↓	favorable
Male rats	Stokes et al.[39]	2000	plasma TC	T, DHT, AED	plasma TC ↓	favorable

AED, androstenedione; DHEA, dehydroepiandrosterone; DHT, dihydrotestosterone; HDL-C, high-density lipoprotein cholesterol; Mφ, macrophages; T, testosterone; TC, total cholesterol; Tx, thromboxane; VSMCs, vascular smooth muscle cells. *The inhibition of superoxide generation was found to be minimal for T. ↑, ↓ and ↔ indicate an increase, decrease or no change, respectively, in atherogenesis vs. contol animals. † The gender of the animals used was not reported benefit was found by the more recent studies in contrast to the older studies. In part, this might be due to the use of more clinically relevant doses or improvements in study design.

Another important issue relates to the androgen exposure of the tissue(s) studied. Acute effects may be mediated through non-genomic effects such as calcium channels[32] and thus not reflect effects caused by long-term (or chronic) androgen therapy. Therefore, the phenomena seen in these experimental studies may not reflect the clinical outcome in male patients receiving long-term androgen replacement.

More recently, Hayashi and colleagues[16] tested the hypothesis that the beneficial effect of DHEA on atherogenesis is mediated through the conversion to estradiol via aromatase. Despite the fact that they used female animals, their data were consistent with this hypothesis, and also pointed to an endothelium-dependent increase in the synthesis of nitric oxide (NO). If these results are confirmed, it is tempting to speculate that indeed all aromatizable androgens may use this pathway and that local estrogen synthesis at the vascular level may in part be responsible for the atheroprotective effect of androgens seen in these experimental animal studies. This mechanism of action, if also of biological importance for testosterone in men, may counteract the seemingly deleterious effects of testosterone, but this still remains to be investigated. Non-aromatizable androgens (e.g. dihydrotestosterone and synthetic compounds) may therefore work through different mechanisms.

The lack of intact sympathetic and parasympathetic nerve fibers to the vascular smooth muscle cells in ring preparations should also be kept in mind when evaluating these data. For instance, it has been shown that estradiol affects the muscarinic receptors of vascular smooth muscle cells. Androgens themselves or by conversion into estrogen may have similar influences.

The route of androgen administration in terms of vascular effects is also an issue that needs much more study. In our study of fat-fed male rabbits[15], testosterone was given either orally or intramuscularly, and despite the fact that an antiatherogenic effect was observed for both modalities, the serum concentrations obtained and thus the exposure of vascular tissue to testosterone differed between groups. This might be important regarding the accumulation of cholesterol[15]. Attention should be paid to the influence of route of administration of androgens on cardiovascular risk factors.

CONCLUSIONS

Experimental animal studies continue to be used to investigate the effect of androgen therapies on atherogenesis in an attempt to predict the likely effects of such therapies on the health of aging men. Such studies are of particular importance in that they may reveal the underlying mechanisms behind the gross effects on vascular pathology. Regrettably, these studies vary much in experimental design and differ with respect to species and even gender. The data point to an atherosclerotic effect of androgens in female monkeys[12,13] and rabbits[5,14], but the the lack of studies of androgen replacement therapies in male monkeys is a concern.

Until these issues are resolved it is difficult to extrapolate the current data to man considering androgen replacement or supplementation. Nevertheless, animal models may be useful in screening drugs for potential beneficial effects in humans and in elucidating mechanisms of action of sex hormones on the vasculature. Further animal research (particularly mechanistic and secondary prevention studies) are likely to be useful in studying both the 'classic' and the 'designer' androgens.

References

1. Anitschkow N. Über die atherosklerose der aorta beim Kaninchen und über deren entstehungsbedingungen. *Beitr path Anatomie allgem Pathol* 1914;59:306–48

2. Sirek OV, Sirek A, Fikar K. The effect of sex hormones on glycosaminoglycan content of canine aorta and coronary arteries. *Atherosclerosis* 1977;27:227–33

3. Copeman HA, Papadimitriou JM, Watson IG. Hormonal effects on prevention or regression of atheroma. *Adv Exp Med Biol* 1984;168: 51–84

4. Toda T, Toda Y, Cho BH, Kummerow FA. Ultrastructural changes in the comb and aorta of chicks fed excess testosterone. *Atherosclerosis* 1984;51:47–57

5. Fischer GM, Bashey RI, Rosenbaum H, Lyttle CR. A possible mechanism in arterial wall for mediation of sex difference in atherosclerosis. *Exp Mol Pathol* 1985;43:288–96

6. Gordon GB, Bush DE, Weisman HF. Reduction of atherosclerosis by administration of dehydroepiandrosterone. A study in the hypercholesterolemic New Zealand white rabbit with aortic intimal injury. *J Clin Invest* 1988;82:712–20

7. Wojcicki J, Tustanowski S, Samochowiec L. Endocrine function in atherosclerotic rabbits. *Pol J Pharmacol Pharm* 1989;41:109–13

8. Arad Y, Badimon JJ, Badimon L, *et al.* Dehydroepiandrosterone feeding prevents aortic fatty streak formation and cholesterol accumulation in cholesterol-fed rabbit. *Arteriosclerosis* 1989;9:159–66

9. Fogelberg M, Björkhem I, Diczfalusy U, Henriksson P. Stanozolol and experimental atherosclerosis: atherosclerotic development and blood lipids during anabolic steroid therapy of New Zealand white rabbits. *Scand J Clin Lab Invest* 1990;50:693–6

10. Eich DM, Nestler JE, Johnson DE, *et al.* Inhibition of accelerated coronary atherosclerosis with dehydroepiandrosterone in the heterotopic rabbit model of cardiac transplantation. *Circulation* 1993;87:261–9

11. Larsen BA, Nordestgaard BG, Stender S, Kjeldsen K. Effect of testosterone in atherogenesis in cholesterol-fed rabbits with similar plasma cholesterol levels. *Atherosclerosis* 1993;99:79–86

12. Adams MR, Williams JK, Kaplan JR. Effects of androgens on coronary artery atherosclerosis and atherosclerosis-related impairment of vascular responsiveness. *Arterioscler Thromb Vasc Biol* 1995;15:562–70

13. Obasanjo IO, Clarkson TB, Weaver DS. Effects of the anabolic steroid nandrolone decanoate on plasma lipid and coronary arteries of female cynomolgus macaques. *Metabolism* 1996;45:463–8

14. Bruck B, Brehme U, Guel N, *et al.* Gender-specific differences in the effects of testosterone and estrogen on the development of atherosclerosis in rabbits. *Arterioslcer Thromb Vasc Biol* 1997;17:2192–9

15. Alexandersen P, Haarbo J, Byrjalsen I, *et al.* Natural androgens inhibit male atherosclerosis: a study in castrated, cholesterol-fed rabbits. *Circ Res* 1999;84:813–19

16. Hayashi T, Esaki T, Muto E, *et al.* Dehydroepiandrosterone retards atherosclerosis formation through its conversion to estrogen: the possible role of nitric oxide. *Arterioscler Thromb Vasc Biol* 2000;20:782–92

17. Bhargava KP, Dhavan KN, Saxena RC. Enhancement of noradrenaline pressor responses in testosterone-treated cats. *Br J Pharmacol* 1967;31:26–31

18. Fischer GM, Swain ML. Effect of sex hormones on blood pressure and vascular connective tissue in castrated and non-castrated male rats. *Am J Physiol* 1977;232: H617–21

19. Wolinsky H. Effects of androgen treatment on the male rat aorta. *J Clin Invest* 1972;51: 2552–5

20. Greensberg S, George WR, Kadowitz PJ, Wilson WR. Androgen-induced enhancement of vascular reactivity. *Can J Physiol Pharmacol* 1974;52:14–22

21. Baker PJ, Ramey E, Ramwell PW. Androgen-mediated sex differences of cardiovascular responses in rats. *Am J Physiol* 1978;235:H242–6

22. Nakao J, Change WC, Murota SI, Orimo H. Testosterone inhibits prostacyclin production by rat aortic smooth muscle cells in culture. *Atherosclerosis* 1981;39:203–9

23. Karanian JW, Sintetos AL, Moran FM, *et al*. Androgenic regulation of vascular responses to prostaglandins. In Herman AG, Vanhoutte PM, Denolin H, Goossens A, eds. *Cardiovascular Pharmacology of the Prostaglandins*. New York: Raven Press, 1982:245–58

24. Bronson RE, Claaman SD, Traish AM, Kagan HM. Stimulation of lysyl oxidase (EC 1.4.3.13) activity by testosterone and characterization of androgen receptors in cultured calf aorta smooth muscle cells. *Biochem J* 1987;244:317–23

25. Wakasugi M, Noguchi T, Kazama YI, *et al*. The effects of sex hormones on the synthesis of prostacyclin (PGI2) by vascular tissues. *Prostaglandins* 1989;37:401–10

26. Masuda A, Mathur R, Halushka PV. Testosterone increases thromboxane A_2 receptors in cultured rat aortic smooth muscle cells. *Circ Res* 1991;69:638–43

27. Hölmang A, Björntorp P. The effects of testosterone on insulin sensitivity in male rats. *Acta Physiol Scand* 1992;146:505–10

28. Weyrich AS, Rejeski WJ, Brubaker PH, Parks JS. The effects of testosterone on lipids and eicosanoids in cynomolgus monkeys. *Med Sci Sports Exerc* 1992;24:333–8

29. Mohan PF, Jacobson MS. Inhibition of macrophage superoxide generation by dehydroepiandrosterone. *Am J Med Sci* 1993;306:10–15

30. Fujimoto R, Morimoto I, Morita E, *et al*. Androgen receptors, 5 alpha-reductase activity and androgen-dependent proliferation of vascular smooth muscle cells. *J Steroid Biochem Mol Biol* 1994;50:169–74

31. Schror K, Morinelli TA, Masuda A, *et al*. Testosterone treatment enhances thromboxane A2 mimetic induced coronary artery vasoconstriction in guinea pigs. *Eur J Clin Invest* 1994;24(Suppl 1):50–2

32. Yue P, Chatterjee K, Beale C, *et al*. Testosterone relaxes rabbit coronary arteries and aorta. *Circulation* 1995;91:1154–60

33. Farhat MY, Wolfe R, *et al*. Effect of testosterone treatment on vasoconstrictor response of left anterior descending artery in male and female pigs. *J Cardiovasc Pharmacol* 1995;25:495–500

34. Chou TM, Sudir K, Hutchison SJ, *et al*. Testosterone induces dilation of canine coronary conductance and resistance arteries *in vivo*. *Circulation* 1996;94:2614–19

35. Taniguchi S, Yanase T, Kobayashi K, *et al*. Dehydroepiandrosterone markedly inhibits the accumulation of cholesteryl ester in mouse macrophage J774–1 cells. *Atherosclerosis* 1996;126:143–54

36. Mohan PF, Benghuzzi H. Effect of dehydroepiandrosterone on endothelial cell proliferation. *Biomed Sci Instrum* 1997;33:550–5

37. Hutchison SJ, Sudhir K, Chou TM, *et al*. Testosterone worsens endothelial dysfunction associated with hypercholesterolemia and environmental tobacco smoke exposure in male rabbit aorta. *J Am Coll Cardiol* 1997;29:800–7

38. Furutama D, Fukui R, Amakawa M, Ohsawa N. Inhibition of migration and proliferation of vascular smooth muscle cells by dehydroepiandrosterone sulfate. *Biochim Biophys Acta* 1998;1406:107–14

39. Stokes KI, Benguzzi HA, Cameron JA. Physiological responses associated with sustained delivery of T, DHT, and AED in male rats. *Biomed Sci Instrum* 2000;36:209–14

31 Androgens and hemostasis

Ulrich H. Winkler, MD

INTRODUCTION

Androgen deficiency is associated with an increased incidence of cardiovascular disease. There is evidence linking both venous and arterial thromboembolic disease in hypogonadic males to their low basal fibrinolytic activity. Hypogonadism in males is associated with an enhancement of fibrinolytic inhibition via increased synthesis of the plasminogen activator inhibitor (PAI-1). Administration of androgen reduces PAI-1 activity, leading to an increase in fibrinolytic activity. However, reports of thrombotic diseases in men abusing anabolic steroids suggest the presence of a prothrombotic mechanism which may change the net effect from anti- to prothrombotic in a dose-dependent way. There appears to be an individual threshold dose above which thrombogenic effects on platelets and vasomotion may overcome the profibrinolytic effects on PAI-1. In addition, several other metabolic mechanisms need to be taken into account. Androgens affect the plasma lipoprotein profile, in particular by reducing plasma triglyceride levels, and also influence the insulin/insulin-like growth factor-1 (IGF-1) system. Hypertriglyceridemia and insulin resistance are both associated with low fibrinolytic activity and increased PAI-1 levels. Plasma levels of lipoprotein(a) (Lp(a)) respond favorably to androgen treatment in both men and women. In women estradiol may modulate testosterone effects on hemostasis. Androgen medication, for example danazol, in premenopausal women

reduces PAI-1 activity, suggesting an improvement in fibrinolytic activity.

Information on the effects of androgens on the hemostasis system is limited, possibly owing to the effects of changes in other sex steroids. There are numerous effects of synthetic androgens on the synthesis and release of hemostatic factors, most importantly an increase in the inhibitors of coagulation and a decrease in the inhibitors of the fibrinolytic system. The use of androgens in patients with congenital deficiencies of coagulation factors or previous cardiovascular incidents has yielded disappointing results. Nonetheless, the ability of androgens to reduce fibrinolytic inhibition and Lp(a) levels would in theory reduce the risk of cardiovascular disease.

HEMOSTATIC EFFECTS OF ANDROGENS IN MEN

The rate of mortality from cardiovascular disease (CVD) before the age of 50 years is at least twice as high in men as in women. Besides the well-known beneficial effects of estrogens, deleterious effects of androgens may play a role in this condition[1]. In both animal models and experimental studies androgens have been shown to have significant effects on the extracellular matrix, namely the collagen/elastin ratio[2], extracellular nitric oxide (NO) production[3] and the prostaglandin metabolism in platelets and endothelial cells[4]. These mechanisms may have marked indirect effects on hemostatic function: an increase of blood pressure[2], vascular tone[3] and platelet aggregability[5] would translate into rather unfavorable prothrombotic effects and might – as shown in mice – exaggerate the impact of thrombotic stimuli *in vivo*[6].

On the other hand there is evidence of a positive correlation of androgen levels and fibrinolytic activity. Fibrinolytic activity is physiologically determined by the activity of free tissue-plasminogen activator (t-PA), a serine protease that converts plasminogen to the active fibrinolytic protease plasmin. Regulation of fibrinolytic activity mainly depends on the release of t-PA from the endothelial cells into the circulation and the amount of PAI-l present in the circulation[7]. The latter may be released from endothelial cells or synthesized by hepatic cells. High levels of PAI-1 have been shown to significantly reduce fibrinolytic activity (as measured by means of stimulation tests) and to be associated with an increased risk of post-surgical thrombosis[8] and a poor prognosis after myocardial infarction (MI)[9-10]. The androgen-associated reduction of PAI-1 is therefore likely to be favorable with respect to CVD: fibrinolytic activity and reactivity is increased and a potential risk factor of venous or arterial thrombotic disease is reduced. However, it should be noted that this mechanism only operates as long as t-PA release is not altered. If t-PA activity is also reduced, a reduction of PAI-1 levels would have no net effect on the fibrinolytic activity.

Clearly, the effects of androgens on the hemostatic system are rather complex, and factors such as dose of the androgen, agonistic or antagonistic effects of additional steroids and state of the hemostatic system prior to treatment are of crucial importance for the net clinical effect[11]. Clinical and experimental work in hypogonadic men, patients with coagulation inhibitor deficiencies or predisposition to CVD and weight-lifters abusing anabolic steroids have contributed to our understanding of androgenic effects[12].

Hypogonadism

Given the gender difference in CVD it is puzzling that atherosclerosis is associated with low rather than high testosterone levels in males[13]. Moreover, male survivors of MI have elevated rather than low levels of estrogens[14]. These data suggest that male hypogonadism may be associated with metabolic changes predisposing to atherogenesis and ischemic heart disease. There is evidence that reduced fibrinolytic activity contributes to this risk in hypogonadic males[15]. The underlying mechanism is the inverse relationship of testosterone and PAI-1 in this range of testosterone concentration[16]. Thus with low testosterone levels, high PAI-1 concentrations will constitute a rather high threshold of fibrinolytic activation. The release of very high quantities of t-PA is required to overcome immediate inactivation by PAI-1 and eventually result in actual plasmin generation.

PAI-1 over-expression has long been recognized as a risk marker associated with a high incidence of thromboembolic disease after hip surgery[8] and a poor prognosis in young survivors of MI[9,10], and intravascular, mainly prothrombotic, as well as extravascular atherogenetic pathomechanisms have been postulated[17]. In fact, hypogonadic men appear to suffer from a high incidence of thromboembolic disease[15].

Testosterone

Supraphysiological doses of testosterone have been investigated as a hormonal male contraceptive treatment. Anderson and colleagues[18] reported on changes from pretreatment baseline of several hemostatic variables during and after up to 52 weeks of intramuscular treatment with a weekly dose of 200 mg testosterone enanthate. Fibrinogen levels decreased by about 15% within 16 weeks of treatment, suggesting a favorable effect on blood viscosity. However, there was a slight increase of hemoglobin concentration and hematocrit as well as white blood cell count. Also, a slight increase of antithrombin III, and a decrease of protein C and S activity were noted. The prothrombin fragment F 1 + 2 was slightly increased. The authors surmised that these changes indicate an increase of coagulatory activity, which may theoretically increase the risk of thrombosis in predisposed patients. The concentration of all these factors returned to pretreatment levels during continued treatment. Furthermore, a decrease of PAI-l activity was observed predominantly during the first months of treatment. While this finding was discussed as evidence of improved fibrinolytic activity and reduced risk of arterial disease, it was concluded that the overall effect of supraphysiological doses of testosterone had no marked prothrombotic effect.

Stanozolol

Anabolic steroids have long been known to enhance hepatic synthesis of some plasma proteins such as fibrinogen and plasminogen[19]. Much interest has focused on the effects on protein C and antithrombin III, inhibitors of the coagulatory enzyme thrombin. Congenital deficiencies of these inhibitors are known predispositions to thromboembolic disease and the capacity of stanozolol and other anabolic steroids to increase plasma levels even in deficient subjects raised some expectations of potential therapeutic effects of androgens on the risk of thromboembolic complications in antithrombin III deficiency[20], protein C deficiency[21], postoperative thrombosis[22] and Raynaud's syndrome[23].

Unfortunately, even though stanozolol proved to increase plasma levels of antithrombin III and protein C in both male and female patients suffering from a congenital deficiency syndrome, the clinical effects were disappointing[20]. A probable explanation is that stanozolol failed to improve the insufficient anticoagulant function. Indirect evidence for this hypothesis has been provided by studies on the effect of

synthetic androgens on reaction products of coagulatory activity. Two recent reports confirmed an increase in plasma concentration and activity of inhibitors under therapy but failed to find a reduction of coagulatory activity as depicted by fibrinopeptide A (FPA) plasma levels[23,24]. Interestingly, the effects of stanozolol as well as danazol[25] differ from those reported for supraphysiological doses of testosterone[18], suggesting that the anabolic effects of stanozolol and even danazol were much more pronounced. While testosterone enanthate reduced fibrinogen levels as well as protein C and S levels, stanozolol and danazol were associated with increases, stressing once more the issue of dose and anabolic potency of androgens.

The enhancement of fibrinolytic activity[26] by synthetic androgens has been confirmed by studies in patients with defective fibrinolysis[27,28]. Stanozolol has been shown to decrease the plasma levels and activity of PAI-1, thus increasing the fibrinolytic activity by reduction of the inhibitory threshold[29]. However, the clinical use of androgens for the prevention of thromboembolic disease was limited by early reports on thrombotic complications of high-dose stanozolol[30]. These clinical data suggested a dose dependency of the net effects of androgens: low doses of stanozolol may improve the fibrinolytic activity but high doses may have predominantly procoagulatory effects[10]. Further support for this concept has been derived from studies in male abusers of anabolic steroids.

Anabolic steroids

In general, weight-lifters and other young male athletes should carry very few risk factors for CVD. Athletes themselves tend to believe that in spite of potentially adverse effects on lipids[31] and carbohydrates[32] the abuse of anabolic steroids would not be harmful. However, after a first report on a case of MI in a 22-year-old weight-lifter using anabolic steroids[33], several other cases of ischemic heart disease, stroke and arterial and venous thromboembolism have been published[11]. The absence of classical risk factors, the youth of these men and the apparent lack of atherosclerotic lesions suggested a thrombotic rather than atherogenic pathomechanism, raising questions on the prothrombotic effects of high-dose androgens[34]. There are several reports suggesting that an increased platelet aggregability *in vivo* might mediate a prothrombotic effect of high-dose androgens: platelet aggregability was significantly increased in abusers of anabolic steroids when compared to their fellow male weight-lifters who did not use androgens[35]. Platelet aggregability is largely dependent on arachidonic acid metabolism, and an effect of high-dose androgens on both platelet[5] and vascular cyclo-oxygenase activity[36] has been demonstrated. Thus, high-dose anabolic steroids are capable of increasing vascular tone and reactivity, (i.e. blood pressure), and platelet aggregability (i.e. blood coagulability). These effects are clearly prothrombotic and in opposition to the antithrombotic effects of androgens operating through upregulation of the fibrinolytic action.

In summary, the numerous cases of arterial thrombotic disease in abusers of androgens clearly indicate that at least in some individuals the net effect of high-dose anabolic steroids on lipids, carbohydrates, platelets and vascular function may be prothrombotic, that is it may overcome the antithrombotic effects on the fibrinolytic capacity. The dose dependency of the male response to androgens provides further evidence for the concept of an individual predisposition to thrombotic diseases.

HEMOSTATIC EFFECTS OF ANDROGENS IN WOMEN

Among the most important factors that may modulate the hemostatic as well as all metabolic effects of steroid hormones is gender and the hormonal milieu. In principle, the hormonal milieu may modulate the effects of a certain steroid by lowering the impact of the competing steroid on a particular target cell (the effects on bioavailability and receptor expression) or by competing at the protein level of protein synthesis, either directly or via secondary messengers. Examples of the latter are the modulation of lipid profiles or vascular tone in estrogen versus estrogen/progestin–androgen combinations in women[37]. Thus the effects of androgens on the hemostatic system in women may be quite different from those in men.

Recently the interrelationship of the fibrinolytic system with Lp(a) has gained considerable interest. Lp(a) is an independent risk factor of CVD in male high-risk populations and possibly also in postmenopausal women[38]. There is a remarkable homology of Lp(a) with the proenzyme of the fibrinolytic system, plasminogen. Atherothrombotic effects of Lp(a) may be mediated by competitive binding at plasminogen binding sites both on the endothelium and within the fibrin matrix of fresh clots[39]. Additionally, an Lp(a)-induced upregulation of endothelial PAI-1 synthesis may increase the threshold of fibrinolytic inhibition[40]. The relative contributions of each of these mechanisms are still not clear. In an animal model increased Lp(a) serum levels were shown to be associated with inhibition of the fibrinolytic response and atherogenesis[41]. The finding of decreased Lp(a) concentration in HRT is therefore considered beneficial. Androgens such as stanozolol and danazol have been shown to reduce the serum Lp(a) concentration markedly[42]. While estrogen replacement alone, as well as in combination with progesterone derivatives, appears to reduce Lp(a) only by up to 20%[43], tibolone was reported to reduce Lp(a) in longitudinal studies by 50%[44,45]. However, comparative trials on the differential effects of these preparations are still rare. Moreover, several reports on hormonal effects on Lp(a) have noted that these effects appear to depend on the pretreatment Lp(a) level, i.e. the effects were most pronounced in women with markedly elevated pretreatment values[42,44,45].

CONCLUSIONS

Data on the hemostatic effects of androgens are scarce. There is evidence of a dose response with regard to the effects on blood pressure, platelet aggregability, hemoglobin, platelet and red cell count and coagulatory activation, suggesting a safe dose range in physiological or moderately supraphysiological doses and increasing risks in predisposed subjects with increasing doses of anabolic steroids. Testosterone therapy at moderate doses seems to be associated with a more antithrombotic profile with an increase of coagulation inhibitors and a decrease of fibrinogen as well as the inhibitor of fibrinolysis, PAI-1.

Studies addressing the net effect of androgen administration to the aging male need to take into account potential confounders such as the pretreatment risk profile with regard to the hemostatic system as well as the lipid and carbohydrate metabolism, particularly the pretreatment Lp(a) and IGF-1 levels.

References

1. Kalin MF, Zumoff B. Sex hormones and coronary disease: a review of clinical studies. *Steroids* 1990;55:330–52

2. Fischer GM, Swain ML. Effect of sex hormones on blood pressure and vascular connective tissue in castrated and noncastrated male rats. *Am J Physiol* 1977;232:H616–21

3. Meyers P, Guerra GJR, Harrison D. Release of NO and EDRF from cultured bovine aortic endothelial cells. *Am J Physiol* 1989;256: H1030–7

4. Rosenblum VI, El-Sabban F, Nelson GH, Allison TE. Effects in mice of testosterone and dihydrotestosterone on platelet aggregation in injured arterioles and *ex vivo*. *Thromb Res* 1987;45:719–28

5. Pilo R, Aharony D, Raz A. Testosterone potentiation of ionophore and ADP induced platelet aggregation: relationship to arachidonic acid metabolism. *Thromb Haemost* 1981;46:538–42

6. Uzonava AD. Gonadal hormones and pathogenesis of occlusive arterial thrombosis. *Am J Physiol* 1978;234:H454–9

7. Shih GC, Haijar KA. Plasminogen and plasminogen activator assembly on the human endothelial cell. *Proc Soc Exp Biol Med* 1993;20:258–64

8. Juhan-Vague I, Valadier J, Alessi MC, Aillaud MF. Deficient t-PA release and elevated PA inhibitor levels in patients with spontaneous or recurrent deep venous thrombosis. *Thromb Haemost* 1987;57:67–70

9. Hamsten A, Walldius G, Szamosi A, *et al.* Plasminogen activator inhibitor in plasma: risk factor for recurrent myocardial infarction. *Lancet* 1987;ii:3–9

10. Hamsten A, Wiman B, Defaire U, Blombäck M. Increased plasma levels of a rapid inhibitor of tissue plasminogen activator in young survivors of myocardial infarction. *N Engl J Med* 1985;313:1558–63

11. Mammen EF. Androgens and antiandrogens. *Gynecol Endocrinol* 1993;7:79–86

12. Winkler UH. Effects of androgens on haemostasis. *Maturitas* 1996;24:147–55

13. Cauley J, Kuller L, Gutai J. Prospective study of the relationship between sex hormones and coronary artery disease. *CVD Epidemiol Newslett* 1986;39:23

14. Sewdarsen M, Jialal I, Vythilingum S, Desai R. Sex hormone levels in young Indian patients with myocardial infarction. *Arteriosclerosis* 1986;6:418–21

15. Bennet A, Sié P, Caron P, *et al.* Plasma fibrinolytic activity in a group of hypogonadic men. *Scand J Clin Lab Invest* 1987;47:23–7

16. Caron P, Bennet A, Camare R, *et al.* Plasminogen activator inhibitor in plasma is related to testosterone in men. *Metabolism* 1989;38:1010–15

17. Sawdey M, Loskutoff DJ. Regulation of murine type 1 plasminogen activator inhibitor gene expression *in vivo*. Tissue specificity and induction by lipopolysaccharide, tumor

necrosis factor-alpha and transforming growth factor-beta. *J Clin Invest* 1991;88:1346–53

18. Anderson RA, Ludiam CA, Wu FCW. Haemostatic effects of supraphysiological levels of testosterone in normal men. *Thromb Haemost* 1995;74:693–7

19. Barbosa J, Seal US, Doe RP. Effects of anabolic steroids on haptoglobin, orosomucoid, plasminogen, fibrinogen, transferrin, ceruloplasmin, α2-antitrypsin, ß-glucuronidase and total serum protein. *J Clin Endocrinol* 1971; 33:388–98

20. Winter JH, Fenech A, Bennett B, Daylas AS. Prophylactic antithrombotic therapy with stanozolol in patients with familial antithrombin III deficiency. *Br J Haematol* 1984;57: 527–37

21. Broekmans AW, Conrad J, van Weyenberg RG, *et al.* Treatment of hereditary protein C deficiency with stanozolol. *Thromb Haemost* 1987; 57:20–4

22. Blamey SL, Mcardle BM, Burns P, *et al.* A double-blind trial of intramuscular stanozolol in the prevention of postoperative deep vein thrombosis following elective abdominal surgery. *Thromb Haemost* 1984;51:71–4

23. Jayson MI, Holland CD, Keegan A, *et al.* A controlled study of stanozolol in primary Raynaud's phenomenon and systemic sclerosis. *Am J Rheum Dis* 1991;50:41–7

24. Douglas JT, Blamey SL, Lowe GDO, *et al.* Plasma beta-thromboglobulin, fibrinopeptide A and Bß 15-42 antigen in relation to postoperative DVT, malignancy and stanozolol treatment. *Thromb Haemost* 1985;52:235–8

25. Ford I, Li TC, Cooke ID, Preston FE. Changes in haematological indices, blood viscosity and inhibitors of coagulation during treatment of endometriosis with danazol. *Thromb Haemost* 1994;72:218–21

26. Kluft C, Preston FE, Malia RG, *et al.* Stanozolol-induced changes in fibrinolysis and coagulation in healthy adults. *Thromb Haemost* 1984;51:157–64

27. Kluft C, Bertina RM, Preston FE, *et al.* Protein C, an anticoagulant protein, is increased in healthy volunteers and surgical patients after treatment with stanozolol. *Thromb Res* 1984;33:297–304

28. Tengborn L. The effects of stanozolol on various types of defective fibrinolysis. *Fibrinolysis* 1984;1:29–32

29. Verheijen JH, Rijken DC, Chang GT, *et al.* Modulation of rapid plasminogen activator inhibitor in plasma by stanozolol. *Thromb Haemost* 1984;51:396–7

30. De Stefano V, Leone G, Teofili L, *et al.* Transient ischemic attack in a patient with congenital protein-C deficiency during treatment with stanozolol. *Am J Hematol* 1988;29: 120–1

31. Hurley BF, Seals DR, Hagberg JM, *et al.* High density lipoprotein cholesterol in bodybuilders vs. powerlifters: negative effects of androgen use. *J Am Med Assoc* 1984;252: 507–13

32. Cohen JC, Hickman R. Insulin resistance and diminished glucose tolerance in powerlifters ingesting anabolic steroids. *J Clin Endocrinol Metab* 1987;64:960–3

33. McNutt RA, Ferenchick S, Kirlin PA, Hamlin NJ. Acute myocardial infarction in a 22-year-old world class weightlifter using anabolic steroids. *Am J Cardiol* 1988; 62:164

34. Ferenchick GS. Anabolic/androgenic steroid abuse and thrombosis: is there a connection? *Med Hypotheses* 1991;35:27–31

35. Ferenchick GS, Schwartz D, Ball M, Schartz K. Androgen-anabolic steroid abuse and platelet aggregation: a pilot study in weight lifters. *Am J Med Sci* 1992;303:78–82

36. Greenberg S, Georg WR, Kaclowitz PJ, Wilson WR. Androgen-induced enhancement of vascular reactivity. *Can J Physiol Pharmacol* 1973;52:14–22

37. The writing group for the postmenopausal estrogen/progestin interventions trial. Effects of estrogen or estrogen/progestin regimens on heart disease risk factors in postmenopausal women. *J Am Med Assoc* 1995;273:199–203

38. Cremer P, Nagel D, Labrot B, *et al.* Lipoprotein Lp(a) as predictor of myocardial infarction in comparison to fibrinogen, LDL cholesterol and other risk factors: results from the prospective Göttingen Risk Incidence and Prevalence Study (GRIPS). *Eur J Clin Invest* 1994;24:444–53

39. Edelberg JM, Pizzo SV. Lipoprotein (a): the link between impaired fibrinolysis and atherosclerosis. *Fibrinolysis* 1991;5:135–43

40. Etingin OR, Hajjar DP, Hajjar KA, *et al.* Lipoprotein(a) regulated plasminogen activator inhibitor-1 expression in endothelial cells: a potential mechanism for thrombogenesis. *J Biol Chem* 1991;266:2459–65

41. Lawn RM, Wade DP, Hammer RE, *et al.* Atherogenesis in transgenic mice expressing human apolipoprotein(a). *Nature* 1992;360: 670–2

42. Soma MR, Meschia M, Bruschi F, *et al.* Hormonal agents used in lowering lipoprotein(a). *Chem Phys Lipids* 1994;67–8: 345–50

43. Kim CJ, Jang HC, Cho DH, Min YK. Effects of hormone replacement therapy on lipoprotein(a) and lipids in postmenopausal women. *Arterioscler Thromb* 1994;14:275–81

44. Haenggi W, Riesen W, Birkhäuser MH. Postmenopausal hormone replacement therapy with tibolone decreases serum lipoprotein(a). *Eur J Clin Chem Clin Biochem* 1993;31:645–50

45. Rymer J, Crook D, Sidhu M, *et al.* Effects of tibolone on serum concentrations of lipoprotein(a) in postmenopausal women. *Acta Endocrinol Copenhagen* 1993;128:259–62

32 Androgens and blood pressure in men

Guy Lloyd, MBBS, MRCP

INTRODUCTION

Hypertension in men is a major public health issue, with a rate nearly double that of premenopausal women (Figure 1). Hypertension confers a significantly elevated risk of cardiovascular disease, with the risk of myocardial infarction being doubled and that of stroke increasing fourfold. Strategies to prevent hypertensive disease have led to a decline in hypertensive mortality over the last 20 years, but despite this hypertension was responsible for over 17 000 deaths in the USA for the year 1997 alone. Ethnic groups, in particular those of Afro-Caribbean origin, are particularly at risk and in some populations 30% of hypertensive males die as a result of their blood pressure[1].

Treatment of hypertension is successful in controlling the risk of stroke but has been less successful in reducing the risk of coronary disease. This was particularly evident in the early randomized controlled trials. In a Medical Research Council trial men and women with systolic blood pressure up to 209 mmHg were randomized to either diuretics or β-blockade, or placebo. Stroke was reduced by 25% but coronary events by only 19%, confined to the patients treated with diuretics[2]. Recent studies using newer drugs such as calcium channel antagonists in high-risk populations have confirmed a cardiac benefit[3,4]. Sadly, the evaluation of newer and potentially cardioprotective agents, such as inhibitors of angiotensin converting

enzyme, is problematic because of the ethical constraints in randomizing hypertensive subjects to placebo treatment.

The choice of antihypertensive agent may be less important than the absolute risk of disease at baseline and the efficacy of the intervention (in terms of blood pressure changes). Guidelines now focus on achieving an optimal blood pressure of below 140/85 with more aggressive targeting of diabetic subjects who are at special risk[5].

Whilst much research energy has been directed to assessing the impact of estrogen and other female sex hormones on cardiovascular disease, adrenal and testicular androgens continue to have an enigmatic relationship with cardiovascular diseases. The attraction of female sex hormones as cardioprotective agents, based on the low incidence of disease in premenopausal women compared to age-matched males, together with a (less convincing) increase in the disease following the menopause, is intuitive. The corollary of this relationship – that androgens are harmful, perhaps due to adverse effects on plasma lipids – has also achieved widespread acceptance. However, in men plasma androgen levels do not show a rapid and steep decline analogous to the menopause. There is no acute 'deficiency syndrome' analogous to the situation in menopausal women, although some time-trends are now acknowledged. Men show an

351

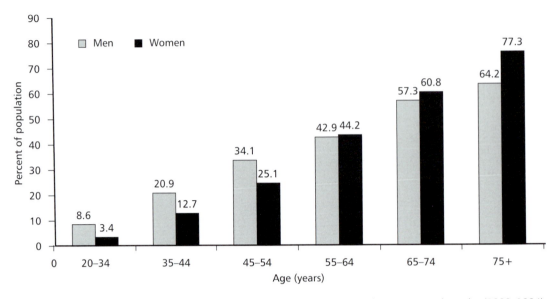

Figure 1 The percentage of the American population with hypertension according to age and gender (1988–1994). Note the lower incidence of hypertension among premenopausal women. Reproduced with permission from reference 1

age-dependent decrease in sex hormones, particularly testosterone. This decline predates the decline in women, starting as early as 21 years and continues in a linear manner into old age[6].

Cross-sectional studies show lower (not higher) plasma androgen levels in patients with coronary artery disease[7], indicating that androgens, far from being deleterious, may share a role with estrogen in the maintenance of vascular integrity in men. Thus, the age-dependent decline in plasma testosterone levels may be an important co-factor in the development of cardiovascular diseases such as hypertension and atherosclerosis. This chapter covers the relationship between androgens and blood pressure in both experimental and *in vivo* settings, and discusses whether androgens may modulate cardiovascular risk in men.

RELATIONSHIP BETWEEN ANDROGENS AND HYPERTENSION

Animal models

Much of our understanding of the influence of androgens on blood pressure is derived from the salt-sensitive, spontaneous hypertensive (Sprague-Dawley) rat model of hypertension. In this model testosterone clearly has a pivotal role in mediating blood pressure. Males develop significantly higher arterial blood pressure than females, but when castrated this difference is lost in both sexes (Figure 2). Furthermore subcutaneous testosterone implants resulting in physiological male plasma concentrations in females raises their blood pressures to those of non-castrated males. Adding back testosterone to castrated animals results in equal blood pressure to intact animals while treatment with estrogen in non-castrated animals results in lower pressures[8]. Interestingly, the renin–angiotensin system appears to be a major determinant of this hormone-dependent gender dimorphism: enalapril treatment equally reduces blood pressure across male, female, castrated and testosterone-replaced animals[9]. In the same model intact males and ovariectomized females treated with testosterone have a significantly lower incremental renal sodium excretion in response to increases in blood pressure compared to castrated males or intact females[10]. This androgenic influence on

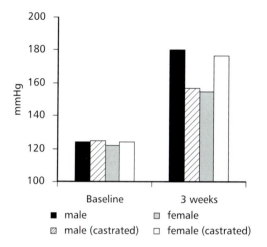

Figure 2 The influence of modifying endogenous sex hormones on blood pressure in the Sprague-Dawley salt-sensitive rat model. Reproduced with permission from reference 8

blood pressure is receptor-mediated, as it can be inhibited by the androgen receptor antagonist flutamide[11]. Finasteride however, an inhibitor of 5α-reductase, does not antagonize this hypertensive response. This suggests that a direct testosterone/receptor effect is responsible, rather than a conversion to the active metabolite dihydrotestosterone as with many 'testosterone effects' such as benign prostatic hypertrophy and male pattern baldness.

Animal models have also helped explain how testosterone might regulate cardiac hypertrophy in response to hypertension. Morano and colleagues[12] report that in spontaneously hypertensive rats the reduction in blood pressure seen in response to castration was linked to an increased expression of the β-myosin heavy chain gene, while testosterone replacement (3 mg/day of dihydrotestosterone) favors the expression of α-heavy chain gene. This switch in gene regulation would be expected to lead to cardiac hypertrophy[12]. This phenomenon has been observed in an alternative model based on the denervated rat model (Wistar strain). Subcutaneous testosterone propinate treatment (0.5 pg/kg) after castration resulted in increased blood pressure in the rats and a

significantly increased left ventricular weight at necropsy, when compared to intact animals[13].

Available evidence from limited animal models therefore suggests that testosterone should have a negative influence on blood pressure and the left ventricular reaction to hypertension. Epidemiological evidence from male populations and studies in human subjects suggest an alternative hypothesis.

Blood vessel behavior

Endothelial dysfunction is seen in most hypertensives and may represent an early stage in the pathophysiology of their condition. Estrogen administration improves the function of the endothelium in both women[14] and men[15] but the effect of androgens is unclear. When testosterone at doses ranging from sub- to grossly supraphysiological is introduced into the coronary arteries of men during angiography, it causes a dose-dependent increase in vessel diameter and coronary blood flow, similar to that seen with estradiol administration[16]. This suggests that testosterone improves endothelial function. Conversely, in female-to-male transsexuals, testosterone treatment reduced flow-mediated forearm blood flow, an endothelium-dependent process[17]. Similarly, surgically or chemically castrated prostate cancer patients have an enhanced brachial artery reactivity, suggesting enhanced nitric oxide release[18]. However, it is well recognized that all vessels may not exhibit the same behavior.

In the classic aortic ring system testosterone relaxes preconstricted rabbit arterial rings[19]. In this landmark study the relaxation was significantly greater in the coronary artery rings than in the aortic rings, perhaps explaining the negative findings in the forearm investigations outlined above. What is fascinating about these experiments is that the testosterone-dependent vasodilatation did not seem to be acting through any of the well-recognized pathways for sex steroid action. The dilatation was not dependent on an intact endothelium nor was it

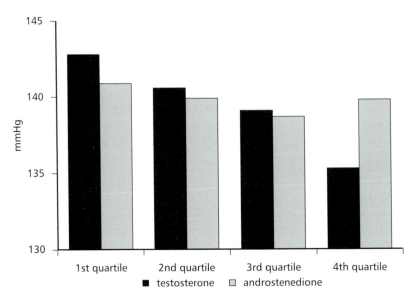

Figure 3 The relationship between increasing quartiles of testosterone and andro-stenedione and systolic blood pressure in the Rancho–Bernardo study. Figure reproduced with permission from reference 22

influenced by nitric oxide synthase inhibitors; the dose-dependent contraction in response to calcium was unchanged, suggesting that calcium antagonism was not responsible; and testosterone receptor blockade did not affect the response suggesting a direct effect on the arterial wall (see Chapter 14).

Effects of DHEAS and adrenal androgens on blood pressure

The effects of the endogenous adrenal androgens androstenedione and dihydroepiandro-stenedione sulfate (DHEAS) on blood pressure is unclear and the literature is divided, as is often the case with androstenedione. Schunkert and colleagues[20] examined a group of 646 men. In this population DHEAS concentrations in middle-aged men were significantly higher in the hypertensive individuals. This was also associated with, but independent of, higher levels of aldosterone. Furthermore, in patients with established hypertension, low levels of DHEAS are associated with a reduction in diurnal blood pressure variation, generally considered to be an indication of adverse

outcome[21]. Other studies have however failed to note any relationship between androstene-dione and blood pressure.

Testosterone

In the Rancho–Bernardo study with 1132 men a negative association was seen between plasma testosterone levels and blood pressure[22] (Figure 3). The relationship with lower plasma testosterone was true across all the quintiles of blood pressure and was independent of other factors including obesity. No relationship was seen with estrogens or adrenal androgens. In a small study of hypertensive men, hypertension was associated with reduced levels of both total and free testosterone[23]. In contrast, the women in this study showed a positive correlation with testosterone, suggesting that the effects of testosterone on blood pressure may be gender-dependent. In another small study of 30 men and 30 women, plasma testosterone did not correlate with blood pressure in men although once more a positive relationship was seen in women[24]. In a small group of men evaluated for the association between blood pressure and erectile dysfunction, testosterone levels were lower in the hypertensive men, although conventional measures of erectile dysfunction were similar in both groups[25]. Further studies of varying designs have also supported the association[23,26].

Data from the Multiple Risk Factor Intervention Trial substudy[27] suggests that the reduction in testosterone levels with time may not be directly related to the development of hypertension. In 66 participants in the study mean total testosterone declined by a mean 41 ng/dl. When analyzed using multivariate analysis the change in testosterone levels was associated with a rise in triglyceride and a fall in high density lipoprotein (HDL)-cholesterol, but not with changes in either systolic or diastolic blood pressure[27].

In a cross-sectional study of women attending an endocrine clinic for menstrual irregularity, an elevated testosterone level (> 30 ng/dl) predicted central obesity and to some extent hypertension. The odds ratio for systolic and diastolic blood pressure is 2.4 (1.0–6.2) and 2.7 (0.8–8.8), respectively. The combination of hyperandrogenemia and obesity was a powerful predictor of the presence of hypertension[28].

There is, therefore, a discrepancy between the findings in animal models and those observed in human subjects. The animal studies are heavily dependent on the relationship between salt and hypertension through the renin–angiotensin system, while in human subjects other factors may be equally or more important. It may be that the modulations in endothelial function equal or outweigh other hypertensive influences resulting in a much more complicated relationship between testosterone and blood pressure.

EXOGENOUS ANDROGENS AND BLOOD PRESSURE

Testosterone and derivatives

Studies designed to investigate the influence of androgen administration on blood pressure in healthy men are rare. Whitworth and co-workers[29] carried out a small trial in which a synthetic androgen (testosterone undecanoate, 120 mg/day) was administered to 14 normotensive males. No increase in blood pressure or plasma volume was noted with this large dose over 5 days. However, the study was small and might not have had the statistical power to detect any changes. Similarly, a randomized crossover study of 20 men treated with intravenous testosterone in either physiological (twice normal) or supraphysiological doses (six times normal) found no obvious effects on blood pressure[30]. Administration of 'physiological' doses of testosterone by various regimens including depot and transdermal to obese men resulted in no change in blood pressure but improved insulin sensitivity[31].

Anabolic androgenic steroids

In contrast to the findings with testosterone, the high doses of anabolic androgenic steroids used in sport do seem to increase blood pressure. In an early randomized control trial of 13 athletes given methandrostenolone, a small but significant increase in blood pressure was observed, although clinical hypertension developed in only one individual[32]. In an observational Dutch study, self-administration of anabolic steroids was associated with elevated blood pressure, an effect sustained at an average of 5 months of follow-up[33]. In a randomized trial of 21 weight-lifters, testosterone enanthate resulted in a reversible 10 mmHg increase in systolic blood pressure[34]. Conversely, Palatini and colleagues[35] demonstrated no overall effect of steroid abuse on blood pressures measured in the clinic setting. However, a reduction in nocturnal dipping was observed, and this loss of day/night variability on 24 h blood pressure monitoring is an early hypertensive change[35]. Nandrolone also appears to induce a rise in diastolic blood pressure that reverts to normal within 6 weeks[36], and the effects of other steroids appear to be relatively short-lived after stopping therapy[37].

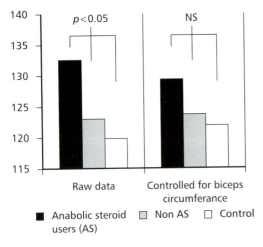

Figure 4 The effect of anabolic steroid use and exercise training on systolic blood pressure before and after controlling for biceps circumference. Reproduced with permission from reference 38

One important covariate that must be considered is changes in body habitus associated with anabolic steroid use, particularly an increase in the circumference of the arm, which may influence blood pressure measurement. Riebe and colleagues[38] found that systolic and diastolic pressures both at rest and after various forms of exercise were raised compared with non-users and sedentary controls (Figure 4). However, after the inclusion of biceps size in the statistical model, these differences were no longer significant[38].

Left ventricular hypertrophy (LVH) is a common finding among patients with hypertension and predicts an adverse prognosis. Among athletes in training left ventricular hypertrophy is also a common finding and relates to increased myocardial work. *In vitro* work in hypertensive rats has demonstrated that treatment with anabolic steroids results in a decrease in myocardial compliance[39]. This absence of an influence on experimental LVH has also been observed with other steroids such as nandrolone[40]. Indirect evidence for an additive effect of steroids on LVH comes from the retrospective arm of a study by Dickerman and

colleagues[41], where LVH on echocardiography was found in 43% of body-builders compared with 100% of those who used anabolic steroids in addition to exercise. In a further study by di Bello and co-workers,[42] there was a trend towards highest left ventricular mass among steroid users, although that was not statistically significant. However other observational studies have failed to replicate these findings[43-45]. All studies appear to agree that diastolic relaxation of the left ventricle is not affected by the presence of LVH, whether or not steroids are used.

Anabolic steroids seem to induce hypertension and may increase LVH; their use should therefore be discouraged. Users should be monitored closely for the development of hypertension, and if it develops all steroid use should cease. Clearly anabolic derivatives of testosterone should never be used for the purposes of physiological replacement.

CONCLUSIONS

The relationship between androgens and hypertension remains unclear. Evidence from existing animal models suggests that testosterone administration has the potential to induce hypertension and increase the hypertrophic response of the left ventricle to hypertension. Conversely, *in vivo* testosterone appears to act as a coronary and possibly peripheral vasodilator acting primarily through nitric oxide release and the modulation of endothelial function. Certainly testosterone levels appear to be lower in patients with both hypertension and coronary artery disease and it remains an attractive hypothesis that sex steroids in both sexes are important in maintaining vascular integrity. However, the large number of covariates including weight, smoking and lipid changes makes the epidemiological evidence difficult to evaluate. Administration of 'physiological' dose testosterone to hypogonadal men or those more loosely classified as being 'andropausal' does not seem to be associated with any hypertensive effect and can be considered 'safe', although in hypertensive subjects suitable monitoring should continue. The abuse of anabolic steroids in sport may induce small, reversible rises in blood pressure and close observation of these individuals is prudent. If hypertension develops, then subjects should

be strongly advised to stop using these drugs, especially because of the potential role of these steroids in mediating the development of LVH. For men with hypertension the cornerstone of therapy remains the evidence-based strategies of aggressive blood pressure reduction and risk-factor modulation.

References

1. American Heart Association. *2001 Heart and Stroke Statistical Update*. Dallas, TX: AHA, 2000
2. The MRC Working Party. Medical research council trial of treatment of hypertension in older adults: principal results. *Br Med J* 1992; 304:405–12
3. Staessen J, Fagard R, Thijs L, *et al*. Randomised double-blind comparison of placebo and active treatment for older patients with isolated systolic hypertension. The Systolic Hypertension in Europe (Syst-Eur) Trial Investigators. *Lancet* 1997;350:757–64
4. Wang J, Staessen J, Gong L, Liu L. Chinese trial on isolated systolic hypertension in the elderly. Systolic Hypertension in China (Syst-China) Collaborative Group. *Arch Intern Med* 2000;160:211–20
5. Ramsay L, Williams B, Johnston G, *et al*. Guidelines for management of hypertension: report of the third working party of the British Hypertension Society. *J Hum Hypertens* 1998;13:569–92
6. Zumoff B, Strain G, Kream J, *et al*. Age variation of the 24-hour mean plasma concentrations of androgens, estrogens and gonadotrophins in normal adult men. *J Clin Endocrinol Metab* 1982;54:534–8
7. English K, Mandour O, Steeds R, *et al*. Men with coronary artery disease have lower levels of androgens than men with normal coronary angiograms. *Eur Heart J* 2000;21: 890–4
8. Crofton J, Share L. Gonadal hormones modulate deoxycorticosterone-salt hypertension in male and female rats. *Hypertension* 1997;29: 494–9

9. Reckelhoff J, Zhang H, Srivastava K. Gender differences in development of hypertension in spontaneously hypertensive rats. Role of the renin–angiotensin system. *Hypertension* 2000;35:480–3
10. Reckelhoff J, Zhang H, Granger J. Testosterone exacerbates hypertension and reduces pressure-natriuresis in male spontaneously hypertensive rats. *Hypertension* 1998;31:435–9
11. Reckelhoff J, Zhang H, Srivastava K, Granger J. Gender differences in hypertension in spontaneously hypertensive rats, role of androgens and androgen receptor. *Hypertension* 2000;34:920–3
12. Morano I, Gerstner J, Ruegg J, *et al*. Regulation of myosin heavy chain expression in the hearts of hypertensive rats by testosterone. *Circ Res* 1990;66:1585–90
13. Cabral A, Vasquez E, Moyses MR, Antonio A. Sex hormone modulation of ventricular hypertrophy in sinoaortic denervated rats. *Hypertension* 1988;11:I-93–I-97
14. Collins P, Rosano G, Sarrel P, *et al*. 17 beta-Estradiol attenuates acetylcholine-induced coronary arterial constriction in women but not men with coronary artery disease. *Circulation* 1995;92:24–30
15. New G, Timmins K, Duffy S, *et al*. Long-term estrogen therapy improves vascular function in male to female transsexuals. *J Am Coll Cardiol* 1997;29:1437–44
16. Webb C, McNeill J, Hayward C, *et al*. Effects of testosterone on coronary vasomotor regulation in men with coronary heart disease. *Circulation* 1998;100:1960–6
17. McCredie R, McCrohon J, Turner L, *et al*. Vascular reactivity is impaired in genetic

females taking high-dose androgens. *J Am Coll Cardiol* 1998;32:1331–5

18. Herman S, Robinson J, McCredie R, *et al*. Androgen deprivation is associated with enhanced endothelium-dependent dilatation in adult men. *Arterioscler Thromb Vasc Biol* 1997;17:2004–9

19. Yue P, Chatterjee K, Beale C, *et al*. Testosterone relaxes rabbit coronary arteries and aorta. *Circulation* 1998;91:1154–60

20. Schunkert H, Hense H, Andus T, *et al*. Relation between dehydroepiandrosterone sulphate and blood pressure levels in a population-based sample. *Am J Hypertens* 1999;12:1140–3

21. Barna I, Feher T, de Chatel R. Relationship between blood pressure variability and serum dehydroepiandrosterone sulphate levels. *Am J Hypertens* 1998;11:532–8

22. Khaw K, Barrett-Connor E. Blood pressure and endogenous testosterone in men: an inverse relationship. *J Hypertens* 1988;6:329–332

23. Hughes J, Mathur R, Margolius H. Sex steroid hormones are altered in essential hypertension. *J Hypertens* 1989;7:181–7

24. Lundberg U, Wallin L, Lindstedt G, Frankenhaeuser M. Steroid sex hormones and cardiovascular function in healthy males and females: a correlation study. *Pharmacol Biochem Behav* 1990;37:325–7

25. Jaffe A, Chen Y, Kisch E, *et al*. Erectile dysfunction in hypertensive subjects. Assessment of potential determinants. *Hypertension* 1996;28:859–62

26. Simon D, Charles M, Nahoul K, *et al*. Association between plasma total testosterone and cardiovascular risk factors in healthy adult men: The telecom study. *J Clin Endocrinol Metab* 1997;82:682–5

27. Zmuda J, Cauley J, Glynn N, *et al*. Longitudinal relation between endogenous testosterone and cardiovascular risk factors in middle-aged men. A 13-year follow-up of former Multiple Risk Factor Intervention Trial participants. *Am J Epidemiol* 1997;146:609–17

28. Ayala C, Steinberger E, Sweeney A, *et al*. The relationship of serum androgens and ovulatory status to blood pressure in reproductive-age women. *Am J Hypertens* 1999;12:772–7

29. Whitworth J, Scoggins B, Andrews J, *et al*. Haemodynamic and metabolic effects of short term administration of synthetic sex steroids in humans. *Clin Exper Hypertens A* 1992;14:905–22

30. White C, Ferraro-Borgida M, Moyna N, *et al*. The effects of pharmacokinetically guided intravenous testosterone administration on electrocardiographic and blood pressure variables. *J Clin Pharmacol* 1999;39:1038–43

31. Marin P, Krothiewski M, Bjorntorp P. Androgen treatment of middle-aged, obese men: effects on metabolism, muscle and adipose tissues. *Eur J Med* 1992;1:329–36

32. Freed D, Banks A, Longson D, Burley D. Anabolic steroids in athletics: crossover double-blind trial on weightlifters. *Br Med J* 1975;31:471–3

33. Lenders J, Demacker P, Vos J, *et al*. Deleterious effects of anabolic steroids on serum lipoproteins, blood pressure and liver function in amateur body builders. *Int J Sports Med* 1988;9:19–23

34. Giorgi A, Weatherby R, Murphy P. Muscular strength, body composition and health responses to the use of testosterone enanthate: a double blind study. *J Sci Med Sport* 1999;2:341–55

35. Palatini P, Giada F, Garavelli G, *et al*. Cardiovascular effects of anabolic steroids in weight-training subjects. *J Clin Pharmacol* 1996;12:1132–40

36. Kuipers H, Wijnen J, Hartgens F, Willems S. Influence of anabolic steroids on body composition, blood pressure, lipid profile and liver function in body builders. *Int J Sports Med* 1991;12:413–18

37. Hartgens F, Kuipers H, Wijnen J, Keizer H. Body composition, cardiovascular risk factors and liver function in long-term androgenic-anabolic steroids using bodybuilders three months after drug withdrawal. *Int J Sports Med* 1996;6:429–33

38. Riebe D, Fernhall B, Thompson P. The blood pressure response to exercise in anabolic steroid users. *Med Sci Sports Exerc* 1992;24:633–7

39. LeGros T, McConnell D, Murray T, *et al.* The effects of 17 alpha-methyltestosterone on myocardial function *in-vitro. Med Sci Sports Exerc* 2000;32:897–903

40. Phillis B, Irvine R, Kennedy J. Combined cardiac effects of cocaine and the anabolic steroid, nandrolone, in the rat. *Eur J Pharmacol* 2000;398:263–72

41. Dickerman R, Schaller F, McConathey W. Left ventricular wall thickening does occur in elite power athletes with or without anabolic steroid use. *Cardiology* 1998;90:145–8

42. di Bello V, Giorgi D, Bianchi M, *et al.* Effects of anabolic-steroids on weight-lifters' myocardium: an ultrasonic videodensitometric study. *Med Sci Sports Exerc* 1999;31:514–21

43. Salke R, Rowland T, Burke E. Left ventricular size and function in body builders using anabolic steroids. *Med Sci Sports Exerc* 1985;17:701–4

44. Thompson P, Sadaniantz A, Cullinane E, *et al.* Left ventricular function is not impaired in weight-lifters who use anabolic steroids. *J Am Coll Cardiol* 1992;19:278–82

45. Yeater R, Reed C, Ullrich I, *et al.* Resistance trained athletes using or not using anabolic steroids compared to runners: effects on cardiorespiratory variables, body composition and plasma lipids. *Br J Sports Med* 1996; 30:11–4

33 Androgens and arterial disease

Carolyn M. Webb, PhD, and Peter Collins, MD, FRCP, FESC

ANDROGENS AND ARTERIAL DISEASE

Historically androgens have been considered a risk factor for coronary artery disease in men, since postmenopausal women have a lower incidence of coronary heart disease and myocardial infarction than men of a similar age. However, there has been no direct evidence linking physiological concentrations of androgens to an increased incidence of coronary heart disease and myocardial infarction, and recent evidence suggests that the reverse may be true. In a study examining the effect of risk factors (including estradiol and testosterone) on predicting myocardial infarction in males who had not had a previous myocardial infarction, Phillips and co-workers[1] raised the possibility that hypotestosteronemia in men may be a risk factor for coronary atherosclerosis. Serum total and free testosterone levels were negatively correlated with degree of risk of coronary artery disease and with risk factors for myocardial infarction. These findings have been confirmed by other studies[2,3]. Decreased total and free testosterone levels have been shown to be associated with ischemic stroke in men[4], further implicating testosterone in the pathophysiology of vascular diseases. Declining levels of the androgen dehydroepianedrosterone sulfate (DHEAS) has been associated with an increased risk of vascular disease[5]. Confusion arises from data concerning the use of high doses of androgens (anabolic steroids) to increase muscle mass and athletic performance, where there is a well-documented increase in incidence of cardiovascular events[6].

Androgens and the coronary and peripheral circulations

Testosterone is known to affect the coronary circulation in animals[7,8] and humans[9]. In men with coronary artery disease, physiological concentrations of testosterone infused directly into the coronary arteries induced coronary dilatation and enhancement of coronary blood flow (Figure 1)[9]. There was no effect on vasomotor or flow responses to acetylcholine before versus after testosterone administration, indicating a possible endothelium-independent mechanism.

The direct effects of testosterone on coronary arteries, increasing blood flow, may explain the observed effects of testosterone administration on signs of exercise-induced myocardial ischemia. Reports from the 1940s suggest that testosterone therapy in men has a beneficial effect on angina pectoris[10-13]. This was confirmed and extended in the 1970s in a double-blind study carried out in 50 men who had ST segment depression after exercise[14]. It was shown that, after 4–8 weeks' treatment with testosterone or placebo, there was a

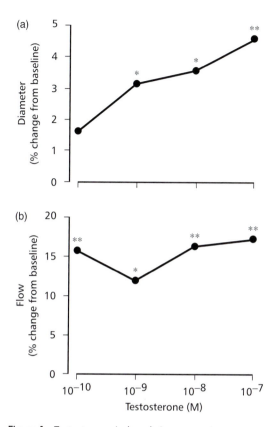

Figure 1 Testosterone-induced increases in coronary artery diameter (a) and blood flow (b). *$p < 0.05$ and **$p < 0.01$ compared with baseline. Reproduced with permission from Lippincott, Williams & Wilkins 'Effects of testosterone on coronary vasomotor regulation in men with coronary heart disease'. *Circulation* 1999;100(16): 1690–6[9]

significant decrease in the exercise-induced extent of ST segment depression by testosterone when compared to placebo. The mechanism by which testosterone decreased post-exercise ST segment depression was not established. This study may have been confounded by the fact that the presence of significant coronary artery disease was not confirmed. Recent studies have demonstrated an acute and longer-term beneficial effect of testosterone on myocardial ischemia in men with established coronary artery disease[15–17]. In the studies performed by both Rosano and Webb and their colleagues, acute intravenous testosterone or placebo was given in a cross-over design to men withdrawn from cardioactive medication, and the study of

Webb and colleagues[16] included men with baseline testosterone levels below or at the lower end of the normal range. Both studies showed an enhancement in exercise time to myocardial ischemia 30 min after testosterone infusion; however, the study of Rosano and co-workers[15] also showed a benefit on total exercise time and rate-pressure product (an indicator of myocardial work). Transdermal testosterone patches, given for 12 weeks in addition to current antianginal medication, has been shown to significantly increase time to 1 mm ST segment depression on the electrocardiogram in men with coronary artery disease[17]. Interestingly, the magnitude of the response was greater in men with lower baseline testosterone levels.

Acute testosterone-induced increases in flow-mediated brachial artery diameter changes have been demonstrated in men with coronary artery disease, suggesting that in this vascular bed testosterone may have a beneficial effect on endothelium-dependent responses (Figure 2)[18]. This differs from a recent study which has suggested an improvement in vasoreactivity in men undergoing treatment for prostatic cancer who were orchidectomized or given antiandrogen therapy compared to controls[19]. In this publication the endothelium-dependent dilatation response of the control group was only 2–3%, an unusually low value, and interestingly this response was not significantly associated with cholesterol levels. This is different from similar reports by these investigators[20,21]. Also, hormone withdrawal may not necessarily be expected to have inverse effects to hormone supplementation, especially in a different population of men such as those with coronary heart disease. As is shown with the varying effects of steroid hormones on lipid levels, extrapolation of hormonal effects outside study parameters cannot be assumed[22].

Androgens and atherosclerosis

Large doses of testosterone can increase coronary artery atheroma progression in female

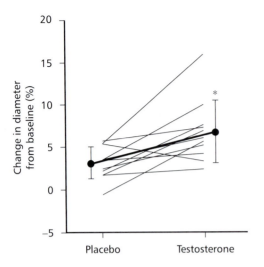

Figure 2 Flow-mediated reactivity in individual patients 60 min after an intravenous infusion of 2.3 mg of testosterone. *Bold line* indicates mean change from baseline, *p = 0.005. Reproduced with permission from Excerpta Medica Inc., 'Testosterone enhances flow-mediated brachial artery reactivity in men with coronary artery disease'. *Am J Cardiol* 2000;85:269–72

animals but preserve endothelial function in coronary arteries in these animals[23]. A study in rabbits demonstrated a sex-specific atheroprotective effect of testosterone in male animals, independent of changes in lipid profile[24]. Intimal thickening in the proximal aortic arch was significantly inhibited by testosterone in these male animals.

There is no evidence that physiological levels of testosterone increase the risk of myocardial infarction, in contrast to data from men taking high doses of anabolic steroids who are known to be at increased risk for myocardial infarction and stroke[6]. High doses of androgens have been associated with advanced atheroma progression[23], and detrimental effects on plasma lipid profile[25] and hemostatic factors[26,27].

Androgens and vasoreactivity: lessons from studies in women

There is evidence from studies in women that testosterone may have favorable effects on arterial endothelial function. Preliminary evidence indicates an increase in flow-mediated

dilatation of the brachial artery induced by testosterone implants in postmenopausal women already receiving hormone replacement therapy (12 women were taking a cyclical progestin in addition to a non-standardized estrogen)[28]. In female-to-male transsexuals, high-dose androgen treatment is associated with impaired vascular reactivity in the brachial artery[29]. Compared to untreated age- and cigarette smoking-matched controls (nine of 12 subjects in each group were smokers), transsexuals had the same endothelium-dependent responses, but significantly impaired response to the endothelium-independent vasodilator glyceryl trinitrate. These studies highlight the importance of dose of androgen treatments in determining a beneficial or detrimental vasomotor effect.

Androgens and atherosclerosis

The influence of androgens on atherogenesis in women is unclear and relatively unexplored. Endogenous androgens, DHEAS in particular, have been shown to correlate with a lower risk of carotid artery atherosclerosis in women[30,31], but not coronary atherosclerosis[32]. There is evidence to suggest that premenopausal women with coronary artery disease, a relatively rare disease in women before the menopause, may have decreased DHEAS levels[33], indicating that DHEAS may in some way be atheroprotective.

Sex differences in foam cell formation, known to play a key role in atherogenesis, have recently been identified. Lipid loading of macrophages isolated from women were not affected by the androgen dihydrotestosterone, whereas macrophages from men showed a dose-dependent and androgen receptor-mediated increase in macrophage cholesteryl ester content[34].

CONCLUSION

Contrary to previous assumptions, physiological levels of androgens appear to be associated with arterial health in men. Findings of recent studies indicate the need for further investigation of the cardiovascular effects of androgens in men.

References

1. Phillips GB, Pinkernell BH, Jing TY. The association of hypotestosteronemia with coronary artery disease in men. *Arterioscler Thromb* 1994;14:701–6

2. Chute CG, Baron JA, Plymate SR, *et al*. Sex hormones and coronary artery disease. *Am J Med* 1987;83:853–9

3. English KM, Mandour O, Steeds RP, *et al*. Men with coronary artery disease have lower levels of androgens than men with normal coronary angiograms. *Eur Heart J* 2000;21:890–4

4. Jeppesen LL, Jorgensen HS, Nakayama H, *et al*. Decreased serum testosterone in men with acute ischemic stroke. *Arterioscler Thromb Vasc Biol* 1996;16:749–54

5. Barrett-Connor E. Sex differences in coronary artery disease. Why are women so superior? The 1995 Ancel Keys Lecture. *Circulation* 1997;95:252–64

6. Bagatell CJ, Bremner WJ. Androgens in men – uses and abuses. *N Engl J Med* 1996;334:707–14

7. Yue P, Chatterjee K, Beale C, *et al*. Testosterone relaxes rabbit coronary arteries and aorta. *Circulation* 1995;91:1154–60

8. Chou TM, Sudhir K, Amidon TM, *et al*. Testosterone-induced coronary conductance and resistance vessel relaxation *in vivo*: potential mechanisms of action. *J Am Coll Cardiol* 1995;14A(abstr)

9. Webb CM, McNeill JG, Hayward CS, *et al*. Effects of testosterone on coronary vasomotor regulation in men with coronary artery disease. *Circulation* 1999;100:1690–6

10. Hamm L. Testosterone propionate in the treatment of angina pectoris. *J Clin Endocrinol* 1942;2:325–8

11. Sigler LH, Tulgan J. Treatment of angina pectoris by testosterone propionate. *NY State J Med* 1943;43:1424–8

12. Walker TC. The use of testosterone propionate and estrogenic substance in the treatment of essential hypertension, angina pectoris and peripheral vascular disease. *J Clin Endocrinol* 1942;2:560–8

13. Lesser MA. Testosterone propionate therapy in one hundred cases of angina pectoris. *J Clin Endocrinol* 1946;6:549–57

14. Jaffe MD. Effect of testosterone cypionate on postexercise ST segment depression. *Br Heart J* 1977;39:1217–22

15. Rosano GMC, Leonardo F, Pagnotta P, *et al*. Acute anti-ischemic effect of testosterone in men with coronary artery disease. *Circulation* 1999;99:1666–70

16. Webb CM, Adamson DL, de Ziegler D, Collins P. Effect of acute testosterone on myocardial ischemia in men with coronary artery disease. *Am J Cardiol* 1999;83:437–9

17. English KM, Steeds RP, Jones TH, *et al*. Low-dose transdermal testosterone therapy improves angina threshold in men with chronic stable angina: a randomized, double-blind, placebo-controlled study. *Circulation* 2000;102:1906–11

18. Ong PJL, Patrizi G, Chong WCF, *et al*. Testosterone enhances flow-mediated brachial artery reactivity in men with coronary artery disease. *Am J Cardiol* 2000;85:14–17

19. Herman SM, Robinson JT, McCredie RJ, *et al*. Androgen deprivation is associated with enhanced endothelium-dependent dilatation in adult men. *Arterioscler Thromb Vasc Biol* 1997;17:2004–9

20. Celermajer DS, Sorensen KE, Gooch VM, *et al*. Non-invasive detection of endothelial dysfunction in children and adults at risk of atherosclerosis. *Lancet* 1992;340:1111–16

21. Celermajer DS, Cullen S, Deanfield JE. Impairment of endothelium-dependent pulmonary artery relaxation in children with congenital heart disease and abnormal pulmonary hemodynamics. *Circulation* 1993;87:440–6

22. Hulley S, Grady D, Bush T, *et al*. Randomized trial of estrogen plus progestin for secondary prevention of coronary heart disease in postmenopausal women. *J Am Med Assoc* 1998;280:605–12

23. Adams MR, Williams JK, Kaplan JR. Effects of androgens on coronary artery atherosclerosis

and atherosclerosis-related impairment of vascular responsiveness. *Arterioscler Thromb Vasc Biol* 1995;15:562–70

24. Bruck B, Brehme U, Gugel N, *et al.* Gender-specific differences in the effects of testosterone and estrogen on the development of atherosclerosis in rabbits. *Arterioscler Thromb Vasc Biol* 1997;17:2192–9

25. Thompson PD, Cullinane EM, Sady SP, *et al.* Contrasting effects of testosterone and stanozolol on serum lipoprotein levels. *J Am Med Assoc* 1989;261:1165–8

26. Ajayi AA, Mathur R, Halushka PV. Testosterone increases human platelet thromboxane A2 receptor density and aggregation responses. *Circulation* 1995;91:2742–7

27. Heller RF, Meade TW, Haines AP, *et al.* Inter-relationships between factor VII, serum testosterone and plasma lipoproteins. *Thromb Res* 1982;28:423–5

28. Worboys S, Kotsopoulos D, Teede H, *et al.* Evidence that parenteral testosterone therapy may improve endothelium-dependent and independent vasodilation in postmenopausal women already receiving estrogen. *J Clin Endocrinol Metab* 2001;86:158–61

29. McCredie RJ, McCrohon JA, Turner L, *et al.* Vascular reactivity is impaired in genetic females taking high-dose androgens. *J Am Coll Cardiol* 1998;32:1331–5

30. Bernini GP, Sgro M, Moretti A, *et al.* Endogenous androgens and carotid intimal–medial thickness in women. *J Clin Endocrinol Metab* 1999;84:2008–12

31. Bernini GP, Moretti A, Sgro M, *et al.* Influence of endogenous androgens on carotid wall in postmenopausal women. *Menopause* 2001;8:43–50

32. Herrington DM, Gordon GB, Achuff SC, *et al.* Plasma dehydroepiandrosterone and dehydroepiandrosterone sulfate in patients undergoing diagnostic coronary angiography. *J Am Coll Cardiol* 1990;16:862–70

33. Slowinska-Srzednicka J, Malczewska B, Srzednicki M, *et al.* Hyperinsulinaemia and decreased plasma levels of dehydroepiandrosterone sulfate in premenopausal women with coronary heart disease. *J Intern Med* 1995;237:465–72

34. McCrohon JA, Death AK, Nakhla S, *et al.* Androgen receptor expression is greater in macrophages from male than from female donors. A sex difference with implications for atherogenesis. *Circulation* 2000;101:224–6

34 Androgenic influences on ventilation and ventilatory responses to O_2 and CO_2 during wakefulness and sleep

Koichiro Tatsumi, MD

INFLUENCE OF TESTOSTERONE ON BREATHING DURING WAKEFULNESS

Gender differences in ventilation and ventilatory control have been described[1,2] but the extent to which these are due to female or male sex hormones is unclear. While the effects of the female sex hormones have been extensively investigated, relatively few studies have examined the role of the male hormone testosterone[3,4]. White and colleagues[3], reported that testosterone raised both resting ventilation and metabolic rate in hypogonadal men. As end-tidal partial pressure of carbon dioxide (PCO_2) did not change with treatment, he proposed that the increased metabolic rate underlies the increase in ventilation. In contrast, Matsumoto and co-workers[4], found no change in metabolic rate after testosterone treatment. The reason for conflicting results is unclear. In the more controlled environment of experimental animals, resting ventilation and PCO_2 production increased but end-tidal PCO_2 was unchanged after neutered male cats were treated with testosterone, implying that effective alveolar ventilation did not change[5], in agreement with the results

of White and colleagues[3]. However, in guinea pigs the action of castration induces hypoventilation[6].

The effects of testosterone on hypoxic and hypercapnic ventilatory responses are also poorly understood. White and colleagues[3] reported an augmented hypoxic ventilatory response (HVR) after testosterone replacement in hypogonadal men, whereas Matsumoto and co-workers[4] found that HVR decreased after such treatment. Likewise, the effect of testosterone on the hypercapnic ventilatory response (HCVR) has been inconsistent: a decrease was shown in one study[7] but no change was seen in others[3,4,8]. Returning to experimental animal models of respiratory function, testosterone treatment of neutered male cats[5] raised HVR (Figure 1). Testosterone also augmented HCVR in animals.

An increased metabolic rate has been shown to be an important determinant of HVR[2,9,10]. Therefore, the increased metabolic rate may have contributed to the elevation in HVR observed in one human[3] and one animal[5] study,

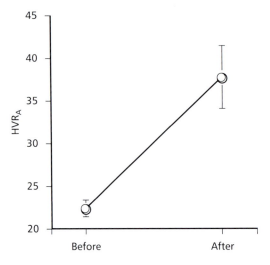

Figure 1 The ventilatory response to hypoxia shape parameter A (HVR$_A$) was increased by testosterone treatment ($n = 8$)

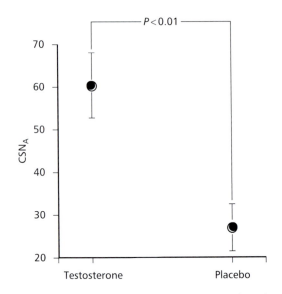

Figure 2 The carotid sinus nerve response to hypoxia shape parameter A (CSN$_A$) was greater in the testosterone-treated compared with the placebo-treated animals ($n = 8$)

although in neither case were the investigators able to correlate change in HVR with those of either oxygen consumption or CO_2 production. This, however, does not rule out the possibility that increased metabolic rate was responsible for the rise in HVR.

Other possible explanations for the increase in HVR are that testosterone might affect either the carotid body (Figure 2). In the anesthetized experimental cats, the ventilatory and carotid sinus nerve (CSN) responses to hypoxia were determined simultaneously after either testosterone or placebo treatment[5]. Testosterone increased both HVR (Figure 1) and CSN responsiveness to hypoxia (Figure 2)[11,12], indicating that the increase in HVR with testosterone treatment was dependent on increased peripheral chemoreceptor responsiveness. Further studies using hormone receptor blockers are required to determine whether the effects of testosterone are direct or steroid receptor-mediated and, in turn, whether such receptors are located in tissues involved in ventilatory control.

Metabolic rate seems to increase with testosterone and numerous studies indicate an association of increased HVR with increased metabolic rate, as mentioned above[2,9,10].

However, it is uncertain whether this explains the increased carotid body responsiveness in an animal study, because previous studies show that an elevation in metabolic rate produced by passive hindlimb stimulation fails to raise carotid body responsiveness to hypoxia[13,14].

In both the human[3] and the animal[15] study, testosterone levels attained after treatment varied among individuals over a very wide range. None of the changes in the physiological parameters (ventilation, metabolic rate, HVR or HCVR) induced by testosterone administration correlated with either the absolute or relative changes in serum testosterone level. One could expect the exaggerated effects by the high serum testosterone obtained. However, White and colleagues[3] discovered that in one patient who had a normal testosterone level, at baseline the addition of exogenous testosterone had no effect on metabolism or chemosensitivity. This suggests a 'plateau' effect where increasing testosterone levels beyond the normal range may have no further effect than is seen with replacement in hypogonadal men.

The mechanism of steroid hormone action is largely mediated via specific receptors. Even though the ultimate effects of androgens on cellular constituents are tissue specific (the production of the tissue specific proteins), the steps of androgen action are common to many organs, including (1) the binding of testosterone or its metabolite, 5α-dihydrotestosterone to specific cytoplasmic receptor proteins that are transferred to nuclei; (2) an interaction of the receptor–steroid complexes with chromatin that is accompanied by a synthesis of RNAs; and (3) the translation of steroid-specific RNAs, resulting in formation of hormone-specific proteins to alter target cell functions. In the middle way of these steps, there seem to be two major factors regulating androgenic actions in individual tissues: (1) the steroid recognition mechanism including the serum androgen concentration and steroid-binding specificity of the androgen receptors; and (2) the structure of chromatin which receptor–steroid complexes bind, where they presumably activate genes for androgen-specific proteins.

Recent studies have demonstrated that androgenic stimulation of responding genes depends on the nuclear uptake of the receptor–steroid complex. The longer the complex is retained in the nucleus, the shorter the lag period and the greater the magnitude of the response, although a certain threshold nuclear androgen receptor concentration must be exceeded and should be present for an extended period of time before a stimulation of androgen-responsive genes occurs[15]. Therefore the failure to find a direct relationship between serum total testosterone levels and respiratory responses (ventilation, metabolic rate, HVR or HCVR) is not unexpected.

INFLUENCE OF TESTOSTERONE ON BREATHING DURING SLEEP

Ventilatory control in the sleeping state may be partly androgen dependent. Hypoventilation and sleep apnea with desaturation are seen more frequently in men than women[16,17]. A potential beneficial role of female hormones such as progesterone in explaining some of the gender and menopausal differences in disordered breathing during sleep is mentioned in the next section. An alternative possibility to explain the gender differences in sleep-disordered breathing is that androgens or the ratio of androgen to progesterone may be implicated. This has been suggested by several early case reports. In one instance the patient with hypogonadism was the only subject in a group of obese males who did not experience sleep-disordered breathing and desaturation[18]. This led them to speculate that decreased testosterone level may protect an individual from respiratory dysrhythmias during sleep. In the other cases, both a male patient with primary hypogonadism and a 54-year-old female with the anemia of chronic renal failure developed the obstructive sleep apnea syndrome after testosterone administration. Apneas and symptoms improved with discontinuation of androgen and recurred with its resumption[8,19].

Subsequently, effects of testosterone on breathing during sleep have been studied systematically by two groups[3,4]. These groups studied respiratory rhythm during sleep in hypogonadal men both on and off testosterone-replacement therapy and presented similar results. The total number of disordered breathing events (apnea + hypopnea) per hour of sleep increased significantly following androgen administration, suggesting that androgen is likely to be one of many factors that are important in the development of dis-ordered breathing during sleep. However, this was a highly variable event with some subjects demonstrating large increases in apnea and hypopnea when androgen was replaced, whereas others had little change in respiration during sleep.

Although testosterone could be important in the development of disordered breathing during sleep, neither the site of action nor the mechanism by which this effect is mediated is understood. Several possibilities should be considered. Johnson and co-workers[19], observed an increase in supraglottic resistance following androgen replacement to facilitate the development of obstructive sleep apnea in a woman who was known to snore mildly prior to initiation of hormone replacement therapy. They suggested that she was particularly predisposed to development of obstructive sleep apnea, because of existing subclinical upper airway compromise or other factors. In contrast, White and colleagues[3] reported that upper airway dimensions, evaluated by the anatomy (computed tomography) and airflow resistance of the upper airway, were unaffected by testosterone in four male subjects. However, they pointed out that the two subjects who increased their dysrhythmic episodes during sleep tended to have a higher supraglottic resistance and lower mean pharyngeal airway size than the other two subjects. This may in part explain interindividual variation of the increase in sleep disordered breathing by testosterone replacement.

Another possibility is that enhanced HVR in a subject with a small airway may lead to more prominent sleep disordered breathing. Testosterone seems to increase HVR[3,5] although this has been inconsistent[4]. White and colleagues[3] found no correlation between the change in HVR induced by testosterone during wakefulness and the changes in breathing rhythm during sleep. However, they suggested the association between these two variables, since most subjects demonstrated an increase in both variables. At high altitude increased HVR may act to drive CO_2 tensions below levels required to sustain regular breathing and make ventilatory control unstable, resulting in increased apnea and hypopnea[20,21]. This might be analogous to those increases seen in the condition after testosterone treatment. The interactions between unstable ventilatory control induced by augmented HVR and decreased upper airway patency may induce more disordered breathing during sleep[22,23].

INTERACTIONS BETWEEN TESTOSTERONE AND FEMALE HORMONES

There is evidence that the individual cellular effects of either androgen or estrogen may be modified by the presence of the other sex steroids. The synergistic action of these hormones has been demonstrated in at least one system[24], but in most other tissues their effects appear to be antagonistic. The anti-estrogenic effect of androgens has been observed in human prostate and rat liver[25,26] and this effect has been indicated to be mediated by an androgen receptor mechanism in breast cancer cells; i.e. androgens do not inhibit estrogen action by interfering with the formation, activation, nuclear binding or nuclear processing of estrogen–receptor complexes[27]. It has also been reported that androgens prevent the estrogen-dependent augmentation of cytoplasmic progesterone receptor in human breast cancer cells[28]. However, there is a possibility that these effects are tissue specific. The interaction of androgen and estrogen in the tissues involving the respiratory control system remains to be established.

Progesterone also appears to act as an antiandrogen. Progesterone therapy has been reported to improve obstructive sleep apnea in some but not all patients[29]. Furthermore, high dosages of progesterone have been reported to suppress gonadal function[30] and have induced in some patients with obstructive sleep apnea symptoms of hypogonadism such as diminished libido[29]. Therefore, administration of progesterone seems to diminish serum testosterone levels.

CONCLUSION

Androgens administration may increase resting ventilation, matabolic rate, and hypoxic and peripheral chemoreceptor responsiveness to hypoxia in awake state. In contrast, androgen may cause or act to accentuate apnea and hypopnea during sleep. Neither the site of action nor mechanism by which these effects are mediated is understood.

References

1. Regensteiner JG, Pickett CK, McCullough RE, *et al.* Possible gender differences in the effect of exercise on hypoxic ventilatory response. *Respiration* 1988;53:158–65

2. White DP, Douglas NJ, Pickett CK, *et al.* Sexual influence on the control of breathing. *J Appl Physiol* 1983;54:874–9

3. White DP, Schneider BK, Santen RJ, *et al.* Influence of testosterone on ventilation and chemosensitivity in male subjects. *J Appl Physiol* 1985;59:1452–7

4. Matsumoto AM, Sandblom RE, Schoene RB, *et al.* Testosterone replacement in hypo-gonadal men: effects on obstructive sleep apnoea, respiratory drives and sleep. *Clin Endocrinol* 1985;22:713–21

5. Tatsumi K, Hannhart B, Pickett CK, *et al.* Effects of testosterone on hypoxic ventilatory and carotid body neural responsiveness. *Am J Respir Crit Care Med* 1994;149:1248–53

6. Hohimer AR, Hart MV, Resko JA. The effect of castration and sex steroids on ventilatory control in male guinea pigs. *Respir Physiol* 1985;61:383–90

7. Strumpf IJ, Reynolds SF, Vash P, Tashkin DP. A possible relationship between testosterone, central control of ventilation and the Pickwickian syndrome (Abstract). *Am Rev Respir Dis* 1978;117:abstr.183

8. Sandblom RE, Matsumoto AM, Schoene RB, *et al.* Obstructive sleep apnea syndrome induced by testosterone administration. *N Engl J Med* 1983;308:508–10

9. Regensteiner JG, Woodard WD, Hagerman DD, *et al.* Combined effects of female hormones and metabolic rate on ventilatory drives in women. *J Appl Physiol* 1988;66:808–13

10. Weil JV, Byrne-Quinn E, Sodal JE, *et al.* Augmentation of chemosensitivity during mild exercise in normal man. *J Appl Physiol* 1972;23:813–19

11. Nishino T, Lahiri S. Effects of dopamine on chemoreflexes in breathing. *J Appl Physiol* 1981;50:892–7

12. Vizek M, Pickett CK, Weil JV. Increased carotid body hypoxic sensitivity during acclimatization to hypobaric hypoxia. *J Appl Physiol* 1987;63:2403–10

13. Aggarwal D, Milhorn HT Jr, Lee LY. Role of the carotid chemoreceptors in the hyperpnea of exercise in the cat. *Respir Physiol* 1976;26:147–55

14. Davies RQ, Lahiri S. Absence of carotid chemoreceptor response during hypoxic exercise in the cat. *Respir Physiol* 1973;18:92–100

15. Janne OA, Bardin CW. Androgen and anti-androgen receptor binding. *Ann Rev Physiol* 1984;46:107–18

16. Block AJ, Boysen PG, Wynne JW, Hunt LA. Sleep apnea, hypopnea and oxygen desaturation in normal subjects. A strong male predominance. *N Engl J Med* 1979;300:513–17

17. Guilleminault C, van den Hoed J, Mitler MM. Clinical overview of the sleep apnea syndrome. In Guilleminault C, Dement WC, eds. *Sleep Apnea Syndrome.* New York: Alan R Liss Inc. 1978:1–12

18. Harman E, Wynne JW, Block AJ, Malloy-Fisher L. Sleep disordered breathing and oxygen desaturation in obese patients. *Chest* 1981;79:256–60

19. Johnson MW, Anch AM, Remmers JE. Induction of the obstructive sleep apnea syndrome in a woman by exogenous androgen administration. *Am Rev Respir Dis* 1984;129:1023–5

20. Berssenbrugge A, Dempsey J, Skatrud J. Hypoxic versus hypocapnic effects on periodic breathing during sleep. In West J, Lahiri S, eds. *High Altitude and Man.* Bethesda, MD: Am Physiol Soc, 1984;115–127

21. Skatrud JB, Dempsey JA. Interaction of sleep state and chemical stimuli in sustaining rhythmic ventilation. *J Appl Physiol* 1983;55:813–22

22. Cherniack NS. Sleep apnea and its causes. *J Clin Invest* 1984;73:1501–6

23. Onal E, Lopata M, O'Connor T. Pathogenesis of apnea in hypersomnia-sleep apnea syndrome. *Am Rev Respir Dis* 1982;125:167–74

24. Tokarz RR, Harrison RW, Seaver SS. The mechanism of androgen and estrogen synergism in the chick oviduct. *J Biol Chem* 1979;254:9178–84

25. Huggins C, Hodges CV. Studies on prostatic cancer. I. The effects of castration of estrogen and of androgen injection on serum phosphatases in metastatic carcinoma of the prostate. *Cancer Res* 1941;1:293–7

26. Roy AK, Milin BS, McMinn DM. Androgen receptor in rat liver: hormonal and developmental regulation of the cytosol cytoplasmic receptor and its correlation with the androgen dependent synthesis of α2-globulin. *Biochim Biophys Acta* 1974;354:213–32

27. MacIndoe JH, Etre LA. An antiestrogenic action of androgens in human breast cancer cells. *J Clin Endocrinol Metab* 1981;53: 836–42

28. Horwitz KB, Costlow ME, McGuire WL. MCF-7: a human breast cancer cell line with estrogen, androgen, progesterone, and glucocorticoid receptors. *Steroids* 1975;26: 785–95

29. Hensley MJ, Saunders NA, Strohl KP. Medroxyprogesterone treatment of obstructive sleep apnea. *Sleep* 1980;3:441–6

30. Southern AL, Gordon GG, Vittel J, Altman K. Effect of progestagens on androgen metabolism. In Martini L, Motta M, eds. *Androgens and Antiandrogens*. New York, Raven Press, 1977:263–79

35 The role of androgens in respiratory function

Anne M. Spungen, EdD

INTRODUCTION

This section will review the muscles of breathing, the effect of endogenous and exogenous testosterone or anabolic steroid agents on peripheral skeletal muscle, and the animal and limited human literature of the effect of anabolic steroid administration on respiratory function. Only 'androgens', testosterone or any of its synthetic anabolic steroid derivatives, will be discussed in this section. Other anabolic agents, such as β-2 agonists or growth hormone, which also promote anabolism but are not androgens, will be excluded from discussion.

MUSCLES OF BREATHING

The muscles of breathing comprise three main groups: the diaphragm, intercostal/accessory muscles and the abdominal wall group. These muscles are unique from the other skeletal muscles in three aspects: (1) they are both involuntary and voluntary; (2) they overcome resistive and elastic loads rather than inertial loads; and (3) they must contract regularly without prolonged rest for an entire life[1]. The respiratory muscles work as either prime movers or stabilizers of the chest wall to promote inspiration and exhalation. The inspiratory muscles of breathing function in a coordinated effort to enlarge the thoracic cavity, creating a negative intrapleural pressure and inflating the lung. The diaphragm

is the primary muscle responsible for inspiration during quiet breathing (tidal breathing). Exhalation during quiet breathing is largely passive. The inspiratory action of the diaphragm is dependent on its configuration and the presence of abdominal resistance. In patients with pulmonary compromise, the diaphragm may flatten, weakening its ability to inspire. The diaphragm is innervated at cervical level 3, 4 and 5 (Figure 1). The accessory muscles include the scalenes, sternocleidomastoids and trapezius; these muscles contribute minimally to inhalation during tidal breathing. DeTroyer et al.[2] has speculated that the scalenes may play an active role by stabilizing the rib cage during quiet breathing. In cases of cervical paralysis, such as seen in those with tetraplegia, the pectoralis major has been shown to participate in exspiration[3]. The intercostal muscles are primarily responsible for forced efforts of inhalation (external intercostals) and exhalation (internal intercostals); these muscles are innervated at thoracic level 1 to 12 (Figure 1) and are recruited to assist with deep inspirations and forceful exhalations. The abdominal wall group consist of the recti, external and internal obliques and the transverse abdominis. These muscles primarily contract to participate in exhalation at higher levels of ventilation, such as during exercise or stress and during explosive

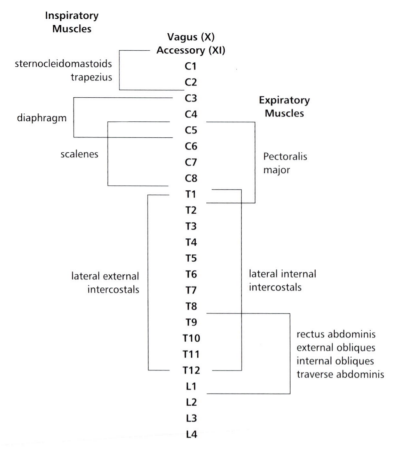

Figure 1 The innervation of the muscles of breathing

exhalation (cough), and they are relatively inactive during quiet breathing. The abdominal wall group is innervated at thoracic level 1 to lumbar level 2.

Morgan and colleagues[1] describe three major etiologies responsible for respiratory failure and muscle fatigue manifesting themselves in three ways: (1) lack of central neurological drive; (2) mechanical disorders of the chest wall; and (3) failure of the muscles to generate the required force, that is fatigue. Anabolic therapies are postulated to have the most significant impact on the third mechanism, muscle fatigue, by their effect to strengthen respiratory muscles. Following is a discussion of the mechanisms of anabolic therapies and their effect on respiratory muscles.

EFFECTS OF TESTOSTERONE ON SKELETAL MUSCLE

Testosterone administration increases muscle protein synthesis in normal men[4]. Hypogonadism in non-elderly men is associated with reductions in lean body and muscle mass, with testosterone replacement therapy increasing lean body tissue and muscle strength[5–9]. Mauras and colleagues[8] addressed the specific effects of androgens on body composition and protein metabolism in six healthy men (23.2 ± 0.5 (SE) years of age). Gonadal suppression was achieved with a long-acting gonadotropin releasing factor analog (Lupron, TAP Pharmaceuticals, IL, USA) to produce pre-pubertal levels of serum testosterone. After 10 weeks of suppressive therapy, all subjects demonstrated a decrease in fat-free mass and an increase in fat mass; muscle strength of the legs was decreased[8]. Thus, in men with hypogonadism or in young men who were chemically ablated for endogenous androgens, muscle mass and strength were clearly deficient.

Normal aging is associated with a decline in serum testosterone levels[10,11]. It has been controversial as to whether the fall in serum testosterone levels with advancing age is due to chronic illness or medication use. Gray and colleagues[10] conducted a cross-sectional survey of a population of men aged 39 to 70 years who were either completely healthy ($n = 415$) or who had a medical condition or were on prescription medications ($n = 1294$). The less healthy men had 10 to 15% lower levels of androgens than those who were healthy. However, regardless of health status, the percentage rate of change of total testosterone, free testosterone or major androgens and metabolites declined in a similar manner[10]. As part of the Baltimore Longitudinal Study, Harman and co-workers[11] performed serum testosterone measurements in a population of men ($n = 890$) over 20 years. The incidence of hypogonadism, using total testosterone criteria, increased from 20% of men over the age of 60 to 30% over 70 and 50% over 80. Because of the potential of testosterone replacement to prevent or partially reduce the age-related changes in body composition, muscle strength, functional impairment and quality of life, such hormonal therapy may be indicated in those men with the lowest serum testosterone concentrations.

Several reports have studied testosterone replacement in elderly men[12–15]. Urban and colleagues[12] investigated the effects of physiological testosterone administration for 4 weeks in six healthy older men (67 ± 2 (SE) years of age). Leg muscle strength increased, as did fractional synthetic rate of muscle protein by a stable-isotope infusion technique. Other reports have generally noted an increase in lean body tissue, muscle strength and decreased fat mass

in response to testosterone replacement therapy[13–15]. Secondary causes of androgen deficiency, such as hypogonadal men with acquired immunodeficiency syndrome (AIDS) and a wasting myopathy, have been shown to correlate with testosterone levels and respond to androgen therapy[9,16,17].

Individuals with spinal cord injury occupy the lowest end of the activity spectrum and have been considered to be a model of immobilization and premature aging[18,19]. The level of pulmonary impairment is closely related to the level of spinal cord lesion. Chronic spinal cord injury is associated with a continuous loss in lean body tissue mass[19]. Tsitouras and colleagues[20] noted that persons with spinal cord injury had significantly lower levels of serum total and free testosterone compared with able-bodied subjects. In larger groups of subjects, Bauman and co-workers[21] found that those with spinal cord injury also had lower serum total testosterone levels, which declined at 9% per decade compared with 5% per decade in the able-bodied controls.

Supraphysiological administration of testosterone has been demonstrated to have a pronounced effect on muscle mass. Bhasin and colleagues[22] administered 600 mg of testosterone enanthate or placebo weekly for 10 weeks. Even in the absence of strength training, supraphysiological testosterone doses produced increased muscle mass of the arms and legs, associated with increased strength; this effect was further augmented with strength training[22]. Anabolic steroid therapy in the higher dose ranges would be expected to have a similar effect on muscle mass to that seen with supraphysiological testosterone administration.

EFFECTS OF ANABOLIC STEROIDS ON THE DIAPHRAGM

Several animal studies have been performed to investigate the effect of synthetic anabolic steroid and/or testosterone administration on respiratory muscles. In a study of healthy postpubescent female and male rats, Bisshop and co-workers[23] investigated the effect of 5 weeks of low-dose (1.5 mg/kg) and high-dose (7.5 mg/kg) nandrolone decanoate (a testosterone derivative administered IM with a moderately high anabolic-to-androgenic ratio) on histochemical, contractile and fatigue properties of the diaphragm. In the nandrolone decanoate-treated groups compared with the control group, the cross-sectional area of type IIx/b fibers was increased ($p < 0.05$), whereas type I and type IIa fibers were not statistically different. Time-to-peak tension and half-relaxation time decreased in the two treatment groups ($p < 0.05$ and $p < 0.01$, respectively), whereas maximal twitch tension, maximal tetonic tension and the ratio did not change significantly with treatment. Force-frequency curves and fatigue properties were not effected by nandrolone decanoate treatment. A significant gender bias was not found for any of the diaphragm properties measured. The significant changes in muscle function found in this study were consistent with diaphragm muscle hypertrophy. Prezant and colleagues[24] investigated the use of testosterone propionate (2.5 mg/day; 5 days/week) in healthy male and female rats during short-term (2.5 weeks) and long-term (10 weeks) administration. In females, but not males, testosterone treatment produced significant increases in body weight, costal diaphragm weight and contractility and significant decreases in fatigue resistance indexes. One explanation for the lack of a significant finding in male rats was that the dose of testosterone administered was too low to elicit an effect. In both sexes, no significant difference in fiber type proportions or areas was observed, regardless of treatment duration or the baseline circulating androgen level. When all rats were analyzed together, significant improvements were found for diaphragm contractility and fatigue resistance. The authors noted that these were healthy, normally breathing animals and that in a more compromised breathing model, greater testosterone-related changes may occur.

Van Balkom and colleagues[25] studied the effect of anabolic steroid administration on respiratory muscle function in pulmonary compromised animal models. One study was designed to investigate whether anabolic steroid administration could block the loss of diaphragm force caused by long-term use of methylprednisolone. Adult male rats were administered low-dose methylprednisolone (0.2 mg/kg/day for 9 months) with saline or with saline and nandrolone decanoate (1 mg/kg/week IM during the final 3 months). The methylprednisolone-only group experienced a marked reduction in diaphragm force (10%). This effect was completely antagonized in the group that received nandrolone decanoate. In a similar study by these same investigators, using an emphysematous hamster model, the addition of nandrolone decanoate in a clinically relevant dose completely reversed myosin heavy chain type IIa and IIx diaphragm muscle atrophy caused by the glucocorticoid agent. In both *in vitro* and *in vivo* rat studies, anabolic steroid agents have been demonstrated to competitively displace corticosteroids from their cytoplasmic receptors in muscle[26]. At low stimulation frequencies in the emphysematous hamsters, the improvement in force generation in the diaphragm from the anabolic steroid addition was to the level of the control animals[27].

Compared with other skeletal muscles, the diaphragm has a higher cytosol androgen receptor density[28] and participates in continuous cyclic contraction, theoretically increasing its potential to benefit from anabolic steroid administration. These animal studies lend support to the concept that anabolic steroid administration may significantly impact respiratory skeletal muscle fatigue. Patients with pulmonary compromise, such as from emphysema, chronic obstructive pulmonary disease (COPD), tetraplegia and other neuromuscular disorders, may benefit from anabolic steroid administration. To date, there is a scarcity of investigation performed in this area. However, it may be speculated that anabolic steroid therapy has the potential to improve diaphragmatic strength and endurance in patients with respiratory failure.

EFFECTS OF ANABOLIC STEROIDS ON PULMONARY FUNCTION

Only a few studies exist in humans that have investigated the role of anabolic steroids to improve respiratory muscle function and/or general pulmonary function. Patients with chronic obstructive pulmonary disease (COPD) often experience moderate to severe weight loss in association with decreases in pulmonary function and their general ability to breathe. Ferreira and co-workers[29] investigated the effect of oral anabolic steroids on body mass index (BMI), lean body mass, anthropometric measures, respiratory muscle strength, and functional exercise capacity in subjects with COPD in a prospective, randomized, double-blind, placebo-controlled study. The study group received testosterone (250 mg IM) and oral stanozolol (12 mg/day) for 27 weeks. The control group received placebo injection and an oral placebo tablet. Seventeen of 23 subjects completed the study (10 in the treatment group and 7 controls). Anabolic treatment was associated with increases in BMI, lean body mass, and anthropometric measures of arm and thigh circumference, with no significant changes in endurance exercise capacity. A trend was evident in the treatment group for maximal inspiratory mouth pressure (PI_{max}) to increase by an average of 41%, but this was not statistically different from the control group (who demonstrated a 20% increase in PI_{max}). The authors reported that administration of an oral anabolic steroid for 27 weeks to malnourished male subjects with COPD was free of clinical or biochemical side-effects.

In another study, by Schols and colleagues[30], 217 patients with COPD participated in a placebo-controlled, randomized trial investigating the physiological effects of nutritional intervention alone for 8 weeks or combined with an anabolic steroid, nandrolone decanoate, injected IM over 8 weeks (on days 1, 15, 29 and 43 at doses of 25 mg in women or 50 mg in men). Maximal inspiratory mouth pressure improved for the nutrition-only and the anabolic steroid plus nutrition groups in the first 4 weeks of treatment. After week 8 of treatment, only those in the nandrolone decanoate plus nutrition group were significantly greater from the placebo group for maximal inspiratory pressure ($p < 0.03$). The nutrition group had a significant weight gain that was predominantly due to an expansion of fat mass ($p < 0.03$). In contrast, the weight gain in the nandrolone decanoate plus nutrition group resulted from more favorable relative changes in fat-free mass, as well as other measures of muscle mass ($p < 0.03$).

Pulmonary complications are a major cause of morbidity and mortality among individuals with cervical spinal cord lesions, primarily due to paralysis of the muscles of respiration. Strengthening of the remaining intact respiratory musculature may reduce these complications and improve pulmonary function. An open-label pilot study was performed to investigate the effect of 1 month of treatment with oxandrolone (an anabolic steroid with the highest anabolic-to-androgenic ratio) on weight gain and pulmonary function. Ten healthy adult male subjects with complete motor tetraplegia of greater than 1-year duration participated in this study. Spirometry, maximal inspiratory and expiratory pressures and resting self-rating of dyspnea (Borg Scale) were measured at baseline and repeated again at the end of 1 month of oxandrolone therapy (20 mg/day). On average, the subjects gained 1.4 ± 1.5 kg, a $2 \pm 2\%$ increase in weight ($p = 0.01$). A significant $9 \pm 2\%$ improvement was found in the combined measures of spirometry ($p < 0.005$). Maximal inspiratory pressure improved by an average of $10 \pm 7\%$ ($p < 0.001$). Maximal expiratory pressure improved by $9 \pm 13\%$ (non-significant). Subjective self-rating of dyspnea decreased by an average of $37 \pm 28\%$ ($p < 0.01$). In healthy subjects with tetraplegia, the use of oxandrolone was associated with significant improvements in weight and pulmonary function, and a subjective reduction in breathlessness[31]. In the absence of any clinical studies, it may be speculated that anabolic steroid administration be considered in the therapy of individuals with tetraplegia in an effort to strengthen respiratory musculature during respiratory insufficiency precipitated by intercurrent infectious pulmonary illness.

SUMMARY

The respiratory musculature may have an augmented potential to respond to anabolic steroid therapy compared with other skeletal muscles to improve in size, strength, and contractility and delay the onset of fatigue. For the pulmonary compromised patient, there is an obvious need for further investigation in this area. Studies to determine the optimal dosing regimens of anabolic steroids combined with nutrition and/or exercise training are needed. Potential applications to accelerate ventilator weaning are also of considerable importance.

References

1. Morgan MDL, Silver JR, William SJ. The respiratory system of the spinal cord patient. In: Bloch RF, Basbaum M, eds. *Management of Spinal Cord Injury*. Baltimore: Williams & Wilkins, 1986:78–116

2. DeTroyer A, Kelly S, Zin WA. Mechanical action of the intercostal muscles on the ribs. *Science*. 1983;220:87–8

3. DeTroyer AD, Estenne M. The expiratory muscles in tetraplegia. *Paraplegia* 1991;29: 359–63

4. Griggs RC, Kingston W, Jozefowicz RF, et al. Effect of testosterone on muscle mass and muscle protein synthesis. *J Appl Physiol* 1989;66:498–503

5. Forbes GB, Reina JC. Adult lean mass declines with age: some longitudinal observations. *Metabolism* 1970;19:653–63

6. Brodsky IG, Balagopal P, Nair KS. Effects of testosterone replacement on mucle mass and muscle protein synthesis in hypogonadal men. *J Clin Endocrinol Metab* 1996;81:3469–75

7. Bhasin S, Storer TW, Berman N, et al. Testosterone replacement increases fat-free mass and muslce size in hypogonadal men. *J Clin Endocrinol Metab* 1997;82:407–13

8. Mauras N, Hayes V, Welch S, et al. Testosterone deficiency in young men: marked alterations in whole body protein kinetics, strength, and adiposity. *J Clin Endocrinol Metab* 1998;83:1886–92

9. Grinspoon S, Cororan C, Lee K, et al. Loss of lean body mass and muscle mass correlates with androgen levels in hypogonaldal men with acquired immunodeficiency syndrome wasting. *J Clin Endocrinol Metab* 1996;81:4051–58

10. Gray A, Feldman HA, McKinlay JB, et al. Age, disease, and changing sex hormone levels in middle-aged men: Results of the Massachusetts Male Aging Study. *J Clin Endocrinol Metab* 1991;73:1016–25

11. Harman SM, Metter EJ, Tobin JD, et al. Longitudinal effects of aging on serum total and free testosterone levels in healthy men. *J Clin Endocrinol Metab* 2001;86:724–31

12. Urban RJ, Bodenburg YH, Gilkison C, et al. Testosterone administration to elderly men increases skeletal muscle strength and protein synthesis. *Am J Physiol* 1995;269:E820–26

13. Tenover JS. Effects of testosterone supplementation in the aging male. *J Clin Endocrinol Metab* 1992;75:1092–98

14. Snyder PJ, Peachey H, Hannoush P, et al. Effect of testosterone treatment on body composition and muscle strength in men over 65 years of age. *J Clin Endocrinol Metab* 1999;84:2647–53

15. Wang C, Swerdlof RS, Iranmanesh A, et al. Transdermal testosterone gel improves sexual function, mood, muscle strength, and body composition parameters in hypogonadal men. *J Clin Endocrinol Metab* 2000;85:2839–53

16. Berger JR, Pall L, Hall CD, *et al.* Oxandrolone in AIDS-wasting myopathy. *AIDS* 1996;10: 1657–62

17. Bhasin S, Storer TW, Asbel-Sethi N, *et al.* Effects of testosterone replacement with a nongenital, transdermal stystem, Androderm, in human immunodeficiency virus-infected men with low testosterone levels. *J Clin Endocrinol Metab* 1998;83:3155–62

18. Bauman WA, Spungen AM. Disorders of carbohydrate and lipid metabolism in veterans with paraplegia or quadriplegia: A model of premature aging. *Metabolism* 1994;43:749–56

19. Spungen AM, Wang J, Pierson Jr RN, *et al.* Soft tissue body composition changes from immobilization determined from a mono-zygotic twin model: One with spinal cord injury. *J Applied Physiol* 2000;88:1310–15

20. Tsitouras PD, Zhong YG, Spungen AM, *et al.* Serum testosterone and insulin-like growth factor-I/growth hormone in adults with spinal cord injury. *Horm Met Res* 1995;27:287–92

21. Bauman WA, Zhong YG, Spungen AM. Depressed serum testosterone levels in sub-jects with SCI. *J Spinal Cord Med* 2001; 24:S20

22. Bhasin S, Storer TW, Berman N, *et al.* The effects of supraphysiological doses of testos-terone on muscle size and strength in normal men. *N Engl J Med* 1996;335:1–7

23. Bisschop A, Gayan-Ramirez G, Rollier H, *et al.* Effects of nandrolone decanoate on res-piratory and peripheral muscles in male and female rats. *J Appl Physiol* 1997;82:1112–8

24. Prezant DJ, Valentine DE, Gentry EI, *et al.* Effects of short-term and long-term androgen treatment on the diaphragm in male and female rats. *J Appl Physiol* 1993;75:1140–9

25. Van Balkom RH, Dekhuijzen PN, Folgering HT, *et al.* Anabolic steroids in part reverse glucocorticoid-induced alterations in rat diaphragm. *Appl Physiol* 1998;84:1492–9

26. Mayer M, Rosen F. Interaction of anabolic steroids with glucocorticoid receptor sites in rat muscle cytosol. *Am J Physiol* 1975;229:1381–6

27. Van Balkom RH, Dekhuijzen PN, van der Heijden HF, *et al.* Effects of anabolic steroids on diphragm impairment induced by methyl-prednisolone in emphysematous hamsters. *Eur Respir J* 1999;13:1062–9

28. Eggington S. Effects of an anabolic hormone on aerobic capacity of rat striated muscle. *Pflugers Arch* 1987;410:356–62

29. Ferreira IM, Verreschi IT, Nery LE, *et al.* The influence of 6 months of oral anabolic steroids on body mass and respiratory muscles in undernourished COPD patients. *Chest* 1998;114:19–28

30. Schols AM, Soeters PB, Mostert R, *et al.* Physiologic effects of nutritional support and anabolic steroids in patients with chronic obstructive pulmonary disease. A placebo-controlled randomized trial. *Am J Respir Crit Care Med* 1995;152:1268–74

31. Spungen AM, Grimm DR, Strakhan M, *et al.* Treatment with an anabolic agent is associated with improvement in respiratory function in persons with tetraplegia: a pilot study. *Mt Sinai J Med* 1999;66:201–5

Section VIII

Central nervous system/psyche

John E. Morley, MB, BCh

It is the complex interaction of neurons within the central nervous system that allows modern man to manipulate his environment and to achieve happiness. This section highlights the changes in the central nervous system that occur with aging and how they impact on the quality of life. In particular, the differences in central nervous system aging in the male compared with the female are highlighted.

Memories are the most powerful component of the human psyche. The chapter on cognitive changes highlights the fact that by 85 years of age one-quarter of men will have dementia. Many more will have minor cognitive impairment. The good news for men is that Alzheimer's disease is more common in females than males. Unfortunately, vascular dementia is more common in males! This section highlights the other causes of dementia and their treatment. It also points out the importance of the early recognition of delirium and the need to distinguish delirium from dementia.

With aging, the decline in testosterone results in a waning of libido. This coupled with the decline in erectile function can lead to a marked decline in sexual activity with aging. Recently, it has been recognized that some of these changes are particularly important issues for quality of life of the older homosexual. A simple 10-question screener for low testosterone in older males, the ADAM, is provided.

Two chapters examine the problem of depression and its management in older men. While men become depressed less often than women, they are more likely to commit suicide. Depression in older persons can present atypically as weight loss or memory dysfunction. For this reason, use of the Geriatric Depression Scale to screen for depression is recommended. While behavior therapy remains the cornerstone of treatment of depression in all, except the most cognitively impaired, a large number of newer antidepressants are available to compliment the psychological approaches. In addition, the increasing use of St. John's Wort by people with minor levels of dysphoria is discussed.

The decline in testosterone with age appears to play a role in the decrease in cognition seen in older men. There is increasing evidence that testosterone replacement may enhance some of this age-associated cognitive decline. Testosterone also appears to play an important role in the modulation of mood and enthusiasm for life.

Sleep disorders are highly prevalent in older persons. Again, men suffer from these less commonly than females. However, sleep apnea is very common in overweight older males. It presents with daytime somnolence. It has been associated with an increased prevalence of dementia and myocardial infarction. Sleep apnea is a totally reversible disorder and as such needs to be screened for in all older males. Appropriate sleep hygiene techniques remain the cornerstone of management of insomnia. Numerous drugs are available for the treatment of insomnia but it is stressed that they should be used only short-term for insomnia and not for prolonged periods of time.

Overall, this section highlights the importance of paying attention to the disorders of the central nervous system in the aging male. The potential role of testosterone in enhancing central nervous system function in the older male is an area of intense investigation. Screening for cognitive problems, depression, sleep apnea and low testosterone states is mandatory in the older male. Numerous treatments are available for each of these conditions.

36 Changes in libido/sex life

Syed H. Tariq, MD

INTRODUCTION

Decline in sexual activity, interest and desire has been reported by a number of investigators[1-5]. Advanced age has a significant negative effect on sexual desire, but there is no difference in sexual enjoyment and satisfaction between young and older persons[6]. About 50% of older adults express sexual desire in the ninth decade and about 15% are sexually active[7]. Pfeiffer and colleagues[8] reported that in their study 95% of men aged 46 to 50 years had weekly intercourse, a figure which decreased to 28% at the age of 66 to 71. Kinsey and co-workers[9] reported a reduced frequency of intercourse to once every 10 weeks by age 80. Sexual activity is reported to decrease in older married couples from 53% at the age of 60 to 24% over the age of 76[10]. In one study of older adults between the ages of 80 and 102 years who were sexually active, 83% of men were reported touching and caressing without intercourse and 72% of men indulged in masturbation[11]. Janus and Janus[12] reported a decrease in the frequency of masturbation after the age of 65 years.

Erectile dysfunction affects about 10 to 20 million men in the USA[13]. Kinsey and colleagues[9] reported an increase in erectile dysfunction with age, reaching 27% at the age of 70 years, 55% at the age of 75 years and about 75% at the age of 80 years.

In the USA there are about 3.5 million gay people over the age of 60[14,15]. Older gay men are a diverse population, with many aging successfully, living healthy and satisfying lives[16].

All older gay persons have in common, at least in the USA, an experience of living in a society where the gay life-style is oppressed, with a concomitant failure to recognize that loving relationships exist between those of the same gender. Most older homosexual men will not reveal their sexual feelings in public, but they face similar problems with relationships as older heterosexual men experience. Older homosexual men suffer additional problems of stress while hiding their sexual preferences or trying to find a partner – especially in nursing homes. Gay-oriented long-term care facilities are currently not available. However a support group called 'Gay and Lesbians Older and Wiser' (GLOW) has been established in Ann Arbor, Michigan[17]. The GLOW service is provided by a university-based geriatric clinic, staffed by professional social workers who provide social support. The GLOW initiative and others have shown that older gay men who are integrated into the gay community develop extended relationships, thereby building up a surrogate family[18,19].

Recent advances have made it possible to understand the effects of aging on sexuality and of disease and drugs on sexual/erectile dysfunction. Today there are more treatment options available that are non-invasive and are efficacious. The media are playing a major role in advertising the newly available commercial products that place the burden on the primary care physician to identify and treat sexual problems. Patients expect physicians to help maintain quality of life in the seventh decade and beyond. Men with erectile dysfunction have an impaired quality of life compared with healthy individuals as sexual activity contributes to the quality of life of couples or individuals[20].

THE PHYSIOLOGY OF PENILE ERECTION

Sexual activity consists of libido and potency. Libido comprises sexual desire/drive, thoughts and fantasies, satisfaction and pleasure, while potency is the ability to attain and maintain erection and to ejaculate. Penile erection is obtained in three different ways. The first pathway is through local genital stimulation affording afferent sensations in the sensory receptors of the penile shaft and glans penis that are carried to the spinal cord by the somatic pudendal nerve. The sensory perception is then carried to the higher centers, and efferent impulses leave the spinal cord via the sacral parasympathetic center to the pelvic plexus and the cavernous nerves into the corpus cavernosum. The second pathway is psychogenic stimulation, which occurs through visual or auditory stimuli; this is more complex and less well understood. The third type of penile erection is seen during rapid eye movement (REM) sleep, the physiology of which is not known.

In the flaccid state sympathetic activity causes vasoconstriction of the arteries, arterioles, and sinusoidal spaces within the corpora cavernosa. During erection the adrenergic-induced vasoconstriction of the sinusoidal spaces is overcome by the vasodilatation of the parasympathetic nervous system. Vasodilatation leads to an increase in arterial blood flow causing an increased pressure in the cavernosal spaces, which occludes the venous system and leads to penile erection. After ejaculation or termination of the erotic stimuli, the sympathetic nerve terminals release catecholamines, which cause contraction of the smooth muscles around the sinusoids and arterioles, resulting in a decrease in blood inflow and expulsion of blood out of the sinusoidal spaces, resulting in a flaccid state.

A number of neurotransmitters play an important role in penile erection. Nitric oxide is released during sexual stimulation by endothelial cells and cavernous nerves. Nitric oxide, along with other agents such as prostaglandins E_2 and E_1, vasoactive intestinal peptide, neuropeptide Y and acetylcholine, causes smooth muscle relaxation and penile erection. Smooth muscle contraction is caused by prostaglandin F_2, substance P, histamine and norepinephrine.

PHYSIOLOGICAL CHANGES WITH AGE IN THE MALE

There are four stages in the cycle of sexual response – excitement, plateau, orgasm and resolution. Masters and Johnson[21] described changes in these cycles with aging. During the excitement phase there is delay in erection, decrease in erectile strength and decrease in scrotal congestion and testicular elevation with advanced age. There is a prolongation of the plateau phase along with a decrease in pre-ejaculatory secretion. The orgasmic phase is shorter, with diminished prostatic and urethral contractions and a decrease in ejaculatory force. The ejaculation time is longer compared to that of young adults with longer periods of coitus. In the resolution phase there is rapid detumescence and rapid testicular descent. The refractory period is also prolonged with age. The sensitivity of the penis to stimulation decreases with age and it takes longer to achieve erection[22]. Erection becomes more dependent on physical stimulation of the penis and less responsive to visual, nongenital and psychologic stimulation. Although penile rigidity decreases with age it generally remains adequate for vaginal penetration, although in some men the capability for penetration is lost[9].

Nocturnal penile tumescence is impaired and is considered as an indicator of erectile dysfunction. Schiavi and colleagues[6] reported that, in married couples or those in stable relationships between the ages of 45 and 75, sexual desire, arousal, coital frequency and prevalence of erectile problems correlated with nocturnal penile tumescence measures. Furthermore in healthy older men there are decreases in frequency and degree of erection obtained during sleep[23–25].

In normal older adults there are individual variations in circulating testosterone levels, which are not associated with individual variations in sexual drive or behavior[26]. With the onset of middle-age there is a gradual decrease in sexual desire or libido[27,28]. Libido in men is linked to testosterone[29] and when testosterone is replaced in hypogonadal men there is an increase in sexual thoughts and sexual desire[30–32]. In men, similar to the menopause in women, partial endocrine deficiencies occur (andropause, secondary hypogonadism, ADAM, PADAM). These are characterized by decreases in total and bioavailable testosterone but often without a concomitant increase in luteinizing hormone levels[33–36]. Schiavi and colleagues[6] reported that bioavailable testosterone is related to sexual desire but not to coital frequency. The mechanism of action of androgen on sexual drive is yet to be determined in humans, but there are data from animal studies that indicate that the median preoptic hypothalamus area and associated limbic structures are involved in sexual behavior[37].

Other agents that have been suggested by others to be involved in sexual desire and arousal in men are estrogen, prolactin and endogenous opiate peptides[38,39]. Elevated prolactin levels can be associated with low sexual desire independently from androgen levels and probably act as a direct effect or via reduced central dopaminergic activity.

PSYCHOLOGICAL PROBLEMS

Sexual problems can be attributed to psychological problems in both young and older adults.

Psychological conditions such as depression and psychosocial stresses (such as divorce, death of spouse, loss of social status, loss of job, health-related family problems) are prevalent in older adults and contribute to sexual problems[39]. Sexual dissatisfaction is also related to marital relationship problems, which vary from interpersonal problems and inadequate communication of sexual needs to poor sexual techniques. Other issues such as problems of commitment, power struggle, and lack of trust may all reflect dissatisfaction on the partner's behalf and may relate to sexual problems[39–41]. Older men may develop 'widower's syndrome', which is characterized by failure to achieve erection after the death of their spouse[42,43].

EVALUATION OF THE DECREASE IN SEXUAL DRIVE/LIBIDO

A thorough and careful history will help to differentiate difficulties in achieving erection from a decreased desire for sex or decreased libido. A detailed history with the partner will help uncover some of the problems within a relationship. Risk factors for erectile dysfunction can also be assessed in the history, such as vascular disease, hormonal problems (thyroid, diabetes) neurological dysfunction, medication, past surgery, or trauma; and psychological and social factors, including evaluation for depression. A detailed examination of medication is important, since a number of medications are associated with decreased libido (Table 1). The standard depression assessment tools such as the Beck Depression Inventory or Yesavage Geriatric Scale can be used. Tools are also available to screen the patient for androgen deficiency such as that developed by Saint Louis University, the Androgen Deficiency in Aging Males (ADAM) questionnaire (Table 2). A positive answer to question 1 or 7 or any other 3 questions is considered to indicate a high likelihood of having low levels of testosterone. The ADAM questionnaire has a sensitivity of 88% and

Table 1 Drugs that may affect sexual desire in men

Drugs that may increase sexual desire
Androgens (in androgen deficit states)
Baclofen (possible anti-anxiety effect)
Benzodiazepines (anti-anxiety effect)
Haloperidol (indirect effect due to improved
  sense of well-being)

Drugs that may decrease sexual desire
Antihistamines/barbiturates/benzodiazepines
Tricyclic antidepressants
Diuretics
  Spironolactone
  Hydrochlorothiazide
  Acetazolamide
  Methazolamide
Antihypertensives
  Reserpine
  Propranolol
  Clonidine
  Alpha-methyldopa
  Prazosin
Cimetidine
Hormones
  Estrogen
  Medroxyprogesterone
Clofibrate
Digoxin
Lithium

Table 2 Saint Louis University ADAMS Questionnaire

1. Do you have a decrease in libido (sex drive)?
2. Do you have a lack of energy?
3. Do you have a decrease in strength and/
   or endurance?
4. Have you lost height?
5. Have you noticed a decreased 'enjoyment
   of life'?
6. Are you sad and/or grumpy?
7. Are your erections less strong?
8. Have you noticed a recent deterioration in your
   ability to play sports?
9. Are you falling asleep after dinner?
10. Has there been a recent deterioration in your
    work performance?

Adapted from: Validation of a screening questionnaire for androgen deficiency of aging males. Morley JE, et al. *Metabolism* 2000;49(9):1239–42

a specificity of 60%, validated in 310 Canadian physicians. There is a clear improvement in the ADAM questionnaire results after treatment with testosterone[44].

Physical examination should include an assessment of secondary sexual characteristics and a detailed search for vascular and neurological problems. Local penile shaft examination is also important to rule out Peyronie's disease.

Laboratory evaluations will help to look for the etiology of erectile dysfunction, such as tests for diabetes, renal function, lipid profile, thyroid function tests, prolactin levels and penile brachial pressure index. The single most important test for a decrease in sexual drive or libido is to check total testosterone and bioavailable testosterone (non-sex hormone-bound testosterone). Most cross-sectional studies[34,45–48] have demonstrated that levels of testosterone decrease with age, although the

Baltimore Longitudinal Aging Study failed to find a decrease in testosterone in cross-sectional data[49]. Morley and Kaiser[50] have demonstrated a fall in testosterone levels of 100 ng/dl/decade in a longitudinal study of older males in the New Mexico Process Study of Aging. Just as free testosterone level declines with aging, a number of studies have reported a decline in bioavailable testosterone with aging[34–36,51,52]. Bioavailable and free testosterone decline earlier than the total testosterone with aging[53]. A decline in bioavailable testosterone is seen in 50% of men by 50 years of age[35]. Luteinizing hormone levels fail to increase appropriately in response to the decreasing testosterone levels with age, suggesting failure of the hypothalamic–pituitary axis and hence secondary hypogonadism[34,35,54–56].

TREATMENT OF DECREASED SEXUAL DRIVE

The choice of treatment in men with a decrease in sexual drive or libido is guided by the possible cause and the treatment options available. If the history suggests any marital discord or psychiatric problems such as depression or anxiety, appropriate counseling should be provided or medical treatment should be offered for depression. This is discussed elsewhere in this section. If the decrease in sexual desire is related to the use of medication it should be stopped. If the problem is secondary to testosterone deficiency, then testosterone replacement therapy is indicated. A number of options are available for the administration of testosterone.

Intramuscular injections

Intramuscular injections of testosterone enanthate or cypionate are the two available forms. Injections of either 100 mg or 200 mg can be given every 7 to 21 days, but are normally given every 14 days. They are cheap compared to other preparations but are contraindicated in patients who are on warfarin therapy.

The administration of injectable preparations results initially (in about 72h) in supraphysiological levels of serum testosterone followed by a steady decline over the next 10–14 days. This decline frequently results in a very low nadir immediately before the next injection. This phenomenon translates in wide swings in mood and well-being – the roller-coster effect – which is disconcerting and upsetting to both patients and their partners.

Transdermal preparations

Three transdermal preparations are available. Testoderm (Alza Pharmaceuticals, Palo Alto, CA) is a patch that is applied to the scrotum (with a prerequisite of shaving). Absorption is good and achieves a normal physiological level of circulating testosterone and is successfully used in older persons[57,58]. The initial dose of Testoderm is 6 mg/day, applied to the scrotal skin for 22 to 24 hours. Serum levels are determined after 3–4 weeks of daily application. If the desired levels are not achieved in 6–8 weeks of therapy another form of testosterone should be considered. The second transdermal preparation is Androderm (SmithKline Beecham, Pittsburgh, PA), which is placed on any area of the skin except the scrotum and is associated with higher levels of allergic reactions[59,60]. It is applied for 24 hours.

Table 3 Effects of testosterone replacement in older hypogonadal men

Increase in libido
Increase in visual-spatial cognition
Increased facial recognition
Increased beard growth
Gynecomastia
Increased hematocrit
Increase in muscle mass
Increase in muscle strength
Increase in protein synthesis
Increase in bone mineral density
Decrease in hip fracture
Decrease in leptin (decrease in visceral fat)
Decrease in atherosclerosis (minimal effects on lipids)(?)
Enhanced potency(?)
Worsening of metastatic prostate cancer

The third transdermal preparation is a gel called Androgel™ (Unimed Pharmaceuticals, Chicago, IL). It has the advantage of not being visible and maintains patient privacy.

Testosterone pellets

Testosterone pellets are a slow-release preparation, lasting for 3 months, implanted under the skin. The major disadvantage is difficulty in removing the pellets.

Oral preparations

Oral androgen preparations (Ondrol®, Androl®) have become popular due to their convenience (i.e. dose flexibility, self-administration, possibility of immediate discontinuation). However, they demand special consideration as they undergo rapid hepatic and intestinal metabolism. Thus special precautions may be necessary to acheive adequate serum androgen levels.

Oral preparations are potentially toxic to the liver, with the exception of testosterone undecanoate (Ondrol), which is not available in the USA, and is absorbed through the lymphatics. It can be used as an alternative to intramuscular injections for testosterone replacement therapy.

The major side-effect of testosterone replacement therapy is an increase in hematocrit levels independent of erythropoietin[61], which can lead to cerebrovascular accident. This effect of increase in hematocrit is also seen in nursing-home patients[62]. The myth that testosterone has deleterious effects on the prostate comes from studies in which patients with metastatic prostate cancer were treated with testosterone[63]. Retrospective studies have failed to show an increase in prostate cancer or benign prostatic hypertrophy in men treated with testosterone[64]. Other effects of testosterone replacement are shown in Table 3.

References

1. Bachman GA. Sexual issues at menopause. *Ann N Y Acad Sci* 1988;87:87–94, 123–33
2. Kaiser FE. Sexuality and impotence in aging men. *Clin Geriatr Med* 1991;7:63–72
3. Kellet JM. Sexuality in later life. *Rev Clin Gerontol* 1993;3:309–14
4. Ludeman K. The sexuality of older persons: review of the literature. *Gerontologist* 1981; 21:203–8
5. Morley JE, Kaiser FE. Sexual function with advancing age. *Med Clin North Am* 1989; 73:1483–5
6. Schiavi RC, Schreiner-Engel P, Mandeli J. Healthy aging and male sexual function. *Am J Psychiatry* 1990;147:766–71
7. Mulligan T, Katz G. Erectile failure in the aged: evaluation and treatment. *J Am Geriatr Soc* 1988;36:54–62
8. Pfeiffer E, Verwoerdt A, Wang HS. Sexual behavior in aged men and women. *Arch Gen Psychiatry* 1968;19:735–58
9. Kinsey AC, Pomeroy WB, Martin CE. *Sexual Behavior in the Human Male*. Philadelphia: WB Saunders, 1948
10. Marsiglio W, Donnelly D. Sexual relations in later life: a national study of married persons. *J Gerontol* 1991;46:S338–S344
11. Catalan J, Hawton K, Day A. Couples referred to a sexual dysfunction clinic. Psychological and physical morbidity. *Br J Psychiatry* 1990;156:61–7
12. Janus SS, Janus CL. *The Janus Report on Sexual Behavior*. New York: John Wiley & Sons, 1993
13. NIH consensus development panel on impotence. *J Am Med Assoc* 1993;270:83–90
14. Dawson K. Serving the older gay community. SIECUS, Report, 5–6, November 1982
15. Gwenwald M. The sage model for serving older lesbians and gay men. *J Social Work Hum Sexuality* 1984;2(2/3):53–61
16. Quam JK, Whiteford GS. Adaptation and age-related expectations of older gay and lesbian adults. *Gerontologist* 1992;32:367–74
17. Slusher MP, Mayer CJ, Dunkle RE. Practice concepts: gay and lesbians older and wiser (GLOW): a support group for older gay people. *Gerontologist* 1996;36:118–23
18. Bell AP, Weinberg MA. *Homosexuality. A study of Diversity among Men and Women*. New York: Simon and Schuster, 1978
19. Francher JS, Henkin J. The menopausal queen: adjustment to aging and the male homosexual. *Am J Orthopsychiatry* 1973;43: 670–4
20. John M, Moon T, Brannan W. The effect of age, ethnicity and geographic location on impotence and quality of life. *Br J Urol* 1995;75:651–5
21. Masters WH, Johnson VE. *Human Sexual Response*. Boston: Little, Brown, 1970
22. Edward AE, Husted J. Penile sensitivity, age, and sexual behavior. *J Clin Psychol* 1976;32: 697–700
23. Kahn E, Fisher C. REM sleep and sexuality in the aged. *J Geriatr Psychiatry* 1969;2: 181–99
24. Karacan I, William RL, Thornby JI. Sleep related penile tumescence as a function of age. *Am J Psychiatry* 1975;132:932–7
25. Schiavi RC, Schreiner-Engel P. Nocturnal penile tumescence in healthy aging men. 1988;43:M146–M150
26. Schiavi RC, White D. Androgens and male sexual function. A review of human studies. *J Sex Marital Ther* 1976;3:214

27. Pardridge WM, Gorski RA, Lippe BM. Androgens and sexual behavior. *Ann Intern Med* 1982;96:488–501

28. Verwoerdt A, Pfeiffer E, Wang HS. Sexual behavior in senescence. Patterns of sexual activity and interest. *Geriatrics* 1969;24:137–54

29. Segraves RT. Hormone and libido. In Leiblum SR, Rosen RC, eds. *Sexual Desire Disorders*. New York: Guildford Press, 1988:271

30. Davidson JM, Kwan M, Greenleaf WJ. Hormonal replacement and sexuality. *Clin Endocrinol Metab* 1982;11:599–623

31. Kwan M, Greenleaf WJ, Mann J. The nature of androgen on men's sexuality: A combined laboratory/self reported study on hypogonadal men. *J Clin Endocrinol Metab* 1983;57:557

32. Skakkeoaek NE, Bancroft J, Davidson DW. Androgen replacement with oral testosterone undecanoate in hypogonadal men. A double blinded control study. *Clin Endocrinol* 1981;14:49

33. Kaiser FE, Morley JE. Gonadotropin, testosterone, and the aging male. *Neurobiol Aging* 1994;15:559–63

34. Kaiser FE, Viosca SP, Morley JE. Impotence and aging: clinical and hormonal factors. *J Am Geriatr Soc* 1988;36:511–19

35. Korenman SG, Morley JE, Mooradian AD. Secondary hypogonadism in older men: its relationship to impotence. *J Clin Endocrinol Metab* 1990;71:963–9

36. Tenover JS, Matsumoto AM, Plymate SR. The effect of aging in normal men on bioavailable testosterone and luteinizing hormone secretion: response to clomiphene citrate. *J Clin Endocrinol Metab* 1987;65:1118–26

37. Everitt BJ, Bancroft J. Of rats and men: the comparative approach to male sexuality. *Ann Rev Sex Res* 1991;2:77

38. Bancroft J. Endocrinology of sexual function. *Clin Obstet Gynecol* 1980;7:253

39. Cole MJ. *Psychological Approach to Treatment*. Edinburgh: Churchill Livingstone, 1993

40. Kaplan HS. *The New Sexual Therapy*. New York: Brunner/Mazel, 1974

41. LoPiccolo J, Stock W. Treatment of sexual dysfunctions. *J Consult Clin Psychol* 1986;54:158–67

42. Dunn ME. Psychological perspectives of sex and aging. *Am J Cardiol* 1988;61:24H–26H

43. Morley JE, Korenman SG, Mooradian AD. UCLA geriatric rounds: sexual dysfunction in the elderly male. *J Am Geriatr Soc* 1987;35:1014–22

44. Morley JE, Charlton E, Patrick P, et al. Validation of a screening questionnaire for androgen deficiency in aging males. *Metabolism* 2000;49:1239–42

45. Gray A, Feldman HA, McKinlay JB. Age, disease, and changing sex hormone levels in middle-aged men: results of Massachusetts Male Aging Study. *J Clin Endocrinol Metab* 1991;73:1016–25

46. Gray A, Berlin JA, McKinlay JB. An examination of research design effects on association of testosterone and male aging: results of meta-analysis. *J Clin Epidemiol* 1991;44:671–84

47. Deslypere JP, Vermeulen A. A Leydig cell function in normal men: effect of age, life style, residence, diet, and activity. *J Clin Endocrinol Metab* 1984;59:955–62

48. Baker HW, Burger HG, De Kretser DM. Changes in the pituitary–testicular system with age. *Clin Endocrinol (Oxf)* 1976;5:349–72

49. Harman SM, Tsitouras PD. Reproductive hormones in aging men. Measurement of sex steroids, basal luteinizing hormone and Leydig cell response to human chorionic gonadotropin. *J Clin Endocrinol Metab* 1980;51:35–40

50. Morley JE, Kaiser FE. Longitudinal changes in testosterone, luteinizing hormone and follicular stimulating hormone in healthy older males. *Metabolism* 1997;46:410–14

51. Baker HW, Hudson B. Changes in the pituitary–testicular axis with age. *Clin Endocrinol* 1983;25:71–83

52. Nakin HR, Calkins JH. Decreased bioavailable testosterone in aging normal and impotent men. *J Clin Endocrinol Metab* 1986;63:1418–20

53. Nahoul K, Roger M. Age-related decline of plasma bioavailable testosterone in adult men. *J Steroid Biochem* 1990;35:293–9

54. Vermeulen A, Deslypere JP, De Meirleir K. A new look to the andropause: altered function of the gonadotrophs. *J Steroid Biochem* 1989;32:163–5

55. Tennekoon KH, Karunanayake EH. Serum FSH, LH, and testosterone concentrations in presumably fertile men: effect of age. *Int J Fertil* 1993;38:108–12

56. Kaufman JM, Deslypere JP, Giri M. Neuroendocrine regulation of pulsatile luteinizing hormone secretion in elderly men. *J Steroid Biochem Mol Biol* 1990;37:421–30

57. Jankowsky JS, Oviatt SK, Orwoll ES. Testosterone influences spatial cognition in older men. *Behav Neurosci* 1994;108:325–32

58. Orwoll ES. Osteoporosis in men. *Endocr Rev* 1995;16:87–116

59. Arver S, Dobs AS, Meikle AW. Improvement of sexual function in testosterone deficient men treated for 1 year with a permeation enhanced testosterone transdermal patch. *J Urol* 1996;155:1604–8

60. Meikle SW, Arver S, Dobe AS. Pharmacokinetics and metabolism of a permeation enhanced testosterone transdermal system in hypogonadal men: influence of application site – a clinical research center study. *J Clin Endocrinol Metab* 1996;81:1832–40

61. Sih R, Morley JE. Testosterone replacement in older hypogonadal men: a 12 month randomized controlled trial. *J Clin Endocrinol Metab* 1997;82:1661–7

62. Drinka PJ, Jochen AL. Polycythemia as a complication of testosterone replacement therapy in nursing home men with low testosterone levels. *J Am Geriatr Soc* 1995; 43:899–901

63. Fowler JE, Whitemore WF. The response of metastatic adenocarcinoma of the prostate to exogenous testosterone. *J Urol* 1981;126: 372–5

64. Hajjar RR, Kaiser FE, Morley JE. Outcome of long-term testosterone replacement in older hypogonadal males: a retrospective analysis. *J Clin Endocrinol Metab* 1997;82:3793–6

37 Depression

Margaret-Mary G. Wilson, MRCP

'The agony they do not show,
the suffocating sense of woe ...'

Lord Byron (1788–1824)
Prometheus, Works: 1832

The pervading trend of global consumerism threatens the positive concept of durability by emphasizing the hazards of antiquity. The perception of aging by modern society is affected by this trend. Western cultures propagate the impression that the aging process is merely the descent along a gradual slope that inevitably leads to death. Viewed in this manner, it is not surprising that depression is erroneously considered a natural reaction to the aging process. Available evidence indicates that this bias exists even among healthcare professionals[1]. Such attitudes pose obstacles to the provision of adequate, well co-ordinated care to a segment of the population at risk from a life-threatening disease.

In the USA one million people over the age of 65 years are diagnosed with major depression and five million others experience depressive symptoms. Annual healthcare costs related to depression are estimated at 43 billion dollars. Within the next two decades these figures are expected to increase by more than 50%[2–4]. The prevalence of depression among community-dwelling older adults ranges from 1 to 3%, with depressive symptoms occurring in 8–16% of this population[5,6]. Although similar figures are reported for the younger segment of the community-dwelling population, older adults are more likely to commit suicide as a result of depression than younger adults[7]. Across the life cycle depression occurs in men at half the frequency with which it occurs in women. Similarly, older men are less likely than older women to be diagnosed with depression. However, following diagnosis the incidence of recurrent episodes is similar between the genders[8]. Gender differences have also been observed in the frequency of suicide, which is higher in men. This gender difference increases with age and peaks among the oldest old[9]. However, suicide attempts, the majority of which are unsuccessful, occur with greater frequency among women[10]. Older, white men commit suicide at a higher rate than any other cohort in society. However, the rate of suicide among African-American men is rising at a faster rate. Between 1980 and 1986, suicide rates among white men increased by 23% compared with an increase of 42% among African-American men[9]. Several explanations have been proffered for the gender and age-related variations in the frequency of suicide. Older men are more likely to use more violent methods of suicide, such as hanging and gunshots. The higher rates of substance abuse and the relatively lean social support systems of older men constitute additional risk factors for suicide in the depressed older man[10,11].

The relatively high prevalence of depression in the institutionalized setting may be a reflection of the significant medical co-morbidity associated with depression in the older adult[12,13].

Major depression is diagnosed in approximately 30% of long-term care residents, with a similar frequency between the genders[4,14]. The older man is less likely than the older woman to report depressive symptoms or seek psychiatric help. However, available data indicate that depression is a marker for increased use of hospital services among older men. A similar relationship does not occur in older women[9,15]. These characteristics may jeopardize prompt clinical detection and treatment of depression in the older man, thereby increasing the risk of morbidity and mortality associated with this disease.

PATHOPHYSIOLOGY

The pathophysiology of depression has not been fully elucidated. Even less well understood are the observed age and gender differences in the manifestations of depression. The role of neurotransmitters has been extensively explored. Current theories implicate a reduction in central nervous system serotoninergic activity. Decreased levels of 5-hydroxyindoleacetic acid (5-HIAA) have been identified in the cerebrospinal fluid (CSF) of depressed persons. Bryer and colleagues[16] measured the concentrations of CSF monoamine metabolites in patients with a recent cerebrovascular infarct. They found significantly lower concentrations of 5-HIAA in the subgroup of patients with depression compared with non-depressed patients. They also demonstrated a significant correlation between 5-HIAA levels and the distance of the infarct from the frontal lobe. Additional studies of post-stroke patients identified a correlation between depression and the anatomical location of the infarct. Review of these studies supports a lateralized effect, but restricts this correlation to the left hemisphere only[17–19]. More recent studies in support of these findings show that left anterior hemisphere lesions are significantly associated with a higher incidence of depression. However, this association was restricted to one month following the stroke, after which anatomic correlation to depressive symptoms can no longer be demonstrated[20]. Neurochemical imaging studies showed that among patients with left hemisphere strokes, 5-hydroxytryptamine receptor binding was significantly lower in the left temporal cortex of depressed patients[21]. These studies lend credence to the occurrence of depression as a biochemical response to structural brain injury. The location of the injury and its consequent impact on the neuronal circuits may determine the extent of the mood disorder. Among older adults, 85% of persons with ischemic white matter changes on magnetic resonance imaging (MRI) suffered from depression. Depressed persons with leuko-encephalopathic changes identified on MRI also demonstrated greater apathy and manifested with fewer cognitive symptoms of depression. The increased frequency of these lesions in older men may be relevant to the age and gender differences observed in the clinical manifestations of depression[22].

Functional imaging studies may ultimately provide a more unified theory regarding the pathogenesis of depression. Positron emission tomography (PET) studies have identified hypometabolic areas in caudate and frontal cortical regions in depressed persons[23,24]. These findings have proved consistent using both glucose metabolism and cerebral blood flow as physiologic variables. More recent studies using this modality have been able to correlate PET findings with disease activity, familial traits and therapeutic response. Pre-frontal and subgenual hypometabolism have been identified in groups of non-depressed persons with a history of familial depression[25]. Additionally, depressed persons with areas of caudate hypometabolism manifest with increased caudate metabolism following initiation of antidepressant therapy. The presence of anterior cingulate hypometabolism has been found by some workers to be a marker for a poor response to therapy[24,26].

Earlier theories implicated dysregulation of the hypothalamic–pituitary–adrenal (HPA) axis as a central theory in the pathogenesis of depression. This was based on the observation that persons with hypercortisolism were found, in some studies, to have an increased incidence of depression[27]. Consequently, age-related dysregulation of the HPA axis was proffered as a possible explanation for depression in the elderly[28]. Definitive evidence in support of this theory is lacking. Furthermore it fails to provide an explanation for age- and gender-related differences in the manifestations of depression.

Neuroendocrine theories are favored as most logical in terms of defining gender differences in the manifestations of depression. Such theories appear to be validated by the occurrence of mood disturbances in association with the menopause and menstruation. However, the validity of biological theories as the sole explanation for depression in the older adult is challenged by the persistence of gender differences despite the physiological blunting of gonadal function that occurs with aging[12]. Based on current research, depression is most probably a syndrome that stems from a complex interplay of biological and psychosocial factors.

Cognitive and behavioral theories remain attractive and offer a psychosocial basis for gender differences in the manifestations of late-life depression. With aging, deteriorating functional status and changing social roles may have a negative impact on the older man's self-image, self-esteem and self-worth. As his adult offspring start their own families and spousal illness or bereavement occurs, the older man may place unrealistic expectations on himself if he fails to recognize that his role as primary provider is no longer critical to family cohesion. The inevitable redistribution of leadership roles within the family may be misconstrued by the aging man as a reflection of his inadequacy or failure, rather than the natural progression of social events. Consequently, the older man may develop a dislocation in his 'sense of belonging'. The latter is a recognized psychological concept which has been shown to correlate with depression. A robust sense of belonging is nurtured by

energy, motivation and the perceived possession of shared group characteristics. Retirement, age-related reduction in physical activity and consequent trimming of the older adult's social support mechanisms may have a negative impact on these vital 'sense of belonging' antecedents. A low 'sense of belonging' is significantly associated with an increased frequency of depression, and current data indicate that this may be a better predictor of depression than social isolation or lack of social support[29,30]. Behavioral and cognitive theorists also emphasize the role of age-related distorted thinking in the genesis of depression. Isolated events in which the individual's performance falls short of personal expectations are often regarded as measures of overall ability and a reflection of the person's social standing and value. The dynamic interplay of these psychosocial cognitive processes may transform into a permanent formalized thought scheme which forms the substrate for the interpretation of life events. Insignificant life events, when viewed within this substrate, may assume greater significance and precipitate or perpetuate depression[12,31,32].

There is currently no convincing evidence to indicate that these theories are gender-specific. It is likely that the difference in social roles and thus perceived expectations may affect the magnitude of these changes. As social equality between genders becomes increasingly widespread, it is likely that gender differences may yield to individual variation and idiosyncratic differences. In support of this hypothesis is the lack of a demonstrable gender difference in the prevalence of depression among older African-Americans. Sociologists attribute this observation to the relatively even distribution of social roles relating to employment and child care among this generation of African-Americans.

RISK FACTORS

Recognized risk factors for depression in the older adult include female sex, poverty,

Table 1 Medical illnesses associated with depression

Endocrine/metabolic
Thyroid disease
Cushing's disease
Hypoadrenalism
Diabetes mellitus
Porphyria
Hyperparathyroidism

Central nervous system
Dementia
Parkinson's disease
Cerebrovascular disease
Intracranial neoplasms
Multiple sclerosis
Complex partial seizures

Connective tissue disease
Systemic lupus erythematosus
Rheumatoid arthritis
Temporal arteritis

Miscellaneous
Chronic pain syndromes
Coronary artery disease
Chronic hepatitis
AIDS
Cancer
Chronic obstructive pulmonary disease
Electrolyte abnormalities

inadequate social support and divorce, separation and single marital status. Adverse life events are also effective stressors and may precipitate or perpetuate depression in the older adult[33]. The association of significant co-morbidity, cognitive dysfunction and functional impairment with late-onset depression has been confirmed in several studies which show that depressed older adults are more likely to have a higher burden of physical illness than non-depressed persons[34,35]. Additionally, severity of medical illness has been shown to correlate with an increased risk of depression[36,37]. A wide variety of medical illnesses are associated with depression (Table 1)[33]. The adverse effects of chronic disease on functional status provide a plausible explanation for depressive symptoms in such cases. Conversely, alternative theories suggest that depression may have an immunosuppressive effect, thereby increasing vulnerability to certain illnesses.

In older adults a positive association has been identified between the extent of cortical and subcortical atrophy, number of cortical infarcts, pituitary volume and the risk of depression. Older adults with an increased ventricular-brain ratio are also more likely to be depressed[38]. Similar neuroanatomic correlates have not been identified in younger adults. Additional risk factors for depression include advancing age, low educational achievement, co-existing psychiatric illness and alcohol abuse[37]. The actual mechanism whereby co-morbidity increases the risk of depression is unclear. However, favored theories include the possible adverse effects of such illnesses on psychosocial well-being and self-esteem. The structure of available social support systems may be altered by the perception of a real or imagined increase in the burden of illness[39–41]. It is conceivable that the older adult's perception of self within a re-defined social network may be adversely affected by such changes.

Available evidence indicates that genetics may be a less significant factor in the pathogenesis of depression in the older adult. Relatives of patients who develop late-life major depression have a lower risk of developing depression compared with relatives of depressed middle-aged adults. Additionally, current data do not support genetic theories as a plausible explanation for gender differences in the incidence of late-life depression[42,43]. Previous hypotheses suggested that depression may be transmitted in an X-linked dominant fashion, thus accounting for the higher incidence of depression in women. Related theories suggested that depression and alcoholism may be clinical expressions of the same gene with manifestations determined by gender. This would account for the increased incidence of alcoholism in the male offspring of depressed persons, while the female offspring demonstrated an increased incidence of depression[44]. To date, objective substantiation of these genetic theories is lacking.

Table 2 Summary of DSM IV criteria for the diagnosis of major depression

At least five of the following symptoms over a
two-week period, at least one of which
is either depressed mood or anhedonia:

  Depressed mood
  Anhedonia
  Unexplained weight loss or weight gain
  Insomnia or hypersomnia
  Psychomotor agitation or retardation
  Fatigue
  Persistent feelings of guilt or worthlessness
  Poor concentration
  Recurrent thoughts of death or suicidal ideation

Symptoms result in significant distress or
impairment in social functioning

Symptoms are not due to the direct physiological
effect of any substance or underlying general
medical condition

Symptoms cannot be accounted for by bereavement

CLINICAL FEATURES

The diagnostic criteria for depression are well defined (Table 2). However, self-reporting of depressive symptoms occurs infrequently among older adults. This may be attributed to the perceived stigma of the disease by the elderly. The intrinsic negativism peculiar to the disease is an additional obstacle to self-reported symptomatology. Consequently, depressive illness in the older adult may be shrouded in a mesh of somatic complaints which often defy physical diagnosis despite elaborate investigations. The attribution of such symptoms to a psychological cause is often fiercely resisted by the patient. Data exist to show that patients who manifest with somatic symptoms are often much less likely to admit to a depressed mood[45,46]. Clinical suspicion of depression should be heightened when dealing with the older adult who expresses inappropriate pessimism with regard to their physical illness or functional status. Older adults who experience apparent satisfaction with remaining in the sick role and display helplessness inconsistent with their physical status should be screened

carefully for depression. Such persons usually display behavior counterproductive to the defined therapeutic management plan[47,48]. Non-compliance and poor personal hygiene and self-care should also prompt evaluation for depressive symptoms. Generalized anxiety, irritability and preoccupation with memory and cognitive function may also serve as diagnostic clues to late-life depression. Anxiety, apprehension or panic attacks may be accompanied by physical correlates of inappropriate tachycardia, tremors, lightheadedness or dizziness. These result from inappropriate activation of the autonomic nervous system[49].

Evidence indicates that late-life depression associated with cerebrovascular disease is more likely to present with cognitive impairment, an association that does not occur in younger adults. Proponents of the 'vascular depression' hypothesis postulate that cerebral ischemic disease may cause late-onset depression. Cerebral atherosclerosis, which is a recognized cause of progressive cognitive decline with aging, may provide a common pathophysiological pathway for these two syndromes[33,38]. However, a clear distinction needs to be made between cognitive dysfunction associated with 'vascular depression' and 'pseudodementia'. The latter syndrome refers to the cognitive impairment which is a direct outcome of the patient's depressed mood. Pseudodementia frequently resolves with effective antidepressant therapy. Additionally, patients with pseudodementia often display a characteristic reluctance to undergo any form of cognitive evaluation, despite the fact that they retain good insight into their illness. Poverty of facial expression and bradykinesia, hallmarks of Parkinson's disease, are recognized features of depression and may confound the early diagnosis of depression in older adults. The recognition of depression may be further thwarted by the co-existence of depression in 30% of persons with dementia and Parkinson's disease[50].

Weight loss in the older adult is a prime index of underlying depression. Available data

Table 3 Atypical features of depression in the older adult

Anorexia
Weight loss
Bradykinesia
Memory dysfunction
Irritability
Anxiety
Paranoid delusions
Multiple unexplained somatic complaints
Increased physical and social dependence
Non-compliance with therapeutic regimens
Poor personal hygiene

indicate that depression may be the underlying cause of weight loss and low body weight in one third of older adults with weight problems[51]. Sleep disturbances are another common manifestation of depression in the elderly. The depressed older adult often complains of difficulty in falling asleep at night or frequent awakenings[49]. The peculiarities inherent in the presentation of late-life depression justify the use of the term 'masked depression' in describing this syndrome[52]. Evidence indicates that older adults who present with masked depression exhibit a greater degree of functional impairment and significantly increasing morbidity[53]. Health professionals must be cognizant of the myriad symptoms which may indicate depression, as early detection, particularly in the older man, is crucial (Table 3). Older depressed men have fewer severe melancholic symptoms. Nevertheless, approximately half of these patients will admit to some form of suicidal ideation. Five per cent of older men with depression have active suicidal ideation with a definite plan or a history of attempted suicide[37]. Older men who may be depressed must be directly questioned regarding active and passive suicidal ideation.

The presentation of depression varies with the clinical setting. Hospitalized medically ill patients are less likely to present with delusions and suicidal ideation. However, anhedonia, anxiety, helplessness and pessimism may predominate in this patient population[37]. The intuitive

expectation of differences in the prevalence of depression between cultures and ethnic groups cannot be supported by objective data. Several studies failed to find any significant difference in the prevalence of depression between Caucasian and African-American older adults. However, presenting symptoms may differ between ethnic groups. Older African-Americans are more likely to present with paranoid features, psychomotor disturbance and appetite dysregulation. Older Caucasian Americans report an increased frequency of sleep disturbance, feelings of guilt and suicidal ideation[54].

The diverse manifestations of depression place the diagnostic burden almost exclusively on the discerning health professional. The physician should be sensitive to counter-transference of feelings of helplessness. These may invoke an unjustifiable empathic response thereby resulting in acceptance of the patient's despair as an appropriate response to the perceived physical or psychosocial burden. Depression in the older adult is a persistent and chronic disorder even when it occurs in the setting of an obviously stressful life event. Thus, substituting protracted clinical observation for aggressive intervention merely constitutes harmful paternalistic inactivity in the management of a potentially deadly disease.

DIAGNOSIS

Studies indicate that depression frequently remains undetected in the older adult. In one study non-psychiatric house staff recognized clinical depression in less than 10% of depressed hospitalized older adults[55]. Recognition rates within the community-dwelling population range from 19 to 94%, emphasizing the wide variability in the ability of physicians to recognize depression[56]. Evidence indicates that most older adults opt to receive antidepressant therapy from their primary care physician, rather than to undergo formal evaluation and management by a psychiatrist. Thus, 75% of older depressed adults present initially

Table 4 Depression scales

Self-rating scales
Geriatric Depression Scale[59]
Zung Scale[60]
Center for Epidemiological Studies Depression Scale[61]

Examiner-rating scales
Hamilton Depression Rating Scale[62]
Cornell Scale for Depression in Dementia[63]
Comprehensive Psychopathological Rating Scale[64]

to their primary care physician[3]. However, 75% of depressed older persons who commit suicide have visited a primary care physician in the preceding month, yet eluded diagnosis and treatment[13,57]. Older men are less likely than women to report a depressed mood and more reluctant to attribute dysphoric symptoms to stressful life events[12]. These attributes increase the risk of undertreatment in this cohort of patients.

Clinical diagnosis of depression based on judgement and subjective interpretation of the patient's medical history is unreliable and ineffective in prompting intervention. Studies indicate that health professionals are more likely to intervene if a positive score is identified on a screening instrument[58]. Routine screening is therefore recommended and highly desirable in the development of an effective therapeutic approach toward combating depression. Several self-rating and examiner-rating scales are available (Table 4)[59–64]. Self-rating scales should not be used in persons with impaired cognitive function. The Cornell scale, which utilizes caregivers as surrogate reporters of depressive symptoms, has been well validated as an effective screening tool for depression in persons with dementia[63]. The Geriatric Depression Scale (GDS) is frequently used in clinical geriatric evaluation. This tool should be reserved for persons with minimal impairment of cognitive function. In persons with a Folstein's Mini-mental score above 15, the GDS has a sensitivity of 84% and a specificity of 91%. Evidence indicates that despite the relative paucity of somatic items on the GDS questionnaire,

co-existent medical illness may confound accurate interpretation of the results[36]. Few rating scales have been standardized for use in the acutely ill older adult. However, the GDS is less affected by acute hospitalization and the clinical course of disease compared with other rating scales, such as the Hamilton Depression Rating Scale (HDRS).

Increasing age, psychomotor retardation, somatization and severity of illness compromise the predictive value of rating scales[65,66]. The effects of these multiple confounding factors on the diagnosis of depression are minimized if rating scales are used solely for screening and initial evaluation. Rating scales should not be utilized as a substitute for formal psychiatric evaluation. Health professionals should also be wary of using the rating score to refute the diagnosis of depression in cases where clinical suspicion of depression is substantial.

MANAGEMENT

Antidepressant therapeutic options include psychosocial and biological modalities. The latter comprise pharmacological and biological treatments. Therapeutic outcome measures, as these relate to remission and relapses, should be defined for each patient, prior to initiating therapy.

Pharmacotherapy

Treatment with antidepressant therapy should be initiated in the older man with severe depression. Selective serotonin reuptake inhibitors (SSRIs) have emerged as the drugs of first choice in the management of depression. These agents are comparable in efficacy to tricyclic antidepressants (TCAs), but have a more favorable side-effect profile. Several classes of antidepressants are available which may be suitable for use in the older man (Table 5). However, the choice of antidepressant should be individualized with due consideration given to the side-effect profile. Monotherapy is preferred

Table 5 Pharmacotherapy in older men: comparison of selected medications

Drug	Advantages	Disadvantages
Tricyclic antidepressants Desipramine Nortryptiline Protryptiline Amoxapine	inexpensive once daily dosing	anticholinergic side-effects multiple drug interactions delirium cardiotoxic
Selective serotonin reuptake inhibitors Sertraline Paroxetine Fluoxetine Citalopram	safer in overdosage once daily dosing	sexual dysfunction nausea seizures headache cytochrome P450 interactions
Serotonin antagonist reuptake inhibitors Trazodone Nefazodone	few drug interactions once daily dosing	sexual dysfunction priapism possible cardiotoxicity
Serotonin–norepinephrine reuptake inhibitors Venlafaxine	favorable side-effect profile	hypertension sexual dysfunction hyperlipidemia multiple daily dosing
Mirtazapine	appetite stimulant	sexual dysfunction blood dyscrasias dependence potential
Dopamine reuptake inhibitors Bupropion	safer in overdose minimal cardiotoxicity	seizures
Alternative therapy St John's wort	favorable side-effect profile	lack of regulatory oversight and uniform standardization insufficient objective data

and treatment should be initiated using the lowest beneficial dose. Physicians should be aware that older adults may not exhibit significant improvement for 6–12 weeks after initiation of therapy. Thus, objective evaluation of clinical response should be deferred for a corresponding period[67]. Drug compliance must be closely monitored, as 70% of patients take less than 50% of their medication[41]. Patients who fail to respond to initial therapy with adequate doses of one antidepressant should be switched to another antidepressant of a different class. Referral to a psychiatrist should be considered if the patient fails to respond to or tolerate two different antidepressants, or if suicidal ideation is suspected.

The risk of recurrence of depression increases from 50% after the first episode of major depression to 90% after the third recurrent episode. Thus, older men who exhibit a satisfactory response to pharmacotherapy should be continued on full dose maintenance therapy for 6–9 months after remission from a first episode. Following recurrent episodes maintenance therapy should be continued for at least one year. This strategy has been shown to reduce the risk of a relapse by 80%[2]. When the decision is made to discontinue an antidepressant, gradual tapering of the dose is recommended to reduce the risk of withdrawal symptoms. These often include anxiety, headache, myalgia and flu-like symptoms[68]. However, older men with

Table 6 Complications of ECT therapy in older men

Cardiovascular
Cardiac arrhythmias
Hypertension
Cardiac ischemia
Hypoxia

Neurological
Amnesia
   retrograde
   antegrade
Headache
Delirium
Gait instability

Table 7 Conditions associated with an increase in the morbidity of ECT

Elevated intracranial pressure
Severe cardiovascular disease
Severe pulmonary disease
Recent cerebral hemorrhage/infarction
Unstable cerebral vascular malformation
Anesthetic risk (ASA ≥ 4)

ASA; American Society of Anesthesiologists

an initial onset of depression very late in life have a risk of relapse which equals that of men with recurrent episodes of depression. In these groups of patients it may be prudent to continue life-long full dose maintenance therapy[69].

Electroconvulsive therapy

Evidence indicates that electroconvulsive therapy (ECT) is underused in the management of depression[33]. However, this therapeutic modality is utilized more often in the treatment of older men than in their younger counterparts. This is attributed to the reluctance of older men to undergo pharmacotherapy for depression[12]. ECT is a safe and effective form of antidepressant therapy; studies show a 75–80% efficacy rate in the treatment of medically ill depressed older adults. Specific indications for the use of ECT include refractory, psychotic or life-threatening depression[70–72]. Cardiovascular and neuropsychiatric complications occur most often, although serious complications are infrequent (Table 6). ECT causes death in 2–4 persons/100 000 treatments[73]. As ECT may be lifesaving in certain situations, there are no absolute contraindications to this procedure. However, the American Psychiatry Association (APA) task force considers certain conditions to be indicators of increased risk (Table 7)[74].

With the rising cost of medication ECT is becoming increasingly cost-effective. Older adults frequently undergo ECT as an outpatient procedure, eliminating the cost of acute hospitalization which was associated with its utilization in the past. Maintenance ECT is recommended for patients who respond satisfactorily to the index treatment. Available studies indicate a significant reduction in rehospitalization and relapse rates in patients receiving maintenance ECT compared with patients on maintenance pharmacotherapy[75].

Psychotherapy

Therapeutic intervention with a combination of pharmacotherapy and psychotherapy is the most effective strategy for the treatment of moderate to severe depression in older men. Interpersonal therapy facilitates effective role transition and allows for the definition of realistic expectations. Exploration of the quality of interpersonal relationships and social interaction is also enhanced by this form of therapy. Cognitive therapy is an alternative psychotherapeutic model. Theoretically, this model allows for conceptualization of the psychological reasoning of the depressed adult. Areas of conflict are identified and resolution strategies are developed that may facilitate effective treatment[32,76,77].

CONCLUSION

Depression is the commonest psychiatric disorder in the older adult. Effective intervention is frequently compromised by delayed diagnosis and inadequate treatment. These factors constitute major obstacles to positive outcomes in the management of depression. Health professionals must develop comprehensive treatment strategies to combat depression in older adults. Ideally, these should include efficient screening methods, appropriate psychological intervention and prompt pharmacotherapy where indicated. The aggressive institution of such strategies tailored to the individual patient is a pivotal weapon in battling this deadly disease.

References

1. Callahan CM, Dittus RS, Tierney WM. Primary care physicians' medical decision making for late-life depression. *J Gen Intern Med* 1996;11:218–25
2. Hirschfield RM, Keller MB, Panico S, et al. The National Depressive and Manic-Depressive Association consensus statement on the undertreatment of depression. *J Am Med Assoc* 1997;277:333–40
3. Boswell EB, Stoudemire A. Major depression in the primary care setting. *Am J Med* 1996;101(6A):3–9S
4. Reynolds CF. Depression: making the diagnosis and using SSRIs in the older patient. *Geriatrics* 1996;51(10):28–34
5. Blazer D, Hughes DC, George LK. The epidemiology of depression in an elderly community population. *Gerontologist* 1987;27:281–7
6. Weissman MM, Leaf PJ, Tischler GL, et al. Affective disorders in five United States communities. *Psychol Med* 1988;18:141–53
7. Dorpet T, Ripley H. A study of suicide in the Seattle area. *Compr Psychiatry* 1960;1:349–59
8. Kessler RC, McGonagle KA, Swartz M, et al. Sex and depression in the national co-morbidity survey: 1. Lifetime prevalence, chronicity and recurrence. *J Affect Disord* 1993;29:85–96
9. Meechan P, Salsman L, Satin R. Suicide among older United States residents: epidemiological characteristics and trends. *Am J Public Health* 1991;81:1198–200
10. Blazer DG, Bachar JR, Manton KG. Suicide in later life. *J Am Geriatr Soc* 1986;34:519–25
11. Adamek M, Kaplan M. Firearm suicide among older men. *Psychiatr Serv* 1996;47:304–6
12. Blazer D. Depression and the older man. *Med Clin North Am* 1999;83(5):1305–16
13. Ganzini L, Smith DM, Fenn DS, et al. Depression and mortality in medically ill older adults. *J Am Geriatr Soc* 1997;45(3):307–12
14. Parmelee PA, Katz IR, Lawton MP. Depression among institutionalized aged: assessment and prevalence estimation. *J Gerontol* 1989;44:M22–9
15. Huang B. *Depression and Use of Health Services in the Elderly.* Master of Public Health thesis, University of North Carolina, Chapel Hill, 1998
16. Bryer JB, Starkstein SE, Votypka V, et al. Reduction of CSF monoamine metabolites in post-stroke depression. *J Neuropsychiatry Clin Neurosci* 1992;55:377–82
17. Morris PLP, Robinson RG, Carvalho ML, et al. Lesion characteristics and depressed mood in the stroke data bank study. *J Neuropsychiatry Clin Neurosci* 1996;8:153–9
18. Herrmann M, Bartles C, Wallesch C-W. Depression in acute and chronic aphasia: symptoms, pathoanatomical–clinical correlations and functional implications. *J Neurol Neurosurg Psychiatry* 1993;56:672–8
19. Astrom M, Adolfsson R, Asplund K. Major depression in stroke patients: a 3-year longitudinal study. *Stroke* 1993;24:976–82
20. Shimoda K, Robinson RG. The relationship between post-stroke depression and lesion location in long-term follow-up. *Biol Psychiatry* 1999;45:187–92
21. Mayberg HS, Robinson RG, Wong DF, et al. PET imaging of cortical S_2-serotonin receptors after stroke: lateralized changes and relationship to depression. *Am J Psychiatry* 1988;145:937–43
22. Krishnan KR, Hays JC, Blazer DG. MRI-defined vascular depression. *Am J Psychiatry* 1997;154:519–22

23. Drevets WC, Videen TO, Price JL, *et al.* A functional anatomic study of unipolar depression. *J Neurosci* 1992;12:3628–41

24. Martinot JL, Hardy P, Feline A, *et al.* Left prefrontal glucose hypometabolism in the depressed state: a confirmation. *Am J Psychiatry* 1990;147:1313–17

25. Drevets WC, Price JL, Simpson JR, *et al.* Subgenual prefrontal cortex abnormalities in mood disorders. *Nature* 1997;386:824–7

26. Mayberg HS, Brannan SK, Mahurin RK, *et al.* Cingulate function in depression. *Neuroreport* 1997;8:1056–61

27. McEwen BS. Protective and damaging effects of stress mediators. *N Engl J Med* 1998;338: 171–9

28. Veith R, Raskin M. The neurobiology of aging: Does it predispose to depression? *Neurobiol Aging* 1988;9:101–17

29. Hagerty BMK, Williams RA, Coyne JC, Early MR. Sense of belonging and indicators of social and psychological functioning. *Arch Psychiatr Nursing* 1996;10(4):235–44

30. Hagerty BM, Williams RA. The effects of sense of belonging, conflict, and loneliness on depression. *Nurs Res* 1999;48(4):215–19

31. Vezina J, Bourque P. The relationship between cognitive structure and symptoms of depression in the elderly. *Cogn Ther Res* 1984;8: 29–36

32. Blazer D. *Depression in Late Life*, 2nd edn. St Louis: Mosby, 1993

33. National Institutes of Health Consensus Development Panel on Depression in Late-life. Diagnosis and treatment of depression in late life. *J Am Med Assoc* 1992;268:1018–24

34. Jones BN, Reifler BV. Depression co-existing with dementia: evaluation and treatment. *Med Clin North Am* 1994;78(4):823–40

35. Koenig HG, Meador KG, Cohen HJ, *et al.* Depression in hospitalized patients with medical illness. *Arch Intern Med* 1988;148: 1929–36

36. Koenig HG, Meador KG, Cohen HJ, *et al.* Screening for depression in hospitalized elderly medical patients: taking a closer look. *J Am Geriatr Soc* 1992;40:1013–17

37. Koenig HG, Meador KG, Shelp F, *et al.* Major depressive disorder in hospitalized medically ill patients: an examination of young and elderly male veterans. *J Am Geriatr Soc* 1991;39:881–90

38. Leuchter AF. Brain structural and functional correlates of late life depression. Presented at the *National Consensus Conference on the diagnosis and treatment of depression in late life*, National Institutes of Health, Bethesda, Maryland, 1991

39. Murphy E. Social origins of depression in old age. *Br J Psychiatry* 1982;141:135–42

40. Rodin G. Depression in the medically ill: an overview. *Am J Psychiatry* 1986;143:696–705

41. Beck DA, Koenig HG, Beck JS. Depression. *Clin Geriatr Med* 1998;14(4):765–83

42. Rice J, McGuffin P. Genetic etiology of schizophrenia and affective disorders. In Michels R, ed. *Psychiatry*. Philadelphia: JB Lippincott, 1990

43. Slater EVC. *The Genetics of Mental Disorders*. London: Oxford University Press, 1971

44. Winokur G, Clayton P. Family history studies: II. Sex differences and alcoholism in primary affective illness. *Br J Psychiatry* 1967;113: 973–9

45. Bridges K, Goldberg D, Evans B, Sharpe T. Determinants of somatization in primary care. *Psychol Med* 1991;21:473–83

46. Ban T. Chronic disease and depression in the geriatric population. *J Clin Psychiatry* 1984;45:18–23

47. Fava GA, Zielezny M, Pilowsky I, *et al.* Patterns of depression and illness behavior in general hospital patients. *Psychopathology* 1984;17:105–9

48. Simon RI. Silent suicide in the elderly. *Bull Am Acad Psychiatry Law* 1989;17:83–95

49. Gareri P, Falconi U, De Fazio P, De Sarro G. Conventional and new anti-depressants in the elderly. *Prog Neurobiol* 2000;61:353–96

50. Starkstein SE, Petracca G, Chemerinski E, *et al.* Depression in classic versus akinetic-rigid Parkinson's disease. *Movement Dis* 1998; 13(1):29–33

51. Wilson MMG, Vaswani S, Liu D, *et al.* Prevalence and causes of undernutrition in medical outpatients. *Am J Med* 1998;104: 56–63

52. Reugg RG, Zissok S, Swerdlow NR. Depression in the aged: an overview. *Psychiatr Clin North Am* 1988;11:83–99

53. Broadhead WE, Blazer DG, George LK, *et al.* Depression, disability days, and days lost from work in a prospective epidemiologic survey. *J Am Med Assoc* 1990;264:2524–28

54. Blazer DG, Landerman LR, Hays JC, *et al.* Symptoms of depression among community-dwelling elderly African-Americans and White older adults. *Psychol Med* 1998;28:1311–20

55. Rapp SR, Walsh DA, Parisi SA, *et al.* Detecting depression in elderly medical inpatients. *J Consult Clin Psychol* 1988;56:509–13

56. Callahan CM, Dittus RS, Tierney WM. Primary care physicians' decision making for late life depression. *J Gen Intern Med* 1996;11(4):218–25

57. Centers for Disease Control and Prevention. Suicide among older persons: United States, 1980–1992. *Morbidity and Mortality Weekly Review* 1996;45(1):3–6

58. German PS, Shapiro S, Skinner EA, *et al.* Detection and management of mental health problems of elderly patients by primary care providers. *J Am Med Assoc* 1987;257:489–93

59. Yesavage JA, Brink TL, Rose TL, *et al.* Development and validation of a geriatric depression screening scale: a preliminary report. *J Psychiatr Res* 1983;17:37–49

60. Zung WWK. A self-rating depression scale. *Arch Gen Psychiatry* 1965;12:63–70

61. Radloff LS. The CES-D scale: a self-report depression scale for research in the general population. *J Appl Psychol Measures* 1977;1:385–401

62. Hamilton M. A self-rating scale for depression. *J Neurol Neurosurg Psychiatry* 1960;23:56–62

63. Alexopolous GS, Abrams RC, Young RC, Shamoian CA. Cornell scale for depression in dementia. *Biol Psychiatr* 1988;23:271–84

64. Asberg M, Montgomery SA, Perris C, *et al.* A comprehensive psychopathological rating scale. *Acta Psychiatr Scand* (suppl) 1978;271:5–27

65. Kurlowicz LH. Depression in hospitalized medically ill elders: evolution of the concept. *Arch Psychiatr Nurs* 1994;8:124–36

66. Kitchell MA, Barnes RF, Veith RC, *et al.* Screening for depression in hospitalized geriatric medical patients. *J Am Geriatr Soc* 1982;30:174–7

67. Georgotas A, McCue R. The additional benefit of extending an antidepressant trial past seven weeks in the depressed elderly. *Int J Geriatr Psychiatry* 1989;4:191–5

68. Sussman N, Stahl S. Update in the pharmacotherapy of depression. *Am J med* 1996;101(6A):26–36S

69. Alexopoulos GS. Affective disorders. In Sadavoy J, Lazarus LW, Jarvik LF, eds. *et al. Comprehensive Review of Geriatric Psychiatry* – II. Washington, DC: American Psychiatric Association Press, 1996

70. Rifkin A. ECT versus tricyclic antidepressants in depression: a review of the evidence. *J Clin Psychiatry* 1988;49:3–7

71. Burke WJ, Rubin EH, Zorumski CF, *et al.* The safety of ECT in geriatric practice. *J Am Geriatr Soc* 1987;35:516–21

72. Williams JH, O'Brien JT, Cullum S. Time course of response to electroconvulsive therapy in elderly depressed subjects. *Int J Geriatr Psychiatry* 1997;12:563–66

73. Abrams R. The mortality rate with ECT. *Convuls Ther* 1997;13:125–7

74. American Psychiatric Association. *The Practice of Electroconvulsive Therapy: Recommendations for Treatment, Training and Privileging.* Washington DC: APA Press, 1990

75. McDonald WM, Phillips VL, Figiel GS, *et al.* Cost effective maintenance treatment of resistant geriatric depression. *Psychiatr Ann* 1998;28:47–52

76. Reynolds CF III, Frank E, Perel JM, *et al.* High relapse rate after discontinuation of adjunctive medication for elderly patients with recurrent major depression. *Am J Psychiatry* 1996;153:1418–22

77. Sholomskas A, Chevron E, Prusoff B, *et al.* Short-term interpersonal therapy with the depressed elderly: case reports and discussions. *Am J Psychother* 1983;37:552–65

38 Testosterone, depression and cognitive function

John E. Morley, MB, BCh

'For it is the semen, when possessed of vitality which makes us to be men, hot, well-braced in limbs, well voiced, spirited, strong to think and act'

Aretaeus, *The Cappadocian*, 150 AD

'What is, therefore, the cause that castrates slow down in their whole vitality?'

Galen, *Peri Spermatas*

INTRODUCTION

The above citations from ancient times suggest that testosterone plays a role in behavior. Despite these early anecdotes, with the exception of studies on libido, there are few well-controlled studies examining the effects of testosterone on behavior. This is in contrast to the relatively large literature on estrogen in women, linking it to cognitive behaviors and perhaps to playing a role in Alzheimer's disease[1,2]. While testosterone has been strongly associated with the mythological concept of the aggressive male, studies examining the effects of testosterone on behavior have yielded mixed results. Schaal and colleagues[3] found that high testosterone levels were more likely to be a marker of social success than to be associated with physical aggression. On the other hand, in free ranging adolescent male non-human primates, elevated cerebrospinal fluid levels of testosterone were associated with overall aggressiveness but not impulsivity[4]. Administration of moderately high doses of testosterone for contraception has failed to reveal adverse effects on male sexual and aggressive behavior[5]. In a controlled trial supraphysiologic doses of testosterone failed to increase angry behavior in healthy eugonadal males[6]. In males rendered hypogonadal with a gonadotropin-releasing hormone (GnRH) antagonist there was not only a decrease in sexual desire and fantasies, but also a trend to increased aggression[7]. In contrast, and using a similar approach, Loosen and colleagues[8] found a reduction in outward-directed anger and no change in inward-directed behavior in hypogonadal males, while Burris and co-workers[9] found that hypogonadal men were more angry than eugonadal men and that this anger decreased with testosterone therapy. A 48XXYY hypogonadal male had a reduction in long-standing aggressive fantasies and behaviors towards women[10].

The reason for the inability to find convincing effects of testosterone on aggressive behavior in males is multifactorial. Most studies have utilized total testosterone rather than free or bioavailable testosterone. The effect of testosterone is small, perhaps in the neighborhood of 1%, which would require sample sizes around 1000 males to demonstrate a clearly significant effect. The reported studies have been much smaller than this. Aggressive behaviors tend to cause a decrease in testosterone either directly within the central nervous system or secondary to increases in cortisol. For example, salivary testosterone levels decreased 15 minutes after watching a stressful movie on dental surgery[11]; highly psychologically stressed males had lower testosterone levels than their low stress counterparts[12]; and male internal-medicine residents have markedly decreased testosterone levels[13]. It is possible that there is an optimal level of testosterone related to appropriate aggressive behaviors, and that higher or lower levels may create a U-shaped dose response curve. Finally, in measuring aggression, the environment and the lifetime learning experience will result in greatly modified responses to any given hormone level.

The rest of this chapter will summarize the meager data available on the effects of testosterone on general behavior, depression and memory in the middle-aged and older male.

TESTOSTERONE AND BEHAVIOR IN THE OLDER MALE: AN OVERVIEW

A syndrome of male 'menopause' was first reported in the 1940s (Table 1)[14]. In 1979 Greenblatt and colleagues[15], based on a large clinical experience, suggested that testosterone replacement in the male 'climacteric' improved fatigue, depression, headaches and libido. More recently we reported a screening questionnaire for androgen deficiency in aging males that included a number of psychological symptoms (Table 2)[16]. We used low bioavailable testosterone as our 'gold standard'. The questionnaire was developed in 316 Canadian physicians aged 40 to 82 years of age, and had acceptable reproducibility. The Androgen Deficiency in Aging Males (ADAM) questionnaire had a sensitivity of 88% and a specificity of 60%. Persons with dysphoria were the most likely to produce false positives on the questionnaire. When males with a positive ADAM were treated improvement was seen in 18/21 patients.

Wu, Yu and Chen[17] analyzed the male andropause in males over 50 years of age (Table 1).

They found that a number of psychological symptoms similar to those in the ADAM questionnaire were related to the andropause. These included decreased libido (91%), lack of energy (89%), erection problems (79%), falling asleep after dinner (77%), memory impairment (77%), sad or grumpy mood changes (68%), decreased endurance (66%) and deterioration in work performance (51%). The Massachusetts Male Aging Study examined psychological factors associated with androgen levels in 1709 males aged 39 to 70 years[18]. They found that males with a high 'availability of androgens' were more likely to display a dominant profile with some associated aggressive behavior. They went on to characterize a testosterone deficiency pattern that included 'low dominance'[19] (Table 1).

Overall these studies suggest that the fall in testosterone levels that occurs in older men is associated with a syndrome of behavioral changes in addition to the physical effects of decreased strength, decreased bone mineral density, increased adiposity and decreased hematocrit. The characteristics of the behavioral syndrome of the andropause are decreased enthusiasm for sex, lack of energy, dysphoria, decreased cognition, fatigue, decreased work and sports performance, falling asleep after dinner and low dominance. Besides the ability of testosterone to reverse the effects on libido, its effects on the rest of this complex of symptoms remain to be proven.

DYSPHORIA AND DEPRESSION

Approximately 70% of men receiving testosterone supplementation have an enhanced sense of well-being. Women are more than twice as likely to have major depression than men. Based on these two facts, it seems likely that testosterone may play a role in mood disorders. In the Rancho Bernado study of 856 males aged 50 to 89 years, the relationship of bioavailable testosterone to dysphoria was examined utilizing the Beck Depression

Table 1 Attempts to characterize an Andropause Syndrome which includes behavioral factors

Author:	Werner[14]	Greenblatt et al.[15]	Heinemann et al.[39]	Wu et al.[17]	Morley et al.[16]	Smith et al.[19]
Source:	JAMA	JAGS	Aging Male	Chang-Keng	Metabolism	Clin Endocrinol
Year:	1946	1979	1999	2000	2000	2000
Behavioral factors:	Nervousness	Decreased libido	Decreased general well-being	Decreased libido	Decreased libido	Low dominance
	Decreased libido	Fatigue	Joint pain	Lack of energy	Lack of energy	Headaches
	Decreased potency	Depression	Muscular aches	Erection problems	Decreased strength/endurance	Sleeplessness
	Irritability	Headaches	Excessive sweating	Falling asleep after dinner	Loss of height	
	Fatigue		Sleep problems	Memory impairment	Decreased enjoyment of life	
	Depression		Tiredness	Sad or grumpy	Sad or grumpy	
	Memory problems		Irritability	Decreased work performance	Decreased work performance	
	Sleep disturbances		Nervousness	Decreased endurance	Decreased ability to play sports	
	Numbness and tingling		Anxiety	Loss of pubic hair	Decreased strength of erections	
	Hot flashes		Physical exhaustion	Loss of axillary hair	Falling asleep after dinner	
			Decreased muscular strength			
			Depressive mood			
			Feeling past your peak			
			Feeling burnt out			
			Decrease in beard growth			
			Decreased ability to perform sexually			
			Decreased libido			
			Decreased morning erections			

403

Table 2 The Saint Louis University ADAM Questionnaire

(Circle one)

Yes	No	1.	Do you have a decrease in libido (sex drive)?
Yes	No	2.	Do you have a lack of energy?
Yes	No	3.	Do you have a decrease in strength and/or endurance?
Yes	No	4.	Have you lost height?
Yes	No	5.	Have you noticed a decreased enjoyment of life?
Yes	No	6.	Are you sad and/or grumpy?
Yes	No	7.	Are your erections less strong?
Yes	No	8.	Have you noticed a recent deterioration in your ability to play sports?
Yes	No	9.	Are you falling asleep after dinner?
Yes	No	10.	Has there been a recent deterioration in your work performance?

A 'yes' to 1 or 7, or any other three questions, represents a positive response

Inventory[20]. Bioavailable testosterone was significantly associated with the Beck Depression Inventory ($p < 0.007$) independent of age, weight change and physical activity. In addition, in the 25 men with true depression, bioavailable testosterone was 17% lower than that in the rest of the group. There was no association between total or bioavailable estradiol and dysphoria. Schweiger and colleagues[21], utilizing frequent sampling over a 24-hour period in 15 male depressed patients and 24 control subjects, found the depressed subjects to have lower daytime, night-time and 24-hour mean testosterone secretion. Luteinizing hormone (LH) pulse frequency tended to be decreased in the depressed males.

Booth, Johnson and Granger[22] examined the interaction of social behavior and dysphoria in 4393 men. In males with a below average level of testosterone there was an inverse relationship between testosterone and dysphoria, while in those with above average testosterone levels testosterone was directly related to dysphoria. This supports a parabolic model for the relationship of testosterone to dysphoria. In men with higher testosterone levels the relationship is no longer maintained when antisocial and risk taking behavior as well as protective factors such as marriage and steady employment are taken into account.

Sih and colleagues[23] failed to find an effect of testosterone replacement therapy on dysphoria in older hypogonadal men; they utilized the Geriatric Depression Scale. Grinspoon and co-workers[24] in a large study of HIV-infected males found a higher Beck Depression Inventory score in the hypogonadal compared to eugonadal males. Testosterone therapy resulted in a significant decrease in the Beck Depression score. There was a strong relationship between decreased dysphoria and weight gain. Seidman and Rabkin[25] added testosterone to the treatment regimen of five men for whom treatment with selective serotonin reuptake inhibitors for depression had failed, finding that testosterone augmentation produced a rapid improvement in depressive symptoms.

Overall, the available data support the concept that depression is a stress state that results in a decline in testosterone levels. Whether or not testosterone replacement improves depressive symptoms will require large controlled trials. Preliminary and anecdotal data are suggestive that testosterone may be a useful adjuvant therapy for depression[26].

COGNITION

In rodents androgens have major effects on brain structure and function. The effects of testosterone in enhancing memory retention in mice appear to involve both its aromatization to estrogen and an effect of dehydrotestosterone. The SAMP8 mouse is a spontaneous animal model of Alzheimer's disease[27]. These mice develop early acquisition and retention deficits that are related to overproduction of β-amyloid[28]. SAMP8 mice also develop low testosterone; replacement results in a reversal of their acquisition and memory deficits[29]. This reversal is associated with a rapid reduction in amyloid precursor protein levels in the limbic system. Testosterone also decreases the production of amyloid precursor protein in a cell culture line[30].

While it is recognized that human males and females display different learning abilities for different tasks, a clear relationship between testosterone and memory has been difficult to demonstrate. This is most probably because the relationship between cognitive performance and testosterone levels is non-linear. In general testosterone in younger men has been related to spatial but not verbal cognitive tasks[31,32].

Barrett-Connor and colleagues[33] examined the relationship between sex hormones and cognitive function in 547 men aged 58 to 89 years of age. Males with the best scores on the Blessed Information Memory Concentration Test and the Buschke Selective Reminding Test had high levels of bioavailable testosterone. High levels of bioavailable testosterone were associated with low scores on the Blessed Information Memory Concentration Test and the MiniMental State Examination. Bioavailable testosterone showed a U-shaped relationship to the Spelling 'World' Backwards Test. These findings suggest that an optimal level of sex steroids may exist for older males. Carlson and Sherwin[34] suggested that higher estradiol levels in older males may protect against the decline in explicit memory associated with normal aging. Morley and co-workers[35] reported that across the lifespan bioavailable testosterone was the steroid hormone that best predicted a variety of cognitive performance tests.

Janowsky and colleagues[36] studied a relatively large group of healthy elderly men who received testosterone in a double-blind trial for three months. They found an improvement in spatial cognition, but no effect on verbal and visual memory, motor speed, cognitive flexibility or mood. Sih's group[23], on a battery of cognitive tests which did not include a spatial task, found no effect of testosterone replacement on memory in older men who were treated for a year. Another study found that testosterone enhanced working memory as measured by the Subject Ordered Pointing Test in older men[37] and Wolf and colleagues[38] found that a single injection of testosterone blocked the practice effect in verbal fluency but had no effect on spatial or verbal memory.

While cross-sectional data in older men suggest an effect of testosterone on cognition, the results of testosterone replacement tests have been less conclusive. In many cases, it would appear that there is an optimal level of testosterone for enhancing cognition and that higher and lower levels are less effective. Testosterone may improve spatial and working memory in older persons.

CONCLUSION

Overall, the effects of testosterone on behavior, while significant, are relatively small. Testosterone appears to have effects on mood, dominance, sleep and cognition. Further studies are necessary to determine whether there exists an optimal range of testosterone to produce behavioral effects or whether supraphysiological and physiological levels of testosterone are equally effective.

References

1. Almeida OP. Sex playing with the mind. Effects of oestrogen and testosterone on mood and cognition. [Review] *Arquivos de Neuro-Psiquiatria* 1999;57:701–6
2. LeBlanc ES, Janowsky J, Chan BKS, Nelson HD. Hormone replacement therapy and cognition – systematic review and meta-analysis [Review]. *J Am Med Assoc* 2001;285:1489–99
3. Schaal B, Tremblay RE, Soussignan R, Susman EJ. Male testosterone linked to high social dominance but low physical aggression in early adolescence. *J Am Acad Child Adolescent Psychiatry* 1996;35:1322–30
4. Higley JD, Mehlman PT, Poland RE, *et al.* CSF testosterone and 5-HIAA correlate with different types of aggressive behaviors. *Biol Psychiatry* 1996;40:1067–82

5. Bahrke MS, Yesalis CE IV, Wright JE. Psychological and behavioural effects of endogenous testosterone and anabolic-androgenic steroids. An update [Review]. *Sports Med* 1996;22:367–90

6. Tricker R, Casaburi R, Storer TW, *et al*. The effects of supraphysiological doses of testosterone on angry behavior in healthy eugonadal men – a clinical research center study. *J Clin Endocrinol Metab* 1996;81:3754–8

7. Bagatell CJ, Heiman JR, Rivier JE, Bremner WJ. Effects of endogenous testosterone and estradiol on sexual behavior in normal young men. *J Clin Endocrinol Metab* 1994;78: 711–16

8. Loosen PT, Purdon SE, Pavlou SN. Effects on behavior of modulation of gonadal function in men with gonadotropin-releasing hormone antagonists. *Am J Psychiatry* 1994;151:271–3

9. Burris AS, Banks SM, Carter CS, *et al*. A long-term, prospective study of the physiologic and behavioral effects of hormone replacement in untreated hypogonadal men. *J Androl* 1992;13:297–304

10. Sourial N, Fenton F. Testosterone treatment of an XXYY male presenting with aggression: a case report. *Can J Psychiatry* 1988;33:846–50

11. Hellhammer DH, Hubert W, Schurmeyer T. Changes in saliva testosterone after psychological stimulation in men. *Psychoneuroendocrinology* 1985;10:77–81

12. Francis KT. The relationship between high and low trait psychological stress, serum testosterone, and serum cortisol. *Experientia* 1981;37:1296–7

13. Singer F, Zumoff B. Subnormal serum testosterone levels in male internal medicine residents. *Steroids* 1992;57:86–9

14. Werner AA. Male climacteric: report of 273 cases. *J Am Med Assoc* 1946;132:188–94

15. Greenblatt RB, Nexhat C, Roesel RA, Natrajan PK. Update on the male and female climacteric. *J Am Geriat Soc* 1979;27:481–90

16. Morley JE, Charlton E, Patrick P, *et al*. Validation of a screening questionnaire for androgen deficiency in aging males. *Metab Clin Exp* 2000;49:1239–42

17. Su CY, Yu TJ, Chen MJ. Age related testosterone level changes and male andropause syndrome. *Chang-Ken I Hsueh Tsa Chih* 2000;23:348–53

18. Gray A, Jackson DN, McKinlay JB. The relation between dominance, anger, and hormones in normally aging men: results from the Massachusetts Male Aging Study. *Psychosom Med* 1991;53:375–85

19. Smith KW, Feldman HA, McKinlay JB. Construction and field validation of a self-administered screener for testosterone deficiency (hypogonadism) in ageing men. *Clin Endocrinol* 2000;53:703–11

20. Barrett-Connor E, Von Muhlen DG, Kritz-Silverstein D. Bioavailable testosterone and depressed mood in older men: the Rancho Bernardo Study. *J Clin Endocrinol Metab* 1999;84:573–7

21. Schweiger U, Deuschle M, Weber B, *et al*. Testosterone, gonadotropin, and cortisol secretion in male patients with major depression. *Psychosom Med* 1999;61:292–6

22. Booth A, Johnson DR, Granger DA. Testosterone and men's depression: the role of social behavior. *J Health Soc Behav* 1999;40: 130–40

23. Sih R, Morley JE, Kaiser FE, *et al*. Testosterone replacement in older hypogonadal men: a 12-month randomized controlled trial. *J Clin Endocrinol Metab* 1997;82: 1661–7

24. Grinspoon S, Corcoran C, Stanley T, *et al*. Effects of hypogonadism and testosterone administration on depression indices in HIV-infected men. *J Clin Endocrinol Metab* 2000; 85:60–5

25. Seidman SN, Rabkin JG. Testosterone replacement therapy for hypogonadal men with SSRI-refractory depression. *J Affect Disord* 1998;49:157–61

26. Seidman SN, Walsh BT. Testosterone and depression in aging men [Review]. *Am J Geriat Psychiatry* 1999;7:18–33

27. Flood JF, Morley JE. Learning and memory in the SAMP8 mouse [Review]. *Neurosci Biobehav Rev* 1998;22:1–20

28. Morley JE, Kumar VB, Bernardo AE, *et al*. Beta-Amyloid precursor polypeptide in SAMP8 mice affects learning and memory *Peptides* 2000;21:1761–7

29. Flood JF, Farr SA, Kaiser FE, et al. Age-related decrease of plasma testosterone in SAMP8 mice – replacement improves age-related impairment of learning and memory. *Physiol Behav* 1995;57:669–73

30. Gouras GK, Xu HX, Gross RS, et al. Testosterone reduces neuronal secretion of Alzheimer's beta-amyloid peptides. *Proc Natl Acad Sci USA* 2000;97:1202–5

31. Neave N, Menaged M, Weightman DR. Sex differences in cognition: the role of testosterone and sexual orientation. *Brain Cognit* 1999;41:245–62

32. Moffat SD, Hampson E. A curvilinear relationship between testosterone and spatial cognition in humans: possible influence of hand preference. *Psychoneuroendocrinology* 1996; 21:323–37

33. Barrett-Connor E, Goodman-Gruen D, Patay B. Endogenous sex hormones and cognitive function in older men. *J Clin Endocrinol Metab* 1999;84:3681–5

34. Carlson LE, Sherwin BB. Higher levels of plasma estradiol and testosterone in healthy elderly men compared with age-matched women may protect aspects of explicit memory. *Menopause* 2000;7:168–77

35. Morley JE, Kaiser F, Raum WJ, et al. Potentially predictive and manipulable blood serum correlates of aging in the healthy human male – progressive decreases in bioavailable testosterone, dehydroepiandrosterone sulfate, and the ratio of insulin-like growth factor 1 to growth hormone. *Proc Natl Acad Sci USA* 1997;94:7537–42

36. Janowsky JS, Oviatt SK, Orwoll ES. Testosterone influences spatial cognition in older men. *Behav Neurosci* 1994;108:325–32

37. Janowsky JS, Chavez B, Orwoll E. Sex steroids modify working memory. *J Cognit Neurosci* 2000;12:407–14

38. Wolf OT, Preut R, Hellhammer DH, et al. Testosterone and cognition in elderly men: a single testosterone injection blocks the practice effect in verbal fluency, but has no effect on spatial or verbal memory. *Biol Psychiatry* 2000;47:650–4

39. Heineman AJ, Zimmermann T, Vermeulen A, Thiel C. A new aging male's symptoms (AMS) rating scale. *The Aging Male* 1999;2:105–14

39 Modern antidepressants

Margaret-Mary G. Wilson, MRCP

'He who is of calm and happy nature will hardly feel the pressure of age ...'

Plato (428BC–348BC),
The Republic

Late-life depression is a major contender in the battle to achieve successful aging. Epidemiological studies estimate the prevalence of major depression at 2–5% in community-dwelling older adults[1–4]. Among older adults in the acute care setting, the prevalence of major depression ranges from 30 to 45%[5,6]. Within the nursing-home setting major depression occurs in 15–25% of residents[7]. Additionally, 15–27% of community-dwelling older adults report depressive symptoms or a notably depressed mood[4,8]. Available data indicate a significant increase in morbidity, functional disability and mortality associated with depression in the older adult[9,10]. Efficient screening and early clinical recognition are critical to improving the prognosis of adults with late-life depression. However, prompt initiation of the correct therapeutic strategy maximizes the potential for complete recovery. Current evidence indicates that depression is often under treated in the older adult[11]. The incidence of initiation of pharmacotherapy is less than 1.5% each year, with older depressed men being half as likely to be treated with antidepressants as women[12,13].

A working knowledge of the mechanism of action of available antidepressants is crucial to the implementation of an objective treatment strategy. A favored unitary hypothesis links depression to a central disturbance in the metabolism of the monoamines, norepinephrine, serotonin (5-HT) and dopamine. Animal studies have identified a reduction in the metabolism of 5-HT and norepinephrine in the aging brain. The latter finding may be relevant to the pathogenesis of late-life depression. In support of this pathogenetic theory, effective antidepressant agents tend to result in an increase in 5-HT or norepinephrine neurotransmission. Tricyclic antidepressants affect either norepinephrine alone or both norepinephrine and 5-HT. Similarly, selective serotonin reuptake inhibitors (SSRIs) act primarily to inhibit 5-HT uptake and also exert some inhibitory effect on norepinephrine uptake[12,14,15].

A wide variety of antidepressants with proven efficacy is available (Table 1). However, age-related changes in pharmacodynamics and pharmacokinetics are major determining factors in the use of these medications in the older adult. Furthermore, the paucity of data specifically relating to the safety and efficacy of newer agents in the treatment of depression in the older adult mandates caution. Optimal characteristics of an antidepressant for the older adult include not only a rapid onset of action and optimal efficacy, but limited potential for side-effects and drug interactions (Table 2). Once daily administration and the availability of the pharmaceutical agent in tablet, liquid and parenteral forms enhance patient compliance. Drugs proven to be non-fatal in toxic doses possess the advantage of a reduced risk of death from attempted suicide. Thus, despite

Table 1 Classification and mode of action of selected newer antidepressants

Drug	Mode of action
Selective serotonin reuptake inhibitors	inhibit presynaptic neuronal re-uptake of 5-HT
Fluoxetine	
Paroxetine	
Sertraline	
Fluvoxamine	
Citalopram	
Serotonin antagonist reuptake inhibitors	antagonize 5-HT receptors and block 5-HT reuptake
Trazodone	
Nefazodone	
Serotonin–norepinephrine reuptake inhibitors	inhibit 5-HT and norepinephrine uptake; weak inhibition of dopamine reuptake
Venlafaxine	
Mirtazapine	
Dopamine reuptake inhibitor	inhibits reuptake of norepinephrine and dopamine; negligible effect on 5-HT reuptake
Bupropion	
Alternative herbal therapy	undefined
Hypericum perforatum (St John's wort)	

Table 2 Characteristics of the ideal antidepressant for the older adult

Effective
Minimal side-effects
Low potential for drug interactions
Safe in over-dosage
Once daily administration
Rapid onset
Tablet and liquid formulations

efficacy but with better safety profiles has relegated these older medications to second choice agents in the management of depression (Table 3). SSRIs possess the advantage of exerting a notably reduced effect on histamine, cholinergic and α-adrenergic receptors, thereby minimizing the side-effects that result from blockade of these receptors (Table 4)[16,17].

Evidence indicates that in depression, there is an upregulation of postsynaptic receptors due to a deficiency in 5-HT availability. Post-synaptic upregulation affects both the terminal and the somatodendritic autoreceptors. Animal studies indicate that the administration of SSRIs causes an increase in 5-HT levels owing to blockade of the 5-HT transport pump. This occurs initially in the midbrain raphe, which harbors predominantly neuronal soma. The increase in 5-HT levels leads to downregulation of the somatodendritic receptors, thereby disrupting 5-HT autoregulation. Consequently, the magnitude of neuronal impulse transmission and terminal axonal 5-HT release increases[12]. This sequence of events suggests that SSRIs exert their effect via a cascade mechanism that induces an exponential response when triggered. The delay in the onset of action of SSRIs may be explained by the time required to negotiate this pharmacological cascade.

Fluoxetine

Fluoxetine is the most widely prescribed antidepressant in the USA[18]. Following oral administration fluoxetine is almost completely

the advent of numerous effective newer antidepressants, health professionals must remain cognizant of the fact that the basic principles of geriatric prescribing must still be applied.

SELECTIVE SEROTONIN REUPTAKE INHIBITORS

Selective serotonin reuptake inhibitors (SSRIs) have emerged as first choice antidepressants for the older adult. These agents are equally as effective as tricyclic antidepressants (TCAs) and produce fewer side-effects. Prior to the advent of SSRIs the TCAs and monoamine oxidase inhibitors (MAOIs) were the mainstays of antidepressant drug therapy. However, despite the efficacy of these agents patient compliance was adversely affected by the myriad adverse effects associated with their use. The subsequent development of antidepressants of comparable

Table 3 Comparative side-effect profile of selected newer antidepressants

Drug	Sedation	Orthostatic hypotension	Anticholinergic
Citalopram	+	−	−
Fluoxetine	−	+	−
Fluvoxamine	−	−	−
Mirtazapine	+	−	−
Nefazodone	+	+	+
Paroxetine	−	+	−
Sertraline	+	+	−
Trazodone	++	++	++
Venlafaxine	++	−	−

Table 4 Antidepressant adverse effects related to receptor blockade

Receptor blockade	Adverse effects
Muscarinic	urinary retention
	overflow incontinence
	constipation
	delirium
	blurred vision
	xerostomia
	anorexia
Histamine	sedation
	delirium
	weight gain
α-adrenergic	orthostatic hypotension
	inappropriate tachycardia

absorbed. However, bioavailability is reduced by first-pass metabolism in the liver[19]. Fluoxetine is highly protein bound and has a large volume of distribution. Ultimately, oxidative metabolism and conjugation result in the production of several metabolites. More than 90% of the parent compound is inactivated. However, active metabolites are also produced. Norfluoxetine, the primary demethylated active metabolite, has a half-life ($t_{1/2}$) of 3–20 days, which is longer than the $t_{1/2}$ of fluoxetine, which ranges from 1 to 3 days. Thus, steady state plasma concentrations may not be achieved for 12–42 days. Fluoxetine undergoes renal excretion[20]. The optimal dose of fluoxetine in the geriatric population has not been determined. However, the recommended initial dose in the older adult is 5–10 mg daily[8]. Owing to the long half-life of fluoxetine and the active metabolite norfluoxetine, dosage changes are not justified during the first four weeks of therapy. Subsequently, the dose may be cautiously increased, in small increments, to a maximum daily dose of 40 mg. Owing to the non-linear pharmacokinetic profile of fluoxetine, cautious use is advised in patients with hepatic impairment[8,21].

Earlier studies suggested that fluoxetine may induce a treatment-related suicidal ideation. This appeared to substantiate the hypothesis that initiation of antidepressant therapy may negate passivity just enough to motivate the depressed patient to institute prior suicidal plans. However, re-evaluation of the available data by various groups, including the Food and Drug Administration's Psychopharmacological Drugs Advisory Committee, has failed to demonstrate any scientifically objective causal association between the use of fluoxetine and suicidal ideation[22].

Drug interactions must be given careful consideration when fluoxetine is prescribed. Serotoninergic syndrome is a potentially fatal condition resulting from the use of fluoxetine in conjunction with other serotoninergic agents, notably MAOI, lithium, chlorimipramine and tryptophan. This syndrome, attributed to elevated central nervous system levels of 5-HT, presents with hyperthermia, neuromuscular irritability, delirium and psychomotor agitation. The long half-life of fluoxetine mandates a long wash-out period of about five weeks between cessation of fluoxetine and institution of an MAOI[21,23–25].

Recognized adverse effects of fluoxetine include anxiety, insomnia, headaches and lethargy. Reduced libido and anorgasmia may occur and compromise patient compliance with therapy. Additionally, several cases of hyponatremia resulting from the syndrome of inappropriate antidiuretic hormone (SIADH) secretion have been reported as complications of fluoxetine therapy. Fluoxetine has a relatively lower incidence of gastrointestinal side-effects compared with other SSRIs and may therefore be preferred in patients with coexisting gastrointestinal disease[18,26,27].

Paroxetine

Paroxetine hydrochloride is a highly selective serotonin reuptake inhibitor[28]. Therapeutic efficacy comparable to that of TCAs has been demonstrated in several studies[29,30]. Paroxetine has a predictable half-life of 24 hours and is highly protein bound. Following absorption paroxetine undergoes partial first-pass hepatic metabolism. Renal excretion of inactive metabolites follows subsequent hepatic transformation[12,31]. Effective clearance of paroxetine is markedly impaired by renal insufficiency, therefore dosage reduction is recommended in patients with a creatinine clearance rate of < 60 ml/min. Compared with other SSRIs, paroxetine is the most potent inhibitor of cytochrome P450 (CYP) 2D6, which is involved in the metabolism of a wide range of drugs. Paroxetine also possesses the added disadvantage of high affinity for muscarinic receptor blockade resulting in a corresponding increase in the incidence of anticholinergic side-effects[9,24]. Additional side-effects of paroxetine include nausea, insomnia, diaphoresis, tremors and ejaculatory dysfunction[32]. Recent data indicate that, unlike fluoxetine, paroxetine may cause a notable decrease in anxiety and is less likely to cause psychomotor agitation[33].

Paroxetine is therefore an appropriate choice in the treatment of depressed persons with prominent features of anxiety or agitation. Therapeutic efficacy has been demonstrated in older depressed adults in doses ranging from 10 to 30 mg daily[9].

Sertraline

Available data indicate that sertraline hydrochloride is comparable in efficacy to tricyclic agents, yet has a safer side-effect profile[34]. Sertraline has a half-life of approximately 24 hours. Hepatic methylation produces a weakly active metabolite, N-demethylsertraline, which has a half-life of 66 hours. A steady state is reached after about seven days. Sertraline is non-sedating with minimal cardiotoxicity and anticholinergic potential. Clinically apparent side-effects usually involve the gastrointestinal tract, causing nausea, vomiting and diarrhea. However, the occurrence of these adverse events may be reduced by administration with food[35,36]. A major advantage to the use of sertraline is the reduced potential for drug interactions, as sertraline displays the least CYP 2D6 inhibition compared with other SSRIs[9]. A starting dose of 12.5 mg/day is recommended for older adults. If tolerated, the dose may subsequently be increased in increments of 12.5–25 mg to a maximum of 150 mg/day[17,34].

Fluvoxamine

Fluvoxamine maleate, one of the newer SSRIs, was initially approved for the treatment of obsessive–compulsive disorders. The antidepressant effect of this agent is comparable to those of imipramine, desipramine, amitriptyline and dothiepin. Fluvoxamine is well absorbed following oral administration and has a half-life of 19–22 hours. Following hepatic metabolism 90% of the dose is converted to inactive metabolites. Fluvoxamine is especially beneficial in severely depressed adults with suicidal ideation. The effective dose ranges from 50 to 200 mg daily[37]. Fluvoxamine is relatively well tolerated, although administration of large doses has been associated with an increased incidence of nausea[38].

Citalopram

Citalopram is a selective inhibitor of 5-HT neural transport. This agent is well tolerated by older patients and is of comparable efficacy to older antidepressants[12]. Citalopram is well absorbed orally, is 80% protein bound and has a half-life of 35 hours. Hepatic demethylation results in the production of less active metabolites that undergo both renal and fecal excretion. Available data indicate that it exerts minimal inhibition on CYP 2D6 and consequently has a limited potential for drug interactions. Citalopram has minimal effects on the cardiovascular system and has a much better safety profile than TCAs. This agent may be a suitable choice in the older depressed adult with cardiovascular disease or conditions which may predispose to autonomic instability[12,15].

SEROTONIN ANTAGONIST REUPTAKE INHIBITORS

Serotonin antagonist reuptake inhibitors (SARIs) refers to a recently defined class of antidepressants that mediate their action through a combination of 5-HT$_2$ receptor blockade and 5HT reuptake inhibition. The additional mechanism of 5-HT$_2$ receptor blockade prevents nonspecific activation of receptors by the increase in 5-HT produced by serotonin reuptake inhibition. Indeed, data indicate that the SARIs may have a lower incidence of agitation, anxiety and sexual dysfunction compared with SSRIs[39].

Trazodone

Trazodone is a phenylpiperazine derivative with weak antidepressant activity. It is frequently, although inappropriately, used as an anxiolytic or sedative in older adults[40]. Trazodone inhibits 5-HT reuptake and antagonizes histamine and α_1-adrenoreceptors, resulting in an increased incidence of adverse effects such as drowsiness, dizziness and orthostatic hypotension[41]. Additionally, priapism is an infrequent, but particularly troublesome, side-effect of trazodone which may discourage the use of this agent in older men. Studies have demonstrated impaired clearance of trazodone in older men[42], of which the mechanism underlying is unclear. However, the relatively higher serum levels in older men may further increase the risk of adverse effects. Patient adherence to the prescribed regimen may be negatively affected not only by the weighty side-effect profile, but also by the short half-life of trazodone, which mandates frequent daily dosing. Trazodone is perhaps best considered a second-line agent reserved for older depressed persons unable to tolerate other medication.

Nefazodone

Nefazodone is also a phenylpiperazine derivative that inhibits serotonin reuptake and blocks 5-HT receptors. In contrast to trazodone, nefazodone has minimal α_1-adrenergic receptor blockade with an almost negligible effect on muscarinic and histamine receptors[43]. This may account for the improved side-effect profile associated with the use of nefazodone compared with trazodone. Orthostatic hypotension and sedation occur with much less frequency in persons who use nefazodone. In particular, no cases of priapism have been associated with the use of nefazodone[12,39]. Nefazodone is rapidly absorbed after oral administration, reaching a peak plasma concentration two hours after administration. However, first-pass metabolism reduces bioavailability to approximately 20%. Subsequent hepatic metabolism results in the production of active metabolites[43]. Altered pharmacokinetics in older adults results in plasma concentrations that may be twice as high as levels in younger adults. Older men tend to have lower levels than older women. Available data do not indicate an increased likelihood of adverse effects in older subjects[44,45].

The recommended starting dose in older adults is 50 mg twice a day, with slow incremental titration by 100 mg/day every two weeks. The recommended maximum total daily dose is 600 mg. Nefazodone inhibits the metabolism of drugs metabolized by the CYP 3A3-4 isoenzyme, thereby increasing the potential for drug interactions. Increased levels of benzodiazepines and carbamazepine may result when these drugs are given in combination with nefazodone. Of particular concern is the potentially fatal interaction that may result from cardiac arrhythmias, characteristically torsades de pointes, when nefazodone is taken with terfenadine, astemizole or cisapride. Less serious side-effects of nefazodone include nausea, sedation, constipation and dizziness. The inhibiting effect of nefazodone on post-synaptic 5-HT receptors makes it a useful choice in the depressed anxious patient. Additionally, the preservation of a normal sleep pattern is often useful in the management of depressed persons with insomnia[12,46].

SEROTONIN–NOREPINEPHRINE REUPTAKE INHIBITORS

Venlafaxine

Venlafaxine, the prototypical agent of this group, exerts a greater effect on 5-HT reuptake than norepinephrine reuptake. Studies have shown that venlafaxine does not demonstrate significant binding to 5-HT, norepinephrine, dopamine, muscarinic, cholinergic, α_1-adrenergic or histamine receptors[47]. This accounts for the rarity of side-effects related to blockade of these receptors. Hepatic metabolism results in the production of active metabolites with a half-life of 9–12 hours compared to 3–5 hours for the parent drug. Venlafaxine is excreted through the kidneys[48]. Clinically significant age-related changes in pharmacokinetics have not been documented. Thus dose adjustment for age is not necessary, unless there is evidence of renal or hepatic impairment. The recommended starting dose is 75 mg/day in two or three daily divided doses, which can be increased in small increments to a maximum of 375 mg/day. Venlafaxine is comparable in therapeutic efficacy to TCAs and SSRIs[47,49].

Adverse effects of venlafaxine are more likely to occur at the onset of treatment and tend to subside with continued use. These include anorexia, dry mouth, sleep disturbance, headaches and sweating. At high doses, sexual dysfunction has been reported in 9% of patients. Dose-related diastolic hypertension complicating therapy has been reported in 3–13% of patients, mandating routine blood pressure monitoring in persons on this drug[50].

Mirtazapine

Mirtazapine blocks presynaptic α_2-adrenergic receptors and postsynaptic 5-HT$_2$ and 5HT3 receptors. Mirtazapine has a half-life of 20–40 hours, permitting once daily administration. This drug is extensively metabolized by the cytochrome P450 system and clearance may be notably reduced in persons with hepatic disease. The administration of mirtazapine with drugs that are co-metabolized by CYP 1A2, CYP 2D6 and CYP 3A4 should be avoided to reduce the risk of competitive inhibition and minimize the incidence of unwanted side-effects[51]. Comparative studies have shown that mirtazapine is equally as effective as fluoxetine, amitriptyline, trazodone and chlorimipramine. Studies also show that mirtazapine has fewer anticholinergic side-effects compared with TCAs. Commonly reported unwanted adverse effects associated with the use of mirtazapine include somnolence, dizziness and sexual dysfunction. Paradoxically, other common side-effects, namely increased appetite and weight gain, may serve as a clinical advantage in the older depressed person with anorexia and weight loss[52]. Similarly, the relatively high affinity of mirtazapine for histamine receptors has proven useful in the management of patients with anxiety, agitation and insomnia. Pharmacokinetic studies support dosage adjustments in renal failure. Older adults have also been shown to have relatively higher serum levels. Nevertheless, available evidence does not support dosage adjustment in older adults with normal renal and hepatic function[53]. The recommended starting dose is 15 mg at bedtime with slow titration upwards every two weeks to a maximum of 45 mg/day. Although dose adjustments have not been recommended for the older adult, it is reasonable to start at a lower dose of 7.5 mg at bedtime and titrate upwards after observing for tolerance.

DOPAMINE REUPTAKE INHIBITORS

Bupropion

Bupropion is an aminoketone that exerts its effect by blocking the reuptake of dopamine and norepinephrine. Bupropion has a therapeutic $t_{1/2}$ of 18 hours and undergoes hepatic metabolism and renal excretion[54,55]. Studies indicate that bupropion is an effective activating antidepressant and is well tolerated in older adults. The absence of significant anticholinergic, cardiovascular or sedating side-effects renders this agent a favorable choice for the older patient[54]. There are no reports of sexual dysfunction complicating the use of this agent; this is attributed to the minimal serotoninergic effect associated with its use[56]. A disadvantage to the use of bupropion is the resultant reduction in the seizure threshold. Bupropion is associated with an increased frequency of grand mal seizures. Additionally, it has a low therapeutic

index and requires multiple dosing, thereby increasing the risk of overdosage, which frequently presents with tremors and seizures[57,58].

The recommended starting dose of bupropion is 50 mg orally twice daily for both the immediate release and sustained release preparations. The sustained release preparation may be associated with lower peak plasma levels and a reduction in the frequency of side-effects. The maximum daily dose should not exceed 400 mg/day. Nocturnal dosing should be avoided as this may result in insomnia[59].

ALTERNATIVE THERAPY

With the growing use of alternative and complementary medicine, several therapeutic options are available within the realms of integrative medicine. Some depressed persons may attach negative connotations to conventional antidepressants. Such patients may opt for 'natural remedies' which often do not labor under the traditional stigma of psychiatric medication. According to the 1994 Dietary Supplement Health Education Act, herbal products are classified as foods in the USA and are not subject to the same stringent quality-control regulations as are standard pharmaceuticals. However, patients have unrestricted and unregulated access to these products. The lack of standardization, regulation and sufficient evidence-based information regarding the safety of these products precludes formal prescription of these agents by orthodox health practitioners. Nevertheless, patients may choose to use these preparations of their own volition. Consequently, the onus is on all healthcare providers to become familiar with available integrative therapies in order to function effectively as patient advocates and counselors.

St John's wort (Hypericum perforatum)

Hypericum perforatum is a flowering plant which was traditionally used in medieval

Table 5 St John's wort (*Hypericum perforatum* extract): biologically active ingredients

Hypericin
Pseudohypericin
Monoterpenes
Xanthones
    sitosterol
Quercetin
Catechin

England during the feast of John the Baptist. The term 'wort' is the old English word for plant. *Hypericum* extracts have been used for medicinal purposes for several centuries, mainly as a treatment for vaguely characterized 'nervous conditions' and insomnia[60]. However, over the past decade St John's wort has emerged as an increasingly popular alternative treatment for depression, with annual sales in the USA increasing from $20 million to $200 million between 1995 and 1997[61]. The mode of action is unclear. However, *Hypericum* extract contains several biologically active substances, several of which have been shown to inhibit 5-HT and monoamine oxidase reuptake (Table 5)[62–64]. Current evidence indicates that hypericin is not the primary active antidepressant ingredient, as previously thought. Nevertheless most preparations of St John's wort are still standardized by the hypericin content[65].

A systematic review of a series of randomized controlled trials indicates that St John's wort is more effective than placebo in the treatment of mild to moderate depression. St John's wort resulted in an absolute increase in the response rate that was 23–55% higher than the placebo response. Studies comparing St John's wort with tricyclic antidepressants suggest comparable efficacy[66,67]. Available data indicate that St John's wort is well tolerated in the majority of patients, with side-effects occurring in 2–8% of adults. Nausea, lethargy and skin rash were the most common side-effects reported.

Occasionally photosensitivity complicates the use of St John's wort. It has been shown that patients on tricyclic antidepressants are 33–78% more likely to experience adverse effects[68–70]. To date, there is no published evidence of serious hematological, renal, hepatic or cardiovascular adverse effects complicating the use of St John's wort[71]. The lack of regulatory oversight and stringent standardization criteria constitute major drawbacks to the use of this preparation. Further studies are needed to objectively define the therapeutic role of St John's wort in the management of depression in the older adult.

CONCLUSIONS

Depression is a common problem in older adults and inadequate treatment has grave consequences. The choice of antidepressant – as with all medications prescribed for the older adult – is often based on several factors. These include age-related changes in pharmacodynamics and pharmacokinetics and the kinetic profile of the prescribed agent. Other considerations include cost, dosing intervals, patient compliance, associated medical conditions and drug interactions. Specifically, with regard to antidepressants, the patient's response to previous antidepressant therapy should be considered.

Available evidence indicates that most antidepressants are of comparable efficacy. However, they differ significantly with regard to their side-effect profile. Geriatric health professionals often display justifiable caution in prescribing new drugs as these agents have frequently not been well evaluated in the older population. Antidepressants are one of the few exceptions to this rule. The emergence of newer drugs has not only expanded the armamentarium of pharmacological therapeutic options, but also reduced the risk of adverse effects traditionally associated with the treatment of late-life depression.

References

1. Weissman MM, Myers JK, Tischler GL, *et al.* Psychiatric disorders and cognitive impairment among the elderly in a US urban community. *Acta Psychiatr Scand* 1985;71: 366–79
2. Weissman MM, Myers JK, Tischler GL, *et al.* Affective disorders in five US communities. *Psychol Med* 1988;18:141–53
3. Potter LB, Rogler LH, Moscicki EK. Depression among Puerto Ricans in New York City: the Hispanic Health and Nutrition Examination Survey. *Soc Psychiatry Psychiatr Epidemiol* 1995;30:185–93
4. Blazer D, William CD. Epidemiology of dysphoria and depression in the elderly. *Am J Psychiatry* 1980;137:439–44
5. Kitchell MA, Barnes RF, Veith RC. Screening for depression in hospitalized geriatric medical patients. *J Am Geriatr Soc* 1982;139: 799–802
6. Kirksey DF, Stern WC. Multi-center private practice evaluation of the safety and efficacy of bupropion in depressed geriatric outpatients. *Curr Ther Res* 1984;35:200–10
7. NIH Consensus Development Panel on Depression in Late-Life. Diagnosis and treatment of depression in late life. *J Am Med Assoc* 1992; 268:1018–1024
8. Fernandez F, Levy JK, Lachar BL, *et al.* The management of depression and anxiety in the elderly. *J Clin Psychiatry* 1995;56 (Suppl 2):20–29
9. Hay DP, Rodriguez MM, Franson KL. Treatment of depression in late life. *Clin Geriatr Med* 1998;14(1):33–46
10. Wells KB, Stewart A, Hays RD, *et al.* The functioning and well-being of depressed patients: results from the medical outcomes study. *J Am Med Assoc* 1989;262:914–19
11. Lecrubier Y. Is depression under-recognized and under-treated? *Int Clin Psychopharmacol* 1998;13(5):S1–S2
12. Gareri P, Falconi U, De Fazio P, De Sarro G. Conventional and new anti-depressants in the elderly. *Prog Neurobiol* 2000;61:353–96
13. Blazer D. Depression and the older man. *Med Clin North Am* 1999;83(5):1305–17
14. Brunello N, Langer SZ, Perez J, Racagni G. Current understanding of the mechanism of action of classic and newer anti-depressant drugs. *Depression* 1994;2:119–26
15. Hyttel J. Pharmacological characterization of selective serotonin re-uptake inhibitors. *Int Clin Psychopharmacol* 1994;9:19–26
16. Crimson ML, Dorson PG. Schizophrenia. In Di Piro JT, Talbert RL, Yee GC, *et al,* eds. *Pharmacotherapy: a Pathophysiologic Approach*, 3rd edn. Stamford, CT: Appleton and Lange, 1997:1381
17. Reynolds CF III. Depression: making the diagnosis and using SSRI's in the older patient. *Geriatrics* 1996;51(10):28–34
18. Gram LF. Fluoxetine. *N Engl J Med* 1994; 331:1354–60
19. Bergstrom RF, Lamberger L, Farid NA, *et al.* Clinical pharmacology and pharmacokinetics of fluoxetine: a review. *Br J Psychiatry* 1988; 153(Suppl 3):47–50
20. De Vane CL. Pharmacokinetics of the SSRI. *J Clin Psychiatry* 1992;53:13–20
21. Altamura AC, Moro AR, Percudani M. Clinical pharmacokinetics of fluoxetine. *Clin Pharmacokinet* 1994;26:201–14
22. Damluji NF, Ferguson JM. Paradoxical worsening of depressive symptomatology caused by anti-depressants. *J Clin Psychopharmacol* 1988;8:347–9
23. Beasley CM, Masica DN, Huliginstine JH, *et al.* Possible MAOI interaction. Fluoxetine clinical data and pre-clinical findings. *J Clin Psychopharmacol* 1993;13:312–20
24. Devane CL. Pharmacogenetics and drug metabolism of newer anti-depressant agents. *J Clin Psychiatry* 1994;55(Suppl 12): 38–47
25. Feighner JP, Boyer WF, Tyler DL, Neborsky RJ. Adverse consequences of fluoxetine–MAOI combination therapy. *J Clin Psychiatry* 1990; 51:222–5
26. Harris MG, Benfield P. Fluoxetine. A review of its pharmacodynamic and pharmacokinetic properties and therapeutic use in older patients with depressive illness. *Drugs Aging* 1995;6:64–84

27. Ten-Holt WL, Klaasen CH, Schrijver G. Severe hyponatremia possibly due to inappropriate anti-diuretic hormone secretion, during the use of the anti-depressant fluoxetine. *Ned Tijdschr Geneeskd* 1994;138:1181–3

28. Nemeroff CB. Paroxetine. An overview of the efficacy and safety of a new selective serotonin re-uptake inhibitor in the treatment of depression. *J Clin Psychopharmacol* 1993;13: 10S–17S

29. Dechant KL, Clissold SP. Paroxetine. A review of its pharmacodynamic and pharmacokinetic properties and therapeutic potential in depressive illness. *Drugs* 1991;41:225–53

30. Dunner DL. An overview of paroxetine in the elderly. *Gerontology* 1994;40:21–7

31. Hiemke C. Paroxetine: pharmacokinetics and pharmacodynamics. *Fortshcr Neurol Psychiatr* 1994;62:2–8

32. Masand P, Murray GB, Pickett P. Psychostimulants in post-stroke depression. *J Neuropsychiatry* 1991;3(1):23–7

33. Geretsegger C, Bohmer F, Ludwig M. Paroxetine in the elderly depressed patient: randomized comparison with fluoxetine of efficacy, cognitive and behavioral effects. *Int Clin Psychopharmacol* 1994;9:25–9

34. Cohn CK, Shrivastava R, Mendels J, *et al*. Double-blind multi-center comparison of sertraline and amitriptyline in the elderly depressed patients. *J Clin Psychiatry* 1990; 51:28–33

35. Doogan DP, Caillard V. Sertraline: a new anti-depressant. *J Clin Psychiatry* 1988;49:46–51

36. Auster R. Sertraline: a new anti-depressant. *Am Fam Physician* 1993;48:311–14

37. Wilde MI, Plosker GL, Benfield P. Fluvoxamine. An updated review of its pharmacology and therapeutic use in depressive illness. *Drugs* 1993;46:895–924

38. Wagner W, Plekkenpol B, Gray TE, *et al*. Review of fluvoxamine safety database. *Drugs* 1992;53:7–12

39. Stahl SM. Antidepressants and mood stabilizers. In *Essential Psychopharmacology: Neuroscientific Basis and Clinical Applications*, 3rd edn. New York: Cambridge University Press, 1996

40. Cole JO, Bodkin JA. Antidepressant drug side effects. *J Clin Psychiatry* 1990;51:21–6

41. Beasley CM Jr, Dornseif BE, Pultz JA, *et al*. Fluoxetine versus trazodone: efficacy and activating-sedating effects. *J Clin Psychiatry* 1991;52:294–9

42. Greenblatt DJ, Friedman H, Burstein ES, *et al*. Trazodone kinetics: the effect of age, gender and obesity. *Clin Pharmacol Ther* 1987;42: 193–200

43. Greene DS, Barbhaiya RH. Clinical pharmacokinetics of nefazodone. *Clin Pharmacokinet* 1997;33:260–75

44. Barbhaiya RH, Buch AB, Greene DS. A study of the effect of age and gender on the pharmacokinetics of nefazodone after single and multiple doses. *J Clin Psychopharmacol* 1996;16(1):19–25

45. Robinson DS, Roberts DL, Smith JM, *et al*. The safety profile of nefazodone. *J Clin Psychiatry* 1996;57:31–8

46. Ellingrod Vl, Perry PJ. Nefazodone: a new anti-depressant. *Am J Health Syst Pharm* 1995;52(24):2799–812

47. Schweitzer E, Feighner J, Mandos LA, *et al*. Comparison of venlafaxine and imipramine for the treatment of major depression in outpatients. *J Clin Psychiatry* 1994;55: 104–8

48. Troy SM, Parker VP, Hicks DR, *et al*. Pharmacokinetics and effect of food on the bio-availability of orally administered venlafaxine. *J Clin Pharmacol* 1997;37: 954–61

49. Venlafaxine French Inpatient Study Group. A double-blind comparison of venlafaxine and fluoxetine in patients hospitalized for major depression and melancholia. *Int Clin Psychopharmacol* 1994;9:139–43

50. Ellingrod Vl, Perry PJ. Venlafaxine: a heterocyclic anti-depressant. *Am J Hosp Pharm* 1994;51(24):3033–46

51. Puzantian T. Mirtazapine, an antidepressant. *Am J Health Syst Pharm* 1998;55:44–9

52. Kasper S, Praschak-Rieder N, Tauscher J, Wolf R. A risk-benefit assessment of mirtazapine in the treatment of depression. *Drug Safety* 1997;17:251–64

53. Kehoe WA, Schorr RB. Focus on mirtazapine: a new antidepressant with nonadrenergic and specific serotoninergic activity. *Formulary* 1996;31:455–6

54. Richelson E. Pharmacology of antidepressants: characteristics of the ideal drug. *Mayo Clin Proc* 1994;69(11):1069–81

55. Hsyu PH, Singh A, Giargiari TD, *et al.* Pharmacokinetics of bupropion and its metabolites in cigarette smokers versus non smokers. *J Clin Pharmacol* 1997;37:737–43

56. Stoudemire A. Expanding psychopharmacologic treatment options for the depressed medical patient. *Psychosomatics* 1995;36(2): S19–S26

57. Harris CR, Gualtieri J, Stark G. Fatal bupropion overdose. *J Clin Toxicology* 1997; 35:321–4

58. Spiller HA, Ramoska EA, Krenzelok EP, *et al.* Bupropion overdose: a 3-year multi-center prospective analysis. *Am J Emerg Med* 1994;12(1):43–5

59. Settle EC Jr. Bupropion: general side-effects. *J Clin Psychiatr Monogr* 1993;11(1):33–9

60. Snow JM. *Hypericum perforatum.* Protocol. *J Botanical Med* 1996;2:16–21

61. Canedy D. Real medicine or medicine sideshow? New York Times, 1998;July 23:C1–2

62. Cott JM. *In vitro* receptor binding and enzyme inhibition by *Hypericum perforatum* extract. *Pharmacopsychiatry* 1997;30 (Suppl 2):108–12

63. Teufel-Mayer R, Gleitz J. Effects of long-term administration of *Hypericum* extracts on the affinity and density of the central serotoninergic 5-HT1 A and 5-HT2 A receptors. *Pharmacopsychiatry* 1997;30(Suppl 2): 113–16

64. Muller WE, Rolli M, Schafer C, Hafner U. Effects of *Hypericum* extract (LI 160) in biochemical models of anti-depressant activity. *Pharmacopsychiatry* 1997;30(Suppl 2):102–7

65. Cott JM. In vitro receptor binding and enzyme inhibition by Hypericum perforatum extract. *Pharmacopsychiatry* 1997;30:113–16

66. Gaster B, Holroyd J. St John's wort for depression: a systematic review. *Arch Intern Med* 2000;160:152–6

67. Williams JW, Mulrow CD, Chiquette E, *et al.* A systematic review of newer pharmacotherapies for depression in adults: evidence report summary. *Ann Intern Med* 2000;132(9): 743–56

68. Schrader E, Meier B, Brattstrom A. *Hypericum* treatment of mild to moderate depression in a placebo-controlled study. *Hum Psychopharmacol* 1998;13:163–9

69. Brockmoller J, Reum T, Bauer S, *et al.* Hypericin and pseudohypericin: pharmacokinetics and effects on photosensitivity in humans. *Pharmacopsychiatry* 1997;30 (Suppl 2):94–101

70. Lieberman S. Nutriceutical review of St John's wort for the treatment of depression. *J Women's Health* 1998;7:177–82

71. Woelk H, Burkard G, Grunwald J. Benefits and risks of the *Hypericum* extract LI 160: drug monitoring with 3250 patients. *J Geriatr Psychiatry Neurol* 1994;7(Suppl):S34–S38

40 Sleep disorders

Hosam K. Kamel, MB, BCh, FACP

INTRODUCTION

Sleep disorders are prevalent in older persons[1-5]. In one study of community-dwelling elderly, 37% reported difficulty falling asleep; 29% reported night-time awakening; and 19% reported early morning awakening[3]. About one-half of community-dwelling elderly use sleep medications[6,7]. Epidemiological studies of older persons found an association between sleep complaints and the presence of chronic illness, mood disturbance, decreased physical activity and physical disability, but little association with increased age[8-12]. This suggests that other factors, other than age *per se*, account for the presence of sleep disorders. Sleep apnea and periodic limb movements in sleep, two primary sleep disorders, increase in prevalence with age. Older women are more likely than older men to report sleep complaints[13]. Self-reported sleeping difficulties are more common in older African-Americans, particularly women and those with depression and chronic illness[14].

AGE-RELATED CHANGES IN SLEEP

Aging is associated with multiple changes in sleep patterns (Table 1). While stages 1 and 2 (the lighter stages of sleep) increase or remain the same, stages 3 and 4 (the deeper stages of sleep) have been shown to decrease with advancing age. Rapid eye movement (REM) sleep occurs earlier during the sleep cycle, with the percentage of REM sleep remaining the same[15]. Older persons have decreased sleep efficiency (time asleep over time in bed),

Table 1 Age-related changes in sleep

Decrease in stages 3 and 4 sleep
Increased night-time awakenings
Increased sleep latency (time to fall asleep)
Decreased sleep efficiency (time asleep over time in bed)
Increased daytime napping
Earlier morning awakening
Earlier onset of REM sleep in night
Decreased total REM sleep

REM, rapid eye movement

decreased sleep time and an increased sleep latency (time to fall asleep). Additional findings include earlier bedtime and earlier morning awakening, more arousals during sleep and more daytime napping compared to younger individuals. After a period of sleep deprivation, older adults show less daytime sleepiness, less evidence of decline in performance measures, and recover their normal sleep structure more quickly than younger persons. Older persons, however, have more sleep disturbances with jet lag and shift work than younger persons[16].

Melatonin

Melatonin is a hormone that is secreted by the pineal gland and appears to have a role in regulating the circadian and seasonal biorhythms in humans and other mammals. Its synthesis and release are stimulated by darkness and inhibited by light. Thus, the diurnal rhythm of melatonin secretion closely follows the day-night cycle. This circadian rhythm, however, may be affected by changes in environmental lighting. Although plasma melatonin levels undergo a continuous decline after peaking at the age of 2 to 5 years, night-time plasma levels of the hormone remain greater than those during the day throughout the life span[17].

There is evidence that links the age-related decline in melatonin plasma levels to the development of insomnia in later years of life. The administration of melatonin to older adults with insomnia at doses sufficient to raise night-time plasma levels to those of younger adults, restored normal sleep patterns in these individuals[18]. On the other hand, melatonin supplementation had no effect on sleep patterns in older adults who did not have insomnia in spite of the presence of low melatonin plasma levels. It appears that the age-related decline in nocturnal plasma melatonin levels can not,on its own, explain the development of insomnia in all older adults. However, elderly individuals who do develop insomnia are likely to benefit from melatonin supplementation.

EVALUATION OF SLEEP IN OLDER PERSONS

The National Institutes of Health Consensus Statement on the Treatment of Sleep Disorders of Older People suggested three simple questions for clinicians to screen for sleep disorders in older adults[19]. First, is the person satisfied with his/her sleep? Second, does sleep or fatigue intrude into daytime activities? And third, does the bed partner or others complain of unusual behavior during sleep, such as snoring, interrupted breathing, or leg movement?

In general transient sleep disturbances (less than 4 weeks) are usually situational; persistent sleep problems, on the other hand, often require detailed evaluation. To aid the assessment of sleep complaints it is helpful to ask patients to keep a 'sleep log' in which, each morning, they record their time in bed, their estimated amount of sleep, number of awakenings, time of morning awakening and any

symptoms that occur during the night. This should be supplemented by information from bed partners when possible. Patients should have a general physical examination. In addition, all patients with sleep complaints should have their mental status assessed and be screened for depression.

Polysomnography is indicated when a primary sleep disorder, such as sleep apnea or periodic limb movement in sleep, is suspected. Other available methods to assess sleep include a wrist activity monitor, which estimates sleep versus wakefulness based on wrist activity. Another measure of sleep that has been developed for home sleep monitoring is a pressure-sensitive pad that reports signals from respiration and movement. An observational tool for detecting sleep problems and sleep-related breathing disorders has been used in nursing-home residents in the research setting[20]. Ambulatory monitoring devices that measure pulse oximetry, heart rate and respiration are also available and are frequently used in both clinical and research settings.

COMMON SLEEP DISORDERS IN OLDER ADULTS

Insomnia (difficulty in initiating or maintaining sleep) is usually due to a psychiatric, medical or a neurological illness. Excessive daytime sleepiness, on the other hand, is usually due to a primary sleep disorder such as sleep apnea. There is a significant overlap of conditions, however, that cause symptoms of insomnia or excessive daytime sleepiness[6].

Psychiatric disorders and psychological problems

Psychiatric disorders have been reported to be responsible for more than 50% of cases of insomnia. Depression is the commonest condition involved and is characterized by early morning awakening, increased sleep latency and more night-time wakefulness. In depressed older patients with sleep disturbances, treatment of depression has been reported to improve the sleep abnormality, with changes in sleep electroencephalography towards a more normal sleep structure. Anxiety and stress may be associated with difficulty in initiating sleep. Older caregivers report more sleep complaints than do similarly aged healthy adults. In one study about 40% of older women who were family caregivers of adults with dementia reported using a sleeping medication in the previous month[10].

Drugs and alcohol dependency

Drugs and alcohol use account for 10 to 15% of cases of insomnia. Chronic use of sedatives may cause light and fragmented sleep. Most sleeping medications when used chronically lead to tolerance and the potential for increasing doses. When chronic hypnotic use is suddenly stopped, there may be a rebound insomnia that leads to restarting the medication[21]. Alcohol abuse is often associated with lighter and shorter duration of sleep. The use of alcohol to treat insomnia should be discouraged. Although alcohol may cause an initial drowsiness, it can impair sleep later in the night as blood alcohol levels decrease.

Medical problems

Pain from arthritis and other conditions, cough, dyspnea from cardiac or pulmonary illness, gastroesophageal reflux and night-time urination can impair sleep. In addition, sleep can be impaired by certain medications taken near bedtime such as diuretics, stimulating agents (for example caffeine, sympathomimetics and bronchodilators). Certain medications – such as some antidepressants, anti-parkinsonian agents, and antihypertensives (for example propranolol) – can induce nightmares and impair sleep.

Sleep apnea

Sleep apnea refers to a periodic reduction in ventilation during sleep. Patients with sleep apnea often complain of excessive daytime sleepiness. Sleep apnea may be central (simultaneous cessation of breathing efforts and nasal and oral airflow), obstructive (thoracic respirations persist without normal airflow), or mixed. Obstructive sleep apnea is more frequent. In this condition patients usually present with hypersomnolence and are typically unaware of the frequent arousals associated with reductions in ventilation. Patients are often obese and may have morning headache and personality changes. They may also complain of poor memory, confusion and irritability. Other symptoms include loud snoring, cessation of breathing and choking sounds during sleep.

The prevalence of sleep apnea increases with age. The reported prevalence of sleep apnea among older persons varies from 20 to 70% depending on the population studied. The most important predictor of sleep apnea is large body mass. Other predictors identified in community-dwelling elderly people include falling asleep at inappropriate times, male gender and napping. Alcoholism is an important risk factor for sleep apnea, and sleep-disordered breathing is a significant contributor to sleep disturbances in male alcoholics over the age of 40. Finally, there appears to be an association between sleep apnea and dementia. One study[22] of nursing home residents found an association between sleep apnea and dementia, as well as a positive correlation between the severity of sleep disturbances and the severity of dementia. Patients suspected of having sleep apnea should be referred to a sleep laboratory for evaluation. Older patients tolerate the primary treatment of obstructive sleep apnea, nasal continuous positive airway pressure (CPAP), as well as middle-aged patients.

Periodic limb movements in sleep and 'restless legs syndrome'

Periodic limb movements in sleep (PLMS, or nocturnal myoclonus) is a condition of repetitive, stereotypical leg movements occurring in non-REM sleep. The leg movements occur every 20 to 40 seconds and can last much of the night, which may interfere with sleep. The occurrence of PLMS increases with age. One study reported that one-third of community-dwelling elderly had evidence of PLMS. PLMS may present as difficulty maintaining sleep or excessive daytime sleepiness. A bed partner may be aware of the leg movements, or these movements may remain occult until identified in a sleep laboratory.

'Restless leg syndrome' (RLS) is a condition of uncontrollable urges to move one's legs at night. The diagnosis is made based on the patient's description of symptoms, and the sleep complaint is usually difficulty in initiating sleep. There may be a family history of the condition and, in some cases, an underlying medical disorder (for example renal, neurological or cardiovascular disease). The prevalence of RLS also increases with age. Many patients with RLS also have PLMS. In older patients with PLMS or RLS, dopaminergic agents are the initial treatment of choice for both conditions (for example an evening dose of carbidopa/levodopa or pergolide). Some patients may describe a shift of their symptoms to daytime hours with successful treatment of symptoms at night. Benzodiazepines or opiates have also been used for these conditions.

DISTURBANCES IN THE SLEEP–WAKE CYCLE

Disturbances in the sleep-wake cycle may be transient, as in jet lag, or associated with an obvious cause (for example shift work). Some patients have persistent disturbances with either a delayed sleep phase (in which they fall asleep late and waken late) or an advanced sleep phase (in which they fall asleep early and waken early). The advanced sleep phase is particularly common in older individuals. Problems related to an advanced sleep phase may respond to appropriately timed exposure to bright light. Patients with a significant sleep-phase cycle disturbance should be referred to a sleep laboratory for evaluation.

REM sleep behavior disorder

REM sleep behavior disorder is characterized by excessive motor activity during sleep, with the pathologic absence of the normal muscle atonia during REM sleep. The presenting symptoms are usually vigorous sleep behaviors associated with vivid dreams. These behaviors may even result in injury to the patient or the bed partner. This condition is more common in older men than women and may be acute or chronic. Acute transient REM sleep behavior disorders have been associated with toxic-metabolic abnormalities, primarily drug or alcohol withdrawal or intoxication. The chronic form of REM sleep behavior disorder is usually idiopathic or associated with a neurological abnormality (for example drug intoxication, vascular disease, tumor, infection, degenerative disorder, or trauma). Polysomnography is recommended to establish the diagnosis. Clonazepam is the treatment of choice for REM sleep behavior disorder. Environmental safety interventions are also indicated, such as removing dangerous objects from the bedroom, and putting cushions on the floor around the bed.

Changes in sleep with dementia

Demented patients have more sleep disruption and arousal, lower sleep efficiency and a higher percentage of stage 1 sleep with reduction in stages 3 and 4 sleep compared to non-demented older persons. Disturbances of the sleep–wake cycle are common with dementia, resulting in daytime sleep and night-time wakefulness.

MANAGEMENT OF SLEEP DISORDERS

The management of sleep disorders should be guided by knowledge of the probable etiology

Table 2 Pharmacological agents commonly used to treat insomnia

Drug	Therapeutic dose (mg/day)	Time to onset of action (min)	Half-life (h)
Estazolam	1–2	15–30	8–24
Flurazepam	15–30	30–60	10–15
Lorazepam	1–4	30–60	8–24
Temazepam	15–30	45–60	3–25
Trazodone	50–200	30–60	5–9
Triazolam	0.125–0.25	15–30	1.5–5
Zaleplon	5–10	< 30	1
Zolpidem	5–10	30	1.5–4.5

and potential contributing factors. A trial of improved sleep hygiene is usually the recommended initial approach. Short-term hypnotic therapy may be appropriate in conjunction with improved sleep hygiene in some cases of transient, situational insomnia such as during acute hospitalization, and periods of temporary acute stress. In chronic insomnia the clinician should rule out primary sleep disorders and review medications and other medical conditions that may be contributory. Non-pharmacological interventions are usually the best choice for the treatment of chronic insomnia[23,24].

Non-pharmacological interventions to improve sleep in older people

Several non-pharmacological interventions can be quite effective in improving sleep in older persons. Behavioral interventions have been shown to produce multiple therapeutic benefits, including improved sleep efficiency, sleep continuity and satisfaction with sleep, and decreased hypnotic use[23]. Stimulus control[25] and sleep restriction therapy[26] have been shown to be helpful for older persons with insomnia. Cognitive and educational interventions are also important in changing attitudes to sleep. One randomized trial of older individuals with insomnia compared the effectiveness of (1) cognitive behavior therapy (stimulus control, sleep restriction, sleep hygiene and cognitive therapy) (2) pharmacotherapy (with temazepam)

(3) both cognitive therapy and pharmacotherapy, and (4) placebo. All three active treatment groups were effective in short-term follow-up in improving sleep based on sleep diaries and polysomnography; however, subjects were more satisfied with the behavioral treatment and sleep improvements were better sustained over time (up to two years) with behavioral treatment[24].

The effects of exposure to bright light (either natural sunlight or with commercially available light boxes) on sleep in older persons with insomnia have been tested in multiple studies. Positive effects on sleep have been demonstrated with light exposure of various intensities for various durations and at various times during the day. Evening light exposure was particularly useful in older persons with an advanced sleep phase. Even short durations of bright light exposure in the morning have been shown to improve sleep complaints in healthy older people. Another study reported on the beneficial effects in a small sample of women over the age of 65 years of a 'visor' which provided 200 lux to each eye and was worn for only 30 minutes in the evening[27,28].

Bathing before sleep has been demonstrated to enhance the quality of sleep in older people, perhaps because of an increase in body temperature with bathing. Moderate-intensity exercise has also been shown to improve sleep in healthy, sedentary people aged 50 years and older who reported moderate sleep complaints at baseline[29].

Pharmacotherapy for sleep problems in older people

Table 2 lists the commonly used sleeping medications. Benzodiazepines remain the most commonly prescribed agents for sleep. These medications should be used for only short periods, and if used for longer than a week they should not be used for more than three nights a week. Short-acting agents are recommended for problems with sleep maintenance. Short-acting agents are less likely to be associated with falls and hip fractures. Rebound insomnia after cessation of short-acting agents is frequent and can be reduced by tapering the dosage prior to discontinuing the drug. Temazepam has an intermediate half-life and no known active metabolites, and its metabolism is not thought to be affected by aging. However, daytime sedation may occur with this agent. Estazolam is a benzodiazepine with rapid onset and intermediate duration of action, so it may be effective in both initiating and maintaining sleep. This agent has weakly active metabolites and some accumulation may occur. The most common adverse effects are somnolence and hypokinesia. Estazolam is thought to have little effect on daytime psychomotor performance and is likely to cause tolerance. Long-acting agents should not be used in older people because of associated daytime sedation, lethargy, ataxia, falls and cognitive and psychomotor impairment.

Short-acting non-benzodiazepine hypnotics include zolpidem and the more recently available agent zaleplon. Both agents are structurally unrelated to benzodiazepines but they share some of the pharmacological properties such as interacting with the central nervous system γ-amino butyric acid (GABA) receptor complex at benzodiazepine (GABA-BZ) receptors. Zolpidem and zaleplon have a rapid onset of action and should be taken immediately prior to bedtime or after the patient has gone to bed and has been unable to fall asleep. Both have been shown to have little effect on daytime performance of cognitive and psychomotor tests. Low doses of sedating antidepressants such as trazodone or nefazodone at bedtime may also be used as a sleeping aid.

Evidence is mixed regarding the effectiveness of melatonin as a treatment for insomnia. In some studies administration of melatonin to older persons with insomnia decreased sleep latency (time to fall asleep) and wake time after the onset of sleep, and increased sleep efficiency (time asleep over time in bed)[30]. Other studies showed no beneficial effect. These mixed results and the lack of regulatory control over the currently available melatonin products make it difficult for clinicians to recommend the use of melatonin.

References

1. Foley DJ, Monjan A, Simnonsick EM, *et al.* Incidence and remission of insomnia among elderly adults: an epidemiologic study of 6,800 persons over three years. *Sleep* 1999;22 (Suppl 2):S366–72
2. Ganguli M, Reynolds CF, Gilby JE. Prevalence and persistence of sleep complaints in a rural older community sample: the MoVIES project. *J Am Geriatr Soc* 1996;44(7):778–84
3. Prinz PN, Vitiello MV, Raskind MA, Thorpy MJ. Sleep disorders and aging. *N Engl J Med* 1990;323:520–6
4. Ancoli-Israel S. Insomnia in the elderly: a review for the primary care practitioner. *Sleep* 2000;23(Suppl 1):S23–30
5. Pollak CP, Perlick D, Linsner JP. Daily sleep reports and circadian rest–activity cycles of elderly community residents with insomnia. *Biol Psychiatry* 1992;32(11):1019–27
6. Ancoli-Israel S, Poceta JS, Stepnowsky C, *et al.* Identification and treatment of sleep problems in the elderly. *Sleep Med Rev* 1997;1:3–17
7. Jorm AF, Grayson D, Creasey H, *et al.* Long-term benzodiazepines use by elderly people

living in the community. *Aust NZ J Pub Health* 2000;24(1):7–10

8. Polak CP, Perlick D, Linsner JP, et al. Sleep problems in the community elderly as predictors of death and nursing home placement. *J Community Health* 1990;15:123–35

9. Roberts RE, Shema SJ, Kaplan GA, Strawbridge WJ. Sleep complaints and depression in an aging cohort: a prospective perspective. *Am J Psychiatry* 2000;157(1):81–8

10. Bliwise DL. Sleep in normal aging and dementia. *Sleep* 1993;16:40–81

11. Janssens JP, Pautex S, Hillert H, Michel JP. Sleep disordered breathing in the elderly. *Aging (Milano)* 2000;12(6):417–29

12. Foley DJ, Monjan AA, Masaki KH, et al. Associations of symptoms of sleep apnea with cardiovascular disease, cognitive impairment, and mortality among older Japanese American men. *J Am Geriatr Soc* 1999;47(5):524–8

13. Fukuda N, Honma H, Kohsaka M, et al. Gender differences of slow wave sleep in middle aged and elderly subjects. *Psychiatry Clin Neurosci* 1999;53(2):151–3

14. Foley DJ, Monjan AA, Izmirlian G, et al. Incidence and remission of insomnia among elderly adults in a bi-racial cohort. *Sleep* 1999; 22(Suppl 2):S373–8

15. Chiu HF, Wing YK, Chung DW, Ho CK. REM sleep behavior disorder in the elderly. *Int J Geriatr Psychiatry* 1997;12:888–91

16. Moline ML, Pollak CP, Monk TH, et al. Age-related differences in recovery from simulated jet lag. *Sleep* 1992;15(1):28–40

17. Brown GH, Young SN, Gruthler S, et al. Melatonin in human cerebrospinal fluid in daytime: its origin and variation with age. *Life Sci* 1979;25:929–36

18. Wurtman RJ, Zhdanova I. Improvement of sleep quality by melatonin (letter). *Lancet* 1995;346:1491

19. National Institutes of Health Consensus Development Conference Statement: the treatment of sleep disorders of older people. *Sleep* 2001;14:169–77

20. Cohen-Mansfield J, Waldhorn R, Werner P, Billing N. Validation of sleep observations in a nursing home. *Sleep* 1991;13:512

21. Kripke DF. Chronic hypnotic use: deadly risks, doubtful benefits. *Sleep Med Rev* 2000; 4:5–20

22. Ancoli-Israel S, Klanber MR, Butters N, et al. Dementia in institutionalized elderly: relation to sleep apnea. *J Am Geriatr Soc* 1991;39: 258–63

23. Morin CM, Mimeault V, Gagne A. Nonpharmacological treatment of late-life insomnia. *J Psychosom Res* 1999;46(2): 103–16

24. Morin CM, Colecchi C, Stone J, et al. Behavioral and pharmacological therapies for late-life insomnia: a randomized controlled trial. *J Am Med Assoc* 1999;281(11):991–9

25. Schnelle JF, Alessi CA, Al-Samarrai NR, et al. The nursing home at night: effects of an intervention on noise, light and sleep. *J Am Geriatr Soc* 1999;47:430–8

26. Hoch CC, Reynolds CF III, Buysse DJ, et al. Protecting sleep quality in later life: a pilot study of sleep restriction and sleep hygiene. *J Gerontol B Psychol Sci Soc Sci* 2001;56(1): P52–9

27. Kohasaka M, Fukuda N, Kobayashi R, et al. Effects of short duration morning bright light in healthy elderly. II: Sleep and motor activity. *Psychiatry Clin Neurosci* 1998;52:252–3

28. Mihima K, Okawa M, Hishikawa Y, et al. Morning bright light therapy for sleep and behavior disorders in elderly patients with dementia. *Acta Psychiatr Scand* 1994;89: 1–17

29. Alessi CA, Yoon E, Schnle JF, et al. A combined physical activity and environmental intervention in nursing home residents: do sleep and agitation improve? *J Am Geriatr Soc* 1999;47:784–9/789–91

30. Van Reeth O, Weibel L, Olivares E, et al. Melatonin or a melatonin agonist corrects age-related changes in circadian response to environmental stimuli. *Am J Physiol Regul Integr Comp Physiol* 2001;280(5):R1582–92

41 Cognitive changes in aging

Syed H. Tariq, MD, and John E. Morley, MB, BCh

COGNITION AND AGING

Cognition is defined as the various thinking processes through which knowledge is gained, stored, manipulated and expressed. Although many cognitive skills decline with age, the extent and pattern of decline vary both at individual level and according to the type of function. Some individuals age successfully and maintain a similar cognitive function to that of the young, and some functions may even improve with aging. Other individuals may have some intact cognition functions (e.g. long-term memory, complex motor skills) while there is a decline in other areas of cognition (e.g. learning new information). Cognitive function is affected by a number of variables such as demographic factors (age, education), work and leisure activities and individual differences[1,2]. Psychiatric problems such as depression and substance abuse also affect cognition.

In this chapter we will discus the epidemiology of cognitive impairment, different methods involved in studying cognition, normal age-associated cognitive decline and the disease process involved in causing changes in cognition (dementia), diagnostic strategies and available treatments.

EPIDEMIOLOGY OF COGNITIVE IMPAIRMENT IN OLD AGE

The prevalence of dementia is 5% in persons of 65 years of age[3] and increases to 22% between the ages of 85 and 89 years. When persons with mild cognitive impairment are included the prevalence is almost doubled[4]. Alzheimer's disease (AD) is the most common type of dementia and affects 4 million people in the USA, but epidemiologists project that the number of patients with AD will be 14 million by 2040[5,6]. Males less commonly develop AD than do females. Minor cognitive decline is seen in the normal elderly, two out of three of whom have some sort of impairment on psychological testing[7].

CONCEPTUAL ISSUES IN THE STUDY OF COGNITIVE FUNCTION

Studying cognitive impairment is a difficult task. When studying cognition one should bear in mind that cognitive tests are affected by educational level, culture, language use, prior experience, emotional and physical status and measurement error. This makes it difficult to differentiate differences in cognitive score as a result of these factors from those due to disease processes. In epidemiological studies it is very important to consider a wide range of cognition, from the upper end of normal to the lower end of the disease process. Similarly there is a need for uniform measurement of cognition in all subjects along with restrictions on time and subject burden. Published epidemiological data have relied upon cognitive testing at one point in time, which is a direct approach but which is influenced by a number of factors other than disease processes, such as education (which is easily measured) and others which are difficult to define or measure. The way to find cognitive decline is by analyzing changes over a period of time; the timing between tests should, of course, be long enough to provide time for change.

There are a number of problems that limit a change in cognitive function as an outcome in epidemiologic studies. First the test should examine the entire range of cognitive function in the population to be studied. Second, the observed difference in cognitive function is usually very small compared to the entire range of function, necessitating the development of tests that are of sufficient sensitivity to measure small changes and are reliable. Unfortunately reliability data on most of the tests are not available. Third, to measure cognitive change it is important to use the same test at multiple end-points. Some people do well over time because of the learning effect, the size of which may vary among the risk group thereby affecting the outcome[8].

In modeling the association between risk factors and changes in cognitive function, the analytic issues are complicated by the need for time to be considered in the analysis. The methods that are most effective utilize advanced longitudinal analysis. Multiple outcome models, such as multivariate regression methods, including random effect models and generalized estimating equations (GEE), can be used with three or more risk factors over time. These methods can take into account all the observations and estimate the association of risk factor with level of cognitive function and with rates of change. A mixed model of fixed and random effects is the model of choice, when the cognitive scores are approximately within normal limits[9]. It also allows for individual variation, that is, the random effect. The main limitations of this method are that it requires continuous

data and multiple assumptions need to be made. GEE are used when the cognitive scores are not randomly distributed[10,11]. GEE have the same benefits as the random effect models except that they do not allow for differences in individual rates of decline. Another approach is to use a linear regression model and compute the change in cognitive score over time. These linear slopes are then used to determine the outcome variables in another linear regression model. The main limitation is that the individual slopes are treated as true slopes rather than estimates. There is the possibility of 'finding' an association where none, in fact, exists because some of the risk factors are underestimated.

When building models for changes in cognitive function both age and education need to be carefully considered since both are associated with many other potential risk factors[12]. When assessing changes in scores over time one should take into account the differential effects of age and education on the individual's capacity to learn[8]. Use of cognitive decline as a categorical variable – i.e. decline in cognition or no decline – limits the statistical power and gives rise to the possibility of deriving wrong associations by providing cut-off values. Similarly when individuals are combined into groups (persons showing improvement and those showing no improvement) it is possible for an exposure group with more variation to appear to have suffered more decline even though it actually experienced more improvement. When dementia is defined by a certain score rather than by a change in score many other variables are ignored. For example a person with a low level of education may score close to the cut-off point of dementia as compared to one with a high educational status, but a small change in the latter's score may be required to fall into the group of patients with dementia on follow-up. This approach is limited by the way in which the ability to distinguish between the initial level and change is lost.

Sometimes tests are combined to reduce the skewed distribution between the floor and ceiling effects. When selecting a method for combining tests, the investigator should give careful consideration to how different tests are weighted and to what assumption this implies about relationships among the tests[13]. In conclusion advanced statistical and longitudinal designs should be used in any studies aimed at age-associated changes[12].

DECLINE IN COGNITIVE FUNCTIONS WITH AGING, OR PRIMARY COGNITIVE DECLINE

The cognitive domains are intelligence, attention, language, memory, learning, visuospatial ability, psychomotor ability and speed, and executive functions.

Intelligence

Intelligence is a multifactorial construct; intellectual performance peaks at the age of 30 years, plateaus through the fifties and sixties and then declines, but there is a sharper decline in the late seventies[14]. Changes in intelligence as a function of age may be confounded by cohort effects as shown in many cross-sectional studies[15], while longitudinal studies may either overestimate or underestimate changes in intelligence[16]. Three decades ago Horn and Cattell[17] introduced the concept of crystallized and fluid intelligence. 'Crystallized intelligence' represents an individual's accumulated knowledge base, which is obtained and can be expanded throughout his/her life span. 'Fluid intelligence' is the ability to solve new problems from day to day and requires new knowledge and skills. Studies have shown that fluid intelligence deteriorates more with aging as compared to crystallized intelligence[18,19]. Czaja and Sharit[20] compared the abilities of 65 subjects to learn new computer tasks in the age range 25–70 years; the older subjects

made more errors and had longer response times. Similarly, in another study elderly skilled typists did not show any slowing in their motor abilities, but elderly unskilled typists were slower than young unskilled typists, demonstrating the effects of fluid intelligence. Some slowing in central processing may be responsible for the decline in fluid intelligence in old age[21-23].

The Wechsler Adult Intelligence Scale (WAIS) is the standard test used for testing intelligence[24]. There is an earlier onset and age-related decline observed on the verbal subsets of this scale. Hultsch and colleagues[25] examined a non-institutional sample of the population and reported that the age-related decline occurred in the working memory, verbal fluency and world knowledge, when the sample was controlled for differences in individual effects of aging. In a meta-analysis of 65 studies, there was no clear relationship between age and work performance; but these studies did not show the nature of the work and the experience of the individuals performing it[26]. It has also been reported that experience at a job leads to an increase in crystallized intelligence, which can, indeed, increase with age.

Performance speed

Speed of performance is usually not regarded as a cognitive function on its own, but it operates in many aspects of cognition. Performance speed declines as is evident by a decrease in the speed of walking[27] and as shown by the 'finger-tapping test'[28]. Slowing of cognition or reaction time is also recognized by psychological testing with advancing age[21,22,29]. The WAIS has shown that there is more age-related decline in the performance subsets scores as compared to the verbal subsets scores[24,30]. The decline in the performance subset arises not because of motor slowing, but involves perceptual and integrative processes, as is shown by the relationship of P300 event-related latencies and age. The P300 and other evoked potentials directly measure the central processing time[31].

Memory and learning

Memory and learning comprise the general set of functions associated with the acquisition, storage and retrieval of new information. Thirty-one per cent of elderly living in the community without cognitive impairment and 47% of those with cognitive impairment complain of memory problems[32]. This self-reported memory loss can also act as a predictor of impending cognitive decline[32-35].

There are three types of memory and they are affected by age in different ways. Primary memory or working memory is a temporary storage capacity, which is time limited and is maintained only through practice. One example of primary memory is to hold a telephone number in one's mind while one uses it to dial a number or hold a number while one scans for the address. Craik[36] reported that older people might be slower in accessing information from primary stores, though tasks on digit span are performed equally well in the young and old age groups[37].

Secondary memory is the ability to acquire new information and seems to be susceptible to aging. Age-dependent impairment in secondary memory is somewhat more apparent during tasks such as free recall rather than crude recall or recognition[38,39]. Furthermore, episodic memory (e.g. recall of specific words on a list displayed 5 minutes earlier) declines substantially with age, whereas semantic memory (e.g. retrieval from one's vocabulary or general knowledge base) declines modestly[40,41]. If one takes into account educational attainment, decrement in semantic memory almost does not exist[42]. Some investigators reported that explicit memory (conscious attempts to recall specific information) declines more than implicit memory (skills acquired through previous experience)[43,44]. It is hypothesized that

the decreased ability to learn new information might be related to degeneration of the hippocampus, and a decrease in efficacy or abundance of acetylcholine[45]. Numerous age-related differences are found with both the encoding and the retrieval of new information in long-term memory. Older adults are more sensitive to distraction on attention tasks[36], quick pacing of materials[46], and the amount of material presented at one time[47]. When older people are provided with memory encoding strategies they do well on memory performance, provided they continue using these techniques[48]. Perhaps reinforcement paradigms that emphasize rehearsal and use of these new learned skills would prove beneficial. It has been shown that learning in older adults might be less effective because they are more likely to learn peripheral information, while the younger are more task oriented[49]. In addition to encoding, retrieval is also more difficult for older people. It is very difficult to understand whether older adults apply less effort to retrieve information or whether weakly encoded material by definition is difficult to retrieve.

Tertiary or remote memory is a type of memory that is stored and consolidated over time (examples are one's wedding anniversary or birthday or a historical event). Clinicians have long been aware that remote memories are clearer and more readily accessible to older adults than are more recent memories. Elderly people do as well as young on skills learned long ago, for example reading and spelling. In fact the performance of the elderly at these tests generally is consistent with or higher than their previous academic achievement.

Language

Difficulty with spoken language is a common complaint in older individuals[50] and problems in communication are reported by older adults to affect their quality of life[51]. Most of the studies in older adults have reported that peripheral auditory impairment accounts for most of the variance in speech perception scores. This is considered as the primary contributor to the age-related decline in understanding speech[52,53]. Humes and Watson[52] reported that hearing loss accounted for 75% of the variance in identification scores among older subjects listening in a quiet environment; when background noise was added only 50% of the variance could be explained by the person's absolute sensitivity. The input side of language involves perception of the letters and speech sounds that make up words, and comprehension of the meaning of words and sentences. These input-side processes remain remarkably stable in old age, independent of sensory deficits and decline in the ability to encode new information[54]. The technique used to measure the processing of word meanings and their organization in semantic memory is the semantic priming paradigm (e.g. the reduction in the time required to identify a target word). The semantic priming effects are reliably larger for older than younger adults[55]. The semantic selection process during sentence comprehension remains constant across the age groups[54]. Off-line task measures comprehension processes by examining what people remember about the meaning of a paragraph presented earlier. Age differences invariably appear in such tasks[56], but may have less to do with initial comprehension than with the process of encoding and recall of comprehended information[57]. Wingfield and colleagues[58] asked younger and older adults to repeat sentences that were produced at different speaking rates in two levels of semantic context. The first sentences were semantically and syntactically meaningful (e.g. he walked along the path), while the second sentences were intact syntactically but semantically meaningless (e.g. fruitless brown dreams sleep curiously). Performance was significantly poorer for both age groups when sentences did not include semantic information. However when the semantic information was added to the syntax context, older adults performed better than

younger adults[59,60]. Recent studies indicate that at least two cognitive abilities are essential for processing spoken language, which become impaired in old age. First is the ability to maintain perceptual constancy with speech signals that vary because of vocal-tract differences among talkers. Second is the ability to distinguish phonetically similar words. These are referred to as talker normalization and lexical discrimination, respectively. They are part of the earliest stages of speech perception and have been shown to be important for recognizing spoken words[61,62].

Words produced by a man, a woman and a child will have different acoustical properties because of differences in the physical characteristics of the speaker[63]. Sommers[61] has shown that there is a significant age-related reduction in the ability to carry out perceptual normalization of talker differences. In this study both young and older adults were asked to identify words against a background noise. In the first part of the experiment all the words were produced by a single speaker and in the second ten different speakers produced the words. There was no difference in the speech recognition performance with a single speaker, but in the second part of the test both groups performed worse. However, the decline from single to multiple speakers was significantly greater for older adults. The multiple speakers had a greater effect on the perception of speech in the older adults. This finding suggests that one of the factors that may contribute to age-related impairment in understanding speech is a reduced ability to maintain perceptual constancy by compensating for acoustic-phonetic changes that result from differences in speaker (vocal-tract) characteristics.

Lexical refers to the structure of meaning and its representation in words. Intact lexical functions include the ability to access and recognize words on demand. Sommers[61] measured the speech identification score for two types of words as a function of age. The first type comprised lexically 'easy' words. The lexically 'hard' words used as the second type of stimulus were phonetically similar to other common English words. There was no difference in the identification of easy words between the two groups (70%), but the performance on hard words in both groups was poor. The older group exhibited significantly lower scores in the identification of lexically hard words compared to young adults. A multiple regression model indicated that the performance on lexically difficult words was not correlated with a measure of absolute sensitivity. Thus, independently of hearing status, older subjects had greater difficulty in identifying words that were phonetically similar to others stored in their long-term memory.

Visuospatial functioning

Visuospatial function is the ability to perceive objects and subsequently manipulate visual information. The magnification hypothesis model predicts that individual differences (between young and older adults) will increase systematically with the difficulty of the task. When both young and older adults performed visuospatial information tasks, the response times yielded a single principal component with a similar composition in both age samples. For both samples the response time for fast and slow subgroups for the seven tasks (18 conditions) on the corresponding mean of response time for their age group accounted for 99% of the variance. These findings suggest that individual differences in processing time were largely task-independent. The response times of slower individuals are more affected by aging than those of faster individuals.

It is also hypothesized that aging and hemispheric laterality interact to produce relatively greater decrements in older individuals in right hemispheric-dominant (visuospatial) than left hemispheric-dominant (verbal) tasks. Twenty-four early middle-aged

males (mean age 37.6 years) and 24 older males (mean age 71.2 years) – of equal educational status – were given a task. The Shark test is a verbal and visuospatial paired-associated learning task and is sensitive to left and right hemispheric dysfunction, respectively. The subjects were also given the Shipley Institute for Living Scale and the Memory-for-Designs Test. No group differences were present on the Shipley verbal age scale, but the older group had significantly lower Shipley abstraction ages and memory-for-designs scores. They made more errors than the middle-aged group on both the verbal and visuospatial learning tasks. These data do not support the notion of a laterality effect associated with aging.

A cross-sectional analysis of community residents age 65 and older found a decrease in visuospatial ability and speed of execution as age increased. There was also a poor performance among female subjects and those with lower levels of education. A convenience sample of 59 people (35 women and 24 men) with mild dementia of the Alzheimer type, 66 (39 women and 27 men) with mild dementia of the Alzheimer type, and 146 healthy non-demented individuals (90 women and 56 men) was studied. The participants' ages ranged from 51 to 96 years. Severity of dementia was staged by means of the Clinical Dementia Rating. In this sample visuospatial deficit was more apparent in very mild dementia of the Alzheimer type. Individuals with both very mild and mild dementia of the Alzheimer type made more errors involving peripheral figures and rotation of a major figure than did healthy, non-demented individuals.

Executive function

Executive functions are cognitive processes that orchestrate complex, goal-directed activities[64]. The American Psychiatric Association added executive function to its list of cognitive domains that can be used to establish the diagnosis of dementia[65]. Executive function has been associated with the frontal cortex, but is thought to be more a product of the frontal cortico-subcortical system[66]. Impairment in executive function is linked to age-related frontal cortical atrophy and decline in frontal perfusion among healthy people[67,68]. Executive impairment undermines a patient's independence by interfering with the direction, planning, execution and supervision of behavior[69]. The prevalence of executive function impairment is unknown in older adults in the community. It is reported that decline in executive function can be detected in healthy adults as young as 45–65 years of age compared to educationally and sex-matched adults aged 20–35 years[67]. Executive function can be measured by the Wisconsin Card Sorting Test (WCST), Executive Interview (EXIT-25), Mini Mental State Examination (MMSE) and Clock Drawing Task (CLOX). The EXIT-25 correlated with other measures of executive control including the WCST ($r = 0.54$), Trail Marking Part B ($r = 0.64$), the test of sustained attention (time, $r = 0.82$; errors, $r = 0.83$) and Lezak's Tinker Toy Test ($r = 0.57$). The EXIT-25 is more sensitive than MMSE to early cognitive impairment and non-cortical dementia in elderly subjects[70,71]. MMSE is a very familiar instrument[72] but is insensitive in early dementia and poorly educated subjects[73]. The clock drawing task (CLOX), when administered to healthy and demented elderly as an executive function, was closely correlated with EXIT-25 and MMSE[74]. This association persists after adjusting for age and education[75].

Neuropsychological data show that age-related frontal lobe changes are most significant compared to changes in other cortical structures[76]. These changes vary across individuals and are evident after 65 years of age. A recent theory of aging links impairment in executive function to cognitive decline in memory and attention, which in turn is associated with the frontal lobes[77]. Executive memory supervises the content of working memory, where information from long-term memory is integrated with information in the immediate present to plan, initiate and carry out a course of action[78]. Cognitive impairment recognized by the MMSE or by the Dementia Rating Scale is associated with impairment on complex, instrumental activities of daily living[79]. In the early stages of dementia patients under-report difficulties in daily activities, an inaccuracy correlated with cognitive impairment[80]. Executive function plays an important role in daily motor functions of the elderly, and many of them report difficulty on one or more activity of daily living (ADLs). Executive abilities are necessary to recognize, initiate and carry out consequences of actions and may well be the critical skills that regulate the performance of many ADLs, particularly high order ADLs (operation of tools or instruments and tasks that require more steps for successful completion than do the basics ADLs). One study examined the association of cognition and physical function in community dwellers with minor disabilities in East Baltimore with a mean age of 74 years. In this sample it was found that old age, lower educational attainment and African-American race were all associated with poor physical performance. Impairments in executive function – flexibly planning and initiating a course of action – were selectively associated with slower performance of high order tasks such as the instrumental activities of daily living, relative to other domains of cognition[81].

Executive dysfunction also contributes to the care received by older retirees in a retirement community. In one study retired residents in such a community were provided with services at three levels of care: independent living apartments (level 1), residential care where laundry, house-cleaning, meals and supervision of medication were provided (level 2) and skilled nursing units in which residents were provided with assistance in activities of daily living, nurse care and medication (level 3). Several tests (EXIT-25, MMSE [general cognition], Geriatric Depression Scale short form [mood], the Nursing Home Behavior Problem Scale [problem behavior], the Cumulative

Illness Rating Scale [physical disability], age, educational level, and amount of medication prescribed) were used to examine the effect on the need for the perceived level of care given. In this small sample it was found that impaired executive function contributed most to the need, as perceived by the carers, for the variation in care given in this retirement community. The other markers of general cognition, depression and physical illness contributed relatively little additional variation. The strongest contribution to the perceived need for a variation in the level of care given was by EXIT-25, which accounted for 70% of the observed variation. In this sample it was also found that 55% of the residents who scored greater than or equal to 24 on the MMSE failed the EXIT-25 test at 15/50, suggesting that the MMSE test is not as sensitive as the EXIT-25 test[82].

Attention

Attention is the ability to concentrate on tasks. It can be divided into two types, divided attention and sustained attention. Divided attention is the ability to differentiate between two different stimuli, such as different auditory stimuli presented to each ear; this begins to decline in the fourth decade. Sustained attention is the ability to focus on single tasks; examples are series of numbers differing by seven (e.g. 100, 93, 86, 79, 72....) or spelling 'world' backwards. Sustained attention is maintained and does not decline before the age of 80 years.

PRIMARY DEMENTING ILLNESS

Dementia is a general term used to describe a significant decline in two or more areas of cognitive functioning, usually associated with cognitive decline. Dementia is not synonymous with aging because the cognitive changes are progressive and disabling and are not an inherent part of aging. Table 1 provides a list of the possible etiologies of dementia.

Alzheimer's disease

Alzheimer's disease (AD) usually affects people after the age of 60 years; it rarely affects people before this age. The disease process is gradual and progressive; the average life expectancy after the first symptoms apperar is 8–10 years. AD is seen in 6–8% of all persons after the age of 65 years, and the prevalence doubles every 5 years after the age of 60 years, so that at the age of 85 years prevalence has increased to 30%[83–85]. Alzheimer's is a disease characterized by amyloid plaques and neurofibrillary tangles. It has been genetically associated with chromosome 21 (Down's syndrome and beta amyloid gene), chromosomes 14 and 1 and chromosome 19 (apolipoprotein E_4).

The risk factors for Alzheimer's disease are outlined in Table 2. Alzheimer's disease is a major burden on society and in the USA costs about $100 billion each year, the costs being made up of medical expenses, long-term care, home care and lost of productivity of caregivers[86,87]. Alzheimer's disease also causes emotional toll on the caregivers and 50% of sufferers' families develop some form of psychological distress[88].

The Diagnostic and Statistic Manual of Mental Disorders (DSM) IV has developed criteria for the level of dementia in Alzheimer's disease. The cognitive deficit manifested by both memory impairment and at least one of the following cognitive disturbances – aphasia, apraxia, agnosia and disturbance in executive functions – causes impairment in social and occupational function. These symptoms should not arise because of other conditions or drugs that cause impairment in cognition. The onset is gradual and there is a progressive decline in cognition, with sparing of motor and sensory functions, until late in the disease. Memory impairment is present in the early stages of the disease and the person has difficulty learning

Table 1 Disorders that may cause dementia

Primary dementing illness	Secondary dementing illness
Alzheimer's disease	Vascular dementias
Pick's disease	Thrombotic disorders
Frontotemporal dementia	Embolic disease
Huntington's disease	Inflammatory vascular condition
Parkinson's disease	Systemic lupus erythematosus
Progressive supranuclear palsy	Temporal arthritis
Cortical Lewy-body disease	*Metabolic and endocrine disturbances*
Drugs and toxins	Hypothyroidism/hyperthyroidism
Alcohol-induced dementia	Hyoadrenalism/hyperadrenalism
Drug-induced dementia	Hypoparathyroidism/hyperparathyroidism
Intracranial conditions	Hypoglycemia/hyperglycemia
Brain tumors	Vitamin B$_{12}$ deficiency
Brain abscesses	Pellagra
Hydrocephalus	Uremic/dialysis encephalopathy
Subdural hematoma	Aluminum
Trauma to the head	*Psychiatric disorders*
Infections	Depression
Creutzfeldt–Jakob disease	Mania
AIDS	Schizophrenia
Neurosyphilis	
Chronic meningitis	

Table 2 Risk factors and protective factors for Alzheimer's disease

Risk factors
Age
Family history
Early age (genetic mutation on chromosomes 1, 14, 21)
Late onset (Apolipoprotein E$^*_4$ allele on chromosome 19)
Down's syndrome
Head trauma
Female gender
Lower educational achievement

Protective factors
Estrogen use
Higher educational level
Anti-inflammatory drug use
Apolipoprotein E$^*_2$ allele
Antioxidant use

activities of daily living as well as social skills are intact until late in the disease. Changes occur in mood and behavior such as personality changes, irritability, anxiety or depression, delusions and hallucinations[89], which is very troubling for the family and frequently leads to nursing home placement[90]. It is very hard to identify dementia in the setting of either delirium or depression and sometimes they coexist in hospital settings[91]. It is very important to differentiate delirium and depression from dementia; Tables 3 and 4 outline the important differences. Dementia is a risk factor for delirium and contributes to the higher prevalence of delirium in the elderly[91]. About 50% of initially reversible causes of dementia and depression can lead to irreversible dementia in 5 years[92].

new information and even retaining it for a shorter period. Cognitive impairment may also affect activities of day-to-day living: problems with meal planning, managing medication and finances, use of the telephone and problems in driving. In mild to moderate AD many of the

Pick's disease

Pick's disease is characterized by a preponderance of atrophy in the frontotemporal region, in contrast to Alzheimer's disease, where the distribution is parietal-temporal.

Table 3 Differences between delirium and dementia

Characteristic	Delirium	Dementia
Onset	Sudden	Gradual over months to years
Reversibility	Usually reversible	Irreversible and progressive
Disorientation	Early and profound	Later during the disease
Consciousness	Clouded, fluctuating	Not usually affected
Language	Uses wrong words, vocabulary intact	Worsens with advanced disease
Attention span	Strikingly short	Not affected
Speech	Incoherent	Coherent
Sleep–wake cycle	Hour to hour variability	Day–night reversal
Psychomotor changes	Marked*	None until late

*Hyperactive or hypoactive

Table 4 Differences between depression and Alzheimer's disease (AD)

Characteristic	Depression	AD
Onset	Rapid, relatively short duration	Gradual, long duration
Mood	Flat or depressed (anxious, suicidal)	Apathetic to irritable (memory loss occurs first)
Intellectual function	Don't know answers	Confident but inaccurate answers
Memory loss	Loss of short and long-term memory	Recent memory most impaired
Other symptoms	Impaired concentration	Impaired orientation
Self image	Poor	Normal
Personal and family history	Depression more common	Depression less common

Pick's disease constitutes 5% of all irreversible dementias. In Pick's disease the earliest changes are related to personality, such as socially inappropriate behavior and frontal lobe disinhibition. Patients with Pick's disease have an early onset of language disturbances and Klüver–Bucy syndrome (hyperphagia, emotional blunting, hypersexuality and visual and auditory agnosia), but there is sparing of memory, visuospatial abilities and the ability to calculate[93]. Computed tomography (CT) scan shows frontotemporal atrophy, and histology shows Pick bodies, inflated cells, white matter gliosis, and loss of dendritic spines. There is no known etiology and therefore no specific treatment.

Other frontal lobe degeneration dementias are: frontal lobe degeneration without Pick's pathology, amyotrophic lateral sclerosis, and progressive subcortical gliosis, stroke involving the anterior cerebral artery, multiple sclerosis, hydrocephalus and syphilis.

Dementia with extrapyramidal disorders

Dementia with extrapyramidal disorders is different from Alzheimer's disease or frontal lobe disease. A descriptive term, 'cortical and subcortical dementia', is used to differentiate between the two dementias and is outlined in Table 5.

Huntington's disease

Huntington's disease is an idiopathic degenerative disease characterized by dementia and chorea. It is an autosomal dominant trait with 50% penetration, the gene being located on chromosome 4. The age at onset is usually 35 to 40 years but it can occur after the age of 50 years. It is characterized by dementia and affective disorders, and a considerable number of patients develop a schizophrenic-like disorder[94]. There is atrophy of the caudate

Table 5 Differences between cortical and subcortical dementias

Characteristic	Cortical dementia	Subcortical dementia
Language	Early aphasia	No aphasia
Memory	Both recall and recognition impaired	Recall more impaired than recognition
Abstraction	Impaired	Impaired on difficult tasks
Mood	Normal	Depressed
Personality	Normal	Apathetic
Speech	Affected late	Dysarthric
Posture	Upright	Extended
Co-ordination	Normal but affected late	Impaired
Motor function	Normal	Slow
Site of disease	Hippocampus and associated cortex	Basal ganglion, thalamus, brain stem
Diseases	*AD and FTD	Parkinson's disease, Huntington's disease, progressive supranuclear palsy

*AD, Alzheimer's disease; FTD, frontotemporal dementia

nucleus on both CT scan and positron emission tomography (PET) scan and there is a decrease in levels of γ-amino butyric acid[95]. No specific treatment is available; however the associated psychiatric disorders respond to treatment.

Parkinson's disease

Parkinson's disease is a disease of middle-aged and older adults; 80% of the people affected are between the ages of 60 and 79 years[96]. The prevalence of dementia in Parkinson's disease is 8–80%[97]. Parkinson's disease is manifested by resting tremor, rigidity, bradykinesia and loss of righting reflexes. Intellectual impairment is more common in older patients with akinesa and a prolonged disease course. There is a deficiency of dopamine, with variable loss of epinephrine, serotonin, acetylcholine and selected neuromodulators. Pathologically there is cell loss and gliosis in the substantia nigra, and some portion of Lewy bodies in the remaining neurons. It is reported that some patients with Parkinson's disease have classical Alzheimer's lesions[96,97]. Fetal tissue implants are being investigated as a treatment for the motor symptoms[98].

Cortical Lewy-body disease

A subgroup of patients with dementia has Lewy-bodies (hyaline inclusion bodies) associated with neuronal loss in certain nuclei e.g. nucleus basalis and brain stem nuclei[99]. It has been suggested that in Lewy-body disease there is dopamine deficiency and cholinergic deficiency[97]. The older neuroleptic medications are likely to worsen the motor symptoms of Parkinson's disease and cause psychotic symptoms, but the newer neuroleptic drugs such as clozapine or risperidone may be useful. Persons with Lewy-body dementia tend to present with behavioral symptoms before they develop cognitive symptoms.

Progressive supranuclear palsy

This illness is more common in men than in women, affecting people in their sixth or seventh decade, and the average length of time until death is 5–10 years. Progressive supranuclear palsy is characterized by an extrapyramidal syndrome and dementia. Clinically there is more rigidity in midline structures and erect posture with extension of the neck. It is most often associated with sleep disturbances and depression[100]. Progressive supranuclear palsy involves the subthalamic nucleus, red nucleus, globus pallidus, substantia nigra, and dentate nucleus. Pathologically, there is granulovacuolar degeneration, neurofibrillary tangles and cell loss. A variety of drugs have been used to treat these patients such as L-dopa, amantadine, benztropine and amitriptyline[101–103].

SECONDARY DEMENTING ILLNESS

Vascular dementia

Vascular dementia is the second most common cause of dementia and occurs more often in people aged 55 or older. The criteria for the diagnosis of vascular dementia are multiple cognitive deficit manifested by both memory impairment and one of the following: aphasia, apraxia, agnosia or disturbances in executive functioning along with focal neurological signs that are judged to be etiologically related to the disturbances (DSM-IV). The risk factors for vascular dementia are hypertension and other cardiovascular risk factors[104]. The differences between vascular dementia and Alzheimer's disease are outlined in Table 6.

Recently a neuropathologic classification of vascular dementia has been provided. It is determined by the size of the vessel affected and the region of the brain affected[105]. Small vessel-disease may cause subcortical damage resulting in subcortical dementia or affect the white matter of the frontal lobes, producing a frontal lobe syndrome. Binswanger's disease is also known as subcortical atherosclerotic encephalopathy. It is characterized by multiple small infarcts of the white matter; lacunar infarcts are also seen in Binswanger's disease[105]. In the past it was considered less common but with the availability of sophisticated techniques such as magnetic resonance imaging it is diagnosed more commonly these days.

DRUGS AS A CAUSE OF DEMENTIA

The elderly represent 12% of the population and consume about 30% of all the prescribed medication, and 70% of them use over-the-counter medication[105]. Any drug can potentially cause cognitive or behavioral changes; some drugs are more common as causative agents

than others and can easily be remembered by the mnemonic: 'ACUTE CHANGE IN MS' outlined in Table 7[106–108].

DEMENTIA ASSOCIATED WITH TOXIC SUBSTANCES

Alcoholism is one of the most important health problems in the USA[109]. It has a bimodal distribution with the second peak occurring between the seventh and eight decades of life[110]. Long-term alcohol consumption produces dementia syndrome with frontal lobe dysfunction, and apathy independent of head injury, malnutrition and hepatic failure[111,112]. Alcoholic dementia is usually mild and slowly progressive and may partially remit if abstinence can be maintained for several months[112]. There is evidence that alcohol primarily causes atrophy of white matter because of its toxic effect on myelin. New onset alcoholism may occur in older persons.

Exposure to some metals – e.g. lead, arsenic, mercury, manganese, nickel, bismuth and tin – can cause dementia. Aluminum has been associated with dialysis-induced dementia in patients with long-term dialysis[113]. Patients with dialysis-induced dementia present with personality changes, myoclonus and seizures. Treatment includes reducing the exposure and treating with the chelating agent deferoxamine.

NEOPLASMS CAUSING DEMENTIA

Neoplasms are common in the elderly and must be considered in the differential diagnosis of dementia. Brain tumors may cause different symptoms depending on the location. They can cause changes in mental status, increased intacranial pressure, focal weakness, personality changes, intellectual changes and sensory and visual defects. Dementia occurs in 70% of patient with frontal lobe tumors e.g. meningiomas, gliomas, or metastatic tumors[114,115].

Table 6 Differences between vascular dementia and Alzheimer's disease (AD)

Characteristic	Vascular dementia	AD
Onset	Sudden; may be stroke related	Gradual
Progression	Stepwise; sudden cognitive declines, fluctuates	Gradual decline in cognition and function
Neurologic findings	Focal deficit	No focal deficit
Neuroimaging	One or more infarct(s) in the area affecting cognition	May appear normal
Gait	Disturbed early in dementia	Usually normal
Cerebrovascular history	History of TIA, remote stroke or vascular risk factors	Less common

TIA, transient ischemic attack

Table 7 Drugs associated with dementias

A, Anti-parkinsonian drugs
C, Corticosteroids
U, Urinary incontinence drugs
T, Theophylline
E, Emptying drugs (e.g. metoclopramide)

C, Cardiovascular drugs (Digoxin, clonidine, methyldopa, procainamide)
H, H$_2$ blockers
A, Antimicrobials (rare but case reports exist)
N, Narcotics
G, Geropsychiatric drugs
E, ENT drugs

I, Insomnia drugs
N, NSAIDs

M, Muscle relaxants
S, Seizure drugs

NSAID, non-steroidal anti-inflammatory drug; ENT, ear nose throat drugs (used for respiratory and sinus disorders)

DEMENTIA CAUSED BY INFECTIOUS DISEASES

HIV encephalopathy

Acquired immunodeficiency syndrome is caused by the human immunodeficiency virus, which attacks the immune system and impairs patient response to infections. HIV encephalopathy is the leading infectious cause of dementia[116]. The HIV invades the brain, shortly afterwards causing systemic infection, and remains latent for long periods[117]. HIV encephalopathy has subcortical features such as apathy, impaired concentration and memory,

indifference and poor motivation[118]. The Center for Disease Control (CDC) in a longitudinal study reported no decline in neuropsychological profile among patients with stage 2 or 3 disease for one year, but in another study 25% of the patients developed clinically significant dementia at 9 months and an additional 25% in one year[119,120]. Azidothymidine (AZT) may improve cognitive function in patients with encephalopathy, and methylphenidate or dextroamphetamine may improve apathy, poor motivation and attention deficit[121,122].

Creutzfeldt–Jakob disease

This condition was first described by Creutzfeldt in 1920 and by Jakob in 1921. The incidence is one in one million. It is sporadic in 85% of cases and is caused by a virus-like agent or 'prion' (a proteinaceous infectious agent). About 5 to 10% of cases are familial in nature[123]. An autosomal dominant form is described in families with abnormalities in chromosome 20 in about 10% of cases. The disease typically starts in the sixth or seventh decade of life and is rapidly progressive, with 50% of the patients dying in 6–9 months. Creutzfeldt–Jakob disease (CJD) is particularly common in persons who received growth hormone extracted from the pituitary when they were children. Clinically CJD manifests in three stages. In stage 1 there is fatigue, insomnia, depression, anxiety and unpredictable behavior. In the next stage dementia, myoclonic jerks, cerebellar ataxia, aphasia, blindness and brain stem involvement are seen and in the final stage the patient enters into a vegetative state and coma and finally death. The CT may show cortical atrophy or no significant change, while EEG shows a characteristic pattern, periodic bursts of polyspike and wave activity, enabling the clinician to make a correct diagnosis[124]. Pathological findings include prominent astrocytes and spongiform changes involving the cerebral cortex. CJD has been shown to be infectious, and can be transmitted by corneal grafts[125].

Meningitis

Chronic meningitis – bacterial, parasitic or fungal – may present with a dementia syndrome, cranial nerve palsies and raised intacranial pressure[126]. Diagnosis is made by cerebrospinal fluid examination and treated according to the specific agent identified.

Normal pressure hydrocephalus

The etiology of this disease is not known, but there is a history of subarachnoid bleeding (ruptured aneurysm) in one third of patients. The classical presentation is a triad of dementia, gait abnormality and urinary incontinence. Normal pressure hydrocephalus is associated with depressive symptoms and apathy and rarely with psychosis[127,128]. On CT scan there is ventricular enlargement with disproportionate enlargement of the frontal and temporal horns compared to the posterior and lateral horns. There are no randomized control trials for shunt placement but there are some case studies. Thomsen and Borgeson[129] reported a better outcome if the cause of normal pressure hydrocephalus is known and there is a short history and an absence of gyral atrophy. Persons whose gait improves after removal of 120 ml of cerebrospinal fluid also do better after shunting.

DEMENTIA CAUSED BY HEAD INJURY

Traumatic brain injury causes dementia in both young and older adults. About 500 000 individuals are hospitalized in the USA for head injuries per annum. About 70 000 to 90 000 of these will develop long-term disabilities[130]. Dementia after head injury results from diffuse axonal injury from shearing forces, focal contusion, hemorrhage, laceration and hypoxic insults. Even patients without loss of consciousness after head injury develop cognitive impairment[115]. Traumatic contusion affects the anterior temporal and inferior frontal lobes, while diffuse axonal injury affects the subcortical white matter, the mesencephalon and the diencepahalon. In boxers dementia occurs because of repeated head blows. This dementia is associated with ataxia and is termed dementia pugilistica[131]. Pathological findings include diffuse brain atrophy, ventricular dilatation and deep pigmentation of the substantia nigra. Neuroimaging is important to identify the pathological condition of most dementia secondary to trauma.

EVALUATION

The components of evaluation include history and physical examination and laboratory tests. If theses are inconclusive specialized testing is indicated. History and physical examination are important parts of the diagnostic assessment[132,133]. Historical information should be obtained from the patient, family members, nurses in case of nursing homes and social workers. The history should document the onset of the dementing illness and include a detailed past medical history of any specific diseases, injuries, operations, hospitalizations, psychiatric disorders, alcohol and substance abuse, nutrition and exposure to environmental toxins. It is important to obtain a family history in patients who have symptoms of dementia or depression or any other psychiatric problems. Social history should be obtained, with regard to specific events that may affect the emotional state of the patient. It is very important to obtain a detailed history of medication, both prescription and over-the-counter medication. It is good practice to ask a patient to bring all their medications for each clinic visit. It is important to recognize and treat reversible causes of dementia by adding a complete blood count, battery of chemical tests, and thyroid function test to the history and physical examination[132]. In approximately 90% of cases the diagnosis of Alzheimer's disease is made on general medical and psychiatric evaluation[134]. Tools such as the Functional Activity Questionnaire[135] and Revised Memory and Behavior Problem Check list[136] are two important instruments that help determine lapses in memory and language use, ability to read and retain new information, handle complex information and demonstrate sound judgment.

The physician should also perform a comprehensive physical examination, including a neurological and mental status examination. A brief screening of cognitive function can be used such as the MMSE[72] or Informant Questionnaire on Cognition[137]. Patients with a lower level of education will score low on the MMSE and those with a higher level of education may achieve normal scores even if impaired. It is probably important to consider neuropsychological testing in patients with a higher education level and minimum cognitive impairment. It is also important to look for depression in the elderly population, using a geriatric depression scale, as depression can mimic dementia; use of the Cornell Scale of Depression is recommended for the demented patient[138]. Delirium is also common in elderly hospitalized patients with dementia, thus an episode of delirium should prompt an evaluation for dementia[91,139]. The causes of delirium can be remembered using the mnemonic D-E-L-I-R-I-U-M-S:

Drugs
Emotions (depression)
Low O_2 states (myocardial infarction, pulmonary embolism, CVA)
Infection
Retention of urine or feces
Ictal (seizure)
Undernutrition, dehydration, electrolyte disorders
Metabolic disorders (thyroid, vitamin B_{12}, massive organ failure)
Subdural.

Laboratory evaluation generally includes complete blood count, blood chemistry, liver function tests, serological test for syphilis and determination of thyroid function testing and B_{12} levels[140]. Other laboratory tests should be ordered as indicated by the history and physical examination. Elevated serum homocysteine levels are considered by some to be a sensitive indicator for cognitive impairment[141,142] but in a recent cross-sectional study increased homocysteine levels were found to be very common in centenarians, probably because of vitamin deficiencies and decreased renal clearance, but they were not associated with cognitive impairment[143]. Apolipoprotein E genotyping does not provide sufficient sensitivity or specificity to be used alone as a diagnostic test for Alzheimer's disease[144]. Other laboratory tests should be ordered when indicated by history and physical examination, e.g. HIV testing would be appropriate if the patient has risk factors for HIV infection.

Imaging studies are optional but recommended by most experts. A non-contrast CT scan of the head is adequate in most instances, especially if no reversible causes of dementia can be identified and there are focal neurological signs of short duration. Magnetic resonance imaging (MRI) is better for vascular dementia but white matter changes revealed by T_2-weighted images are not generally related to dementia and should not be overinterpreted[132,133,145]. Vascular dementia is probably over diagnosed[146]. If the initial work-up is negative and there is a progressive cognitive decline a repeat assessment is recommended in six months. Functional imaging studies, such as PET and single-photon emission CT (SPECT), may show the characteristic parietal and temporal deficits in AD or widespread irregular deficits in vascular dementia[147,148], and are usually recommended when CT/MRI is/are negative and the diagnosis of AD is still suspected[149]. Some patients diagnosed with vascular dementia are found on autopsy to have AD. However, cerebrovascular disease may contribute to the severity of the cognitive symptoms of AD[150]. Potentially reversible dementias are uncommon[151].

Table 8 Pharmacological treatment of Alzheimer's disease

Cholinergic inhibitors
Tacrine
Donepezil
Rivastigmine
Galantamine
Cholinergic agonists
Xanomeline*
Milameline*
Antioxidants
Vitamin E (Alpha-tocopherol)
Alpha-lipoic acid*
Hormones
Estrogen
Other potential cognitive enhancers
Gingko biloba
Non-steroidal anti-inflammatory drugs
Acetyl-L-carnitine*

*Investigational

PHARMACOLOGICAL TREATMENT

Cholinesterase inhibitors

Table 8 provides a list of medications used for the treatment of Alzheimer's disease. Tacrine is a centrally acting aminoacridine with reversible non-specific cholinesterase inhibitor activity. In approximately 2000 patients with mild to moderate AD, between 20 and 30% showed an observable improvement compared with those taking placebo, representing on an average six months of deterioration[152]. The side-effects are frequent gastrointestinal distress, cholinergic side-effects, and 30% had elevated levels of serum transaminase[153]. The starting dose is 10 mg four times a day to a maximum of 40 mg four times a day. This drug is no longer recommended for use.

Donepezil, a second-generation cholinesterase inhibitor, has a longer duration of inhibitory activity and greater specificity for brain tissue. There have been eight randomized control trials involving 2664 participants. In selected patients with mild to moderate Alzheimer's disease treated for a period of 12, 24 or 54 weeks, donepezil produced a modest improvement in cognitive function. No improvement was present in patients'

self-assessed quality of life. A 5 mg dose of donepezil was better tolerated than 10 mg in these trials[154].

Rivastigmine is a newer cholinesterase inhibitor and is used in sixty countries. There have been seven randomized control trials involving 3370 participants. Rivastigmine is associated with mild to moderate improvement in Alzheimer's disease. Improvement is seen in cognitive functions, activity of daily living, and severity of dementia with a daily dose of 6 to 12 mg. Adverse effects are mostly cholinergic in nature[155]. Studies have shown rivastigmine to be cost saving as regards the direct cost of caring for patients with AD after 2 years of treatment[156,157].

Galantamine is a specific, competitive and reversible acetylcholinesterase inhibitor and is currently available in Sweden and Austria. Seven randomized control trials have been carried out, with six being phase II or III industry-sponsored multicenter studies. In all these trials 8 mg of galantamine was consistently associated with significant benefits. Galantamine has shown positive effects in trials of three months, five months and six months. There is evidence demonstrating the efficacy of galantamine on global rating, cognitive function, activities of daily living and behavior. The cognitive effects of donepezil, rivastigmine and tacrine are comparable. The main side-effects are cholinergically mediated gastrointestinal side-effects, but the whole side-effect profile is not available[158].

Antioxidants

There has been one randomized control trial of vitamin E[159]. The primary outcome used in this study of 341 participants was survival time to the first of four end-points – death, institutionalization, loss of two out of three basic activities of daily living, or severe dementia, defined as a global Clinical Dementia Rating of 3. There appeared to be some benefit from vitamin E with fewer participants reaching end-point – 58% (45/77) of completers compared with 74% on placebo. However, more participants taking vitamin E suffered a fall (15.6% compared with 5%). It was not possible to interpret the reported results for specific end-points or for secondary outcomes of cognition, dependence, behavioral disturbance and activities of daily living. There is insufficient evidence of the efficacy of vitamin E in the treatment of people with Alzheimer's disease. The one published trial[159] was restricted to patients with moderate disease, and the published results are difficult to interpret, though there is sufficient evidence of a possible benefit to justify further studies. There was an excess of falls in the vitamin E group compared with the placebo group that requires further evaluation. Animal studies suggest that alpha-lipoic acid may be a more effective antioxidant than vitamin E for treating persons with dementia.

Selective monoamine oxidase-B inhibitors

A meta-analysis of 15 trials examined the effect of selegiline on cognition; 12 of them also explored mood and behavioral aspects. The data showed improvement in cognitive function, mood and behavior, although the global rating scale showed no effects of selegiline. The conclusion from the analysis was that selegiline has beneficial effects on patients with Alzheimer's disease but there is still not enough evidence to recommend its use in routine clinical practice[160].

Other agents

Hydergine for dementia

Hydergine is at present used almost exclusively for treating patients with either dementia or age-related cognitive decline. In a meta-analysis of 19 trials, hydergine was well tolerated by 78% of the randomized subjects that were available for analysis. In this review it was concluded that hydergine showed significant treatment effects when assessed by global rating or comprehensive rating scales. There is a limited number of trials available for subgroup analysis to identify significant moderating effects. The main limitations with the randomized control trials was that most of the data were published before 1984 when there were no standardized diagnostic criteria. As a result uncertainty remains regarding the use of hydergine[161].

Gingko biloba extract

In a 52-week, randomized, double-blind, placebo-controlled, parallel-group, multicenter study, mild to severely demented outpatients with Alzheimer's disease or multi-infarct dementia, without other significant medical conditions, received either treatment with gingko biloba extract (120 mg/day) or placebo. Gingko biloba extract was safe and appears capable of stabilizing and, in a number of cases, improving the cognitive performance and the social functioning of demented patients for 6 months to 1 year[162]. In a 26-week trial for the treatment of Alzheimer's disease and multi-infarct dementia a dose of 120 mg/day of gingko biloba extract (Egb) was used. Intent to treat analysis was performed. The primary outcome measures included the Alzheimer's Disease Assessment Scale-Cognitive Subscale (ADAS-Cog), Geriatric Evaluation by Relative's Rating Instrument (GERRI) and Clinical Global Impression of Change. Of 309 patients, 244 (76% for placebo and 73% for Egb) actually reached the 26th week visit for intent to treat analysis. Mean treatment differences favored Egb with 1.3 and 0.12 points, respectively, on the ADAS-Cog ($p = 0.04$) and the GERRI ($p = 0.007$). In the group receiving Egb, 26% of the patients achieved at least a four-point improvement on the ADAS-Cog, compared to 17% with placebo ($p = 0.04$). On the GERRI scale 30% of the Egb group improved and 17% worsened, while the placebo group showed an opposite trend, with 37% of patients worsening and 25% improving ($p = 0.006$). Regarding safety, no differences between Egb and placebo were observed[163].

Other drugs

The use of non-steroidal anti-inflammatory drugs and estrogen for the treatment of Alzheimer's disease is supported by epidemiologic studies but not confirmed by prospective trials. There are no generally accepted benefits of lecithin, chelation therapy and choline. Currently most clinicians use aspirin for cognitive impairment in vascular dementia, though the literature lacks any evidence to support the effectiveness of aspirin for the treatment of this condition. Further research is required to assess the effects of aspirin on cognition, behavior and quality of life[164].

Antidepressants are recommended when depressive symptoms are present. Treatment of depression includes non-pharmacological and pharmacological approaches. The choice of antidepressant should be based on the side-effects profile and the patient's general and medical condition. Selective serotonin reuptake inhibitors (SSRIs), tricyclic antidepressants and monoamine oxidase A inhibitors can be used. All have different side-effect profiles.

In the middle or later stages of dementia about 50% of patients exhibit agitation[165], while psychosis is less common. A meta-analysis has shown that antipsychotic drugs can produce modest improvement in some behavioral symptoms in dementia[166] and may be most effective against psychotic symptoms[167]. Evidence suggests that risperidone and clozapine are effective at very low doses in the treatment of agitation and psychosis in elderly patients[168,169]. Some of the newer atypical antipsychotics are sertindole, quetiapine and ziprazadone. Clinical trials show comparable efficacies among the antipsychotic drugs, therefore clinicians should base the use of such drugs on their side-effect profile. The high potency antipsychotic drugs should be used with caution because they can cause parkinsonian symptoms, sedation, postural hypotension and anticholinergic effects. Tardive dyskinesia and neuroleptic malignant syndrome are reported with typical antipsychotics and risperidone, but not with clozapine[170]. However clozapine can cause anticholinergic effects and requires blood monitoring for agranulocytosis.

Benzodiazepines are also used for the treatment of behavioral symptoms, particularly anxiety, associated with dementia. The short-acting benzodiazepines such as oxazepam and lorazepam are preferred over the long-acting benzodiazepines, but the latter are associated with adverse affects[171]. Other drugs used include the anticonvulsants carbamazepine[172] and valproate[173]; the hydroxytryptophan modulator, trazodone[174]; the tranquilizer buspirone[175]; and SSRIs[176].

NON-PHARMACOLOGICAL TREATMENT

It is important that dementia patients maintain regular exercise and adequate caloric intake[177,178]. Techniques proposed to restore cognitive dysfunction include reality orientation and memory retraining[179]. Individual and group therapies focused on emotional aspects such as pleasant events and stimulation-oriented treatment are examples of psychosocial treatments that may influence depressive symptoms.

Managing patients with Alzheimer's disease is a great challenge and importance should be given to the safety of their environment and functional independence. The most important principle is to keep regular follow-up appointments, review of medication, screening for sleep problems and to identify early behavior and medical problems and work closely with the family or caregivers. It is very important to discuss with the family and patient early in the disease the treatment options, including the need for a 'living will' and advance directives along with discussion of long-term care placement. It is helpful for the family to be aware of the progression of the disease, including memory problems and emotional and behavioral symptoms. Studies have shown that information and emotional support enhances the quality of life for the patient and caregiver and delays placement in long-term

care facilities[180]. Programs should be established to improve patient behavior and mood by regularly attending family events. Environmental modulation is important and moderate stimulation is the best. It is necessary to explain to the family that overstimulation can cause agitation and understimulation can cause withdrawal. For the mildly demented individual it is important to be in contact with the world by electronic media and reminders of time can be achieved by displaying the time and calendars and lists of daily tasks. Close attention should be paid to safety by using electronic alarm guards and door locks to prevent wandering. It is also important to have a discussion with the family regarding driving skills; if the patient is getting lost in familiar surroundings this may be a sign that they should stop driving. Incontinence is also a great burden and frequent toileting and prevention of bedsores need to be addressed. Most family members are unaware of the concept of hospice, which needs to be discussed early in the course of the disease. Finally, the family should know of the available resources, including specialist care-workers such as gerontologists, neurologists and a geriatric psychiatrist, psychologist and social worker.

References

1. Mejia S, Pineda D, Alvarez LM. Individual differences in memory and executive function abilities during normal aging. *Int J Neurosci* 1999;95:271–84
2. Butler SM, Ashford JW, Snowdon DA. Age, education, and changes in the Mini-Mental State Exam score of older women: findings from the Nun Study. *Am J Geriatr Soc* 1996;44:675–81
3. Jorm AF, Korten AE, Henderson AS. The prevalence of dementia: a quantitative integration of the literature. *Acta Psychiatr Scand* 1987;76:465–79
4. Ganguli M, Seaberg E, Belle S. Cognitive impairment and the use of health services in an

elderly rural population: the MoVIES project. *J Am Geriatr Soc* 1993;41:1065–70
5. Advisory Panel on Alzheimer's disease. *Alzheimer's Disease Related Dementias: Acute and Long-term Care Services*. Washington, DC: US Dept of Health and Human Services, NIH Publication 96-4136, 1996
6. Evans DA. Estimated prevalence of Alzheimer's disease in the US. *Milbank Q* 1990;68:267–89
7. Benton AL, Eslinger PJ, Damasio R. Normative observation on neuropsychological tests performance in old age. *J Clin Neuropsychol* 1981;3:33–42

8. Jacqmin-Gadda H, Fabrigoule C, Commenges D. A 5 year longitudinal study of Min-Mental State Examination in normal aging. *Am J Epidemiol* 1997;145:498–506

9. Laird NM, Ware JH. Random-effects models for longitudinal data. *Biometrics* 1982;38: 963–74

10. Liang KY, Zeger SL. Longitudinal data analysis using generalized estimating questions. *Biometrika* 1986;73:13–22

11. Zeger SL, Liang KY. Longitudinal data analysis for discrete and continuous outcomes. *Biometrics* 1986;42:121–30

12. Morris MC, Evans DA, Hebert LE. Methodological issues in the study of cognitive decline. *Am J Clin Epidimiol* 1999;149(9): 789–93

13. Guildford JP, Fruchter B. *Fundamental Statistics in Psychology and Education*, 6th edn. New York: McGraw-Hill Book Company, 1978

14. Cunningham WR. Intellectual abilities and age. In Schaie HW, ed. *Annual Review of Gerontology and Geriatrics*. New York: Springer, 1987:117–34

15. Eisdorfer C, Wilke F. Intellectual changes with advancing age. In Jarvik LF, Eisdorter C, eds. *Intellectual Functioning in Adults*. New York: Springer, 1973:21–9

16. Schaie KW. Internal validity threats in studies of adult cognitive development. In Howe ML, ed. *Cognitive Development in Adulthood: Progress in Cognitive Development Research*. New York: Springer-Verlag, 1988: 241–72

17. Horn JL, Cattell RB. Age differences in fluid and crystallized intelligence. *Acta Psycho biological* 1967;26:107

18. Christensen H, Mackinnon A, Jorm AF. Age differences and interindividual variation in cognition in community-dwelling elderly. *Psychol Aging* 1994;9:381–90

19. Kaufman AS, Horn JL. Age changes on test of fluid and crystallized ability for women and men on the Kaufman Adolescent and Adult Intelligence Test (KAIT) at age 17–94 years. *Arch Clin Neuropsychol* 1996;11:97

20. Czaja SJ, Sharit J. Age differences in the performance of computer-based work. *Psychol Aging* 1993;8:59–67

21. Birren JE, Fisher LM. Aging and slowing of behavior: consequences for cognition and survival. *Nebr Symp Motiv* 1991;39:1–37

22. Fleishmann UM. Cognition in humans and the borderline to dementia. *Life Sci* 1994;55: 2051–6

23. Salthouse TA. The processing-speed theory of adult age differences in cognition. *Psychol Rev* 1996;103:104

24. Wechsler B. *Manual for the Wechsler Adult Intelligence Scale – Revised*. New York: The Psychological Corp, 1981

25. Hultsch DF, Hertzog C, Small BJ. Short-term longitudinal changes in cognitive performance in later life. *Psychol Aging* 1992;7:571–84

26. McEvoy GM, Casico WF. Cumulative evidence of the relationship between employee age and job performance. *J Appl Psychol* 1989; 74:11–17

27. Bohannon RW. Comfortable and maximum walking of adults aged 20–79 years. Reference values and determinants. *Age Ageing* 1997; 26:15

28. Ruff RM, Parker SB. Gender- and age-specific changes in motor speed and eye-hand coordination in adults: normative values for finger tapping and grooved pegboard test. *Percept Mot skills* 1993;76:1219

29. Lorge I. The influence of the test upon the nature of mental decline as a function of age. *J Educ Psychol* 1936;27:100

30. Anderer P, Semlitsch HV, Saletu B. Multichannel auditory event-related brain potentials: effects of normal age on the scalp distribution of N1, P2, N2 and P300 latencies and amplitudes. *Electroencephalogr Clin Neurophysiol* 1996;99:458

31. Gilmore R. Evoked potentials in the elderly. *J Clin Neurophysiol* 1993;12:132

32. Schofield PW, Marder K, Dooneief G. Association of subjective memory complaints with subsequent cognitive decline in community-dwelling elderly individuals with baseline cognitive impairment. *Am J Psychiatry* 1997; 154:609

33. Small GW, La Rue A, Komo S. Mnemonics usage and cognitive decline in age-associated memory impairment. *Int Psychogeriatr* 1997; 9:47

34. Jonker C, Launer LJ, Hooijer C. Memory complaints and memory impairment in older individuals. *J Am Geriatr Soc* 1996;44:44

35. Barker A, Prior J, Roy J. Memory complaints in attenders at a self-referral memory clinic: the role of cognitive factors, affective symptoms and personality. *Int J Geriatr Psychiatry* 1995;10:777

36. Craik FIM. Age differences in human memory. In Birren JE, Schaie KW, eds. *Handbook of the Psychology of Aging*. New York: Van Nostrand Reinhold, 1997;384–420

37. Botwinick J. Intellectual abilities. In Birren JE, Schaie KW, eds. *Handbook of the Psychology of Aging*. New York: Van Nostrand Reinhold, 1997;580–605

38. Craik FIM, Byrd M. Patterns of memory loss in three elderly samples. *Psychol Aging* 1987;2:79

39. Wahlin A, Beckman L. Free recall and recognition of slowly and rapidly presented words in very old age: a community-based study. *Exp Aging Res* 1995;21:251

40. Nilsson L-G, Backman L. The Betula prospective cohort study: memory, health, and aging. *Aging Neuropsychol Cogn* 1997;41:1

41. Perlmutter M. What is memory aging the aging of? *Dev Psychol* 1978;14:330

42. Backman L, Nilsson L-G. Semantic memory functioning across the adult life span. *European Psychologist* 1996;1:27

43. Jelicic M, Craik FIM, Moscovitch M. Effects of aging on different explicit and implicit memory tasks. *Eur J Cogn Psychol* 1996;8:225

44. Schugens MM, Daum I, Spinder M. Differential effects of aging on explicit and implicit memory. *Aging Neuropsychol Cogn* 1997;4:33

45. La Rue A, Bank L. Health in old age: how do physicians' rating and self-rating compare? *J Gerontol* 1979;8:108

46. Monge R, Hultsch D. Paired associate learning as a function of age and length of anticipation and inspection intervals. *J Gerontol* 1971;26:157–62

47. Light LL, Zelinski EM, Moore M. Adult age difference in reasoning from new information. *J Exp Psychol Learn Cognition* 1982;8:435–47

48. Scogin F, Bienas JL. A three year follow up of older adults participating in a memory skills training program. *Psychol Aging* 1988;3:334–7

49. Boyarsky RE, Eisdorfer C. Forgetting in older persons. *J Gerontol* 1988;27:254–8

50. Committee on Hearing and Bioacoustics Working Group on Speech Understanding and Aging (CHABA). Speech understanding and aging. *J Acoust Soc Am* 1988;83:859–95

51. Jacobs-Condit L, ed. *Gerontology and Communication Disorders*. Rockville MD: American Speech-Language-Hearing Association, 1984

52. Humes LE, Watson BU. Factors associated with individual differences in clinical measures of speech recognition among the elderly. *J Speech Hear Res* 1994;37:464–74

53. Humus LE. Speech understanding in the elderly. *J Am Acad Audiol* 1996;7:161–7

54. Madden DJ. Adult age differences in the effects of sentence context and stimulus degradation during visual word recognition. *Psychol Aging* 1988;3:167–72

55. Laver GD, Burke DM. Why do semantic priming effects increase in old age? A meta-analysis. *Psychol Aging* 1993;8:34–43

56. Hartley J. Aging and individual differences in memory for written disclosure. In Light LL and Burke DM, eds. *Language, Memory and Aging*. New York: Cambridge University Press, 1988:36–57

57. Burke DM, Harrold RM. Automatic and effortful semantic process in old age. Experimental and naturalistic approaches. In Light LL and Burke DM, eds. *Language, Memory and Aging*. New York: Cambridge University Press, 1988:100–16

58. Wingfield A, Alexander AH, Cavigelli S. Does memory constrain utilization of top-down information in spoken word recognition? Evidence from normal aging. *Lang Speech* 1994;37:221–35

59. Pichora-Fuller MK, Scheider BA. How young and old adults listen to noise. *J Acoust Soc Am* 1995;97:593–608

60. Hutchinson KM. Influence of sentence context on speech perception in young and older adults. *J Gerontol* 1989;44:36–44

61. Sommers MS. The structural organization of the mental lexicon and its contribution to age-related changes in spoken word recognition. *Psychol Aging* 1996;11:333–41

62. Mullennix JW, Pisoni DB, Martin CS. Some effects of talker variability on spoken word recognition. *J Acoust Soc Am* 1989; 85:365–78

63. Peterson GE, Barney HL. Control methods used in a study of the vowels. *J Acoust Soc Am* 1952;24:175–84

64. Lezak MD. The problem of accessing executive functions. *Int J Psychol* 1981;17:281–97

65. American Psychiatric Association *Diagnostic and Statistics Manual of Mental Disorders*, 4th edn. Washington DC: American Psychiatric Association, 1994

66. Mega MS, Cummings JL. Frontal-subcortical circuits and neuropsychiatric disorders. *J Neuropsychiatry* 1994;6:358–70

67. Daigneault S, Brian CMG. Early effects of normal aging on preservatives and non-preservatives prefrontal measures. *Dev Neuropsychol* 1992;8:99–114

68. Kuhl DE. The effects of normal aging patterns of local cerebral glucose utilization. *Ann Neurol* 1984;15:133–7

69. Fogel BS, Brock D, Goldscheider F. *Cognitive Dysfunction and the Need for Long Term Care: Implication for Public Policy*. Washington, DC: American Association of Retired Persons, 1994

70. Royall DR, Mahurin RK. Bedside assessment of dementia type using qualitative evaluation of dementia (QED). *Neuropsychiatry Neuropsychol Behav Neurol* 1993;6:235–44

71. Royall DR, Mahurin RK, Gray K. Bedside assessment of executive cognitive impairment. The executive interview (EXIT). *J Am Geriatr Soc* 1992;40:1221–6

72. Folstein M, Folstein S, McHugh PR. Minimental state: a practical method for grading the cognitive state of patients for the clinician. *Psychiatry Res* 1975;12:89–98

73. Nelson A, Fogel BS, Faust D. Bedside cognitive screening instruments: a critical assessment. *J Nerv Ment Dis* 1986;174:73–84

74. Royall DR, Cordes JA, Polk Marsha. CLOX: an executive clock drawing test. *J Neurol Neurosurg Psychiatry* 1998;64:588–94

75. Ainslie NK, Murden RA. Effect of education on the clock drawing dementia screen in non-demented elderly persons. *J Am Geriatr Soc* 1993;41:249–52

76. Shaw TG, Mortel KF, Meyer JS. Cerebral blood flow changes in benign aging and cerebrovascular disease. *Neurology* 1995; 34:855–62

77. Dempster FN. The rise and fall of inhibitory mechanism: towards a unified theory of cognitive development and aging. *Develop Rev* 1992;12:45–75

78. Cummings JL. *Subcortical Dementia*. New York: Oxford University Press, 1990

79. Lemsky CM, Smith G, Malec JF. Identifying risk for functional impairment using cognitive measures: an application of CART modeling. *Neuropsychology* 1996;10:368–75

80. DeBettignies FN, Mahurin RK. Insight for impairment in independent living skill in Alzheimer's disease and multi-infarct dementia. *J Clin Exp Neuropsychol* 1990;12:355–63

81. Carlson MC, Linda FP. Association between executive attention and physical performance in community-dwelling old women. *J Gerontol* 1999;54(5):S262–S270

82. Royall DR, Cabello M. Executive dyscontrol: an important factor affecting the level of care received by older retirees. *J Am Geriatr Soc* 1998;46:1519–24

83. Ritchie K, Kildea D. Is senile dementia age related or aging related? Evidence from meta-analysis of dementia prevalence in the oldest old. *Lancet* 1995;346:931–4

84. Bachman DL, Wolf PA, Linn RT. Incidence of dementia and probable Alzheimer's disease in a general population: the Framingham study. *Neurology* 1993;43:515–19

85. Jorm AF. *The Epidemiology of Alzheimer's Disease and Related Disorders*. London, England: Chapman & Hall, 1990

86. National Institute of Aging. *Progress Report on Alzheimer's disease 1996*. Bethesda, Maryland MD: NIH Publication 96-4137, 1996

87. Ernst RL, Hay JW. The US economic and social cost of Alzheimer's disease revisited. *Am J Public Health* 1994;84:1261–4

88. Schulz R, O'Brien AT. Psychiatric and physical morbidity effects of dementia caregiving: prevalence, correlates, and causes. *Gerontologist* 1995;35:771–91

89. Mega MS, Cummings JL. The spectrum of behavioral changes in Alzheimer's disease. *Neurology* 1996;46:130–5

90. Stern Y, Alpert M. Utility of extrapyramidal signs and psychosis as a predictor of cognitive and functional decline, nursing home admission and death in Alzheimer's disease: prospective analysis from the Predictors Study. *Neurology* 1994;44:2300–7

91. Lerner AJ, Hedera P, Koss E. Delirium in Alzheimer's disease. *Alzheimer's Dis Assoc Disord* 1997;11:16–20

92. Alexopoulos GS, Meyers BS. The course of geriatric depression with reversible dementia: a controlled study. *Am J Psychiatry* 1993; 150:1693–9

93. Jung R, Solomon K. Psychiatric manifestation of Pick's disease. *Int Psychogeriatrics* 1993; 5:187–202

94. Caine ED, Shoulson I. Psychiatric syndromes in Huntington's disease. *Am J Psychiatry* 1983;140:727–33

95. Hayden MR, Martin AJ. Positron emission tomography in the earlier diagnosis of Huntington's disease. *Neurology* 1986;36: 888–94

96. Martilla RJ. Epidemiology. In Koller WC, ed. *Handbook of Parkinson's Disease*. New York: Marcel Dekker, 1976

97. Cummings JL. Intellectual impairment in Parkinson's disease: clinical, biochemical and pathologic correlates. *J Geriatr Psychiatr Neurol* 1988;1:24–36

98. Lewin R. Dramatic results with brain graft. *Science* 1987;237:245–7

99. Forstl H, Burns A, Luthert P. The Lewy-body variant of Alzheimer's disease. Clinical and pathological findings. *Br J Psychiatry* 1993; 162:385–92

100. Aldrich MS, Foster NL, White RF. Sleep abnormalities in progressive supra-nuclear palsy. *Ann Neurol* 1989;25:477–581

101. Mendell JR, Chase TN, Engel WK. Modification by L-dopa of case progressive supranuclear palsy. *Lancet* 1970;1:593–4

102. Haldman S, Goldman JW, Hyde J. Progressive supranuclear palsy computed tomography, and response to anti-Parkinson's drugs. *Neurology* 1982;31:442–59

103. Newman GC. Treatment of progressive supra-nuclear palsy with tricyclic antidepressants. *Neurology* 1985;35:1189–93

104. Ermini-Funfschilling D, Stahelin HB. Is prevention of dementia possible? *Zeitschrift Fur Gerontologie* 1993;26:446

105. Roman GC, Tatemichi TK, Erkinjuntti T. Vascular dementia: diagnostic criteria for research studies. *Neurology* 1993;43: 259–60

106. Thompson TL, Moran MG. Psychotropic drug use in the elderly. *N Engl J Med* 1993; 308:134–8

107. Flaherty JH. Commonly prescribed and over the counter medication: causes of confusion. *Clin Geriat Med* 1998;14(1): 101–27

108. Cummings JL. *Dementia: a Clinical Approach*, 2nd edn. Stoneham, MA: Weinemann-Butterworths, 1992

109. West LJ. Alcoholism. *Ann Intern Med* 1984; 100:405

110. Zimberg S. Alcohol abuse among the elderly. In Carstenson B, Edelstein B, eds. *Handbook of Clinical Gerontology*. New York: Pergamon, 1987:57

111. Cutting J. The relationship between Korsakov's syndrome and alcohol dementia. *Br J Psychiatry* 1978;132:240–51

112. Ron MA. Brain damage in chronic alcoholism: a neuropathological, neuroradiological, and psychological review. *Psychol Med* 1977;7:103–12

113. Mach J, Korchik W, Mahowald M. Dialysis dementia, in treatment consideration of Alzheimer's disease and related dementing illness. In Philadelphia MG, ed. *Clinical Geriatric Medicine*. Philadelphia, PA: WB Saunders, 1988:853–68

114. Avery TL. Seven cases of frontal tumor with psychiatric presentation. *Br J Psychiatry* 1971;119:19–23

115. Cummings JL, Benson DF. *Dementia-A Clinical Approach*. Boston, MA: Butterworth-Heinemann, 1992

116. Price RW, Brew B, Sidtis J. The brain in AIDS: central nervous system HIV-1 infection and AIDS dementia complex. *Science* 1987;239:586–92

117. Resnick L, Berger JR. Early blood brain barrier penetration by HIV. *Neurology* 1988; 38:9–14

118. Navia BA, Jordan BD. The AIDS dementia complex. I: clinical features. *Ann Neurology* 1986;19:517–24

119. Selnes OA, Miller E, McArther J. HIV infection: no evidence of cognitive decline during the asymptomatic stages. *Neurology* 1990; 40:204–8

120. Sidtis JJ, Thaller H, Brew BJ. The interval between equivocal and definite neurological signs and symptoms in the AIDS dementia complex. Presented at the *Fifth International Conference on AIDS*, International Development Research Center, Montreal, 1989

121. Yarchoan R, Berg G, Brouwer P. Responses of human immunodeficiency virus-associated neurological disease to 3-azido-3-deoxythymidine. *Lancet* 1987;1:132–5

122. Fernandez F, Adams F. Cognitive impairment due to AIDS, related complex, and its response to psychostimulants. *Psychosomatics* 1988;29:38–46

123. Collings J, Palmer MS. Prion diseases in humans and their relevance to other neurodegenerative diseases. *Dementia* 1993;4: 178–85

124. Brown P, Cathala F, Castaigne P. Creutzfeldt–Jakob disease: clinical analysis of a consecutive series of 230 neuropathologically verified cases. *Ann Neurol* 1986;20: 597–602

125. Gajdusek DC. Unconventional viruses and the origin and the disappearance of kuru. *Science* 1977;197:943–60

126. Mahler ME, Cummings JL. Treatable dementias. *West J Med* 1987;146:705–12

127. Price TRP, Tucker GJ. Psychiatric and behavioral manifestation of normal pressure hydrocephalus. *J Nerv Ment Dis* 1977;164: 51–5

128. Dewan MJ, Blick A. Normal pressure hydrocephalus and psychiatric patients. *Biol Psychiatry* 1985;20:1127–31

129. Thomsen AM, Borgeson SE. Prognosis of dementia in normal pressure hydrocephalus after shunt operation. *Ann Neurol* 1986; 20:304–10

130. Goldstein M. Traumatic brain injury, a silent epidemic. *Ann Neurol* 1990;27:327

131. Corsellis JAN. Post-traumatic dementia. In Katzman R, Terry RD, eds. *Aging: Alzheimer's Disease: Senile Dementia and Related Disorders*. New York: Raven Press, 1973:7

132. Larson EB. Diagnostic tests in the evaluation of dementia. A prospective study of 200 elderly outpatients. *Arch Intern Med* 1986; 146:1917–22

133. Van Creval H. Early diagnosis of dementia: Which tests are indicated? What are their costs? *J Neurol* 1999;246:73–8

134. Rasmusson DX, Brandt J, Steele C. Accuracy of clinical diagnosis of Alzheimer's disease and clinical features of non-Alzheimer's neuropathology. *Alzheimer's Dis Assoc Disord* 1996;10:180–8

135. Pfeffer RI, Kurosaki TT. Measurement of functional activities in older adults in the community. *J Gerontol* 1982;37:323–9

136. Teri L, Truax P, Logsdon R. Assessment of behavior problems in dementia: the revised memory and behavior problems checklist. *Psychol Aging* 1992;7:622–31

137. Mulligan R, Mackinon A, Jorm AF, Michel JP. A comparison of alternative methods of screening for dementia in clinical settings. *Arch Neurol* 1996;53:532–6

138. Alexopoulos GS. Cornell scale for depression in dementia. *Biol Psych* 1988;23(3):271–84

139. Francis J, Kapoor WN. Prognosis after hospital discharge of older medical outpatients with delirium. *J Am Geriatr Soc* 1992;40:601–6

140. American Academy of Neurology. Practice parameter for diagnosis and evaluation of dementia: report of the Quality Standards Subcommittee of the American Academy of Neurology. *Neurology* 1994;44:2203–6

141. Clarke R. Folate, Vitamin B-12, and serum total homocysteine levels confirmed Alzheimer's disease. *Arch Neurol* 1998; 55(1):1449–55

142. McCaddon A. Total serum homocysteine in senile dementia of Alzheimer's type. *Int Geriatr Psychiatry* 1998;13(4):235–9

143. Ravaglia G, Forti P, Maioli F. Elevated plasma homocysteine levels in centenarians are not associated with cognitive impairment. *Mech Ageing Dev* 2001;121:251–61

144. Mayeux R, Saunders AM, Shea S, *et al.* Utility of the apolipoprotein E genotype in the diagnosis of Alzheimer's disease. Alzheimer's Disease Centers Consor- tium on Apolipoprotein E and Alzheimer's disease. *N Engl J Med* 1998;338(8):506–11

145. Scheltens P. Early diagnosis of dementia: neuroimaging. *J Neurol* 1999;246(1):16–20

146. Brust JC. Vascular dementia: still over diagnosed. *Stroke* 1983;14:298–300

147. Herholz K, Adams R, Kesseler J. Criteria for the diagnosis of Alzheimer's disease with positron emission tomography. *Dementia* 1990;1:156–64

148. Kippenhan JS, Barker WW, Pascal S. Evaluation of neural-network classifier for PET scans of normal and Alzheimer's disease subjects. *J Nucl Med* 1992;33: 1459–69

149. Tamaki N. Image analysis in patients with dementia. *Hokkaido Igaku Zasshi* 1996; 71(3):303–7

150. Snowdon DA, Greiner LH. Brain infarction and the clinical expression of Alzheimer's disease. The Nun Study. *J Am Med Assoc* 1997;277:813–17

151. Arnold SE, Kumar A. Reversible dementias. *Med Clin North Am* 1993;77:215–30

152. Schneider LS. Clinical pharmacology of amino-acridines in Alzheimer's disease. *Neurology* 1993;43:S64–S79

153. Watkins PB, Zimmerman HJ, Knapp MJ. Hepatotoxic effects of tacrine administration in patient with Alzheimer's disease. *J Am Med Assoc* 1994;271:992–8

154. Birk JS, Melzer D, Beppu H. Donepezil for mild and moderate Alzheimer's disease. *Source Cochrane Database of Systemic Reviews*. Issue 1, 2001

155. Birk JS, Grimley Evans J, Iakovidou V, Isolaki M. Rivastigmine for Alzheimer's disease. *Source Cochrane Database of Systemic Reviews*. Issue 1, 2001

156. Hauber AB. Saving in the cost of caring for patients with Alzheimer's disease in Canada: an analysis of treatment with rivastigmine. *Clin Therapeutic* 2000;22:439–51

157. Hauber AB. Potential saving in the cost of caring for Alzheimer's disease: treatment with rivastigmine. *Pharmacoeconomics* 2000; 17:351–60

158. Olin J, Schneider L. Galantamine for Alzheimer's disease. *Source Cochrane Database of Systemic Reviews*. Issue 1, 2001

159. Sano M. A controlled trial of selegiline, alpha-tocopherol, or both as treatment of Alzheimer's disease. *N Engl J Med* 1997; 336(17):1216–22

160. Brick J, Flicker L. Selegiline for Alzheimer's disease. *Source Cochrane Database of Systemic Reviews*. Issue 1, 2001

161. Olin J, Schneider L. Hydergine for dementia. *Source Cochrane Database of Systemic Reviews*. Issue 1, 2001

162. Le Bars PL. A placebo-controlled, double blinded, randomized trial of an extract of Ginkgo biloba for dementia. *J Am Med Assoc* 1997;278(16):1327–32

163. Le Bars PL, Kieser M, Itil KZ. A 26-week analysis of a double-blind, placebo-controlled trial of gingko biloba extract Egb 761 in dementia. *Dementia Geriatr Cogn Dis* 2000;11(4):230–7

164. Williams PS, Rands G, Orell M, Spector A. Aspirin for vascular dementia. *Source Cochrane Database of Systemic Reviews*. Issue 1, 2001

165. Patterson MB, Bolger JP. Assessment of behavioral symptoms in Alzheimer's disease. *Alzheimer's Dis Assoc Disord* 1994;8 (Suppl 3):4–20

166. Schneider LS, Pollock VE. A meta-analysis of controlled trials of neuroleptic treatment in dementia. *J Am Geriatr Soc* 1990;28: 553–63

167. Rada RT, Kellner R. Thiothixene in the treatment of geriatric patients with chronic organic brain syndrome. *J Am Geriatr Soc* 1976; 24:105–7

168. Madhusoodanan S, Brenner R, Aruja L. Efficacy of risperidone treatment for psychosis associated with schizophrenia, bipolar disorder or senile dementia in geriatric patients: a case series. *J Clin Psychiatry* 1995;56:514–18

169. Salzman C. Clozapine in older patients with psychosis and behavioral disturbance. *Am J Geriatr Psychiatry* 1995;3:26–33

170. Jesto DV, Eastham JH. Management of late life psychosis. *J Clin Psychiatry* 1996;57 (Suppl 3):39–45

171. Grad R. Benzodiazepines for insomnia in community dwelling elderly: a review of benefits and risks. *J Fam Pract* 1995;41: 473–81

172. Tariot PN, Erb R, Leibovici A, *et al.* Carbamazepine treatment for agitation in nursing home patients with dementia. *J Am Geriatr Soc* 1994;42:1160–6

173. Mellow AM, Solano-Lopez C, Davis S. Sodium valproate in the treatment of behavioral disturbance in dementia. *J Geriatr Psychiatry Neurol* 1993;6:205–9

174. Sultzer DL, Gray KF. A double-blinded comparison of trazodone and haloperidol for treatment of agitation in patients with dementia. *Am J Geriatr Psychiatry* 1997; 5:60–9

175. Sakauye KM, Camp CJ. Effects of buspirone on agitation associated with dementia. *Am J Geriatr Psychiatry* 1993;1:894–901

176. Nyth AL, Gottfries CG. A controlled multicenter clinical study of citalopram and placebo in elderly depressed patients with and without concomitant dementia. *Acta Psychiatr Scand* 1992;86:138–45

177. Broe GA. Health habits and risk of cognitive impairment and dementia in old age. A prospective study on the effect of exercise, smoking and alcohol consumption. *Aust NZ J Pub Health* 1998;22(5):621–3

178. Spinder AA, Renvall MJ, Nichols JF, Ramsdell JW. Nutritional status of patients with Alzheimer's disease: a 1 year study. *J Am Diet Assoc* 1996;96(10):1013–18

179. Baines S, Saxby P. Reality oriented and reminiscence therapy: a controlled cross over study of elderly confused people. *Br J Psychiatry* 1987;151:222–31

180. Mittelman MS, Ferris SH, Shulman E. A family intervention to delay nursing home placement of patients with Alzheimer's disease: a randomized, controlled trial. *J Am Med Assoc* 1996;276:1725–31

Section IX

Musculoskeletal system

Dirk Vanderschueren, MD, PhD

The skeleton is the support system of the body. Aging of the musculoskeletal system, therefore, often results in less self-support. Although age-related bone loss is less in men than in women, osteoporosis is an important problem in terms of both morbidity and mortality in very elderly men. The impact of osteoporosis is discussed in the first chapter by Steven Boonen and Dirk Vanderschueren. Not only bone but also cartilage degenerates in elderly men, in both the axial and the peripheral skeleton. Osteoarthritis resulting in pain and deformities of our joints is, therefore, a considerable health burden. The various aspects of this disease in the peripheral joints and spine, respectively, are discussed in two chapters by Leif Dahlberg and Acke Ohlin. Finally, a practical chapter, written by Greta Dereymaeker and Jan Mievis, is devoted to foot problems of elderly men. Readers are also directed to Section V – Aging and Body Composition, for in-depth discussion of age-related changes in muscle mass.

42 Bone loss and osteoporotic fracture occurrence in aging men

Steven Boonen, MD, PhD, and Dirk Vanderschueren, MD, PhD

OSTEOPOROSIS IN MEN: THE SIZE OF THE PROBLEM

Incidence of osteoporotic fractures in men

In men over the age of 65, the annual hip fracture incidence is 4–5/1000 compared to 8–10/1000 in women[1,2]. Although age-specific incidence rates in men are about half those in women, only about 25–30% of all hip fractures occur in men because of differences in life expectancy[3-5]. In both sexes, the incidence of these fractures rises exponentially with aging, the majority of fractures occurring in men over the age of 80 years. With continued aging of the population, the annual number of fractures in men is expected to rise dramatically in coming decades. Mortality after sustaining a hip fracture is twice as high in men as in women[6]. This difference is only partially explained by differences in comorbidity, suggesting that male gender is a major risk factor for hip fracture-associated mortality. Additionally, almost 50% of men with hip fractures will have to be institutionalized because of the fracture, and up to 80% of those who survive fail to regain their prefracture level of functional independence.

Overall, symptomatic vertebral fractures have similar incidences to those for hip fractures, but occur more in middle-aged men than in the very old. In men, vertebral fractures often result from severe trauma, whereas moderate trauma is more often reported in women. In addition to clinically symptomatic fractures, aging men may develop silent vertebral deformities as revealed by radiological screening. The reported prevalences of these vertebral deformities vary considerably[7]. Their health impact is important, especially in men with multiple severe deformities resulting in disabling back pain.

There are age-related increases not only for hip and spine fractures in men but also for fractures of the proximal humerus, pelvis and ankle. Similarly, the incidence of distal forearm fractures increases with age, although incidence rates remain lower than in women. Importantly, distal forearm fractures in men are also a risk factor for other osteoporotic fractures.

Prevalence of osteoporosis in men

In women, bone densities at either the lumbar spine or the proximal femur of at least 2.5

standard deviations (SD) below the young adult mean are proposed by the World Health Organization (WHO) as thresholds for osteoporosis. These thresholds, however, have hardly been validated as markers for fracture risk in men. It remains unknown, therefore, whether a similar approach can be taken for the diagnosis of osteoporosis in men as in women. A key issue in this regard is whether it would be more appropriate to use gender-specific normative values of bone mass in the evaluation of osteoporosis in men, or whether the same level of absolute bone mass should determine diagnostic categorization in both men and women. This issue is currently quite unclear, and technical, pathophysiological and public-health considerations influence the decision. Not surprisingly, the prevalence of osteoporosis is greater using male-specific ranges. According to male cut-off data from the third National Health and Nutrition Examination Survey (NHANES III), the prevalence of osteoporosis in elderly men is 3–6%[8]. For comparison, the prevalence would be only 1–4% when using female standards.

CLINICAL PRESENTATION OF OSTEOPOROSIS IN MEN

Most fractures occur in older age, in men as in women, and result from the (poorly understood) process of age-related bone loss that has inevitably occurred by that stage of life. This relatively common form of osteoporosis is referred to as 'age-associated' osteoporosis. Fractures resulting from age-associated osteoporosis are most frequent among men over the age of 70. This type of osteoporosis is quite distinct from the unexpected appearance of osteoporosis in a younger man, a syndrome referred to as 'idiopathic' osteoporosis. Idiopathic osteoporosis is much less common than age-associated osteoporosis and will mostly be diagnosed in men between the ages of 30 and 60 years. The diagnosis of 'idiopathic' osteoporosis (in men younger than 70 years) or

'age-associated' osteoporosis (in men older than 70 years) should only be applied if careful screening reveals no potential underlying cause of bone fragility (such as alcohol abuse, glucocorticoid excess or hypogonadism) indicating 'secondary' osteoporosis, a form of osteoporosis seen much more frequently among men than among women.

Age-associated osteoporosis

Aging is the major determinant of fracture incidence, not only in women but also in men. Although men do not experience a well-defined equivalent of the menopause, there is increasing evidence for a relationship between age-related endocrine changes and osteoporosis in men as well. In particular, changes in sex steroid secretion, in the growth hormone–insulin-like growth factor-I (GH–IGF-I) axis, and in the vitamin D–parathyroid hormone (25(OH)D–PTH) system may be associated with osteoporosis and osteoporotic fracture occurrence in men[9]. Recent evidence suggests that bone loss in aging men may be particularly related to declining levels of (bioavailable) estradiol, rather than to other age-associated hormonal changes (such as the partial androgen deficiency associated with normal aging). Even low concentrations of estradiol may be critically important in determining the rate of bone loss, not only in postmenopausal women but also in men[10,11]. However, it remains to be clarified whether and to what extent these hormonal changes act independently of age to increase the risk of skeletal fragility.

Most studies in aging men have addressed the potential impact of hormonal changes on bone density (as a surrogate marker for fracture risk) and have used a cross-sectional design. These studies have reported either the presence or the absence of an association between selected potential endocrine determinants (using different assays) and measurements of bone density (using different methodologies and sites), mostly in a small number of subjects with a wide variation of age ranges. This heterogeneity, in terms of both methodology and study population, and the inconsistent results make it difficult to interpret the findings of these studies. Moreover, some investigations failed to adjust for concomitant changes in body mass index or age, and, thus, do not allow independent associations between hormonal changes and bone loss to be established. Even more important, most studies do not take into account the complex interactions that exist between testosterone, estradiol, IGF-I, sex hormone-binding globulin and/or PTH, which may significantly confound reported associations.

Secondary osteoporosis

If one surveys a typical population of men with osteoporosis, several etiologies will surface frequently. They are alcohol abuse, glucocorticoid excess (either endogenous – Cushing's syndrome – or, more commonly, chronic glucocorticoid therapy) and hypogonadism. In addition, other etiologies are important to consider, including primary hyperparathyroidism, excessive thyroid hormone exposure (hyperthyroidism or overtreatment with thyroid hormone), multiple myeloma and other malignancies, anticonvulsant use, gastrointestinal disorders and high-dose chemotherapeutics.

Glucocorticoid excess is probably the major cause of secondary osteoporosis in men, found in about 20%. The main mechanism in this type of osteoporosis is osteoblast insufficiency. Additionally, glucocorticoids may induce muscular atrophy and secondary hypogonadism.

Numerous reports have clearly documented that male hypogonadism is associated with reduced bone density, especially when present before puberty. The extreme delay of skeletal maturation in men suffering from estrogen deficiency as the result of a mutation in either the estrogen receptor or the aromatase enzyme suggests that part of the androgen action on the male skeleton is mediated by estrogens.

Hypogonadism (either primary or secondary) is reported in 15–20% of cases with spinal osteoporosis. In case–control studies of male fracture patients, varying prevalences of hypogonadism have been reported, but the use of different and insufficiently validated thresholds for both total and free testosterone makes it difficult to compare different studies. These discrepancies emphasize the need to establish cut-offs to define hypogonadism, based on the impact of different degrees of androgen deficiency on the musculoskeletal or other systems.

Alcohol abuse can be revealed in about 15–20% of osteoporotic men, and is probably an underestimated cause of skeletal fragility in men. Bone loss is increased in men with alcohol intake above the median, and recent findings indicate that alcohol abuse may even be associated with an increase in fracture risk.

Finally, a particular secondary cause of osteoporosis in men is idiopathic hypercalciuria. Hypercalciuria (more than 0.1 mmol/kg per day or 4 mg/kg per day), if present, may in part be due to increased intestinal absorption of calcium resulting from alterations in vitamin D metabolism, but the exact underlying mechanism remains to be established. In our experience, the prevalence of hypercalciuria in osteoporotic men may amount to up to 15%.

Idiopathic osteoporosis

Idiopathic osteoporosis is an uncommon syndrome, the estimated incidence being only four new cases per 100 000 persons per year. Nevertheless, the number of men whose osteoporosis remains unexplained after a routine evaluation is approximately 50% in most series. However, many series come from referral centers that tend to attract more unusual patients, and might therefore overestimate the proportion of men with unexplained disease. The diagnosis of idiopathic osteoporosis should be applied only to men under the age of 70 years. By that stage of life, it is more likely that the disease is at least the result of the cumulative effects of the process of age-related bone loss and of factors that affected skeletal health earlier in life (for example, failure to achieve adequate peak bone mass and calcium under-nutrition) but which are no longer identifiable.

The overwhelming majority of patients with idiopathic osteoporosis is symptomatic and presents with fractures. Fractures are most often at the vertebrae, although cortical fractures may occur as well, including stress fractures of the lower extremities or hip fractures. The predominant presenting symptom is back pain. Bone mass measurements in these men reveal markedly reduced bone mineral density. Typically, lumbar spine density T-scores in these men are below -2.5 SD. In our experience, the mean T-score is even less than -3.0. By definition, biochemical screening shows no abnormalities. The natural course of idiopathic osteoporosis is not well documented, but available data seem to indicate that – even with conservative measures – bone loss is not accelerated, suggesting that most of these men failed to reach normal peak bone density.

The pathogenesis of idiopathic osteoporosis is unknown. Both abnormalities in the GH–IGF-I system and alterations in the metabolism or activity of androgens have been suggested as potential etiologies. By no means, however, have they been established as causes.

DIAGNOSIS OF OSTEOPOROSIS IN MEN

The diagnosis of osteoporosis requires assessment of bone mineral density (BMD). In men as in women, diagnostic thresholds have been best validated with dual-energy X-ray absorptiometry (DXA).

There is overall agreement that bone density measurement using DXA should be performed in all men who present with findings that suggest the presence of osteoporosis (such as low trauma fractures or radiographic criteria indicating bone loss), and who are considered to be at increased risk for an atraumatic fracture because

of specific medical conditions (hypogonadism, hyperthyroidism, excessive alcohol intake).

The use of T-scores requires a comparison with measurements in a young reference population. Although fracture risk varies between populations, there is insufficient knowledge at present to recommend that local reference ranges be used. It is recommended, therefore, that the NHANES III database be used as an international reference until further research changes this view. There is some ongoing controversy as to whether gender-specific T-scores should be used or not. Most, but not all, cross-sectional data support the use of female reference values, but some authors propose using young normal mean levels derived from a male reference population. However, in men, the risk of fracture is substantially lower for a bone mineral measurement within their own reference range, so a more stringent criterion seems to be needed to yield the same risk as in women. The most effective approach to the resolution of this problem would be prospective observation in men of the relationship between measures of bone density and future fracture risk. Those data becoming available suggest that absolute BMD rather than gender-specific diagnostic criteria may be more appropriate. For the time being, it might therefore be most appropriate to define osteoporosis in men as a BMD of 2.5 SD or more below the reference range for young women.

In men as in women, spine measurements in older individuals may be confounded by osteoarthritis, whereas the hip is very much less affected. In men over the age of 65–70 years, BMD assessment should therefore include a measurement taken from the hip region.

CLINICAL EVALUATION OF MEN WITH OSTEOPOROSIS

Clinical assessment

The medical history should include a family and a fracture history and should address calcium intake, medications, alcohol intake and tobacco use. The clinical examination should particularly focus on signs of hypogonadism (especially testicular atrophy and span length for early hypogonadism), alcohol abuse and glucocorticoid excess. Body length should be monitored as a marker of osteoporosis. Dorsal kyphosis may indicate severe vertebral deformities. Low body mass index should be considered a risk factor.

Biochemical measures

The biochemical evaluation should include a complete blood count, serum levels of calcium, phosphate, alkaline phosphatase, albumin, creatinine, 25(OH)D and ferritin (to detect hemochromatosis and alcoholic liver disease), liver function tests, and serum protein electrophoresis (to exclude multiple myeloma, in particular in older individuals). A 24-h urine calcium and creatinine excretion level is needed to exclude hypercalciuria (> 300 mg/day). Hypocalciuria (< 100 mg/day) should raise suspicion of markedly reduced dietary calcium absorption (due to vitamin D deficiency, bowel disease or malnutrition).

Measurement of serum intact PTH is indicated whenever serum calcium, phosphate or 25(OH)D levels are abnormal (to detect primary or secondary hyperparathyroidism). In all patients, we would recommend measurement of serum testosterone and thyroid-stimulating hormone (TSH) to exclude hypogonadism and hyperthyroidism, especially in older individuals. Total testosterone should be measured in a morning sample, because testosterone concentrations fluctuate according to a circadian pattern. Some controversy remains whether free testosterone, bioavailable testosterone or sex hormone-binding globulin should be assessed in all patients. Some authors even advocate the routine measurement of estradiol. In men with androgen deficiency, serum levels of luteinizing hormone (LH) and prolactin should be measured to allow differentiation between primary

and secondary hypogonadism and to detect a potential prolactinoma. A 24-h cortisoluria test is indicated whenever there is clinical suspicion of Cushing's disease.

The added value of biochemical markers of bone turnover, such as serum osteocalcin or urinary collagen cross-links, in the clinical management of osteoporotic men remains to be demonstrated. Therefore, the routine measurement of bone markers in men with osteoporosis cannot be recommended.

THERAPEUTIC OPTIONS FOR MEN WITH OSTEOPOROSIS

Life-style measures and dietary recommendations

Whether and to what extent risk-factor modification will reduce fracture rates remains unknown, in men as well as in women. Nevertheless, adequate exercise should be recommended and excessive alcohol intake or smoking discouraged. Medications that potentially increase the risk of falling, such as psychotropic drugs, should be reconsidered, particularly in frail elderly men.

Dietary supplementation of calcium and vitamin D also reduces the rate of bone loss in elderly men with low calcium intake, and may even have an effect on fracture incidence. In line with the recommendations of the National Institutes of Health, dietary calcium intake should be at least 1200 mg/day. In men older than 65 years, a calcium intake of 1500 mg and a vitamin D intake of 800 IU daily are required.

Current pharmacological options

None of the currently available therapeutic options has proven antifracture efficacy as documented in properly designed, randomized, placebo-controlled fracture-endpoint trials. Such studies are difficult to perform because of the low fracture incidence in men. They would require a large study group and long-term follow-up. Therefore, the question arises to what extent data available in women may be extrapolated to men. One possibility is to use bone density as a surrogate marker for fracture risk as primary endpoint, rather than fracture endpoints. Agents with proven antifracture efficacy in postmenopausal women particularly should be considered for use in male osteoporosis, if clinical trials in men document favorable effects on bone mass of similar magnitude to those shown to result in reduced fracture rates in women.

Androgen replacement has been documented to prevent bone loss in hypogonadal men, but the extent to which this type of replacement would be beneficial in normal elderly men with partial androgen deficiency and low bone density remains to be clarified. According to a recent randomized trial, no significant gain in lumbar BMD is observed in older men with borderline low serum testosterone concentrations and low bone density, when compared with calcium supplementation alone. Only in those with low pretreatment testosterone levels will testosterone replacement be associated with a moderate gain in bone density. In addition to information on the potential benefit of androgen replacement in normal elderly men, there is an urgent need for data regarding the long-term safety of this type of therapy.

Parathyroid hormone analogs (such as PTH1–34) have an anabolic action, but have been studied only in small short-term, randomized, placebo-controlled trials, suggesting that these compounds may increase lumbar bone density. Clearly, more studies are required to assess their potential in male osteoporosis. The use of fluoride, another anabolic agent, remains controversial. Dramatic increases can be obtained in vertebral bone mass, but the effectiveness of supplemental fluoride in reducing fracture rates is still uncertain. Fluoride therapy should be further evaluated

in long-term randomized trials before it can be recommended. Similarly, the long-term use of calcitonin cannot be recommended in men with osteoporosis. Pain following vertebral fracture has been reported to be alleviated with calcitonin, and some reports of this benefit have included men, but an additional benefit on lumbar bone density compared to calcium and vitamin D supplements has not yet been documented in men suffering from osteoporosis. Finally, thiazide diuretics may be useful in the treatment of male osteoporosis in those patients who present with hypercalciuria. There are cross-sectional data suggesting a protective effect on fracture incidence, but controlled, prospective information is not available.

In postmenopausal osteoporosis, bisphosphonates have become one of the treatments of choice. Recent evidence suggests that they may be equally useful in male patients. In men suffering from glucocorticoid osteoporosis, bisphosphonate therapy is associated with similar increases in bone density to those in women. More recently, a randomized placebo-controlled trial with alendronate showed significant improvements of both lumbar and femoral bone density in osteoporotic men with or without hypogonadism[12]. The chief entry criteria were a BMD at the femoral neck of at least 2 SD below the mean value in normal young men or a BMD at the femoral neck of at least 1 SD below the mean value in normal young men, and at least one vertebral deformity or a history of an osteoporotic fracture. Over a period of 2 years, the use of alendronate was associated with an increase in lumbar spine BMD of approximately 7% and a gain in total hip BMD of 2.5%. The incidence of vertebral fractures was lower in the alendronate group than in the placebo group (0.8% vs. 7.1%). In line with these radiographic findings, alendronate-treated men showed no decrease in height, whereas men taking placebo lost height significantly. The effects of alendronate were independent of baseline serum free testosterone, suggesting that bisphosphonate therapy may be useful in both androgen-replete and androgen-deficient men. More importantly, the benefits of alendronate therapy in men with osteoporosis were similar to those in postmenopausal women, suggesting that bisphosphonate therapy might be equally effective in men and women with osteoporosis.

MALE OSTEOPOROSIS: A PRACTICAL APPROACH

There is increasing evidence that the approaches developed to diagnose and treat the disorder in women may be equally useful in approaching similar problems in men. Nevertheless, the evaluation and treatment of men suffering from osteoporosis remains a clinical challenge, despite recent advances in the understanding of the male osteoporotic syndrome. In most countries (including the USA), there are currently no approved therapies for male osteoporosis. Moreover, there is some ongoing controversy about the reference values that should be used to derive T-scores, as indicated above.

All men with low bone density should be investigated (both clinically and biochemically) for secondary causes of bone loss, and should be informed regarding life-style measures and dietary calcium intake. In line with recent recommendations from the International Osteoporosis Foundation, we would recommend that the same diagnostic thresholds be used in men – namely a BMD at the hip that lies 2.5 SD below the reference range for young women – until further research changes this view. Because the relationship between BMD and fracture risk seems to be similar in men and women (although the data are scanty), we would recommend treating all men with osteoporosis as defined by female reference values with calcium, vitamin D (when appropriate) and an antiresorptive agent. In view of recent evidence,

bisphosphonate therapy might be the treatment of choice. A BMD measurement value more than 2.5 SD below the young male reference may not warrant antiresorptive treatment (except if there is history of an osteoporotic fracture), but it warrants further investigation to exclude secondary causes of bone loss as well as general recommendations regarding life-style measures and appropriate dietary intake of calcium.

KEY MESSAGES

(1) There is increasing evidence that the approaches developed to diagnose and treat osteoporosis in women may be equally useful in approaching similar problems in men. In particular, bisphosphonates are likely to become an important strategy to increase bone density and reduce fracture risk in osteoporotic men.

(2) In men with osteoporosis, it remains critical to exclude underlying pathological causes as these are much more likely to occur than in women.

(3) The extent to which age-associated endocrine deficiencies contribute to bone loss and fracture predisposition in men remains to be established. In particular, it is not yet clear whether the partial androgen deficiency associated with normal aging has implications for skeletal maintenance.

ACKNOWLEDGEMENTS

Dr S. Boonen and Dr D. Vanderschueren are both Senior Clinical Investigators of the Fund for Scientific Research, Flanders, Belgium (FWO-Vlaanderen). Dr S. Boonen is holder of the Leuven University Chair in Metabolic Bone Diseases, founded and supported by Merck Sharp & Dohme.

References

1. Bilezikian JP. Osteoporosis in men. *J Clin Endocrinol Metab* 1999;84:3431–4

2. Orwoll ES, Klein RF. Osteoporosis in men. *Endocr Rev* 1995;16:87–116

3. Cooper C, Campion G, Melton LJ III. Hip fractures in the elderly: a world-wide projection. *Osteoporosis Int* 1992;2:285–9

4. de Laet CE, van Hout BA, Burger H, *et al.* Bone density and risk of hip fracture in men and women: cross sectional analysis [Published erratum appears in *Br Med J* 1997;315:916]. *Br Med J* 1997;315:221–5

5. Jones G, Nguyen T, Sambrook PN, *et al.* Symptomatic fracture incidence in elderly men and women: the Dubbo Osteoporosis Epidemiology Study (DOES). *Osteoporosis Int* 1994;4:277–82

6. Poor G, Atkinson EJ, Lewallen DG, *et al.* Age-related hip fractures in men: clinical spectrum and short-term outcomes. *Osteoporosis Int* 1995;5:419–26

7. O'Neill TW, Felsenberg D, Varlow J, *et al.* The prevalence of vertebral deformity in European men and women: the European Vertebral Osteoporosis Study. *J Bone Miner Res* 1996; 11:1010–18

8. Looker AC, Orwoll ES, Johnston CC Jr, *et al.* Prevalence of low femoral bone density in older US adults from NHANES III. *J Bone Miner Res* 1997;12:1761–8

9. Boonen S, Vanderschueren D, Geusens P, Bouillon R. Age-associated endocrine deficiencies as potential determinants of femoral neck (type II) osteoporotic fracture occurrence in elderly men. *Int J Androl* 1997;20: 134–43

10. Khosla S, Melton LJ III, Atkinson EJ, *et al.* Relationship of serum sex steroid levels and bone turnover markers with bone mineral density in men and women: a key role for bioavailable estrogen. *J Clin Endocrinol Metab* 1998;83:2266–74

11. Vanderschueren D, Boonen S, Bouillon R. Action of androgens versus oestrogens in male skeletal homeostasis. *Bone* 1998;23: 391–4

12. Orwoll ES, Ettinger M, Weiss S, *et al.* Alendronate for the treatment of osteoporosis in men. *N Engl J Med* 2000;343:604–10

43 Joint disorders

Leif Dahlberg, MD, PhD

INTRODUCTION

A common cause for disability in the elderly population is musculoskeletal disease. This entity includes soft tissue disorders such as non-articular rheumatism, bursitis and tendinitis, gout, and joint disorders such as rheumatoid arthritis (RA) and osteoarthritis (OA). RA, with its prevalence of approximately 1%, is a severely disabling chronic inflammatory arthropathy that can affect all peripheral joints[1]. It is more common in women. RA often shows a symmetric joint distribution with pronounced synovial inflammation and rapid joint destruction. In most cases in RA, an early referral to a rheumatologist is essential for a definitive diagnosis and initiation of anti-inflammatory drug treatment. In contrast, the most prevalent disease that affects joints, OA, can be readily treated by the general practitioner initially. It has been estimated that by 2020 the number of individuals with OA will increase by approximately 50%, owing to the increasing average age of the population[2]. This chapter deals with the definition and diagnosis, pathophysiology, prevention and treatment of joint disorders, mainly knee and hip OA.

DEFINITION AND DIAGNOSIS

The American College of Rheumatology (ACR) has defined osteoarthritis (OA) as 'a heterogeneous group of conditions that leads to joint symptoms and signs which are associated with defective integrity of articular cartilage, in addition to related changes in the underlying bone and at the joint margins'[3]. From this definition it can be concluded that OA is a progressive, age-related disorder that affects all tissues in the joint. It can be regarded as the end state of a multifactorial disease that develops over some 10–20 years.

Osteoarthritis is usually diagnosed by a combination of joint pain and radiographic changes. Accordingly, the main response criteria are merely subjective. This causes problems in OA diagnosis, as well as in the design and interpretation of OA studies[4,5].

CLINICAL MANIFESTATIONS

Osteoarthritis is a non-inflammatory disease with a cyclic pattern. It affects predominantly the knees, hips, spine and hands, but rarely ankles, shoulders, elbows and wrists. Several clinical features, such as tenderness and pain, decreased range of motion and crepitus, often show spontaneous clinical improvement[6]. Although OA usually progresses, this is not absolute. Cohort studies suggest that approximately half of patients show progress as assessed by radiography during a 12–15-year period[7-11]. The risk for deterioration is dependent on the joint site, and is less pronounced in patients in earlier stages of OA.

The prevalence of OA depends on which criteria we include in the definition, symptoms only, or in combination with radiographic changes. It is rare in adults less than 40 years of age. Knee OA is more common than hip

OA and is consistent with more disability[11]. In a recent study from the USA, radiographic knee OA was found in 3.7% of people between ages 25 and 74. Approximately half of these individuals reported knee pain. Conversely, of those that reported knee pain, only 15% had radiographic OA[12]. Knee OA occurs more often in men than in women less than 50 years old, probably because of the greater number of sports injuries in men. After the age of 50, knee OA is more common in women. Hip OA shows no clear gender predisposition.

It should be noted that OA starts years before radiography can detect cartilage changes. Radiography is of value in the decision and planning of a total joint replacement. However, patients with joint pain and normal radiography commonly seek medical advice. Such patients frequently show arthroscopic cartilage pathology[13]. Preradiographic OA is sometimes referred to as 'pre OA' or 'early OA'.

JOINT CARTILAGE

Joint cartilage is a composite tissue in which its major constituent, type II collagen, forms a fibrillar network[14]. The large aggregating proteoglycan (aggrecan), trapped in this fibrillar mesh, creates a swelling pressure counterbalanced by the tensile properties of type II collagen. This allows the cartilage to resist deformation and to dissipate loads, and ensures the compressive stiffness of the joint cartilage. Other matrix molecules, equally as important for the matrix integrity but less abundant, are hyaluronan, small proteoglycans and non-collagenous matrix proteins such as cartilage oligomeric matrix protein (COMP) and fibronectin[15]. There is a continuous turnover of these cartilage matrix constituents. Under physiological conditions, degraded cartilage matrix molecules are replaced by newly synthesized molecules. To withstand the biomechanical forces and keep the functional properties of the articular cartilage intact, the matrix is critically dependent on this finely tuned metabolic balance.

CARTILAGE PATHOPHYSIOLOGY AND NEW PERSPECTIVES ON DETECTION AND TREATMENT OF JOINT DISEASES

A likely prerequisite for successful therapeutic interventions in cartilage disease is that treatment starts before the fibrillar network becomes disrupted and cartilage is lost. By increased knowledge of cartilage metabolism and mechanisms behind the molecular alterations in joint diseases, it will be possible to develop new methods to identify patients in an early progressive phase, before macroscopic cartilage changes occur. Recent studies have shown that degradative biochemical processes are active in OA cartilage[16,17]. The increased proteolytic degradation of type II collagen, aggrecan and COMP involves several of the matrix metalloproteinases, enzymes with potent catabolic actions on connective tissues[14,15]. A metabolic imbalance where degradation outscores repair is suggested in OA[18]. As a result, cartilage is progressively lost, the key feature in OA. Future treatment in OA may include drugs with the capacity to retard disease progression as suggested in OA cartilage culture experiments, where type II collagen degradation was controlled by synthetic enzyme inhibitors[16,19].

In inflammatory joint diseases, there is an up-regulation and release from inflamed synovium of cytokines such as tumor necrosis factor-α and interleukin-1[20]. They play a significant role in the cartilage degradative process. The treatment of patients with RA and ankylosing spondylitis with an interleukin-1 receptor antagonist or an antitumor necrosis factor-α antibody has shown promising clinical results[21,22].

Further support of an altered cartilage metabolism in joint diseases is provided by studies that show a changed release pattern of cartilage-derived matrix molecules into serum and synovial fluid in OA and RA patients[23–25]. Several specific assays for the analysis of such biomarkers of human joint disease are now available[26]. Some molecular markers may have the ability to identify early cartilage abnormality as well as to be of prognostic value[27–29].

Magnetic resonance imaging (MRI) is a non-invasive method that provides new structural information about cartilage[30]. An intravenous injection of a contrast medium (indirect MRI-arthrography) improves the images in traumatic joint disorders, such as labrum tears of the shoulder and cartilage injuries of the knee and fingers[31,32]. To study joint cartilage at a molecular level, it has been experimentally shown that the negatively charged contrast agent, gadolinium-diethylenetriaminepenta-acetate (Gd-DTPA^{2-}), distributes inversely to the negatively charged cartilage matrix proteoglycans[33]. In vivo, Gd-DTPA^{2-} shows a dose-dependent cartilage distribution in healthy volunteers[34]. Patients who receive Gd-DTPA^{2-} intravenously prior to hip or knee replacement show increased distribution of Gd-DTPA^{2-} in cartilage[33]. In the next decade, MRI and molecular markers will most probably become clinically important tools in the diagnosis, prognosis and in vivo monitoring of cartilage integrity in early OA and RA, as well as being used to monitor new treatments[26,30].

RISK FACTORS AND PREVENTION

One significant factor that may account for up to half of OA cases is heredity[35–37]. However, the two main modifiable OA risk factors are obesity and joint injuries[2]. With respect to obesity, it has been shown that it precedes knee OA, that is, obesity is not caused by less physical activity due to knee pain[38]. Obese subjects may have as much as a five-fold risk to develop knee OA. Importantly, weight reduction has been shown to reduce knee OA incidence and progression[2]. Obesity and hip OA are also related[39]. Altered biomechanics is a likely reason for this relationship. However, it seems as if obesity is associated with OA also in unloaded joints, suggesting that systemic factors may contribute to cartilage degradation[40].

A joint injury can be related to an acute major trauma to cartilage, ligaments and meniscus or to iterated minor joint traumas. Athletic activities commonly cause major joint injuries, and studies have shown that as much as 50% of these patients will develop post-traumatic OA in 15–20 years[41,42]. Furthermore, OA patients below the age of 50 operated on by means of high osteotomy of the tibia commonly have a history of knee injury[43].

Iterated minor traumas may cause OA because they exceed the repair capacity of the cartilage. Studies suggest that occupations involving frequent and long duration of kneeling or squatting are consistent with an increased risk of knee OA[2,36,44]. Heavy-laborers and farmers also show a higher than expected risk of hip OA[45,46]. Accordingly to a significant degree, OA is caused by modifiable risk factors[2,44]. This calls for an increased focus on strategies for OA prevention, which should include weight reduction and alterations in ergonomic activities at work. Specific training programs may reduce the risk for ligament and meniscus injuries as well as improve the ability of the cartilage to withstand deterioration.

Other non-drug regimes in OA patients include exercise and patient education. Improved strength and range of motion to reduce pain can be achieved by inexpensive exercise programs[47,48], as shown by an 8-week walking program in patients with OA[49]. Educational self-care programs may reduce the frequency and costs of primary care visits for OA[50]. Exercise and patient education will most certainly become increasingly important OA treatments.

Although frequently used, therapies with ultrasound, laser and transcutaneous nerve stimulation as well as shock-absorbing insoles are less scientifically evaluated, and their use must be considered on a case-by-case basis[51].

DRUG TREATMENTS

No studies have convincingly shown any one OA drug available today to be 'chondroprotective', that is, to inhibit disease progression or to repair cartilage[52]. In human OA, non-steroidal anti-inflammatory drugs (NSAIDs) are the most commonly used pharmacological drugs. Their value as pain killers is undisputed[53]; however, their gastrointestinal side-effects make them less than ideal[54]. Furthermore, an increased risk of OA progression owing to NSAID treatment has been proposed[55]. Their role as first-choice drugs in OA or 'pre-OA' patients can been questioned, and a pure analgesic, such as acetaminophen, is therefore suggested as initial treatment in OA[56,57]. However, in patients who need increased pain reduction, NSAIDs are valuable.

The NSAIDs decrease prostaglandin production by inhibition of the cyclo-oxygenase (COX) enzymes[58]. Recently, several forms of COX have been detected. It is postulated that COX-1 is needed in the protection of the gastric mucosa, and that COX-2 is involved in pathological inflammatory conditions. Accordingly, specific COX-2 inhibitors have been developed and shown in clinical trials to reduce the incidence of peptic ulcers and gastrointestinal bleeding in OA and RA patients, with equally good effect on pain[58]. Specific COX-2 inhibitors will probably be significant new contributors to the treatment of OA and RA over the next several years.

One group of OA drugs, such as glucosamine, chondroitin sulfate, collagen hydrolysate and hyaluronan, can be referred to as 'cartilage extracts'. Recently it was suggested that glucosamine may be a disease modifying drug[59]. Deal and Moskowitz[60] conclude that glucosamine, chondroitin sulfate and collagen hydrolysate are nutraceuticals, and available as health-food supplements. They have not been evaluated by the Food and Drug Administration (FDA), and the number of studies of toxicity and long-term evaluations are limited[60]. A meta-analysis of glucosamine and chondroitin concludes that they may be useful in OA, but further investigations in larger cohorts of patients for longer time periods are needed to prove their usefulness as symptom-modifying drugs in OA[61]. It is suggested that the pros and cons of these agents are described, so that patients can decide whether they wish to proceed with their use[60].

INTRA-ARTICULAR INJECTIONS

Intra-articular injections in knee OA show a strong placebo effect[27]. A study that included a mock injection, involving a complete injection maneuver without anything being injected into the joint, was shown as effective as drug and placebo injections[62]. The variable outcome in studies that examine intra-articular treatment may be due to the extra-articular deposition of approximately one-third of injections[63]. With regard to steroid injections, they have shown to be valuable up to 6 weeks after the injection in OA patients with recurrent joint effusion[64]. However, in contrast to RA, their regular use cannot be recommend in OA.

Hyaluronan is the major macromolecule of synovial fluid. It has been extensively injected into OA joints and is suggested to restore the elastoviscous properties of synovial fluid, to relieve joint pain and to reduce structural damage in the OA joint. However, convincing studies to support these assumptions are lacking[65]. Although some studies show statistically significant improvement in pain variables, the clinical relevance is still doubtful. The reason for beneficial symptomatic effect months after the drug is cleared from the joint is not easily explained. Furthermore, acute local reactions after intra-articular hyaluronan injections for knee OA have been reported[66].

OPERATIVE TREATMENTS

With increased participation in athletic activities, joint injuries may also occur in elderly people. For example, knee meniscus injuries and rotator cuff ruptures of the shoulder may need arthroscopical treatment.

Joint lavage and arthroscopical debridement of loose or degenerated fragments may be beneficial in OA patients[67,68]. Autologous chondrocyte transplantation, perichondrial transplantation and carbon-fiber rods have been used to restore cartilage surface defects mostly in patients with traumatic cartilage lesions, but also in patients with OA[69]. The lack of appropriate control groups makes these studies difficult to evaluate. There is no clear support for surgical cartilage repair in patients with OA lesions[70].

In patients 50–60 years old with early radiographic OA in the medial tibiofemoral compartment, valgus osteotomy of the tibia has a beneficial effect for some 10 years[43].

In patients with more severe OA, joint replacement offers pain relief and increased quality of life for several years[71]. Better patient selection and operative technique, and prophylaxis with antibiotics have improved the survival rate of total joint operations[71]. The infection rate has continuously decreased and is now below 1%. A study that showed beneficial outcome of hip and knee replacement 6 months after surgery indicates that the patient's preoperative functional status predicts the outcome. This may suggest that patients with OA should be operated on in an earlier stage of their disease[72].

ACKNOWLEDGEMENTS

Grant support was provided by the Swedish Medical Research Council (K99–73X), the Swedish Center for Research in Sports, the Medical Faculty of Lund University and the Kock Foundation.

References

1. Fuchs HA, Sergent JS. Rheumatoid arthritis: the clinical picture. In Koopman W, ed. *Arthritis and Allied Conditions*. Baltimore: Williams & Wilkins, 1997:1041–70
2. Felson DT. Epidemiology of osteoarthritis. In Brandt KD, Doherty M, Lohmander LS, eds. *Osteoarthritis*. New York: Oxford University Press, 1998:13–22
3. Altman R, Asch E, Bloch D, *et al*. Development of criteria for the classification and reporting of osteoarthritis. *Arthritis Rheum* 1986;29:1039–49
4. Cushnaghan J, Cooper C, Dieppe P, *et al*. Clinical assessment of osteoarthritis of the knee. *Ann Rheum Dis* 1990;49:768–70
5. Hart DJ, Spector TD, Brown P, *et al*. Clinical signs of early osteoarthritis: reproducibility and relation to X-ray changes in 541 women in the general population. *Ann Rheum Dis* 1991;50:467–70
6. Berkhout B, MacFarlane JD, Cats A. Symptomatic osteoarthrosis of the knee: a follow-up study. *Br J Rheumatol* 1985;24:40–5
7. Hernborg JS, Nilsson BE. The natural course of untreated osteoarthritis of the knee. *Clin Orthop* 1977;98:130–7
8. Dougados M, Gueguen A, Nguyen M, *et al*. Longitudinal radiologic evaluation of osteoarthritis of the knee. *J Rheumatol* 1992;19:378–84
9. Schouten JSAG, van der Ouweland FA, Valkenburg HA. A 12 year follow up study in the general population on prognostic factors of cartilage loss in osteoarthritis of the knee. *Ann Rheum Dis* 1992;51:932–7
10. Spector TD, Dacre JE, Harris PA, Huskisson EC. Radiological progression of osteoarthritis: an 11 year follow up study of the knee. *Ann Rheum Dis* 1992;51:1107–10
11. Dieppe P, Cushnaghan J, Tucker M, *et al*. The Bristol 'OA500 study': progression and impact of the disease after 8 years. *Osteoarthritis Cartilage* 2000;8:63–8
12. Hannan MT, Felson DT, Pincus T. Analysis of the discordance between radiographic changes and knee pain in osteoarthritis of the knee. *J Rheumatol* 2000;27:1513–17
13. Dahlberg L, Lohmander LS, Ryd L. Intraarticular injections of hyaluronan in patients with cartilage abnormalities and knee pain. A one-year double-blind, placebo-controlled study. *Arthritis Rheum* 1994;37:521–8

14. Poole AR. Cartilage in health and disease. In Koopman W, ed. *Arthritis and Allied Conditions*. Baltimore: Williams & Wilkins, 1997: 253–308

15. Heinegård D, Bayliss M, Lorenzo P. Biochemistry and metabolism of normal and osteoarthritic cartilage. In Brandt KD, Doherty M, Lohmander LS, eds. *Osteoarthritis*. New York: Oxford Medical Publications, 1998:74–84

16. Billinghurst RC, Dahlberg L, Lonescu M, *et al.* Enhanced cleavage of type II collagen by collagenases in osteoarthritic articular cartilage. *J Clin Invest* 1997;99:1534–45

17. Caterson B, Flannery CR, Hughes CE, Little CE. Mechanisms involved in cartilage proteoglycan catabolism. *Matrix Biol* 2000;19: 333–44

18. Poole AR. Imbalances of anabolism and catabolism of cartilage matrix components in osteoarthritis. In Kuettner K, Goldberg V, eds. *Osteoarthritis Disorders*. Washington: American Academy of Orthopaedic Surgeons, 1995:247–60

19. Dahlberg L, Billinghurst RC, Manner P, *et al.* Selective enhancement of collagenase-mediated cleavage of resident type II collagen in cultured osteoarthritic cartilage and arrest with a synthetic inhibitor that spares collagenase 1 (matrix metalloproteinase 1). *Arthritis Rheum* 2000;43:673–82

20. Jasin HE. Mechanisms of tissue damage in rheumatoid arthritis. In Koopman W, ed. *Arthritis and Allied Conditions*. Baltimore: Williams & Wilkins, 1997:1017–39

21. Bresnihan B, Alvaro-Gracia JM, Cobby M, *et al.* Treatment of rheumatoid arthritis with recombinant human interleukin-1 receptor antagonist. *Arthritis Rheum* 1998;41: 2196–204

22. Brandt J, Haibel H, Cornely D, *et al.* Successful treatment of active ankylosing spondylitis with the anti-tumor necrosis factor alpha monoclonal antibody infliximab. *Arthritis Rheum* 2000;43:1346–52

23. Saxne T, Heinegård D. Cartilage oligomeric matrix protein: a novel marker of cartilage turnover detectable in synovial fluid and blood. *Br J Rheumatol* 1992;31:583–91

24. Dahlberg L, Ryd L, Heinegård D, Lohmander LS. Proteoglycan fragments in joint fluid: influence of arthrosis and inflammation. *Acta Orthop Scand* 1992;63:417–23

25. Petersson IF, Sandqvist L, Svensson B, Saxne T. Cartilage markers in synovial fluid in symptomatic knee osteoarthritis. *Ann Rheum Dis* 1997;56:64–7

26. Garnero P, Rousseau J-C, Delmas PD. Molecular basis and clinical use of biochemical markers of bone, cartilage and synovium in joint diseases. *Arthritis Rheum* 2000;43:953–68

27. Dahlberg L, Friden T, Roos H, *et al.* A longitudinal study of cartilage matrix metabolism in patients with cruciate ligament rupture – synovial fluid concentrations of aggrecan fragments, stromelysin-1 and tissue inhibitor of metalloproteinase-1. *Br J Rheumatol* 1994; 33:1107–11

28. Sharif M, George E, Shepstone L, *et al.* Serum hyaluronic acid level as a predictor of disease progression in osteoarthritis of the knee. *Arthritis Rheum* 1995;38:760–7

29. Petersson IF, Boegard T, Svensson B, *et al.* Changes in cartilage and bone metabolism identified by serum markers in early osteoarthritis of the knee joint. *Br J Rheumatol* 1998;37:46–50

30. Peterfy CG. Magnetic resonance imaging. In Brandt KD, Doherty M, Lohmander LS, eds. *Osteoarthritis*. New York: Oxford University Press, 1998:473–93

31. Vahlensieck M, Sommer T, Textor J, *et al.* Indirect MR arthrography: techniques and applications. *Eur Radiol* 1998;8:232–5

32. Backhaus M, Kamradt T, Sandrock D, *et al.* Arthritis of the finger joints: a comprehensive approach comparing conventional radiography, scintigraphy, ultrasound, and contrast-enhanced magnetic resonance imaging. *Arthritis Rheum* 1999;42:1232–45

33. Bashir A, Gray ML, Hartke J, Burstein D. Nondestructive imaging of human cartilage glycosaminoglycan concentration by MRI. *Magn Reson Med* 1999;41:857–65

34. Tiderius CJ, Olsson LE, deVerdier H, *et al.* Gd-DTPA^{2-}-enhanced MRI of femoral knee cartilage: a dose-response study in healthy volunteers. *Magn Reson Med* 2001

35. Spector TD, Cicuttini F, Baker J, *et al*. Genetic influences on osteoarthritis in women: a twin study. *Br Med J* 1996;312:940–3

36. Charles ST, Gatz M, Pedersen NL, Dahlberg L. Genetic and behavioral risk factors for self-reported joint pain among a population-based sample of Swedish twins. *Health Psychol* 1999;18:644–54

37. Holderbaum D, Haqqi TM, Moskowitz RW. Genetics and osteoarthritis: exposing the iceberg. *Arthritis Rheum* 1999;42:397–405

38. Felson DT, Anderson JJ, Naimark A, *et al*. Obesity and knee osteoarthritis. The Framingham study. *Ann Intern Med* 1988;109:18–24

39. Cooper C, Inskip H, Croft P, *et al*. Individual risk factors for hip osteoarthritis: obesity, hip injury, and physical activity. *Am J Epidemiol* 1998;147:516–22

40. Cicuttini FM, Baker JR, Spector TD. The association of obesity with osteoarthritis of the hand and knee in women: a twin study. *J Rheumatol* 1996;23:1221–6

41. Roos H, Lauren M, Adalberth T, *et al*. Knee osteoarthritis after meniscectomy: prevalence of radiographic changes after twenty-one years, compared with matched controls. *Arthritis Rheum* 1998;41:687–93

42. Gelber AC, Hochberg MC, Mead LA, *et al*. Joint injury in young adults and risk for subsequent knee and hip osteoarthritis. *Ann Intern Med* 2000;133:321–8

43. Odenbring S, Tjörnstrand B, Egund N, *et al*. Function after tibial osteotomy for medial gonarthrosis below aged 50 years. *Acta Orthop Scand* 1989;60:527–31

44. Cooper C, Coggon D. Physical activity and knee osteoarthritis. *Lancet* 1999;353:2177–8

45. Vingard E, Alfredsson L, Goldie I, Hogstedt C. Occupation and osteoarthrosis of the hip and knee: a register-based cohort study. *Int J Epidemiol* 1991;20:1025–31

46. Axmacher B, Lindberg H. Coxarthrosis in farmers. *Clin Orthop* 1993;287:82–6

47. Minor MA. Exercise in the treatment of osteoarthritis. *Rheum Dis Clin North Am* 1999;25:397–415

48. van Baar ME, Assendelft WJ, Dekker J, *et al*. Effectiveness of exercise therapy in patients with osteoarthritis of the hip or knee: a systematic review of randomized clinical trials. *Arthritis Rheum* 1999;42:1361–9

49. Kovar PA, Allegrante JP, MacKenzie CR, *et al*. Supervised fitness walking in patients with osteoarthritis of the knee. A randomized, controlled trial. *Ann Intern Med* 1992;116:529–34

50. Mazzuca SA, Brandt KD, Katz BP, *et al*. Reduced utilization and cost of primary care clinic visits resulting from self-care education for patients with osteoarthritis of the knee. *Arthritis Rheum* 1999;42:1267–73

51. Cushnaghan J, Forster S. Physical therapy. In Brandt KD, Doherty M, Lohmander LS, eds. *Osteoarthritis*. New York: Oxford University Press, 1998:307–14

52. Brandt KD, Lohmander LS, Doherty M. Prospects for pharmacological modification of joint breakdown in osteoarthritis. In Brandt KD, Doherty M, Lohmander LS, eds. *Osteoarthritis*. New York: Oxford University Press, 1998:Chapter 11

53. Wolfe F, Zhao S, Lane N. Preference for non-steroidal antiinflammatory drugs over acetaminophen by rheumatic disease patients: a survey of 1799 patients with osteoarthritis, rheumatoid arthritis, and fibromyalgia. *Arthritis Rheum* 2000;43:378–85

54. Wolfe MM, Lichtenstein DR, Singh G. Gastrointestinal toxicity of nonsteroidal anti-inflammatory drugs. *N Engl J Med* 1999;340:1888–99

55. Rashad S, Hemingway A, Rainsford K, *et al*. Effect of non-steroidal anti-inflammatory drugs on the course of osteoarthritis. *Lancet* 1989;8662:519–22

56. Hochberg MC, Altman RD, Brandt KD, *et al*. Guidelines for the medical management of osteoarthritis. Part I. Osteoarthritis of the hip. *Arthritis Rheum* 1995;38:1535–40

57. Hochberg MC, Altman RD, Brandt KD, *et al*. Guidelines for the medical management of osteoarthritis. Part II. Osteoarthritis of the knee. American College of Rheumatology. *Arthritis Rheum* 1995;38:1541–6

58. Crofford LJ, Lipsky PE, Brooks P, *et al*. Basic biology and clinical application of specific cyclooxygenase-2 inhibitors. *Arthritis Rheum* 2000;43:4–13

59. Reginster YL, Derasy R, Rovati LC *et al*. Longterm effects of glucosamine sulphate on osteoarthritis progression: placebo-controlled clinical trial. *Lancet* 2001;357:251–6

60. Deal CL, Moskowitz RW. Nutraceuticals as therapeutic agents in osteoarthritis. The role of glucosamine, chondroitin sulfate, and collagen hydrolysate. *Rheum Dis Clin North Am* 1999;25:379–95

61. McAlindon TE, LaValley MP, Gulin JP, Felson DT. Glucosamine and chondroitin for treatment of osteoarthritis: a systematic quality assessment and meta-analysis. *J Am Med Assoc* 2000;283:1469–75

62. Miller JH, White J, Norton TH. The value of intraarticular injections in osteoarthritis of the knee. *J Bone Joint Surg Br* 1958;40B:636–43

63. Jones A, Regan M, Ledingham J, *et al*. Importance of placement of intra-articular steroid injections. *Br Med J* 1993;307: 1329–30

64. Dieppe PA, Sathpatyavongs B, Jones HE, *et al*. Intra-articular steroids in osteoarthritis. *Rheumatol Rehabil* 1980;19:212–17

65. Brandt KD, Smith GN Jr, Simon LS. Intra-articular injection of hyaluronan as treatment for knee osteoarthritis: what is the evidence? *Arthritis Rheum* 2000;43:1192–203

66. Puttick MP, Wade JP, Chalmers A, *et al*. Acute local reactions after intraarticular hylan for osteoarthritis of the knee. *J Rheumatol* 1995; 22:1311–14

67. Ogilvie-Harris DJ, Fitsialos DP. Arthroscopic management of the degenerative knee. *Arthroscopy* 1991;7:151–7

68. Ravaud P, Moulinier L, Giraudeau B, *et al*. Effects of joint lavage and steroid injection in patients with osteoarthritis of the knee: results of a multicenter, randomized, controlled trial. *Arthritis Rheum* 1999;42:475–82

69. Brittberg M, Lindahl A, Homminga G, *et al*. A critical analysis of cartilage repair [Letter; comment]. *Acta Orthop Scand* 1997;68: 186–91

70. Messner K, Gillquist J. Cartilage repair. A critical review. *Acta Orthop Scand* 1996;67: 523–9

71. Robertsson O, Dunbar M, Pehrsson T, Knutson K, Lidgren L. Patient satisfaction after knee arthroplasty: a report on 27 372 knees operated on between 1981 and 1995 in Sweden. *Acta Orthop Scand* 2000;71:262–7

72. Fortin PR, Clarke AE, Joseph L, *et al*. Outcomes of total hip and knee replacement: preoperative functional status predicts outcomes at six months after surgery. *Arthritis Rheum* 1999;42:1722–8

44 Degenerative spine disorders

Acke Ohlin, MD, PhD

INTRODUCTION

The cells of nuclear disc tissue are probably the least well-nourished cells in the human body; oxygen and nutrients as well as metabolites are mainly transported through the endplates of the vertebral bodies into or out from the nucleus. Variations in disc pressure play a major role in this diffusional system at least for the larger molecules: during daily activities, fluid with metabolites is pressed outwards from the nucleus when it is compressed, whereas during rest, an influx of fluid with nutrients to the nucleus will occur[1]. This is probably the reason why the aging process of the disc starts early in life, and why degenerative signs can be observed even in adolescence. Magnetic resonance imaging (MRI) of the spine, even in quite asymptomatic individuals, may reveal significant disc degeneration with hernias in about 30% of cases[2].

When a disc degenerates, the water content is gradually reduced, but also the disc capsule (the annulus fibrosis) shows varying degrees of rupture of the fibrous lamellae. The degenerative process of the disc usually results in an asymptomatic, but somewhat stiffer, old man.

The diagnosis of spondylosis deformans is a radiographic feature without clinical relevance: on plain X-ray films one may observe osteophytes and a reduction of disc height. Elderly men with a poor-appearing radiograph can be quite asymptomatic, whereas younger men with a normal radiograph – and even a normal MRI – may present with disabling back pain.

LOW BACK PAIN

Low back pain is a common disorder in adult men. Almost 80% suffer from low back pain once or more during life. The prognosis is good in the majority of cases. A thorough clinical examination and simple laboratory tests such as hemoglobin level and erythrocyte sedimentation rate (ESR) suffice to exclude severe disease. Increased physical activity is of paramount importance during the initial phase. Routine radiographic examination is not indicated in people under 60 years of age if no signs of other disease are observed within 2 months. A thorough study using the principles of evidence-based medicine on back and neck pain has recently been published[3].

DISC HERNIA

Disc hernias may occur from CII to the sacrum; lumbar disc hernias, however, are by far the most common. The anatomical level of lumbar disc herniation is lower in the young than in the elderly man[4]. Symptomatic disc hernias occur in the thoracic region in about 1%, compared with in the lumbar region, whereas the incidence of cervical disc disease falls somewhere in between.

Disc hernias can be divided into three types: bulging discs, and sequestrated and perforated disc hernias. In the past, disc hernia pain was believed to be due to mechanical factors: stretch and compression on the nerve root. More recently, Olmarker and colleagues[5] demonstrated, in very elegant experiments using pigs, that the chemical influence of agents in the nucleus tissue caused an intense histological reaction in exposed nerve roots. Treatment based on the inhibition of chemical agents in the nucleus tissue is probably realistic for the future.

Patients with a sequestrated disc generally have more intense sciatic pain, often requiring radiographic evaluation. The worst pain is usually experienced by patients with a perforated disc hernia, in accordance with the findings of Olmarker and colleagues[5].

Symptoms and diagnosis

Symptoms vary with the level and usually also the degree of herniation. When the posterior part of the annulus fibrosis is weakened, in most cases just by degeneration, the nucleus may protrude. The patient presents with slight sciatica, and the prognosis is generally excellent. In cases of sequestrated or perforated hernia the clinical symptoms are often more severe, and the prognosis is less certain. In most cases clinical examination reveals the level of the disc hernia.

Hernias at the LV–SI level result in a limited straight leg raising test (SLR), with pain in the buttock lancing to the lateral aspect of the foot. The ankle reflex is often weakened or absent at the affected side. At the LIV–V level, pain radiates to the big toe and weakness of the great extensor is common; the SLR is positive. Patients with a LIII–IV hernia, affecting the LIV nerve, present with pain in the anterior aspect of the thigh, and the patellar tendon reflex is weakened or absent. The SLR is negative but the reverse SLR is positive: the patient is unable to lie prone without flexing his hip.

The level affected by disc herniation is lower in young men than in older men; the LIII–IV hernia rarely occurs in young or middle-aged men[4].

At present, MRI is the most valuable method of neuroradiological examination of disc hernias. However, the method results in a high number of false positives; therefore, a very close comparison of clinical signs and radiographic findings is necessary before surgery.

Treatment

Conservative treatment supported by increased physical activity (i.e. physiotherapy) is of importance in the less severe cases. The natural outcome is usually good: about 80% of cases are symptomless without surgery within 1 year. Patients with severe pain in combination with objective clinical and corresponding neuroradiological findings lasting for more than a month, without signs of improvement, are often good candidates for disc surgery. Patients having SLR less than 40–50° in combination with the above-mentioned clinical and neuroradiological criteria most often benefit from disc surgery, with a high rate of success. Emergency surgery of the degenerative lumbar spine is carried out in cases of cauda equina syndrome, usually caused by a LV–SI massive disc herniation. These patients present with bilateral sciatica and sensory deficit in the perineum, with sphincter dysfunction. The operation should be performed within 24–48 h after the onset of symptoms.

SPINAL STENOSIS

There are many different etiologies of spinal stenosis, but the most frequent is the degenerative type. Degenerative spinal stenosis may occur in the cervical, thoracic or lumbar spine. The lumbar type is by far the most common; cervical stenosis is infrequent and thoracic spinal stenosis is an extremely rare entity.

Disc degeneration is considered the first stage in the pathogenesis of this process in most cases[6]. When disc height is reduced, subluxation of the posterior facet joints results to a varying degree, and osteophytes are formed. These bony spurs can be directed into the spinal canal, or compress the passing nerve roots anterior to the intervertebral joint. Adding to this, a protruding degenerated disc, as well as a folded ligamentum flavum, further reduces the volume for a passing nerve root.

Diagnosis

The symptoms described by the patient are the most important key to diagnosis, since there are seldom any objective signs to be found on examination. The patient complains of a progressively reduced walking endurance, and upon sitting the pain goes away; he can ride a bicycle without problems. All activities with an extended back create pain and reduce function. The most important differential diagnosis is vascular claudication, but hip arthrosis must also be excluded. Radiographic degeneration is usually fairly obvious but, as previously mentioned, in some cases of degeneration the radiograph does not relate to the symptoms. Radiography has some value in cases of concomitant olisthesis. At present, MRI is the method of choice for neuroradiological diagnosis. On MRI a narrowing of the thecal sac is seen; nerve roots compressed in the foramen intervertebrale can be observed, giving important information before surgery.

Treatment

In moderate cases with modest dysfunction, non-steroidal anti-inflammatory drugs (NSAIDs) should be tried. If no significant improvement is obtained, surgery is often indicated, and is successful even in elderly men (< 85 years) without other health problems.

The surgical procedure usually includes a narrow laminectomy (the removal of the spinous processes and the medial parts of the laminae) at one or more levels, respecting the facet joints and their capsules. The passing nerve roots are then decompressed. In rare cases with obvious

segmental instability, a posterolateral fusion with or without segmental stabilization may also be indicated. About 75% of cases operated on benefit significantly from their surgery.

FRACTURES

After major trauma, all types of fracture with or without neurological deficit may occur; these are extremely rare, however, among elderly men. Low-energy trauma is the major cause of vertebral fractures in men over 50 years of age. The lifetime risk of having a spinal fracture in 45-year-old men is 8.6%, compared with 15.4% in women of the same age. The risk of spine fracture at the age of 80 years is 4.7% for men and 8.7% for women[7]. The prevalence of radiographic vertebral deformities, as a marker of vertebral osteoporosis, is equally frequent among men and women: 12% in both genders at the age of 50–79 years[8]. Clinically, the problem of vertebral fractures in the elderly is predominant among women.

Treatment

In simple wedge compression fractures the treatment is analgesics and early mobilization. Secondary prophylaxis with, for example, bisphosphonates is currently being investigated.

The odontoid fracture is a typical fracture in the elderly man, occurring perhaps after a fall. Symptoms are neck pain with restriction of motion. Almost all fractures of this type are without any neurological sign. Fracture of the base of the odontoid process is the most common[9]. Operation is recommended for men older than 50 years, using either anterior screw fixation of the odontoid process or posterior atlantoaxial fixation and fusion. Halovest treatment i.e. having a metallic ring or halo attached to the skull bone which is linked by metallic bars to a vest, is often very complicated in people older than 70 years.

Burst fractures of the lumbar spine seldom create neurological symptoms, and they can most often be treated conservatively with brace and analgesics; healing can be expected within 2–3 months. In elderly men, especially with concomitant steroid medication, any simple vertebral fracture may result in osteonecrosis of the vertebral body. The anterior part of the vertebral body becomes necrotic and disintegrated owing to infarction. Lumbar spine instability because of necrosis or other etiologies may, again, be followed by neurological deterioration. Operation is usually the only treatment to recommend.

INFLAMMATORY DISORDERS

Rheumatoid arthritis and ankylosing spondylitis also affect elderly men. The most common severe spinal manifestations are atlantoaxial instability in rheumatoid arthritis and kyphosis in ankylosing spondylitis. In the advanced stages, posterior atlantoaxial stabilization or spinal osteotomy, respectively, is recommended.

TUMORS

Primary spine tumors are very rare. However it has been estimated that more than 80% of patients with carcinoma will develop skeletal metastases (diagnosed by autopsy) before death[10]. Tumors in males that typically spread to the spine are cancers of the prostate gland, kidney and lung, but lymphoma and myeloma also often result in spinal metastases.

The first most common symptom is pain. Weakness, usually in the lower extremities, is the alarming symptom owing to compression of the spinal cord. Bowel and bladder dysfunction are also common at this stage. If not earlier, the patient now attends the emergency room. The treating physician should have an idea of the process of deterioration prior to this stage. In a study by Galasko and colleagues[11] it was shown that only a small percentage of patients with spinal instability due to malignancy were referred to appropriate specialists in a timely manner.

Diagnosis

History of a known tumor along with spine pain with or without neurological symptoms must arouse suspicion in the mind of the physician. Diagnostic tools are X-radiography, computed tomography and bone scan, but MRI is today the most important method for diagnosis.

Treatment

In radiosensitive tumors without evidence of great mechanical instability or spinal cord compression, radiotherapy or other oncological treatment is the first choice[12]. Patients with severe pain due to spinal instability and/or severe neurological deficit often gain great benefit from surgery, including decompression and stabilization. In cases with a life expectancy shorter than 3 months, patients seldom benefit from surgery; one exception is collapse of a single cervical vertebra, in which case surgical reconstruction results in low morbidity.

The current methods of stabilizing the spine include posterior multisegmental fixation with screws, hooks and rods. Anteriorly, vertebral body replacement with or without further stabilization may be performed, and sometimes the two approaches are used simultaneously.

References

1. Urban JPG. Nutrition of the intervertebral disc. *Clin Orthop* 1977;129:104–14
2. Boden SD, Davis DO, Dina TS, *et al.* Abnormal magnetic resonance scans of the lumbar spine in asymptomatic subjects. *J Bone Joint Surg (A)* 1990;72:403–8
3. Nachemson AL, ed. *Back Pain, Neck Pain.* Stockholm: The Swedish Council on Technology Assessment in Health Care, 2000
4. Spangfort EV. The lumbar disc herniation. A computer-aided analysis of 2504 operations. *Acta Orthop Scand* 1972;142(Suppl):1–95

5. Olmarker K, Rydevik B, Nordborg C. Autologous nucleus pulposus induces neurophysiologic and histologic changes in porcine cauda equina nerve roots. *Spine* 1993;18: 1425–32

6. Kirkaldy-Willis WH, Paine KWE, Cauchoix J, McIvor G. Lumbar spine stenosis. *Clin Orthop* 1974;99:30–50

7. Kanis JA, Johnell O, Oden A, *et al.* Long term risk of fracture in Malmo. *Osteoporosis Int* 2000;11:669–74

8. O'Neill TW, Falsenberg D, Varlow J, *et al.* The prevalence of vertebral deformity in European men and women: the European Vertebral Osteoporosis Study. *J Bone Miner Res* 1996;11:1010–18

9. Anderson LD, Alonzo RT. Fractures of the odontoid process of the axis. *J Bone Joint Surg (A)* 1974;56:1663–74

10. Abrams, *et al. Cancer* 1950;3:74–85

11. Galasko CSB, Norris HE, Crank S. Spinal instability secondary to metastatic cancer. *J Bone Joint Surg (A)* 2000;82A:570–6

12. Wannenmacher M, Eble MJ, Rieden K. Möglichkeiten und Wertigkeit der Strahlentherapie ossärer Metastasen. *Der Chirurg* 1992;63:923–30

45 Common foot problems in elderly men

Greta Dereymaeker, MD, PhD, and Jan Mievis, MD

HALLUX RIGIDUS

This is a painful affliction of the first meta-tarsophalangeal (MTP) joint associated with painful motion and proliferative bone, resulting in increased bulk about the joint and loss of dorsiflexion (Figure 1).

It is much more common in men than in women, and is probably the most common deformity of the forefoot in the elderly man.

Pathophysiology

It begins with changes in the articular cartilage of the MTP joint, especially the metatarsal head dorsally. This causes pain and swelling and synovitis about the joint. As this progresses, there is bony proliferation, particularly dorsal and dorsolateral. This ridge causes impingement between the base of the proximal phalanx and the metatarsal ridge, especially in dorsiflexion. The dorsiflexion movement is especially restricted and plantar flexion is painful owing to irritation of the extensor hallucis and digital nerves over the dorsal and lateral osteophytes. As cartilage degeneration persists, the joint space disappears, and the joint becomes more rigid and may eventually stiffen up completely. The overall alignment of the joint itself is rarely altered.

Risk factors

These include a square, flattened first metatarsal head; osteochondritis of the metatarsal head; a long first metatarsal or hallux; high position of the first metatarsal; a pronated or flat foot; intra-articular fractures; crush injury; and repetitive microtrauma due to, for example, soccer, gout or rheumatoid arthritis. It is hypothesized that most of these conditions place increased stress across the first MTP joint and predispose it to arthrosis.

Diagnosis

Clinically there is thickening about the first MTP joint, restriction of dorsiflexion and pain by forced dorsiflexion and plantar flexion. Radiographically there is degeneration of the first MTP joint. The lateral view shows dorsal osteophytes and, eventually, loose bodies in the joint. Anteroposterior radiographs show the extent of the lateral osteophyte and the remaining joint space. When gout is the under-lying cause, bone cysts are often present.

Treatment

Conservative treatment consists of non-steroidal anti-inflammatory drugs (NSAIDs)

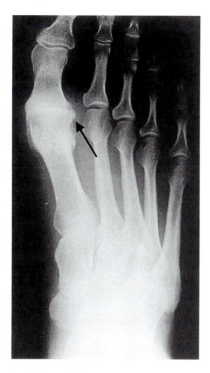

Figure 1 Hallux rigidus joint space narrowing: arrow indicates dorsolateral osteophytes

much destruction of the joint for a cheilectomy to be of use. This can be judged by radiographic examination, indicating virtually no remaining joint space. Arthroplasty (type Keller or Mayo) is chosen in low-demand patients. Arthroplasty using an implant is rarely indicated in men, as arthrodesis gives good results in up to 93% of cases.

GOUT

Gout has been known since antiquity, and is caused by an alteration in purine metabolism so that sodium urate crystals precipitate into the synovial fluid, resulting in an inflammatory reaction and periarticular destruction.

Gout occurs more frequently in men than in women, and about 50–75% of initial attacks involve the big toe, most often leading to hallux rigidus. Gout can also occur in the plantar fascia or Achilles tendon, and in any of the joints of the foot. The ankle joint is more afflicted than other hindfoot joints.

to diminish inflammation, a shoe of adequate size and an orthotic device, a rocker bar that stiffens the sole of the shoe to facilitate dorsiflexion, or an orthopedic insole. Intra-articular injection of a steroid may give temporary relief, but repeated injections can accelerate the process. Operative treatment should be considered if symptoms are sufficiently bothersome. There are several types of surgical technique. The technique used depends on the degree of deformity and subsequent pathological anatomical changes. For grades I and II, cheilectomy is the treatment of choice when the main problem is impingement against the dorsal osteophytes, and there is still enough, good quality, remaining cartilage. The cheilectomy removes the dorsal 20–30% of the metatarsal head. For grades III and IV an arthrodesis is usually indicated, when there is too

Diagnosis

The onset is sudden: the big toe joint becomes swollen and extremely painful. There is rubor, calor, dolor and tumor. The pain is not related to a static problem, and there will also be pain at rest or at night. Diagnosis is best made by identification of sodium urate crystals, but can be inferred on the basis of clinical examination. Biochemical examination of the serum uric acid level will most often confirm the clinical diagnosis.

Treatment

An attack is self-limiting but can recur. Medical therapy is necessary. Orthopedic treatment as suggested for hallux rigidus will support the medical treatment. If severe degeneration of the MTP joint is present, an arthrodesis of the MTP joint will be the final solution.

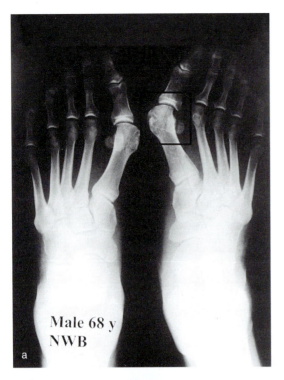

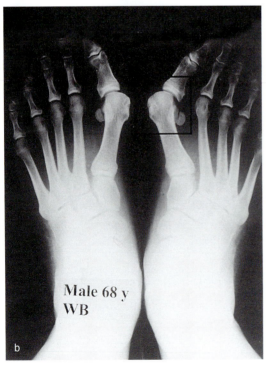

Figure 2 Severe hallux valgus deformity in 68-year-old man: (a) non-weight-bearing; (b) weight-bearing. Note aggravation of dislocation at metatarsophalangeal (MTP) joint

HALLUX VALGUS

This is a subluxation of the first MTP joint with lateral deviation of the big toe and medial deviation of the first metatarsal (Figure 2).

Hallux valgus is much more frequent in women than in men. In our out-patient clinic the ratio is 20 : 1.

Pathophysiology

The deformity occurs at the MTP and metatarsocuneiform joints. The most stable MTP joint is one with a flat surface, and the most unstable is one with a rounded head. The congruent MTP joint is more stable than an incongruent or subluxed joint. The setting of the metatarsocuneiform joint is also important for stability; for example, a horizontal setting tends to resist an increase in the intermetatarsal angle, whereas an oblique setting is less stable. The pathophysiology depends on the nature of the deformity. In the congruent joint, the basic deformity consists of an enlarged medial eminence. In the incongruent joint there is a progressive deformity with attenuation of the medial joint capsule and contracture of the lateral capsule. While this is occurring, the sesamoid sling, which is anchored laterally by the insertion of the adductor hallucis muscle, remains in place as the metatarsal head moves medially. The abductor hallucis muscle slides beneath the medially deviating metatarsal head, so there is loss of stabilization of the head by the intrinsic muscles, and, as the abductor hallucis rotates beneath the metatarsal head, it will rotate the proximal phalanx into pronation since it is connected to it proximally. The smaller toes are under increasing pressure as the hallux drifts laterally. Subluxation or dislocation of the other MTP joints can arise.

Risk factors

Hallux valgus occurs almost exclusively in people who wear shoes. Women wear 'less physiological' shoes than do men: higher heels put more stress on the hallux, as does a smaller toe-box. However, the fact remains that there are many people who wear fashionable shoes who do not develop a hallux valgus. So there must be predisposing intrinsic factors. These include heredity, pes planus, pes planovalgus, hyperpronated foot, metatarsus primus varus, hypermobility of the metatarsocuneiform joint, joint hyperelasticity, metatarsus adductus, and the setting of the MTP and metatarsocuneiform joints.

Diagnosis

Patients complain of a painful bunion, metatarsalgia caused by subluxation of the smaller MTP joints as the hallux drifts laterally, and calluses underneath the medial aspect of the first metatarsal head and smaller MTP joints. In elderly patients it is important to check the circulatory and sensory status of the foot preoperatively. If there is any doubt, a Doppler scan and transcutaneous oxygen measurement should be performed. Radiographs should be taken to see whether the joint is degenerative or not, and to define the degree of hallux valgus deformity and the position of the sesamoids and other MTP joints.

Treatment

Conservative treatment is to provide insoles; orthoses can relieve pain but fail to correct the deformity. Adequate shoes with a broad toe-box and without high heels put less stress on the hallux. If there is an associated pes planus a corrective custom-made insole is necessary.

Surgical treatment is the only way to treat and correct the hallux valgus deformity. There are various surgical techniques, depending upon the degree of deformity, degeneration of the joint, contracture of the soft tissue especially the lateral capsule, and associated smaller-toe deformities. In general, reconstructive surgical

procedures give good results. It is the aim of this surgery to realign the bony structures by osteotomy and to rebalance the muscular and soft tissues, while preserving the MTP joint for as long as possible. Once the deformity is too severe, the long-term results of reconstructive surgery will be less successful and the MTP joint will need to be fused to achieve a stable, pain-free forefoot.

In women, an overall success rate of 90% can be attained by surgery, especially with respect to recurrence of the deformity; in men this rate is only about 50%. It is not known why the results are worse in men than in women. However, men usually wait longer before seeking surgical treatment, as the hallux valgus deformity is not very painful or disabling in itself. It is the painful metatarsalgia or rigid, subluxating, hammer toes of the decompensated forefoot caused by very severe hallux valgus that will urge them to seek treatment.

HAMMER TOES

In a hammer toe there is a flexed proximal interphalangeal joint, an extended or flexed distal interphalangeal joint and an extended MTP joint. This deformity can range from a mild and easily correctable to a rigid and fixed deformity.

It is more frequent in women than in men.

Etiology

Shoes play an important role, especially pointed shoes and high-heeled shoes. This explains why hammer toes are among the most common deformities of the foot. The condition may also be caused by muscle imbalance in association with neuromuscular disorders such as cerebral palsy, Charcot–Marie–Tooth disease and myelodysplasia. Other causes are a contracture of the flexor tendon or insufficiency of the volar plate of the MTP joint.

Prevention

Adequate footwear should be sufficient.

Diagnosis

This is clinical. Painful callosities or hard corns will appear on the dorsal side of the proximal interphalangeal joint, underneath the MTP heads or at the tip of the toe. The rigidity of the flexion contracture must be evaluated as this is important for treatment, as is assessment of the alignment and stability of the MTP joint. Therefore, the patient should be examined while both sitting and standing. A flexible hammer toe can be passively corrected to a neutral position, whereas a rigid one cannot.

Treatment

Pain and rigidity will determine whether conservative or surgical treatment is indicated, as well as the specific surgical procedure needed. If the MTP joint is subluxed or dislocated, this deformity should be corrected simultaneously. Circulatory and sensory status must be checked. Risk factors such as diabetes must be ruled out.

Conservatively, it is most important to wear well-fitted shoes with a high, wide toe-box, a soft sole and soft upper portion of the toe-box; the shoe needs to be long enough and of laced-up type. Locally one can wear toe-caps. Insoles with a metatarsal arch support can relieve pressure. Daily stretching to keep the toes flexible should be started.

Surgery technique depends on the rigidity of the proximal interphalangeal joint and alignment of the MTP joint. It can consist of a flexor to extensor tendon transfer, extensor lengthening or tenotomy, proximal interphalangeal fusion in the rigid deformity and realignment of the MTP joint.

KERATOTIC DEFORMITIES OF THE SMALLER TOES

A corn is an accumulation of keratotic layers of epidermis over a bony prominence, such as medial or lateral phalangeal condyles or rigid proximal interphalangeal joints.

Etiology

The condition can result from extrinsic pressure from footwear. The lateral aspect of the fifth toe is the most common site of a hard corn. Limited joint mobility occuring in the elderly diabetic patient with neuropathy is certainly one of the risk factors.

Diagnosis

This is clinical. Most commonly the condition is found on the lateral aspect of the fifth toe, over the dorsal aspect of the distal interphalangeal or proximal interphalangeal joint or on the tip of a claw, hammer or mallet toe. 'Kissing' corns occur between two fairly rigid toes, especially between the first and second toes.

Treatment

Adequate footwear is important, which should be broad-toed, soft-soled and with a large toe-box. Local measures, for example using a pumice stone after bathing or a silicone toe-cap, can be helpful. Operative treatment is indicated whenever conservative treatment fails. Surgical procedures under local anesthesia such as partial condylectomy or Keller arthroplasty at the level of the fifth toe may be used to relieve the pressure and pain.

SUBCALCANEAL PAIN SYNDROME

This condition presents with pain in the region of the plantar tuberosity of the heel.

Subcalcaneal pain syndrome is more often seen in the aging man who is mildly obese, active in sports (running or jogging) or performing laboring work. No data exist regarding the frequency versus that in women. A static deformity such as a mild flat foot or cavus foot may always have been present without any previous complaints. A short Achilles tendon is often associated.

Pathophysiology

The pain has been attributed to pull of the plantar fascia, which may be associated with microtrauma to the plantar fascia near its attachment, leading to attempted repair and chronic inflammation. This syndrome has also been attributed to nerve entrapment, or irritation of the lateral calcaneal nerve or the nerve to the abductor digiti quinti.

A bony heel spur may occur as an osteophyte at the level of the medial plantar tuberosity or at the origin of the short-toe flexors but not in the plantar fascia. Heel spurs are noted in only about 50% of cases of subcalcaneal pain syndrome, and cannot be considered the etiology of the syndrome.

Diagnosis

The patient's history will indicate that the pain is along the medial plantar side of the foot at the bottom of the heel, starting at the tuberosity and spreading 3–5 cm distal in the plantar fascia. It is worse upon first arising in the morning, with some relief after a few steps. However, the pain may increase after prolonged activity. Periods of inactivity are usually followed by an increase in pain as activity is started again. Night pain is seldom present, unless there is an underlying inflammatory disease (gout or Bechterew).

Clinical examination indicates the type of foot, which is important because it influences the mechanics of the foot and thus the function of the plantar fascia. A flexible flat foot will place increased stress upon the origin of the plantar fascia and calcaneus with ambulation, to maintain a stable arch during gait. A cavus foot puts too much pressure on the heel and allows insufficient shock absorption. There is acute tenderness along the plantar medial side of the

calcaneus and/or distally 3–5 cm of the plantar pedis over the plantar ligament. The tarsal tunnel and sensory status of the foot must be checked. Subtalar and ankle joints should be examined for motion and/or painful mobility.

Radiographs will provide information about the osseous structures. Standing lateral radiographs will also give information about the biomechanics of the foot.

Ultrasound examination can confirm inflammation or lesions in the plantar fascia.

A technetium-99 bone scan will provide evidence of an inflammatory abnormality in this area. About 60% of patients show increased uptake at the plantar tuberosity of the calcaneus. A positive scan correlates with more severe heel pain and better response to local infiltration. A normal scan suggests a non-inflammatory lesion such as simple trauma or nerve entrapment.

Results of laboratory studies are most often normal. However, when the pain is bilateral or persistent and severe, a severe systemic disorder should be considered. Biological investigation with rheumatests, measurement of uric acid levels and HLA-B27 should be part of the work-up.

Treatment

This begins with relative rest, anti-inflammatory medication and use of an orthotic device. A custom-made insole with a deep, soft heel-cup and good support of the medial arch will cushion the heel and relieve pressure. Activities are restricted within the pain level. If a specific area is tender, one to three steroid injections may be given. It is important not to inject into the fat septa because this can cause fat necrosis and increased vulnerability to pressure periostitis. Physical therapy consists of stretching the plantar fascia and Achilles tendon, and strengthening and anti-inflammatory physiotherapy. A below-knee splint with the ankle at a right angle and the toes in 5–10° of dorsiflexion may be used to prevent contractures of the plantar fascia during the night. Immobilization in a plaster of Paris walking boot is used for 4 weeks if other measures fail. These conservative measures should be continued for 9–12 months. Ultra (extra) short wave therapy (ESWT) gives good results in about 60% of cases. Release of the plantar fascia is only done in patients who fail to respond to conservative measures; it gives good results in well-selected patients.

ACQUIRED FLAT FOOT

A flat foot can be congenital or acquired. This chapter discusses the acquired flat foot caused by posterior tibial tendon dysfunction, as this is still often under- or misdiagnosed. Other causes of a painful flat foot are arthrosis of the talonavicular or tarsometatarsal joints, post-trauma following Lisfranc, calcaneal or navicular fractures, neuromuscular disorders or rheumatoid arthritis.

Pathophysiology

The tibialis posterior (PT) is the most powerful inverter of the foot. Owing to the insertions of the PT on the midtarsal bones, applied muscle force moves these bones together, which makes the midfoot rigid. So when the PT is insufficient or lost, the ligaments on the medial side will gradually elongate. Causes of PT dysfunction are direct injury, pathological rupture, idiopathic rupture and PT dislocation.

Diagnosis

Patients present with pain, and will have noticed a gradual arch loss. In more chronic cases the medial pain may diminish in favor of lateral hindfoot and sinus tarsi pain. Fitting normal shoes becomes difficult. Secondary arthritis symptoms can arise.

The clinical examination will show that there is forefoot abduction and valgus of the hindfoot. The function of the PT is tested as follows. The patient is asked to rise on the toes on both feet (double heel rise) and on one foot (single heel rise). Failure or decreased calcaneal inversion on the involved side or incomplete rising up on one foot is a sign of PT dysfunction. Then, the insufficiency of the first metatarsal is assessed. The heel of the foot is taken with one hand and brought passively into varus. In a normal foot, the metatarsal remains on the ground and rises up in PT dysfunction. Finally the flat foot becomes rigid.

Among the imaging methods, magnetic resonance imaging (MRI) has become routine, but the clinical examination is more important. Nevertheless, a precise diagnosis cannot be made until the tendon has been exposed surgically.

Treatment

If the problem is synovitis or tendinitis, aggressive conservative treatment with cast immobilization and anti-inflammatory medication is indicated. If the problem is a long-standing rigid or supple foot, an orthotic device is necessary.

If conservative measures fail to relieve the synovitis, or if it tends to recur, early synovectomy of the tendon is indicated becaus otherwise the tendon will become non-functional.

OSTEOARTHRITIS

Osteoarthritis is a progressive breakdown of the joint cartilage due to aging or other factors such as trauma and rheumatoid arthritis (Figure 3).

Degenerative joint disease usually occurs in middle-aged and elderly men, but it can occur in younger people as the end stage of post-traumatic conditions or avascular necrosis. The most commonly affected sites in the foot are the first MTP joint, the tibiotalar joint (Figure 3), the talonavicular joint and the first metatarsocuneiform joint.

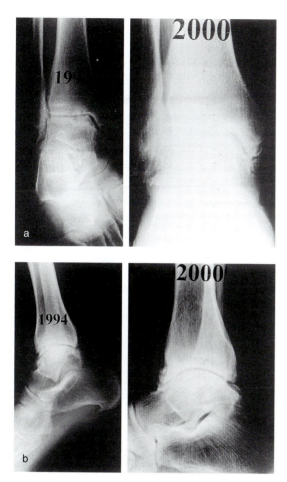

Figure 3 Tibiotalar arthrosis: (a) anteroposterior view; (b) lateral view

Pathophysiology

The degeneration of cartilage in aging men is described in a preceding chapter ('Joint disorders') by Leif Dahlberg.

Diagnosis

General symptoms are morning stiffness, with pain relief after a few steps and aggravation by prolonged walking and standing. Damp-weather ache is common. Swelling, locking and a feeling of giving way may also be present.

Clinically, the joint may be swollen, tender and warm. Motion of the joint is gradually more limited.

Radiographs show diminished joint space, bony proliferations, sclerotic joint margins and subchondral cyst formation (Figure 3).

Risk factors

These include trauma, avascular necrosis, obesity, occupational stress and excessive levels of physical activity.

Treatment

Conservative measures should be begun with stress reduction, anti-inflammatory medication, weight loss, and use of insoles or orthopedic shoes. Surgery should be considered when previous measures fail to relieve pain or when the deformity is not correctable with shoes. Depending on the joints involved, the age of the patient, the foot alignment and previous surgery, an arthrodesis or implant arthroplasty can be done. Arthrodesis at various joints of the foot has been proven to give good, long-lasting results. Recently there has been an increasing tendency towards implants, especially for the ankle joint, considering the better functional results.

ACHILLES TENDON DISORDERS

The etiology of muscle and tendon dysfunction is multifactorial. Upon aging, the connective tissue of the tendons loses quality. Dysfunction varies between peritendinitis, peritendinitis with tendinosis, tendinosis and, finally, tendon rupture. Peritendinitis is defined as an inflammatory process around tendons that possess no sheath, such as the Achilles tendon. Tendinosis points to a degenerative lesion in the tendon tissue, without alteration of the paratenon.

Diagnosis

There is pain, tenderness or swelling over or near to the tendon, most commonly about

5–6 cm above the attachment of the tendon onto the calcaneus. At first this is only after exercise, but as degeneration progresses, this will occur during and after walking, with morning stiffness and impairment of ability. A complete rupture is most often described as a 'pop', and sudden pain that diminishes after a few days. According to the literature, 20% of acute ruptures are missed by physicians. A good test to diagnose a complete rupture is the Thompson squeeze test, in which the patient is prone, and squeezing the calf muscle will not cause plantar flexion of the ankle as the Achilles tendon is ruptured. Sometimes some plantar flexion is maintained, because of the remaining plantar flexors. A gap in the tendon can be felt. If there is bilateral involvement, a systemic disorder should be considered, such as gout, rheumatoid arthritis or Bechterew disease, and also previous local injections, the use of steroids or anabolica, or previous trauma should be investigated. Sudden acute ruptures have recently been described with quinolone treatment.

Risk factors

These include cavus foot, trauma, excessive sport level, local injections, use of steroids, anabolica or some antibiotics, for example Tarivid®, and underlying systemic disease.

Radiographic examination

A complete rupture is a clinical diagnosis. When a peritendinitis or tendinosis is suspected, an ultrasound scan is the first-choice diagnostic tool to differentiate a peritendinitis from a pure tendinitis or a mucoid degeneration, and to indicate the extent of involvement. MRI is especially useful in differentiating inflammatory reactions about the tendon from degenerative changes affecting the structural integrity of the tendon itself. This differentiation is important

in athletes and does not influence the initial conservative treatment.

Treatment

This begins with NSAIDs, physiotherapy, stretching exercises, shock-absorbing heel-cups and heel rise, and immobilization if the other measures fail. Local injections with steroids should be avoided as this can cause ruptures. Peritendinous injections with anti-inflammatory products can be given in cases of peritendinitis. ESWT gives good results in tendinosis, but not in peritendinitis. Surgical treatment is indicated in the patient who has not responded to conservative measures. Surgery can consist of release of the tendon or removal of degenerative tissue. According to the amount of removed tissue, some type of reconstruc-tion of the tendon may be necessary. This gives good results in 70–90% of cases. There is controversy about the procedure to follow in complete acute ruptures. The present authors believe that it is better to repair the tendon, as we see few complications after surgery (especially using the percutaneous surgical technique) and there is less quadriceps waste and quicker functional recovery with a good postoperative regime. Except in cases of rheumatoid arthritis, or severe diabetes or skin problems, conservative treatment is recommended.

POLYNEUROPATHY

Polyneuropathy is a general term indicating a disorder of the peripheral nerves, of any cause.

Etiology

Polyneuropathy can be associated with systemic disease: diabetes, uremia, porphyria, vitamin deficiency, chronic liver disease, amyloidosis, malabsorption or carcinoma; or it can be associated with drugs and environmental factors: isoniazid, amiodarone, *cis*-platinum, hydralazine, vincristine, metronidazole, alcohol or inorganic lead.

Pathophysiology

The loss of protective sensation combined with microtrauma or repetitive trauma leads to skin damage, ulcerations and infections. Patients do not feel that something is wrong until they see or smell it. This can lead to tremendous infections, such as osteomyelitis. Autonomic neuropathy may also contribute to the evolution of Charcot feet, or deformities due to spontaneous fractures.

Diagnosis

When polyneuropathy is suspected, monofilament testing and electromyography should be performed. The foot is carefully inspected for ulcerations, micotic infections, static disorders and bony prominences, and circulatory status established. Radiographs are taken to give an idea of the biomechanical status of the foot and to locate prominences. When osteomyelitis is suspected, an MRI is more sensitive and results in earlier detection than a bone scan.

Treatment

When there is loss of sensation without ulcerations, protective insoles or orthopedic shoes are prescribed to diminish and divide pressure and to support the foot arch. If there are ulcerations, debridement needs to be done to give an idea of the extent and grade of the ulcer. Most important in the treatment of ulcers is to relieve pressure by use of a special temporary shoe, or by total contact casting. If there is a concomitant infection, intravenous antibiotics should be given. It is always important to check whether the vasculatory status is sufficient to promote healing. If not sufficient, vascular surgery may be necessary. Surgical treatment can consist of amputation, debridement, resection of bony prominences or arthrodesis in the case of rigid deformities.

Further reading

1. Dereymaeker G. Management of hallux valgus and metatarsalgia: a comparitive study of various surgical procedures for hallux valgus, based on clinical and radiographic assessment and gait analysis. PhD thesis, Leuven 1996
2. Myerson MS. *Adult acquired flatfoot deformity: treatment of dysfunction of the posterior tibial tendon.* American Academy of Orthopaedic Surgeons Instructional Course Lectures 46. Washington: AAOS, 1997:393–405
3. Rehart S, Peters A, Kerschbaumer F. Arthrodesis of the subtalar joint in adults. Indications, procedures, outcome. *Orthopade* 1999;28:770–7
4. Carden DG, Noble J, Chalmers J, *et al.* Rupture of the calcaneal tendon: early and late management. *J Bone Joint Surg Br* 1987;69:416–20
5. Deutsch AL, *et al.* MRI imaging and diagnostic ultrasound in the evaluation of Achilles tendon disorders. *Foot Ankle Clin* 1997;2:391
6. Hintermann B. Acquired flatfoot deformity associated with insufficiency of the posterior tibial tendon. BVOT, Namur 24 May 2000
7. Graham CE. Painful heel syndrome: rationale of diagnosis and treatment. *Foot Ankle* 1983; 3:261–7
8. Mann RA, Coughlin MJ. *Surgery of the Foot and Ankle*, 6th edn. 167–296
9. Asbury AK. Diseases of the peripheral nervous system. In *Harrison's Principles of Internal Medicine*, 12th edn. 2097–105
10. Sampson SP, Hung GL, Conti SE. The ankle, subtalar joint and surrounding tissues, Chapter 53. Miscellaneous disorders of the foot and ankle, Chapter 54. In Dee R. *Principles of Orthopaedic Practice*, 2nd edn. 985–1006, 1009–37
11. Mankin NOW, Buckwalter. Form and funtion of articular cartilage. Simon SR. *Orthopaedic Basic Science.* Washington: AAOS, 1900;1–43
12. European Instructional Course Lectures, Vol 4. 119–31
13. *Campbell's Operative Orthopaedics*, 9th edn.

Section X

Sensory organs

Frank Ondrey, MD, PhD

The special sense organs including the eye, ear, balance and the gustatory senses are important for achieving higher levels of quality of life when appropriately functioning. The function in all of these organs gradually decreases over time and it is important to take conservation measures to preserve maximal function as one ages. The ability for humans to age gracefully and with dignity is maximized when our special senses function well into advanced age.

46 Aging and the eye

Ali R. Djalilian, MD, and Hamid R. Djalilian, MD

INTRODUCTION

Visual function is an important determinant of the quality of life in older individuals. An older patient with visual impairment is at significantly greater risk for injuries and accidents[1]. Furthermore, loss of vision can lead to the loss of independence by losing the ability to drive and perform activities of daily living. Visually impaired patients may subsequently become depressed and socially isolated.

The incidence of visually significant eye diseases rises dramatically with increasing age. In the USA, the most common age-related conditions responsible for visual loss in the elderly are macular degeneration, glaucoma and cataract. This chapter deals primarily with these three visually significant disorders, although less threatening age-related conditions such as presbyopia, dry eyes and vitreous degeneration are also briefly discussed (Table 1)[2]. Diabetic retinopathy, which is another important cause of blindness in both older and younger patients, will not be discussed and the reader is referred to other excellent reviews[3].

PRESBYOPIA

One of the earliest signs of aging in the eye is loss of accommodation. This occurs universally and is manifested by the inability to focus at near distance. The person will initially try to compensate by holding reading material further from the eye, but eventually is no longer able to read fine print. The typical age of onset is 40–45 years, with progressive loss of accommodation continuing until the age of 60–65 years when essentially all accommodation is lost. Physiologically, presbyopia is thought to be due to the gradual hardening of the lens, which limits its flexibility. Specifically, the lens can no longer change its shape to increase its power,

Table 1 Typical age-related changes in the eye[2]

Structure	Age-related change
Eyelids	increased laxity, atrophy of orbit fat leading to enophthalmus, prolapse of orbital fat leading to dermatochalasis, levator dehiscence causing ptosis
Lacrimal gland	decreased tear production in part due to declining sex hormones
Cornea	arcus senilis (lipid deposit in peripheral cornea), gradual decrease in endothelial cells
Lens	gradual hardening leading to loss of accommodation, loss of clarity and increased yellowish color, increase in size (anterior–posterior diameter)
Vitreous gel	gradual condensation and collapse leading to posterior vitreous detachment, floaters
Retina	gradual decrease in number of photoreceptors and ganglion cells, accumulation of unmetabolized debris (drusen)

which is necessary for focusing on near objects. Although frustrating for the patient, presbyopia is benign, and readily treatable with the use of reading glasses or bifocals.

DRY EYES

Advancing age is associated with a physiological decrease in tear production. Dry eye symptoms are one of the most common ocular complaints in older patients. At least 10% of patients over the age of 65 develop some degree of symptoms related to dry eyes[4]. The most commonly reported symptoms are grittiness and foreign body sensation (like feeling sand in the eye). Other complaints may include burning, photophobia and intermittent blurry vision. Women are affected more often than men partly due to declining levels of sex hormones, which appear to be important for tear production[4,5]. Besides inadequate production, dry eye symptoms may also be due to increased evaporation of tears. Increased evaporation occurs typically when there is increased exposure (inadequate blink, or lid retraction) or insufficient oil film resulting from plugging of the meibomian glands (as in patients with blepharitis).

Moderate to severe dry eyes can be vision threatening. Autoimmune diseases such as Sjögren's syndrome can lead to immunological destruction of the lacrimal gland, as well as the salivary glands. Sjögren's syndrome can occur primarily, or secondary to collagen vascular diseases such as rheumatoid arthritis or lupus. Patients with severe tear deficiency are at risk for developing corneal ulcers, infections and perforations with ultimate loss of the eye.

Dry eyes are treated symptomatically with ocular lubricants. A number of preparations are available over the counter. Patients who require the use of artificial tears more than four times a day are best served by using preservative-free drops, which limits the toxicity due to the preservative. These patients may also benefit from occlusion of the punta,

using plugs or cauterization. Immunomodulatory therapy appears to be important for patients with inflammation associated with dry eyes. The role of hormonal therapy in dry eyes is currently under investigation[5,6].

VITREOUS DEGENERATION

The vitreous gel that normally fills the posterior cavity (Figure 1) gradually begins to liquefy in late middle-age. Functionally, degeneration of the vitreous has no effect on the eye, since the vitreous is primarily important during the development of the eye. In most people the vitreous continues to condense, and eventually separates posteriorly from the retina. This is known as a posterior vitreous detachment. Patients with vitreous condensation or detachment will frequently notice a few floaters, which represent opacities in the vitreous. While irritating to the patient, if stable and only a few in number, these vitreous floaters do not require any specific treatment beyond regular examination of the retina.

Occasionally, as the vitreous detaches from the retina it may cause a tear in the retina. Patients may experience a sudden increase in the number of floaters owing to hemorrhage from the tear. Traction on the retina by the vitreous can also cause the patient to experience light flashes. Any patient who experiences an increase in floaters or recurrent light flashes requires an urgent dilated examination of the retina, since untreated retinal tears can lead to the development of a retinal detachment. Most retinal tears can be treated readily with laser. Patients with high degrees of nearsightedness, family history of retinal detachment, or a history of eye surgery or trauma are at greater risk for developing such tears.

CATARACT

A cataract is by definition any opacity of the crystalline lens. It is the third most common

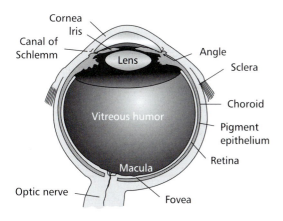

Figure 1 Schematic diagram of the human eye

cause of visual impairment among the elderly in the USA, and the leading cause of blindness worldwide. The incidence rises significantly with increasing age. The Framingham Study found a 17.6% incidence in people under the age of 65, 47.1% in 65–74 year olds and 73.3% in those older than 75 years[7,8]. In addition to age, exposure to ultraviolet light, smoking, low intake of antioxidants, medications (e.g. steroids) and systemic diseases (e.g. diabetes) are known risk factors for the development of cataracts. Decreased estrogen levels in females may also contribute to the development of age-related cataracts.

Diagnosis

In the early stages, cataracts do not cause any visual symptoms. However, as the lens opacity increases, there is a gradual decline in the visual acuity. Typically, in age-related cataracts the distance vision is affected more than the near vision. In addition to blurry vision, patients frequently complain of glare, especially in bright lights. Driving at night can become very difficult for some patients owing to scattering of the light from oncoming cars.

Diagnosis can be readily made by examination. Although the slit lamp is the standard tool for examining the lens, in the primary-care setting a direct ophthalmoscope may also be used to detect changes in the lens opacity.

Adequate visualization of the lens can be difficult in an undilated pupil. The most common finding is a yellowish discoloration of the lens. The view of the fundus is likewise degraded according to the degree of lens opacification. Patients with diabetes or a history of steroid use are prone to developing a posterior subcapsular cataract. These patients may see better under dim light, which allows the pupil to dilate.

Treatment

The treatment for a visually significant cataract is surgical removal. However, the timing of surgery depends mainly on the patient's lifestyle and the extent to which their vision prevents them from participating in their usual activities. For many patients, the ability to drive has the most significant impact on their decision. Before surgery, some of these patients may benefit from tinted glasses or an antireflective coating to reduce their glare symptoms from the cataract. Except in unusual situations, delaying cataract extraction generally does not put the eye at any significant risk.

The earlier techniques for cataract extraction involved removing the whole lens in one piece, which required a 10–12-mm incision. The latest techniques employ an incision which is only 3–4 mm in length, and the lens is fragmented into small pieces using ultrasound before it is aspirated from the eye (phacoemulsification). Unlike the earlier techniques, phacoemulsification does not require the cataract to be 'ripe', and surgery can be done any time the patient feels functionally impaired by the cataract. Placement of an intraocular lens is now a standard part of modern cataract surgery. Adequate anesthesia can be achieved in most patients with the use of only topical drops, although some patients or surgeons may prefer to have a retrobulbar or peribulbar injection. Using these latest techniques, cataract surgery has excellent visual results with low complication rates and minimal stress to the patient.

Although the visual impairment due to cataracts is treatable, life-style modifications may play an important role in preventing or delaying the onset of cataracts. These include the use of ultraviolet protection outdoors, adequate dietary intake of fruits and vegetables high in antioxidants, and avoiding smoking. In the USA, cataract is still an important cause of visual impairment either due to lack of access or because patients may consider their visual decline to be a natural part of aging. Primary-care physicians can make a significant difference by educating their patients, and ensuring that all aging patients receive regular eye examinations.

GLAUCOMA

Glaucoma is the second most common cause of blindness in the USA and the leading cause of blindness among African-Americans. Nearly 10% of African-Americans over age 70 have glaucoma, compared with 2–3% of Caucasians. Fewer than half of all patients with glaucoma in the USA have been diagnosed, and the rest are unaware of their disease[9]. Therefore, the role of primary-care physicians is of utmost importance in detecting and managing patients with glaucoma.

Normally, aqueous humor is produced by the ciliary body, which passes through the pupil and drains through the trabecular meshwork into Schlemm's canal (Figure 2). Any resistance to the outflow of aqueous through the trabecular meshwork can lead to increased intraocular pressure (IOP). This elevated pressure can be transmitted to the optic nerve, resulting in damage to the nerve fibers. The mechanism of this damage may be mechanical or ischemic, or programmed cell death.

Risk factors

The most important risk factors for the development of glaucoma are increased IOP, age, family history and race. Previously, an elevated IOP (> 22 mmHg) was thought to be a prerequisite for the diagnosis of glaucoma. It is

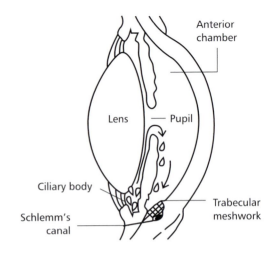

Figure 2 Schematic diagram of the anterior segment, demonstrating the flow of aqueous humor from the ciliary body to the trabecular meshwork

now known that a specific IOP cannot be relied on for the diagnosis of glaucoma. Generally, the range of IOP in 'normal' adult subjects is 10–22 (i.e. 95% of patients without glaucoma fall into this range). However, up to one-fifth of patients with glaucoma will have an IOP of less than 22 ('low tension glaucoma'). Likewise, many patients with an IOP of greater than 22 will never develop glaucoma[10]. Therefore, there is no cut-off pressure, and each patient will vary as to the pressure their eye can withstand. Nonetheless, the higher is the IOP the greater is the likelihood that the patient will have glaucoma. Similar to the case with blood pressure, patients are usually unaware and cannot feel the elevation in their IOP. The exception is when the IOP increases very suddenly (such as acute angle closure).

Age is also a consistent risk factor for development of glaucoma. The prevalence in patients under 40 is about 0.1%, while in those over the age of 70 it may be as high as 2–3%[11]. Racial differences are also striking, with African-Americans having a five times higher chance of developing glaucoma and losing vision, compared with Whites. Having a first-degree relative with glaucoma likewise increases the risk significantly. Hypertension, diabetes and myopia

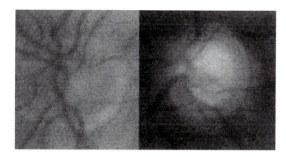

Figure 3 A normal optic nerve (left) from a patient with light pigmentation and a cup-to-disk ratio of 0.3. The optic nerve from an African-American patient with glaucoma and a cup-to-disk ratio of 0.75 (right)

(nearsightedness) have also been identified as associated risk factors for glaucoma.

Diagnosis

Besides intraocular pressure, the diagnosis of glaucoma relies heavily on examination of the optic nerve. One of the characteristic findings is an increase in the central depression (cup) of the optic nerve head (Figure 3). Although there is no absolute number, the risk of glaucoma is generally less when the cup-to-disk ratio is below 0.5 (i.e. the diameter of the cup is less than one-half the diameter of the disk). Actual progression in the cup-to-disk ratio over time is definitive evidence for the presence of glaucoma. Other optic nerve findings include vertical elongation or notching of the cup, thinning of the neural rim or displacement of vessels to the margin.

In addition to the optic nerve, examination of the visual field is an integral part of the diagnosis and the follow-up of glaucoma. The visual loss in glaucoma begins primarily in the periphery and progresses gradually towards the center. Thus, the patient may have significant damage from glaucoma and not realize it, because good central vision can be maintained until the final stages. Patients with severe field loss who have less than 20° remaining in their better eye are legally considered blind. These patients are at significant risk for accidental injuries. If untreated, most of these patients will eventually lose their central vision as well.

Classification

In general, glaucoma is classified into open angle and closed angle. Open angle refers to all cases in which the anterior chamber angle (between the iris and cornea) is open, and aqueous can readily reach the trabecular meshwork. In this case the resistance to outflow is within the structure of the trabecular meshwork. In closed-angle glaucoma, the peripheral iris has come forward to close the angle, and is preventing the flow of aqueous from reaching the trabecular meshwork. In the USA, more than 90% of cases are of the open-angle type. Closed-angle glaucoma can develop gradually (chronic) or acutely. In acute-angle closure, the initial event is usually pupillary block, whereby the aqueous cannot flow into the anterior chamber and is trapped behind the iris. This trapped aqueous then pushes the peripheral iris forward, which subsequently closes the angle (Figure 4). Patients will usually present with acute pain, redness and decreased vision. Since acute elevation of intraocular pressure may also cause nausea and vomiting, patients with angle closure have presented with clinical pictures that were mistakenly diagnosed as myocardial ischemia, or appendicitis. Patients with intermittent acute-angle closure may also complain of intermittent halos and blurriness, owing to edema of the cornea.

In patients with narrow angles, medications with anticholinergic or sympathomimetic effects (for example over-the-counter cold medications) can induce an attack of angle closure by causing the pupil to dilate. The warning label seen on many medications regarding patients with glaucoma refers only to this subset of patients with narrow angles, and otherwise the great majority of patients with open-angle glaucoma should have no problem with such medications. Asian patients and patients with hyperopia are most likely to have narrow angles. The risk of angle closure also increases with

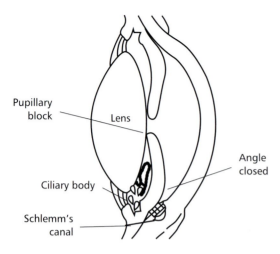

Figure 4 Schematic diagram of the anterior chamber in angle closure due to pupillary block. Aqueous humor is trapped behind the iris and pushes it forward to close the angle

age owing to enlargement of the lens in the anterior–posterior direction. In patients with a narrow angle, shining a pen-light parallel to the iris from the lateral side may cast a shadow on the medial iris.

Overall, acute-angle closure occurs very infrequently in Caucasians and African-Americans. When it does occur, the intraocular pressure should be lowered immediately with medications. The definitive treatment for acute-angle closure or markedly narrow angles is to create a bypass for the aqueous to reach the anterior chamber. This is commonly done in the clinic by making a hole in the peripheral iris using a laser (peripheral iridotomy).

Treatment

The medical treatment of glaucoma is currently aimed at lowering the intraocular pressure. Although this does not cure glaucoma, it can significantly slow the progression of the disease. Topical drops are the mainstay of treatment. The most important consideration for the primary-care physician is awareness of the potential systemic side-effects due to these medications. Currently, the most widely used

medications are beta-blockers such as timolol or levobunolol, which decrease the production of aqueous. Beta-blockers are actually the most likely drops to have significant systemic side-effects, including bronchospasm, bradycardia, depression and impotence. The other topical medications including alpha-adrenergic agonists (bromonidine (Alphagan®)), carbonic anhydrase inhibitors (dorzolamide (Trusopt®), brinzolamide (Azopt®)) and prostaglandin analogs (latanoprost (Xalatan®)) are much less likely to cause any significant systemic problems. Cholinergic agonsits (pilocarpine), which are used less frequently these days, may cause headaches and other cholinergic side-effects. Oral medications such as carbonic anhydrase inhibitors (acetazolamide (Diamox®)), methazolamide (Neptazane®) are not tolerated well by most patients and cannot be used for long-term therapy. In addition to malaise, anorexia and paresthesia, the use of oral carbonic anhydrase inhibitors may occasionally lead to the development of kidney stones.

When medical treatments fail to control the IOP adequately then surgical therapy is considered. Laser trabeculoplasty is an office procedure in which a laser is used to induce structural changes in the trabecular meshwork. In most patients this causes a mild to moderate reduction in the IOP, but the effect usually degrades over the course of several years. The most common surgical technique is a trabeculectomy, whereby a small section of the trabecular meshwork is removed in the operating room. The aqueous then drains through this hole and is collected in a 'bleb' under the conjunctiva, from where it is absorbed into the venous system. In most cases the trabeculectomy is done superiorly; thus, the fluid drains under the superior conjunctiva and is hidden by the upper lid. An important consideration in patients who have undergone a trabeculectomy is that any eye infection such as conjunctivitis should be treated aggressively (with topical antibiotics), given the risk of bacteria entering the eye through this hole and causing an endophthalmitis. An alternative technique to trabeculectomy is using a tube with one end in the anterior chamber and the other end (usually a plate) buried under the conjunctiva.

In patients with established glaucoma, severe loss of vision is rare if the condition is diagnosed early and the patient is compliant with the therapy. The most common reason for loss of vision due to glaucoma is not failure of therapy, but instead delay in the diagnosis. As mentioned earlier, nearly half of all the patients with glaucoma are unaware of their disease. Primary-care physicians play a critical role by referring patients for regular eye examinations, particularly those with risk factors including African-Americans and patients with a family history of glaucoma. In those with established glaucoma, one should remain aware of the side-effects from the medical therapy, while working to control disorders such as diabetes and hypertension that may potentially exacerbate the glaucoma through vascular problems.

MACULAR DEGENERATION

Age-related macular degeneration (AMD) is the leading cause of visual loss among Americans of age 65 or older. Its prevalence increases significantly with age. In a US population-based study, the incidence of late AMD was 0.1% among people 43–54 years old compared with 7.1% among those 75 years or older[12]. The most important risk factors identified besides age include family history, smoking, hypertension and low dietary intake of antioxidants. It is more common among white races, and probably more common among females. Increased exposure to sunlight, and having light-colored irises may also be potential risk factors.

The pathological basis of AMD is the gradual loss of function in the center of the retina, namely, the macula. The macular region includes the central foveal area, which provides the sharp visual acuity necessary for tasks such as reading, driving and recognizing faces (Figure 1). The primary cells affected by AMD appear to

be the retinal pigment epithelial cells, which are in close contact with the photoreceptors and are important for maintaining their health.

Diagnosis

Clinically, AMD can be divided into early and late stages. During the early stage, the visual acuity is relatively well maintained. The initial and most characteristic finding is the presence of drusen in the macula (Figure 5). Drusen are small yellow extracellular deposits of unmetabolized debris from retinal pigment epithelial cells. The prevalence of ophthalmoscopically identifiable drusen increases with age, especially after the sixth decade. Eyes without drusen are generally not considered to have AMD. Typically, drusen do not affect the vision significantly; however, larger and more extensive drusen seem to be associated with an increased risk of central visual acuity loss. In addition to drusen, pigment abnormalities are also a common sign of early AMD[13].

The late stage of AMD is divided into dry (atrophic) and wet (exudative) forms. The dry form, which represents 90% of cases, involves gradual loss and atrophy of retinal pigment epithelium and photoreceptors in the macular region. Patients experience a slow decline in their central vision. While in many cases a small area of central acuity may be relatively preserved, patients can still be functionally limited in their ability to read or drive owing to blind spots or distortions. Patients who develop 'geographic atrophy', involving the foveal region, experience more severe loss of vision.

Exudative or wet AMD represents only 10–15% of cases, but it accounts for more than 80% of cases with severe visual loss. The hallmark of the exudative form is the presence of neovascularization. The new blood vessels arise from the choroids and grow under the macula, and can cause leakage, hemorrhage and ultimately scarring (Figure 5). Compared with dry AMD, the visual loss is more acute and devastating. The symptoms noted by the patient may be

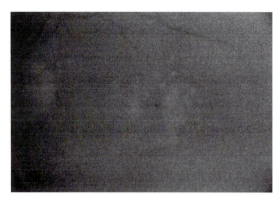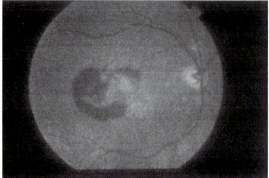

Figure 5   A patient with early macular degeneration demonstrating multiple drusen in the macula (left). A patient with exudative macular degeneration and hemorrhage due to neovascularization (right)

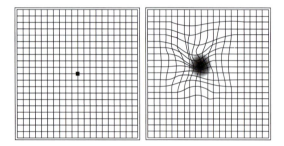

Figure 6   Amsler's grid as seen normally (left) and as seen by a patient with exudative macular degeneration (right)

distortions, whereby straight lines appear as curved, or the presence of a new blind spot. The use of a grid pattern (Amsler's grid) may help patients to recognize these changes earlier (Figure 6). Patients who develop these changes require urgent evaluation for possible treatment. If left untreated, many of these cases lead eventually to scarring of the macula with irreversible and severe loss of central vision.

Treatment

Unfortunately, at this time there is no effective treatment to prevent the development or the progression of AMD. The only therapies available are for patients with wet AMD. Laser photocoagulation, the gold standard, can be used in 10–15% of cases in which the neovascular lesions are small and well defined. However, recurrences are common after laser treatment.

Furthermore, in many cases where the neovascularization involves the fovea, the laser treatment actually destroys most or part of the patient's central vision. Therefore, laser treatment only benefits a small subset of patients with wet AMD. Many new treatments such as photodynamic therapy and transpupillary thermotherapy are under investigation for patients with exudative AMD. Likewise, surgical procedures such as submacular surgery and retinal translocation are also under study. These therapies are likely to provide some benefit to the majority of cases of exudative AMD that are currently untreatable[13].

At present there is no proven treatment for dry AMD. A number of observational studies have found an association between low dietary intake of foods containing antioxidants and the risk of developing AMD[14]. In other studies, lutein, zeaxanthin and zinc have been suggested to be protective against visual loss from AMD[15]. Currently, there are no definitive data proving or disproving that dietary supplement of vitamins or minerals can slow the progression of AMD. This subject is under investigation in the Age-Related Eye Disease Study sponsored by the National Eye Institute[16]. This study has enrolled 3640 patients 55–80 years old to study the clinical course of AMD as well as cataracts. It will attempt to identify factors that influence their development and progression, and evaluate the potential efficacy of high-dose vitamins and zinc in arresting or retarding their progression.

The natural history of AMD is not of relentless progression. While usually bilateral, it is frequently asymmetric with variable and unpredictable progression. Many patients experience only mild to moderate changes in their visual function. Patients with severe loss of central vision usually maintain their peripheral vision, which allows them to ambulate. All patients should be encouraged to seek low-vision services that can provide them with various aids and optical devices, along with training for visual rehabilitation.

A very important consideration for all physicians is to be aware of depression in patients with recent loss of vision from AMD. Losing the ability to drive and perform certain activities of daily living has a profound impact on the person's ability to function independently. Many patients will go through a period of grievance that may result in clinical depression. While most patients eventually learn to adjust to their visual impairment, they may require treatment for the depression in the meantime. The social and family support network plays a critical role in this adjustment process.

Currently, AMD remains a significant public-health problem. Controlling risk factors such as smoking and hypertension while encouraging diets high in fruits and vegetables are the primary preventive measures at this time. With advances in genetics and molecular biology, future treatments may provide the ability to institute preventive therapies long before the onset of the disease.

SUMMARY

Visual impairment is a significant problem in the elderly. At least one-third of all patients over the age of 65 have problems with their vision. The leading causes of blindness among older Americans are macular degeneration, glaucoma, cataract and diabetic retinopathy. More than half of the visual loss in these patients is preventable or treatable. Physicians can maximize their patients' quality of life by enquiring about their visual health, recommending regular eye examinations and referring those with decreased vision.

References

1. Ivers RG, Cummings RG, Mitchell P, Attebo K. Visual impairment and falls in older adults: the Blue Mountain Eye Study. *J Am Geriatr Soc* 1998;46:58–64
2. Faye EE, Stuen CS, eds. *The Aging Eye and Low Vision: a Study Guide for Physicians*, 2nd edn. New York: The Lighthouse Inc., 1995:7
3. Flynn HW, Smiddy WE, eds. *Diabetes and Ocular Disease. Past, Present, and Future Therapies.* Ophthalmology Monographs 14. The Foundation of the American Academy of Ophthalmology, San Francisco, California 2000
4. Schein OD, Munoz B, Tielsch JM, *et al.* Prevalence of dry eye among the elderly. *Am J Ophthalmol* 1997;124:723–8
5. Mathers WD, Stovall D, Lane JA, *et al.* Menopause and tear function: the influence of prolactin and sex hormones on human tear production. *Cornea* 1998;17:353–8
6. Nelson JD, Helms H, Fiscella R, *et al.* A new look at dry eye disease and its treatment. *Adv Ther* 2000;17:84–93
7. Lee DA, Higginbotham EJ, eds. *Clinical Guide to Comprehensive Ophthalmology*. New York: Thieme, 2000
8. Liebowitz HM, Kruege DE, Maunder LR, *et al.* The Framingham Eye Study Monograph: an ophthalmologic and epidemiologic study of cataract, glaucoma, diabetic retinopathy, macular degeneration and visual acuity in a general population of 2631 adults. *Surv Ophthalmol Suppl* 1980;24:335–610
9. Quigley HA. Open angle glaucoma. *N Engl J Med* 1993;328:1097–106

10. Leisgang TJ. Glaucoma: changing concepts and future directions. *Mayo Clin Proc* 1996; 71:689–94

11. Chaudhry I, Wong A. Recognizing glaucoma: a guide for the primary care physician. *Postgrad Med* 1996;99:247–64

12. Klein R, Klein BE, Linton KL. Prevalence of age related maculopathy. The Beaver Dam Eye Study. *Ophthalmology* 1992;99:933–43

13. Fine SL, Berger JW, Maguire MG, Ho AC. Drug therapy: age-related macular degeneration. *N Engl J Med* 2000;342:483–92

14. Mares-Perlman JA, Lyle BJ, Klein R, *et al*. Vitamin supplement use and incident cataracts in a population-based study. *Arch Ophthalmol* 2000;118:1556–63

15. Mares-Perlman JA, Klein R, Klein BE, *et al*. Association of zinc and antioxidant nutrients with age-related maculopathy. *Arch Ophthalmol* 1996;114:991–7

16. Age-related Eye Disease Study Research Group. The Age-Related Eye Disease Study: a clinical trial of zinc and anti-oxidants – AREDS report No 2. *J Nutr* 2000;130:1516S–19S

47 Aging and inner ear dysfunction

Emiro Caicedo, MD, Diego Preciado, MD, George Harris, BS and Frank Ondrey, MD, PhD

INTRODUCTION

As humans age, there is a gradual dysfunction of nearly all organ systems. It is said that communication is both what the message is and the manner in which it is interpreted. Hearing is a key part of this communication in man. However, cochlear dysfunction is often an overlooked entity which can seriously affect the quality of life as one ages. It is estimated by the National Institutes of Health (NIH) in the USA that between 40 and 50 million Americans will experience a disorder of communication during their lifetime, the vast majority of which is hearing loss. While not completely debilitating, hearing problems may result in fear, anxiety, and may also bring up feelings of one's own mortality and aging. This chapter is designed to give the physician a point of reference for diagnosis and treatment of hearing and balance disorders that are more common as one ages.

AUDITORY PERCEPTION AND COCHLEAR ANATOMY

Hearing relies upon several chief components to maintain quality of life in people of all ages. The ear has three basic parts: the external ear, the middle ear and the inner ear.

The external ear includes the pinna (or auricle), and the external auditory meatus (the auditory canal). The pinna has a limited function to direct sound into the auditory canal. The auditory canal curves somewhat upward, and is about 25 mm long. Inside the outer portion of the canal are modified sweat glands that secrete cerumen (wax), and small hairs line this portion. The inner portion of the canal is hairless and smooth, and is lined by portions of the temporal bone. The medial border of the auditory canal is the tympanic membrane (TM) at the annulus.

The TM marks the beginning of the middle ear. The middle ear is normally an air-filled space. Within the middle ear lie the ossicles: the malleus, the incus and the stapes. The last of these, the stapes, contacts the fluid-filled portion of the cochlea, via the oval window. The middle ear contacts the nasopharynx via the eustachian tube.

The inner ear contains the bony and membranous labyrinth, forming the cochlea and vestibule. The bony portion begins where the stapes contacts the vestibule via the oval window, the vestibule leads into the scala vestibuli, which spirals its way through the cochlea for $2\frac{3}{4}$ turns; it then passes through the helicotrema (where it begins to return back down the cochlea), and continues to spiral as the scala tympani, until it reaches the round window. The membranous portion of the cochlea is the cochlear duct (scala media), which is bordered by three structures: the basilar membrane, Reissner's membrane, and the stria vascularis. All three chambers (the scala vestibuli, scala media, and scala tympani) are filled with fluid. The scala vestibuli and the scala tympani are filled with perilymph. The components of perilymph are quite similar to cerebrospinal fluid. On the other hand, the scala media contains endolymph, which has a high K^+ concentration (145 mM) and a low Na^+ concentration (2 mM, similar to intracellular fluid). The stria vascularis is the blood and oxygen supply to the cochlea.

HEARING MECHANICS

When the TM is induced to move inward by sound waves reaching it from the surroundings, movement of the ossicles results in transduction of that wave into motion of the stapes footplate at the oval window. The fluid in the vestibule is displaced, resulting in a pressure wave that travels down the scala vestibuli, through the helicotrema, and continues to the scala tympani, where it displaces the round (cochlear) window. The resulting pressure wave is transmitted to the basilar membrane of the cochlea. The basilar membrane contacts both scalae and the organ of Corti. The organ of Corti is the means by which the oscillations of the basilar membrane result in mechanical displacement of the hair cells' stereocilia, which then either depolarizes or hyperpolarizes the hair cell. Depolarization of the hair cell results in firing of specific branches of the cochlear portion of the vestibulocochlear nerve (CN VIII). The displacement of the basilar membrane results in the movement of the organ of Corti, and with it the movement of the stereocilia of the inner and outer hair cells relative to the tectorial membrane. The stereocilia of the hair cells are not of one set length, but instead progressively lengthen, establishing an axis of polarization (a sense of direction). Simply put, when the stereocilia of the hair cell are deflected toward the taller stereocilia, the cell depolarizes and fires. When deflected away,

the cell hyperpolarizes. There are 15000 outer hair cells and 3500 inner hair cells. Most neural supply is to inner hair cells (usually multiple afferents per cell). The place theory of hearing states that the basilar membrane affects the organ of Corti differently at different places along the cochlea. It is possible to map the portion of the cochlea stimulated by different frequencies, from 20 Hz near the apex (wide region) to about 20 000 Hz near the base (narrow region).

The neural pathway for these signals is as follows: the hair cells in the cochlea synapse with cells of the spiral ganglion (located in the wall of the cochlea) and become the cochlear nerve. This portion of CN VIII may enter either the dorsal or ventral cochlear nucleus of the pons. Here the fibers synapse and head to either the contralateral side or directly ascend to the midbrain. In the midbrain, they synapse with the inferior colliculus, where they may cross via the commissural neurons, and head to the medial geniculate body, where they synapse again and follow the auditory radiations to the auditory center in the superior temporal gyrus, under the lateral fissure of the brain.

The vestibular (or balance) system is closely linked with the hearing system. The main organ of balance is the vestibular labyrinth. There are three canals, the superior, the posterior and the horizontal semicircular canals, and two otolith organs (the utricle and saccule). They are continuous with each other and are filled with endolymph, while they are surrounded by perilymph. The sensory epithelium of the semicircular canals contains a ridge in which hair cells are embedded. The vestibular branch of CN VIII innervates these hair cells. The stereocilia of the hair cells are embedded in a structure called the cupula, which moves when the head is experiencing angular acceleration in some plane, but because the cupula has the same specific gravity as the endolymph, it does not move in response to linear acceleration (like gravity). Instead the sensory epithelium in the otolith organs (the utricle and the saccule), called the macula utriculi and sacculi, have hair cells in a gel mass that contains many small stones of calcium carbonate. These stones increase the specific gravity of the epithelium, known as the otolithic membrane, and are responsive to linear acceleration.

CN VIII is responsible for carrying the information from these hair cells to the brain. The pathway is multileveled. Inputs from the semicircular canals travel in the vestibulocochlear nerve (the cell bodies are in the vestibular ganglion in the mastoid) to the vestibular nuclei in the floor of the fourth ventricle. There are four vestibular nuclei on each side: the superior, the inferior, the lateral and the medial, where the incoming neurons may synapse; other fibers continue to the cerebellum.

From the above description and redundancy of eighth nerve pathways in the brain, one quickly realizes that peripheral disorders of both the end organs (vestibule and cochlea) should be much more common than central disorders of hearing and balance from cortical or brainstem pathologies. Clearly this is the case. It is rare for central nervous system processes to manifest themselves as a simple hearing or balance problem[1].

OBJECTIVE TESTING OF HEARING FUNCTION

Audiometric testing

Formal audiometry in a sound booth is a part of the physical evaluation for any symptom referable to the ear including problems with hearing, tinnitus and imbalance. A basic understanding of the audiogram is most helpful for any caretakers of patients presenting otologic symptoms. An audiogram can be ordered by any physician and is performed by an audiologist with a masters or PhD degree in a hearing science that allows the individual to become licensed to administer complete audiograms. These facilities may be part of hospitals, clinics, or otolaryngology offices, or free standing. An overview of the basic portions of the audiogram is provided in this

section to assist non-otolaryngists with the basic interpretation of audiograms.

Components of an audiogram

The audiogram is arranged on a series of horizontal and vertical axes (Figure 1). The horizontal axes represent the threshold, in decibels (dB), that a pure tone is recognized by the examinee. The vertical axes represent the frequency, in Hz, that the tones are typically presented, from 125 to 8000 Hz. Tones are typically presented at the frequencies designated along the upper portion of the axes. Frequencies can be tested above 8000 Hz in special situations, but not routinely. Typically tones are presented at a reasonably high level at first, to help the patient recognize the sound of the tone, then they are presented at decreasing levels until the threshold value is reached for that frequency. The presentation level of each tone is varied in 5 dB increments until the patient's threshold is ascertained. The test/ retest reliability of this system is typically less than 15 dB variance. The speech frequencies most important for normal conversation are in the 500 to 4000 Hz range, and patients with deficits in this range will have conversational difficulties, particularly in noisy environments like restaurants. Hearing loss is typically rated as mild, moderate, severe and profound. Mild hearing loss is that which occurs from a 21–40 dB loss from the threshold. Losses greater than 40 dB but less than 60 are rated as moderate, severe from 61–80 dB, and profound losses are greater than 80 dB. Presenting tones accurately above 80 dB can be a challenge for some audiometers.

If there are abnormalities in the pure tones tested by air conduction testing, the audiologist will then screen the bone conduction thresholds to test for abnormalities in the conduction system to the cochlea. Air conduction thresholds may be in error for any reason that would affect the sound transmission through the ossicles. At the level of the external ear canal, plugging of the canal with cerumen or a

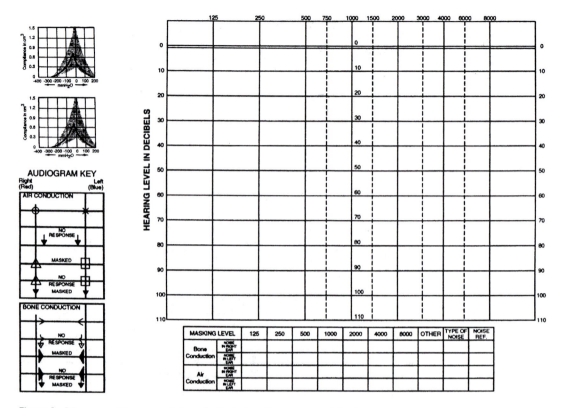

Figure 1 Diagrammatic representation of a typical audiogram report sheet

foreign body may affect perception. At the level of the TM, scarring, perforation or prior surgery are common reasons why air conduction may be affected. At the level of the middle ear, abnormalities of the ossicles including sclerosis, fibrosis, and trauma and disconnection may affect air conduction. In the middle ear, the presence of fluid or negative pressure are common causes of conductive hearing losses. Fixation of the stapes footplate to the oval window membrane, as observed in otosclerosis, will also affect conduction. This type of audiometric testing is performed with a microphone that sits directly over the mastoid air cells and transmits sound by bypassing the middle ear structures. A simpler screen for middle ear disturbances would be testing for sound lateralization with a Weber test with a 512 Hz tuning fork. Lateralization of the perceived sound to one ear when the vibrating

tuning fork is placed on the forehead will indicate a conductive loss in the ear to which the sound lateralizes. A Rinne test can then be followed up to examine whether bone conduction is greater than air conduction in the affected ear. Testing for conductive losses and severe asymmetric losses can be complicated by hearing the sound in the better functioning ear. The trained audiologist can compensate for these asymmetries by use of the technique of masking the better hearing ear. A discussion of masking is beyond the scope of this text.

Speech audiometry

A second form of testing that comprises a complete audiogram would be the testing of speech and word recognition. In this testing spondaic words are read to a patient at levels 25 dB above the average of 500, 1000, and 2000 Hz.

The level of presentation is modulated until a patient scores 50% of the words correctly. This would be the speech reception threshold. Next a standard word list consisting of 25 or 50 items is read to the patient at a level about 30 dB above the threshold, the items are then scored and a percentage of words repeated correctly is determined. If a significant asymmetry exists between the right and left ears (a 20% point or greater difference) the cause must be established, particularly if pure tone differences are small. Causes for this asymmetry could be retrocochlear lesions including acoustic neuroma.

Immitance audiometry

Tympanometry is the most common immitance measure utilized and is routinely tested. Typically a seal is developed over the ear canal and a pressure gradient from −400 to +200 kP of water is delivered during a 220 Hz tone. This test measures the volume of the ear canal and the compliance of the TM, as well as its integrity. It can therefore indicate negative pressure within the middle ear, scarring or perforations of the TM, or eustachian tube dysfunction. The tympanograms are classified as type A (normal), B (flat) or C (negative pressure)[2].

OTHER TESTS

Acoustic reflexes

A test is utilized on occasion to measure the phenomenon of loud sounds causing a reflex contraction of the stapedial muscle. Reflexes should be bilateral when the tone is presented to either ear. If they are absent then one may be experiencing a pathology of the eighth cranial nerve, like acoustic neuroma.

Auditory evoked potentials

This test has several names including acoustic brainstem response (ABR) and brainstem auditory evoked response (BAER). In this test tones are presented to the patient by ear canal microphone and then auditory thresholds are established from scalp electrode recordings similar to those used in electroencephalography (EEG). These tests are helpful when the patient cannot cooperate for standard testing. Additionally, they are highly sensitive measures for screening for acoustic neuromas.

Caveats in testing hearing function in the elderly

Typically hearing function decreases with age, therefore it is important for the audiologist to take the time necessary to establish accurate thresholds in patients who are experiencing decreased hearing as a function of their age. Additionally, the specialized tests, including the ABR, acoustic reflexes and some of the word discrimination tests, are less accurate when hearing levels and thresholds decline significantly.

SENSORINEURAL HEARING LOSS (SNHL)

In the aging patient, the cause of hearing loss is most frequently due to deterioration of peripheral and/or central auditory pathways. There is a relatively large differential diagnosis associated with sensorineural hearing loss (SNHL). Diseases from several categories can cause hearing loss and must be ruled out for optimal patient care. The most common causes are detailed within this chapter, but for reasons of developing a clear differential refer to Table 1.

Establishing causes of hearing loss

One must develop a clear differential diagnosis for hearing loss associated with aging. It is easy to attribute all hearing loss in males over fifty to presbycusis, but other diseases associated with hearing loss must be excluded. Therefore, a thorough history should be established.

Table 1 Causes of hearing loss

Category	Examples
Developmental/hereditary	Waardenburg's, Alport's, Usher's syndrome, Mondini deformity
Infectious	bacterial labrynthitis, herpes, cytomegalovirus, syphilis, Lyme disease
Toxicity	aminoglycosides, diuretics, salicylates, platinum
Trauma	head trauma, blast injury, noise, perilymph fistula, radiation
Neurologic	multiple sclerosis, vertebral basilar insufficiency, atherosclerosis
Immune	Cogan's syndrome, Wegener's granulomatosis, autoimmune inner ear disease
Bone disorders	Paget's disease, otosclerosis
Neoplasms	acoustic neuroma, meningioma, metastases, primary malignancy of temporal bone
Presbycusis	
Endolymphatic hydrops	
Sudden SNHL	

Important questions about the hearing loss would include the length of symptom onset, presence of tinnitus and its character, and any sudden or fluctuating changes in hearing or balance as well as any precipitating or associated events for the same. A past medical history of any diseases that would be associated with hearing loss including diabetes, thyroid dysfunction, atherosclerosis, immune diseases, or other metabolic disease (otosclerosis, Paget's disease) should be taken. A family history of hearing loss in parents or older relatives to establish a potential familial pattern of presbycusis onset and progression is often helpful. Further family history of syndromic and congenital diseases associated with loss of hearing should be questioned. Whether or not the patient experienced significant otitis media as a child or young adult and experienced some level of hearing dysfunction secondary to these infections should be established. A history of toxic medicine exposures including aminoglycoside antibiotics, cancer chemotherapy agents, trauma to the temporal bone, or previous otologic surgery as part of the medical history should be established. Clearly, occupational exposures in males over the age of fifty need to be established. Regulations for hearing conservation in the workplace are more recent developments and most workers in factories have experienced levels of industrial noise in excess of current guidelines. The use of power tools, rifle hunting, smoking, and combat noise exposure should be established as part of the social history. Once these items are clearly addressed, examination of the ear can proceed. Abnormalities of the pinna, ear canal, and TM may guide the physician to a diagnosis associated with any of a number of the conditions aforementioned. Once examination is concluded an audiogram should be performed. If a gradual sloping onset of symmetric hearing loss above 2 kHz is demonstrated with good discrimination scores, the patient likely has presbycusis, provided that the patient has described a gradual onset to his symptoms, and the TM is normal in appearance. Occasionally, a 'notch' is noted in the audiogram at a particular frequency and this may signify a significant noise induced loss at that frequency. Asymmetries in pure tone hearing, conductive hearing, and speech discrimination will require further work up to establish an underlying cause. Clearly an entity such as an acoustic tumor should not be missed because an unusual hearing loss was attributed to an entity such as combat noise exposure.

Presbycusis

Decreased hearing normally occurs as a function of aging. After the age of 40, the average threshold of the highest frequency speech sounds (4 kHz) is already beyond the normal range in the male population. At the age of 60, all of the speech frequencies demonstrate at

Table 2 Age adjusted normalized hearing thresholds for men at various frequencies

Mean age (years)	Hearing thresholds (dB) at the indicated frequency (kHz)			
	0.5	1.0	2.0	4.0
25	10	5	5	10
27.5	10	10	10	15
30	15	10	10	20
32.5	15	10	10	20
35	15	10	15	25
37.5	15	15	15	30
40	15	15	20	30
42.5	20	15	20	35
45	20	20	20	40
47.5	20	20	25	40
50	20	20	25	45
52.5	25	25	30	50
55	25	25	30	50
57.5	25	25	35	55
60	25	30	35	55
62.5	30	30	40	60
65	30	30	40	65
67.5	30	35	45	65
70	30	35	45	70
72.5	35	40	50	70
75	35	40	50	75
77.5	35	40	55	75
80	40	45	55	80
82.5	40	45	60	80
85	40	50	60	80
87.5	45	50	65	85
90	45	50	65	85

least a mild hearing loss, on average (Table 2). Typically, people develop compensation mechanisms so that communication is not affected as aging causes mild losses. The classic hearing complaint of an aging male patient would be that he is experiencing difficulty understanding conversation with females or children when in situations with a significant background noise (e.g. restaurant dining). At this point it would not be unusual for the affected individual to have abnormal auditory thresholds in the moderate to severe range at the frequencies associated with speech (0.5–4 kHz).

Presbycusis is the most common cause of hearing loss in the elderly population. Presbycusis is defined as the hearing loss that is caused by the degenerative changes of aging. These changes can be pathologically demonstrated in several areas of the cochlea and can involve hair cell loss neuronal loss and decreased blood supply through cochlear microvasculature. It is defined as SNHL that is usually symmetric and presents in patients over the age of 60. It is characterized by a slowly progressive hearing loss, which is worse at frequencies above 2000 Hz. Although the exact pathophysiology remains ill-defined, it appears to be a multifactorial process related to hereditary factors, diet, metabolism, noise exposure, and stress. It may also result from heart disease, high blood pressure, diabetic vascular conditions, or other circulatory problems involving perfusion of the nerve or any of the related structures, including the auditory centers in the brain, i.e. stroke[3,4]. Studies have failed to clearly link any of these factors individually to presbycusis.

Efforts to prevent presbycusis need to be investigated further.

Aural rehabilitation

Aural rehabilitation in the form of hearing aids helps most elderly people with presbycusis. Currently, there are numerous strategies under development for the further improvement of hearing aid technology. Typically, most hearing losses can now be treated with hearing aids that fit within the ear or ear canal. Many of these hearing aids also come in both digital and programmable variations that allow the end user to customize their aid for different listening environments. Certain strategies, such as opening the venting of the ear mold, and digitizing the signal, may be useful in selectively amplifying the high frequencies. If the hearing loss is profound enough to not be helped even with the most powerful hearing aid, cochlear implantation remains as an option. The passage of the 'Americans with Disabilities Act' has provided for enhanced quality of life for hearing impaired individuals with the addition of FM listening assistance devices for public gatherings at theaters, churches and public forums.

TINNITUS

Definition

Tinnitus (from the Latin *tinnire*, which means to ring or to tinkle) is the perceived sensation of sound in the absence of acoustic stimuli. Tinnitus is a manifestation of malfunction in the processing of auditory signals involving both perceptual and psychological components and should be differentiated from auditory hallucinations, which are considered to be a symptom of psychiatric or neurological disorders[5]. Auditory hallucinations are more complex sounds such as voices or music. An abnormal neural activity of the auditory pathway is erroneously interpreted as true sound by the central auditory system of the patient suffering from tinnitus. A majority of tinnitus cases can be related to cochlear dysfunction, which could involve central modifications[6].

Tinnitus is not a recent entity, it has been reported as early as 2500 BC in Egyptian papyri which refer to 'the treatment of the bewitched ear'[7]. Over 10% of the US population have a complaint of tinnitus. Approximately, 20% of these individuals relate their tinnitus as being severe enough to importantly decrease their quality of life. The age range of patients suffering tinnitus is between 40 and 80 years; however tinnitus may occur at any age. The prevalence of tinnitus has been shown to increase with age, and males and females are affected equally[8].

Causes of tinnitus

Various hypotheses have been studied as to mechanisms that could underlie tinnitus but none has yet to be determined. Researchers have tracked the origin of tinnitus using positron emission tomography (PET). They found activated sites in the temporal lobe opposite to the affected ear and unexpectedly they found that the hippocampus was activated too. This hippocampal activation could explain the adverse psychological effects that patients with tinnitus often experience[9]. When talking about tinnitus we must keep in mind that it is a symptom not an illness.

Some causes of tinnitus are[5]:

(1) Inner ear pathology associated with hearing impairment: noise induced hearing loss, presbycusis, Meniere's disease, etc.

(2) middle ear pathology often associated with hearing impairment: chronic suppurative otitis media, otosclerosis

(3) cerumen in the ear canal

(4) drug ingestion

(5) cardiovascular or neurological disorders

(6) emotional response to stimulus furthered by stress or depression, and

(7) neoplasm: acoustic neuroma, temporal lobe tumors.

Table 3 Causes of tinnitus[8]

Objective tinnitus
Clonic muscular contractions
   Tensor veli palatini muscle spasm
   Levator veli palatini muscle
   Tensor tympani muscle spasm
Patulous eustachian tube
Vascular disease
   Arterial bruits
      carotid stenosis
      high-riding carotid artery
      persistent stapedial artery
      vascular loop
Arteriovenous aneurysm
Arteriovenous fistula
Arteriovenous shunt
Bening intracranial hypertension
Carotid occlusive disease
Eagle's syndrome
Glomus tumor
Paget's disease
Venous hum
   Dehiscent jugular bulb

Subjective tinnitus
Acoustic neuroma
Anxiety
Autoimmune disease
   Arthritis
   Cervical spondylosis
   Multiple sclerosis
Bell's palsy
Chronic suppurative otitis media
Cranial nerve VII compression
Depression
Ear wax impaction
Foreign body in auditory external canal
Head trauma
Heavy metals
   Arsenic
High-output anemia
Hypertension
Iatrogenic secondary to ear surgery
Lyme disease
Metabolic
   Diabetes mellitus
   Hypothyroidism
   Hyperthyroidism
   Hyperlipidemia
   Trace metal deficiency
      copper
      iron
      zinc
   Vitamin deficiency
Middle ear cholesteatoma or inflammation
Noise-induced hearing loss
Otosclerosis

(continued)

Table 3 *(continued)*

Perilymph fistula
Pharmacologic agents
   Aminoglycoside antibiotics
   Antipsychotic drugs
   Aspirin and aspirin-containing compounds
   Carbamazepine
   Heterocyclic antidepressants
   Lithium
   Loop diuretic
   Non-steroidal anti-inflammatory drugs
   Quinine containing compounds
   Tetracycline antibiotics
Presbycusis
Temporal lobe neoplasms
Temporomandibular joint disorders

Classification

There are several ways to classify tinnitus. A common classification is objective versus subjective tinnitus. The objective tinnitus refers to a tinnitus that a physician can hear placing a stethoscope over the patient's external auditory canal or by placing his ear against the patient's ear. An identifiable cause is usually found when objective tinnitus is present. Consequently, a successful treatment will be implemented. Table 3 shows the causes of objective tinnitus. On the other hand subjective tinnitus cannot be heard by the physician. It is more common and less understood than objective tinnitus. Table 3 also lists the causal factors associated with subjective tinnitus[8]. Additionally, tinnitus can be classified in accordance with time of presentation. Chronic tinnitus lasts for more than three months without signs of spontaneously resolving. A distinction should be made between chronic tinnitus occurring after acute tinnitis and chronic tinnitus of insidious onset. Tinnitus sounds may be continuous or intermittent, fluctuating or non-fluctuating in loudness[10].

Patient evaluation

A complete history is necessary in the work-up of a patient with tinnitus. It is crucial to address age of onset and whether the tinnitus began gradually or suddenly. Characteristics of the tinnitus must be obtained. These include pitch (high or low), location of the tinnitus, pattern (continuous, intermittent or pulsatile), and intensity. Associated symptoms such as hearing loss, vertigo, aural fullness and otorrhea should be explored. Approximately one-third to one-half of patients seeking help for tinnitus are depressed. Mood disorders, especially major depression, are related to patients suffering tinnitus[8]. Consequently, tinnitus patients should be asked about depressive symptoms. Past medical history of cardiovascular, neurological and metabolic disorders (i.e. diabetes mellitus, hypothyroidism, hyperthyroidism, and hyperlipidemia) is important in the evaluation. Drug ingestion (acetyl salicylates and quinine) should be ruled out. An essential part of the history is the family history, past head trauma, previous ear surgery, prior ear infections, and an exposure to ototoxic drugs (e.g. aminoglycosides and loop diuretics).

A complete otoneurologic and head and neck examination must be done. Inspection of auricle, external auditory canal and tympanic membrane is important. Pneumatic otoscopy and tuning fork tests should be done. Auscultation of the mastoid tip, neck, ear, and skull needs to be performed. Neurological examination focusing on cranial nerves V, VII and VIII is crucial to detect acoustic neuroma in an early stage. All patients should have their blood pressure evaluated in both arms.

Audiometry should be performed on the patient to evaluate air and bone conduction and speech discrimination. If tinnitus is persistent and annoying the patient should be referred to an ear, nose and throat clinic, tinnitus clinic, or audiology department for further examination.

The information obtained by history, physical examination and initial tests will determine the next step in the patient's evaluation. Arteriogram, MR angiogram or transcranial Doppler should be ordered if a vascular abnormality is suspected. Patients with positive cranial nerve findings in the physical examination and complaints of unilateral constant tinnitus with progression to hearing loss and vertigo should be evaluated for a posterior fossa tumor by MRI. When medical or metabolic problems are suspected a battery of laboratory studies may be required. These studies include hematocrit, complete blood count, fasting blood glucose levels, thyroid function tests, a lipid battery and a serologic test for syphilis. Tinnitus is a symptom in chronic Lyme disease. Patients with suspected history of exposure to *Borrelia burgdorferi* should be tested for antibodies again this bacterium[5].

Management and Treatment

The treatment for tinnitus begins in primary practice with a thorough explanation of the basic physiology and psychological mechanisms involved in the perception of tinnitus. Patients have to be reassured of the benign nature of their problem. Patients who look for medical help are those who can not habituate to their tinnitus. Relevant examination and reassurance typically helps 80% of the patients referred to otolaryngology clinics. The patient has to be informed that there is no cure for tinnitus. First, any reversible otological or medical condition causing tinnitus should be treated. Second, an evaluation of medications the patient is taking is crucial, and an attempt is made to eliminate all agents known to produce tinnitus. Finally, there are three modalities to relieve tinnitus. Masking the tinnitus is one of the measures. Masking of tinnitus means that an external sound is applied to the ear, and the sound completely blocks out the tinnitus. Before masking the tinnitus, three important characteristics of it need to be investigated. These features are pitch and intensity of tinnitus and minimal masking levels. The masking can be performed by using hearing aids, tinnitus maskers or simple measures such as increasing background noise in the environment (i.e. radio). The second modality treatment is drug therapy. The pharmacological treatment of tinnitus has progressed little in the past few decades. Since 1937 the intravenous administration of local anesthetics has been used. Many studies have shown the benefit of using lignocaine but is of limited value due to its instability in vivo and the potentially life-threatening cardiac side-effects, as well as nausea, dizziness and parenthesis. Attempts using oral analogues have been unsuccessful (i.e. tocainide and mexiletene). Some studies have focused in the intratympanic instillation of local anaesthetics but this method of administration has not been shown to increase the number of positive responses and it is accompanied by extreme side effects that affect the vestibular system. The use of anxiolytics, sedatives and hypnotics are probably the most successful therapy in tinnitus. Nortriptyline was found to reduce tinnitus loudness, but the effect was more evident in patients that were depressed. Alprazolam a triazolo-benzodiazepine was reported to be effective in tinnitus, but the highly addictive features limits its clinical use[7].

Vasodilators have been used for treatment of tinnitus with the hypothesis that the increase in blood flow would result in increased oxygenation of peripheral and central auditory structures. Among these drugs are channel antagonists (i.e. nimodipine), B-histine which effectiveness is limited to Meniere's syndrome, and prostaglandin analogues as misoprostol. Ginkgo biloba an extract from the Chinese Maidenhair tree have shown vasodilator effects. This extract has been studied in different clinical trials that have failed to shown any particular efficacy[7,11].

Conclusion

Patients presenting with tinnitus need a thorough examination of current health, an otoaudiological examination and a psychological evaluation. It is important to give a clear explanation to the patient about their tinnitus. Patients should not just be told they will have to live with their tinnitus, although this is basically true, and the physician should spend more time reassuring the patient. Patients who are

depressed or have psychological problems should be identified as such and treated. All patients should be encouraged to join the American Tinnitus Association[8].

BALANCE DISORDERS

Dizziness, disequilibrium, and vertigo are common complaints in the elderly population. The sense of balance depends on a multitude of physiologic systems that need to function cohesively. Interaction of inputs from the vestibular, visual and proprioceptive systems is necessary to maintain a sense of orientation in space. Dizziness may result with impairment of any of these three systems. Therefore, thorough evaluations of visual, neurologic and musculo-skeletal status are necessary before diagnosing vestibular pathology as the source of dizziness. Cardiac dysfunction must also be investigated. Pure labyrinthine dysfunction rarely, if ever, causes syncope. Orthostatic side-effects should also be considered. Lightheadedness on standing is not typical of vestibular dysfunction. Despite the multiplicity of disease states that may cause dizziness in the elderly, a specific cause can be found in up to 85% of patients with appropriate evaluation and work-up[12].

Peripheral vestibular disorders are the most common cause of dizziness in the elderly. Up to 50% of aged patients complaining of disequilibrium have peripheral vestibular pathology. Peripheral vertigo is often distinguishable from central vertigo both on history and/or physical examination. Peripheral vertigo is often positional. It causes rotational nystagmus that has latency, is fatigable, and may be repressed by visual fixation. Central nystagmus more commonly is purely vertical, constant and not repressed by visual fixation. Furthermore, certain types of peripheral vestibular pathologies may be associated with SNHL. Table 4 lists common causes of central and peripheral vertigo in the elderly.

Benign positional paroxysmal vertigo (BPPV) is certainly one of the most common etiologies

Table 4 Common causes of central and peripheral vertigo in the elderly

Peripheral vertigo disorders	Central vertigo disorders
Meniere's disease	Stroke
Benign paroxysmal positional vertigo (BPPV)	Vertebrobasilar insufficiency
Ototoxicity	Intracranial tumors
Perilymphatic fistula	Multiple sclerosis
Vestibular neuronitis	Migraine
Acoustic neuroma	
Oscillopsia	
Temporal bone fracture/trauma	

of peripheral vertigo, even in the elderly. It is characterized by sudden attacks of vertigo precipitated by certain head positions. The attacks are prompted usually by moving the head to the right or left, or by looking upward. Classically, BPPV has been thought to be secondary to otolith deposits onto the cupula of the posterior semicircular canal. Therapy is aimed at redirecting these otoliths into the utricle via head turning treatments called 'Epley repositioning maneuvers'. Other causes of BPPV include previous head trauma, vascular occlusion and ear surgery. It may occur spontaneously in patients aged over 40 years. Other than Epley repositioning maneuvers treatment should consist of symptomatic control and reassurance as BPPV remits in the vast majority of cases.

Meniere's disease is another frequent cause of vertigo in the elderly. It is characterized by episodes of severe vertigo lasting hours, accompanied by aural fullness, hearing loss (typically low-frequency SNHL) and low-pitched tinnitus. The symptom complex occurs in concert and is fluctuating. The disorder is thought to occur secondary to increased pressure within the endolymphatic chamber, and is thus also named endolymphatic hydrops. Although the process is usually unilateral, the other side may become involved in about 15% of patients. The natural history of the disease is of complete remission in about 60% of patients.

Other causes of peripheral vertigo include perilymphatic fistula (PLF), vestibular neuronitis,

and oscillopsia. Patients with a PLF often have a history or preceding trauma or barotraumas. A sneeze or vigorous nose blowing may be the inciting event. PLFs are not typically age related. Vestibular neuronitis typically begins with a viral illness followed by a period of vertigo lasting up to 6 weeks. Severe attacks may last days to weeks. Again, vestibular neuronitis is not thought to be related specifically to aging. Finally, oscillopsia is also known as vestibular ataxia and is described as inability to maintain the horizon level while walking. It is secondary to severe bilateral vestibular dysfunction. It may also result from degeneration of vestibulo-proprioceptive interconnections.

Vestibular function testing is used to help in distinguishing central from peripheral pathologies and to quantify the degree of unilateral or bilateral vestibular dysfunction. Quantitative testing includes electronystagmograms (ENG), rotational testing and posturography. Results of vestibular testing are unfortunately not specific to a particular disorder or condition and are typically normal for patients with central vascular insufficiency or stroke. Also, in the elderly, caloric responses frequently show declines in response, making ENG testing somewhat less sensitive in this population. Often ENG testing is most useful in pinpointing a specific hypofunction in one of the labyrinths, which may guide rehabilitative, medical or surgical therapy. The specific vestibular disorder is not diagnosed with testing alone, but with a compilation of the findings obtained in the clinical history, physical examination and ancillary tests.

Treatment of the elderly patient with vertigo consists of medical, surgical and rehabilitative modalities. The treatment of peripheral vertigo is often the same in the elderly as it is in younger patients. It is important to note, however, that elderly patients have a more difficult time compensating to treatment when compared to younger patients.

Vestibular rehabilitation consists of exercises aimed at developing alternate balance mechanisms to compensate for the vestibular dysfunction. They are most useful in the setting of unilateral vestibular hypofunction. Alternative balance strategies include visual and proprioceptive inputs to stabilize the visual and postural environments. Many of these exercises were introduced by Cawthorne in the 1940s and remain as mainstays of vertigo treatment in the elderly.

Medical therapies mainly consist of vestibular suppressive therapies in the form of antihistamines (such as meclizine) and long-acting benzodiazepenes (such as diazepam). Often medical vestibular ablative therapy is tried when a unilateral vestibular pathology is diagnosed on ENG. Maintenance of balance sensation is easier for patients with unilateral vestibular input compared to disparate bilateral inputs secondary to hypofunction of one the vestibules. For this reason, therapy can be aimed at ablating the pathologic side. The level of hearing in the pathologic side must be taken into account prior to ablation. Recently, topical gentamicin in the middle ear has been used as a vestibulotoxic agent in order to wipe out pathologic vestibular function. Importantly, gentamicin may cause SNHL in about 10–20% of cases. If this risk of hearing loss is not acceptable to the patient, then alternate treatment therapies must be sought. Obviously, ablative therapy is simpler in cases where the hearing has been affected by the pathologic process.

Surgical management of the patient with vertigo is aimed at removing the vestibular input from the dysfunctional side in cases of unilateral vestibular dysfunction. If the hearing has not been affected by the disease process and is stable, then the procedure of choice is vestibular nerve section. Either a middle cranial fossa or occipital craniotomy approach is taken to identify the 7th and 8th nerve complex as it enters the internal acoustic meatus. The vestibular nerve fibers are identified and cut, leaving the cochlear fibers intact. If the hearing has been affected, then the entire labyrinth may be surgically removed, effectively destroying any residual cochlear or vestibular function.

It is important for elderly patients who have undergone these types of surgical ablative treatments to enroll in intensive rehabilitative programs in order to assist with compensation of vestibular function.

Finally, surgery should not be withheld in elderly patients solely on the basis of age if medical therapies have failed and progressive vestibular dysfunction has been identified. Persistent ataxia after treatment is common. Patients should be counseled to move slowly and deliberately, often with the assistance of canes or other devices. Ultimately, the goal of treatment of vertigo in the elderly should be directed at preventing falls, as these are a significant source of morbidities in the elderly[13]. Hip fractures are potential life-threatening complications of falls. Certainly, control of vestibular symptoms in the elderly should be directed at preventing these complications.

References

1. Cummings CW, Fredrickson JM, Harker LA, et al., eds. Ear and Cranial Base. In Otolaryngology Head and Neck Surgery, (vol 4). St. Louis: Mosby, 1993
2. Laufer W, Gabbay MS, Gold S, Katz J, eds. Handbook of Clinical Audiology, 4th edn. Philadelphia: Lippincott, Williams and Wilkins, 1994
3. Shuknecht HF. Pathology of the Ear, 2nd edn. Philadelphia: Lea and Febiger, 1993
4. Schuknecht HF. Further observations on the pathology of presbycusis. Arch Otolaryngol 1964;80:369–75
5. Vesterager V. Fortnightly review: tinnitus – investigation and management. Br Med J 1997; 314:728
6. Norena A, Cransac H, Chery-Croze S. Towards an objectification by classification of tinnitus. Clin Neurophysiol 1999;110:666–75

7. Simpson JJ, Davies WE. Recent advances in the pharmacological treatment of tinnitus. *Trends Pharmacol Sci* 1999;20:12–18

8. Peifer KJ, Rosen GP, Rubin AM. Tinnitus, etiologia and management. *Clin Geriatr Med* 1999;15:193–204

9. Voelker R. Tracking tinnitus. *J Am Med Assoc* 1998;279:574

10. Erlandsson SI, Hallberg LR-M. Prediction of quality of life in patients with tinnitus. *Br J Audiology* 2000;34:11–20

11. Drew S, Davies E. Effectiveness of Ginkgo biloba in treating tinnitus: double blind, placebo-controlled trial. *Br Med J* 2001;322:73–5

12. Koopmann CF, Goldestein JC. Geriatrics otolaryngology. In Johnson JT, Blitzer A, Ossoff R, Thomas JR, eds. *Instructional courses. American Academy of Otolaryngology – Head and Neck Surgery*. St. Louis: Mosby, 1988:21–26

13. Rubenstein LZ, Robins AS, Schulman BL, *et al*. Falls and instability in the elderly. *J Am Geriatr Soc* 1988;36:266–75

48 Smell and taste

Weiru Shao, MD, and Frank Ondrey, MD, PhD

The chemical sensation of food, smoke and dangerous fumes play an important role in our daily life, nutrition and survival. Olfactory and gustatory dysfunction is associated with a broad range of common diseases and anomalies, including Alzheimer's and Parkinson's diseases. In addition, taste and smell show physiologic deterioration as part of the natural aging process. Physicians treat thousands of patients every year for taste and smell dysfunction. For patients such as cooks, professional food and wine tasters, firemen, natural gas workers, chemists and many industrial workers, livelihood or immediate safety is dependent upon a normal gustatory and olfactory function[1,2]. Treating gustatory and olfactory dysfunction should be a priority for these patients. In this chapter, the anatomy, physiology, pathology, evaluation and treatment of taste and smell complaints common to primary-care offices are presented.

OLFACTION

Anatomy and physiology

The olfactory epithelium is located high in the nasal vault with an area of 2–10 cm². It covers the majority of the cribriform plate and superior septum, and some of the superior turbinates. It is a pseudostratified columnar epithelium and consists of olfactory receptor cells, supporting cells, basal cells and Bowman's glands (the primary source of olfactory mucus)[3].

The basal cells are small stem cells in contact with the underlying basement membrane. They have a unique propensity to regenerate into olfactory receptor cells and supporting cells after their damage[4].

Odorants, most of which are hydrophobic, dissolve and bind to odorant binding proteins in the olfactory mucus. The bipolar olfactory receptor cells project cilia to the mucosa, which dramatically increases the surface area of the olfactory epithelium. The odorant–protein complexes then bind to special receptors located primarily on the cilia, leading to action-potential firing of the receptor cells. These receptor cells are first-order neurons that send unmyelinated axons directly into the cranial cavity without synapse. Viruses and toxins may invade the central nervous system directly through these conduits of nerve fibers[4].

The axons of olfactory receptor cells penetrate through small perforations in the cribriform plate of the ethmoid bone to the olfactory bulb (Figure 1), where they synapse with dendrites of second-order neurons such as mitral cells and tufted cells in intricate microscopic structures called 'glomeruli'[3]. About 15 000 olfactory receptor cells converge on one mitral cell or tufted cell in one glomerulus. Numerous periglomerular cells, granular cells and short axon cells interconnect the glomeruli. Consequently, caudal projection of the olfactory signal becomes divergent. Unlike the visual and somatosensory systems, the olfactory system does not demonstrate point-to-point accuracy[5].

The myelinated axons of mitral or tufted cells form the olfactory tract that gives off medial, intermediate and lateral striae. The medial stria projects to the anterior olfactory nucleus, olfactory tubercle, perpiriform cortex and amygdala – part of the limbic system which processes emotion and memory. Through the lateral stria, olfactory information researches the hypothalamus, which controls appetite. The intermediate stria projects to the intermediate olfactory area. Its role in olfactory perception is probably insignificant in the human[6,7].

Pungency is generally not regarded as a smell, but a different sense related to nociception. It is mediated by the trigeminal nerve, and has a threshold much higher than that of normal smell[8,9]. It has its use in the evaluation of olfaction.

Olfactory disorders

The National Institute on Deafness and Other Communication Disorders estimated that more than 2.7 million adults in the USA (1.4% of the population) have chronic olfactory impairment[10]. The most common cited impairments were of ability to detect spoiled food, gas leaks or smoke, and in eating and cooking.

Major olfactory disorders include the following: anosmia (absence of smell), hyposmia (diminished smell sensitivity), dysosmia (distorted smell perception), hyperosmia (abnormally acute smell function) and phantosmia (olfactory hallucination).

The most frequent complaints seen in a primary-care office are anosmia and hyposmia. The etiologies include a multitude of causes (Table 1) or occur as a consequence of normal aging. In diagnosing olfactory disorders, it helps to consider two major categories: conductive vs. sensorineural loss[4]. In conductive loss, the access of olfactory stimuli to the olfactory epithelium is obstructed by conditions such as nasal polyps, thickened or excessive mucus overlying the epithelium, edema within the epithelium due to nasal or paranasal sinus disease, severe septal

Table 1 Medical conditions that affect smell

Nervous
Korsakoff's syndrome
Parkinson's disease
Head trauma
Multiple sclerosis
Intranasal tumors

Endocrine
Adrenal cortical insufficiency
Primary amenorrhea
Pseudohypoparathyroidism
Cushing's syndrome
Hypothyroidism
Diabetes mellitus
Gonadal dysgenesis (Turner's syndrome)
Hypogonadotropic hypogonadism
  (Kallman's syndrome)

Nutritional
Vitamin B_{12} deficiency
Chronic renal failure
Liver disease including cirrhosis

Local
Allergic rhinitis and atopy
Bronchial asthma
Leprosy
Ozena
Sinusitis and polyposis
Sjögren's syndrome

Other
Familial (genetic)
Laryngectomy
Olfactory sarcoidosis

deviation, intranasal tumors, lack of airflow by laryngectomy and others. In sensorineural loss, lesions are located proximal to the olfactory receptor cells. They may include loss of receptor cells from viral invasion, shear injury of receptor cell axons as they penetrate the cribriform plate in head trauma, intracranial mass lesion, environmental and industrial pollutant to the receptor epithelium, radiation injury and so on. Other causes such as adverse drug effects, nutritional deficits, and central nervous system (CNS) degenerative and congenital diseases are often overlooked during the diagnostic work-up[4].

In many cases, there is a combination of conductive and sensorineural losses, as blockage of olfactory stimuli to the receptor cells and damage to the central elements of the olfactory pathway can be presented at the same time.

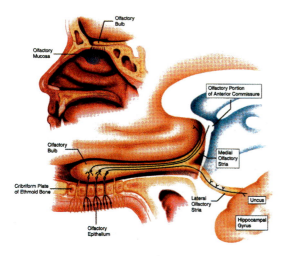

Figure 1 Olfactory pathway. Figure adapted permission from reference 21

Table 2 Examples of medications that affect olfaction[13]

Local anesthetic	cocaine hydrochloride
Antihypertensives	nifedipine, diltiazem, propranolol
Antimicrobials	clarithromycin, ciprofloxacin, ampicillin
Antithyroids	carbimazole, thiouracil
Opiates	codeine, morphine
Antidepressants	amitriptyline, clozapine
Sympathomimetics	amphetamines
Amebicides and anthelmintics	metronidazole, nizidazole
Immunosuppressants	methotrexate, azathioprine
Antirheumatics	gold, colchicine, allopurinol
Antihistamines	loratadine, pseudoephedrine

Nevertheless, the utility in the two diagnostic categories is that we are able to treat many conductive losses, yet the majority of sensorineural losses remain at present untreatable[4]. According to a study of 750 consecutive patients at a major smell and taste center, upper respiratory infection, head trauma, and nasal and paranasal sinus disease account for 60% of cases[11].

Upper respiratory infection

Upper respiratory infection (URI) is one of the most common causes of temporary hyposmia and, rarely, anosmia. Inflammation from URI causes edema in and around the olfactory cleft, and blocks olfactory stimuli from binding to the olfactory receptors. Symptoms typically resolve or lessen in 3–5 days[4]. However, a small group of patients, mostly middle-aged and healthy women, have persistent symptoms. Possible culprits have been suggested to include viral invasion and destruction of the olfactory fibers and other central olfactory components[3]. Only one-third of these patients recover after a number of years[12].

Nasal and paranasal sinus disease

The airstream that carries olfactory stimuli to the olfactory epithelium has been shown to be medial to the anterior portion of the middle turbinate. Because of its close proximity to the anterior ethmoid sinus, the site most prone to sinusitis, anatomical changes in this area such as mucosal swelling and polyposis from chronic infectious or allergic sinusitis can impair olfaction. The progression of symptoms is usually gradual, and prognosis is good if the underlying condition is treated. Relief with a 1–2-week course of oral steroids is diagnostic as well as therapeutic[3].

Medication

Drugs – oral, intravenous or topical – have all been reported to cause olfactory dysfunction (Table 2)[13]. The possible mechanisms are diverse, and may involve altered receptor site binding, diminished cellular renewal at the olfactory epithelium, change of neurotransduction and general CNS toxicity. Sometimes it is almost impossible to differentiate drug effects from the concomitant medical illness that the medication is taken for. Overall, only a small group of patients complain of these olfactory-drug adverse effects, which can be temporary or permanent[3]. Discontinuing the offending medication and changing to another kind may be helpful.

Medical disease

Adrenal insufficiency, hypophyseal insufficiency, hypothyroidism and uremia all affect receptor cell turnover rate, and have all been associated with olfactory dysfunction. Niacin and zinc deficiency can have a similar effect[3]. Intranasal neoplasms, such as inverted papilloma, squamous cell carcinoma, adenocarcinoma and olfactory neuroblastoma may obstruct the olfactory airflow. Intracranial meningiomas, pituitary adenomas and gliomas may cause local neuro-destruction[4]. Approximately 25% of temporal lobe tumors produce an olfactory disturbance[3].

Laryngectomy and other iatrogenic cause

Total laryngectomy results in breathing through a cervical stoma, bypassing the upper airway. The lack of nasal airflow and, hence, lack of intranasal odorants cause a decrease in olfactory perception[3]. It also diminishes retronasal airflow behind the soft palate, reducing the many so-called tastes that are actually smelled, such as chocolate, coffee, tea and meat[8]. Previous nasal and paranasal surgery can affect olfaction by nasal airway obstruction with postoperative adhesions, direct trauma to the olfactory epithelium and axonal damage by cribriform plate fracture[3].

Head trauma

The severity of head injury correlates with olfactory loss, although even minor trauma can produce total anosmia. The mechanism involves shearing of the olfactory receptor axons as they penetrate the cribriform plate. As the body heals over time, the perforations in the cribriform plate may be scarred, which prevents regenerating axons from reaching the olfactory bulb to reinnervate[8,14]. Frontal blows frequently result in olfactory loss; but occipital blows, in themselves less common, are five times more likely to result in total anosmia[12], possibly by a contra-coup mechanism. Olfactory loss is usually immediate, and recovery occurs in less than 10% of patients.

Major recovery, if there is any, usually starts within 3 months and occurs within 6 months. Amnesia following head trauma for more than 24 h indicates poor prognosis[15].

Environmental exposure

Both direct and passive smoking are associated with olfactory loss[16]. The unique exposure of olfactory receptors to the external environment renders them vulnerable to inhaled chemicals. Physiological and anatomical damages, even modification of neurotransmitter levels, can be induced by brief or prolonged exposure to pollutants[14,16].

Congenital

Children begin to discern odors, tastes and pungency at around age 8. Congenital anosmia can be partial to a particular chemical or complete as pan-anosmic. Females are twice as likely as males to be affected. Kallman's syndrome is associated with olfactory bulb ageneis and hypogonadotropic hypogonadism[17]. Congenital anosmia is also associated with Turner's syndrome, premature baldness and vascular headaches in some patients. These patients have been reported to avoid fragrance for fear of overuse[18]. The diagnosis is by exclusion[18].

Psychiatric

In 'olfactory reference syndrome' the patient is so obsessively concerned with minor bodily smell that she/he baths frequently and overuses perfume. Patients with 'Marcel Proust syndrome' often dramatically conjure up memories of odors which interfere with daily routines[3]. In addition, disturbance of the limbic to hypothalamic pathways in depressive states may also lead to olfactory dysfunction[19]. On the other hand, dysfunction itself may affect patients psychologically, as those with dysosmia and dysgeusia are 1.5 times more prone to depression using the Beck Depression Inventory scoring system[10,20].

Neurodegeneration and aging

It has been found that more than 75% of people over the age of 80 have major difficulty detecting and identifying odors[21]. Yet patients with Alzheimer's disease score lower on olfactory tests than do age-matched controls, even when mild levels of dementia are taken into account[22,23]. The presence of relatively high levels of neuritic plaques and neurofibrillary tangles has been noted in olfactory pathways, including the anterior olfactory nucleus, olfactory bulb, prepiriform cortex, prefrontal cortex and the dorsomedial thalamic nucleus. It has been suggested that olfactory dysfunction is among the first signs of Alzheimer's disease[23].

In Parkinson's disease, olfactory dysfunction is also found early in its development. But the dysfunction is unrelated to neurological signs, disease stage or duration[20]. Anosmia is rare in multiple sclerosis[24].

GUSTATION

Anatomy and physiology

The sensation of taste begins with the presentation of a taste stimulus to taste buds that are scattered primarily on the dorsal surface of the tongue, lateral tongue margin and base of the tongue. Taste buds are also found on the soft palate, pharynx, larynx, epiglottis, uvula and upper third of the esophagus. Food stimulates taste buds during chewing and swallowing, and while being pressed on the palate by the tongue[21].

Taste buds are ovoid clusters of receptor cells, supporting cells and precursor cells arranged in segments like those of an orange. Taste receptor cells have a limited life span of around 10 days[1]. They are susceptible to malnutrition, radiation and medications that impair cell renewal[25]. Lingual taste buds are found in taste papillae, which give the tongue its bumpy appearance.

There are four kinds of taste papillae: filiform, fungiform, foliate and circumvallate. The filiform papillae are the most numerous, but they have little role in the human's sense of taste. The fungiform papillae are located mostly on the tip and the edges of the anterior two-thirds of the tongue. The density diminishes towards the center. They are visible as small red dots on the tongue. Each of them contains 1–18 taste buds. The foliate papillae appear deep red from the surrounding mucosa at the posterior lateral sides of the tongue. They are better seen with the mouth wide open and the tongue moved to one side. The circumvallate papillae are slightly elevated and circular. They are located on the rear part of the tongue, with the largest mostly around the midline[25].

The idea of a tongue map – a picture of taste distribution with sweet at the tip of the tongue, sour along the edges, bitter at the back, while salty at all locations – is misleading yet has been tenacious to correction. In 1901, Hänig measured the thresholds for the four basic tastes on the tongue. He noted lower thresholds, although very small differences, to the four tastes on the four loci and generated the tongue map. The truth is that all four primary tastes are independent of each other, and every taste bud has some degree of sensitivity to all four tastes. They can be perceived anywhere on the tongue as long as taste buds are located there[25].

In a taste bud the sensory receptor cells, also called type III cells, taper to form apical microvilli projecting into the taste pore. At the base of the receptor cells there are synaptic vesicles with associated afferent gustatory nerve endings. A single taste bud is innervated by about 50 nerve fibers. Taste stimuli can reach the receptor cells via two means. First, taste elements released during chewing and swallowing reach the microvilli in the taste pore and interact with ion channels (most often salt and acid stimuli) or membrane receptors (bitter stimuli). The subsequent signals lead to activation of the neural synapses at the base of the receptor cells. The biochemical mechanism for sweetness is still unknown, but has been suggested to involve more than one receptor mechanism. Second, blood-borne substances diffuse through capillary walls and stimulate sensitive sites at the base of receptor cells directly. This phenomenon, called venous taste, may be a source of altered taste associated with certain intravenous medication[8,25].

Three nerves carry taste information from taste receptor cells to the brain: facial (cranial nerve, CN VII), glossopharyngeal (CN IX) and, less importantly, vagus (CN X) nerves (Figure 2). Two branches of facial nerve are involved. The chorda tympani nerve innervates the taste buds in the fungiform papillae on the anterior two-thirds of the tongue and some in the foliate papillae[6]. Running along the lingual nerve (CN V_3), which supplies sensation to the same area, the chorda tympani nerve joins the parasympathetic fibers from the submandibular ganglion, which innervates the submandibular and sublingual glands. Coursing cephalad, the nerve reaches the infratemporal fossa between the medial pterygoid muscle and the angle of the mandible, where it leaves the lingual nerve. The chorda tympani penetrates the petrotympanic fissure (Hunguier's canal) of the petrous temporal bone and enters the middle ear at the superior lateral aspect. The nerve is then suspended in the superior quadrants of the middle ear space. The freely suspended section of the chorda tympani nerve is susceptible to damage from middle ear pathology such as ear infection. The nerve exits the middle ear through a bony canaliculus posteriorly, just medial to the fibrous annulus of the tympanic membrane. It then joins the motor portion of the facial nerve in the mastoid. Together they travel towards the internal auditory canal (IAC)[25].

The greater superficial petrosal nerve (GSPN), another branch of the facial nerve, supplies taste to the palate[6]. Nerves that innervate the palatal taste buds travel through the lesser palatine foramina, greater palatine canal, pterygopalatine fossa and pterygoid canal where they become the GSPN. It crosses the foramen lacerum into the middle cranial fossa before it enters the petrous temporal bone at the facial hiatus. The GSPN finally joins the

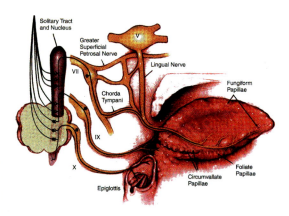

Figure 2 Gustatory pathway. Figure adapted with permission from reference 21

facial nerve at the geniculate ganglion immediately distal to the IAC[25].

The glossopharyngeal nerve innervates the foliate and the circumvallate papillae at the posterior tongue[6]. It runs deep in the tonsillar bed, where it may be vulnerable during difficult tonsillectomy. It eventually enters the jugular foramen and reaches the retro-olivary area of the medulla through the cerebellopontine angle[25].

The superior laryngeal nerve, a branch of the vagus nerve, innervates the taste buds on the laryngeal surface of the epiglottis and possibly the upper third of the esophagus[6]. It also enters the jugular foramen and reaches the medulla. Its role in taste perception is unknown[25].

The taste fibers of all three cranial nerves project to the rostral portion of the nucleus solitary tract in the medulla. From there it further projects to the thalamus, hypothalamus, amygdala and stria terminalis. From the thalamus, it also runs separate projections to the primary gustatory cortex and then secondary cortex on the orbitofrontal surface[6].

Gustatory disorders

Gustatory impairment classification is similar to its olfactory counterpart: ageusia (absence of taste), hypogeusia (diminished taste), dysgeusia (distorted taste) and phantogeusia (more commonly called 'taste phantom')[25].

Gustatory loss (Table 3) seems to be a rare complaint overall. One reason is the multiple peripheral innervation to the gustatory system, which provides a safety net against complete ageusia. Another is the intrinsic self-inhibitory mechanism among gustatory nerves. It has been observed clinically that when a chorda tympani nerve is anesthetized unilaterally by transtympanic membrane injection of lidocaine, tastes innervated by the glossopharyngeal nerve are intensified, with the contralateral bitter taste being the greatest. Painting a topical anesthetic on the contralateral tongue can then abolish the intensified bitterness. This suggests that the taste phantom results from abnormal spontaneous excitation because of the release of active inhibition from the disabled side[25].

'Supertasters' have higher sweet (but not in relation to all artificial sweeteners) and bitter taste sensations for a variety of stimuli than do medium tasters and non-tasters. This is suspected to involve two codominant traits. Supertasters may have more taste buds than medium tasters, and medium tasters more than non-tasters[25]. It is noted that women are more likely than men to be supertasters, and Asians more than Caucasians. Clinically supertasters assign higher bitter intensity scores when given 6-*n*-propylthiouracil than do non-tasters. It is likely that supertasters complain more than do non-tasters of oral pain, involving taste bud areas, connected with mucositis and aphthous ulcers. Supertasters also perceive fat to be more creamy than do non-tasters (fat has no taste or smell). In a sample of postmenopausal women, supertasters had lower body mass indices (weight/height^2) than non-tasters[25].

Chorda tympani injury

Acute or chronic otitis media is the most common middle ear pathology, and has been recognized as an important source of damage to the gustatory system. The chorda tympani nerve is susceptible to inflammatory or direct infectious injury, as it is completely exposed

Table 3 Medical conditions that affect taste

Nervous
Bell's palsy
Damage to chorda tympani
Head trauma
Multiple sclerosis

Endocrine
Adrenal cortical insufficiency
Congenital adrenal hyperplasia
Pseudohypoparathyroidism
Panhypopituitarism
Cushing's syndrome
Cretinism
Hypothyroidism
Diabetes mellitus
Gonadal dysgenesis (Turner's syndrome)

Nutritional
Cancer
Chronic renal failure
Liver disease including cirrhosis
Niacin (vitamin B$_3$) deficiency
Zinc deficiency
Thermal burn

Local
Facial hypoplasia
Glossitis and other oral disorders
Leprosy
Oral Crohn's disease
Radiation therapy
Sjögren's syndrome

Other
Hypertension
Influenza-like infection

traveling through the middle ear cavity[8]. However, chronic otitis media patients actually experience enhanced tastes from some stimuli. This is partly due to increased activity in some nerves as the result of lessened self-inhibition by damaged nerves[25].

During ear surgeries, such as middle ear exploration, stapedectomy, tympanoplasty and mastoidectomy, the chorda tympani nerve may be stretched or cut leading to temporary or permanent taste loss. Although it renders the ipsilateral anterior tongue completely devoid of taste, the most common complaint is not loss of taste but rather a metallic phantom[26,27]. Even washing the ear canal has been reported to produce a similar taste phantom.

Glossopharyngeal trauma

The CN IX, including its lingual and pharyngeal branches, is vulnerable during tonsillectomy[25]. Unfortunately, many tonsillectomy patients have a history of recurrent or chronic ear infection, and may have damaged chorda tympani preoperatively. Because of its insidious nature, the taste change due to chorda tympani damage may be barely noticeable subjectively. Nevertheless, the addition of a glossopharyngeal loss leaves no reserve, such that patients complain of complete loss of taste in the affected tongue area.

Viral injury

Bell's palsy (herpes simplex mononeuritis) and Ramsay Hunt syndrome (herpes zoster oticus) are associated with taste dysfunction as well as unilateral facial paralysis[8]. Interestingly, a natural course of Ramsay Hunt syndrome was carefully documented by Carl Pfaffmann, a pioneer chemosensory researcher who contracted the illness himself. Initially, the affected left side was completely devoid of taste, while the right side produced heightened sense of taste. Daily taste experience was not affected. Over the next 3 years of recovery at the left, the right side taste gradually lessened towards normal[25].

In Lyme disease, about 10% of patients are affected with unilateral or bilateral facial paralysis. Its mechanism is unknown[8,25].

Mass lesion

Temporal bone tumors such as glomus jugulare, facial nerve neuroma and squamous cell carcinoma may affect chorda tympani before facial paresis manifests. Cerebellopontine angle tumors such as acoustic neuroma and meningioma can produce isolated taste loss by involving the nervus intermedius[25].

'Jugular foramen syndrome', also named Vernet syndrome, is the paralysis of all nerves that traverse the jugular foramen (CNs IX, X and XI) from lesions directly involving the skull base at the jugular foramen (glomus jugulare, schwannoma, squamous cell carcinoma).

Symptoms include taste loss from CNs IX and X, ipsilateral vocal cord paralysis and ipsilateral shoulder drop. When a tumor extends deep into the foramen magnum causing ipsilateral tongue paralysis, it becomes Collet–Sicard syndrome. If the tumor compromises the sympathetic trunk in addition to all of the above, it is termed Villaret syndrome. Patients also exhibit Horner's syndrome[25].

Oral cavity and oropharyngeal tumors do not present with taste loss alone. Lack of gag reflex would be more noticeable[25].

Central nervous system

Pontine hemorrhage and damage to the rostral insular cortex may lead to ipsilateral taste loss. Temporal lobe epilepsy occasionally presents a metallic taste prior to a seizure[25].

In head trauma, the incidence of taste loss is 0.4–0.5% by report[25].

Medication

Medications passing through the capillary walls can stimulate taste receptors in taste buds directly. This may be the origin of dysgeusia for many chemotherapy agents[25]. Patients receiving levothyroxine complain of taste loss more frequently, but their taste identification test scores are not lower than those of controls[4].

Some medications have been associated with metallic dysgeusia in some patients. They include tetracycline, lithium, penicilliamine and captopril. Cisplatin and bleomycin are reported to cause hypogeusia, especially at high doses[28].

CLINICAL EVALUATION OF OLFACTORY AND GUSTATORY DISORDERS

To taste or to smell – that is the question

The distinction between taste and smell is vague among the general public. Odorants that are sniffed into the nose are identified as smells without confusion. Yet most people wrongly label odorants entering the nose through the nasopharynx during eating as part of taste[8]. One report showed that of 750 patients complaining of taste loss, fewer than 4% had measurable gustatory deficit; in contrast, 71% had absent or diminished olfactory function[11].

Gustatory loss is much less common than olfactory loss, considering that gustation has multiple innervations over a large area of tongue while olfaction has a single innervation by CN I over a limited area in the olfactory cleft. In addition, olfactory neurons are receptor cells exposed vulnerably to the external environment, while gustatory neurons are buried deep in the taste buds, protected from potential toxins.

True taste loss signifies a loss in the ability to taste saltiness, sweetness, sourness and bitterness[8]. In a primary-care setting, it is often helpful to ask patients whether they can taste the sweetness of sugar, the sourness of grapefruit juice, the bitterness of strong coffee and the saltiness of potato chips. Affirmative answers to all of the above usually preclude general gustatory dysfunction[8]. An olfactory loss should be considered, especially if patients report weak tastes to the above items.

In general, a thorough history and physical examination is necessary as an initial evaluation to smell and taste disorders. Much information and clinical clues are generated from the medical and surgical history alone. A careful examination of the posterior tongue and intranasal mucosa requires special instruments, such as reflective mirror, nasal endoscope and sometimes flexible laryngoscope. Special imaging studies, such as sinus computed tomography, are justified and cost-effective only after physical examination is concluded. They are indispensable in diagnosing sinusitis, examining the integrity of the cribriform plate or locating a posterior mass. Sinus plain X-ray films lack specificity, and are generally discouraged[4]. Early referral to otolaryngology specialists is preferred when symptoms persist.

Olfactory and gustatory tests

In a primary-care office, a rapid and reliable alcohol sniff test (AST) can be used to screen olfactory dysfunction[9]. Developed at the University of California, San Diego, the test involves a standard 70% isopropyl alcohol preparation pad found in most clinics. The pad is opened such that 0.5 cm of the pad is visible. The alcohol pad is then placed beneath the patient's nostrils while the patient inspires twice to become familiarized with the alcohol odor. The pad is then withdrawn and the threshold test is ready to begin. The patient is asked to close the mouth and eyes, breathe normally and indicate when the odor is detected. Active sniffing and deep inspiration are discouraged. The alcohol pad is placed 30 cm below the nose and, with each expiration, is moved 1 cm closer to the nares until the patient detects the presence of the odor. The distance from the anterior nares to the alcohol pad is measured in centimeters where the odor is first detected. The procedure is repeated four times and the mean distance defines the threshold. A distance of more than 10 cm at mid-chest is found in normosia, 5–10 cm in hyposmia and less than 5 cm in anosmia (private communication with the authors).

The mechanism of the AST is that odor thresholds for alcohol are two or more orders of magnitude lower than the trigeminal pungent threshold for the same stimulus. In anosmia, alcohol odor stimulates the trigeminal nerve only when it is very close to the nose. The test is simple and takes only 5 min. Note that the AST is not designed to rule out malingering.

For more accurate and objective information, there are seven smell and taste tests used by special chemosensory centers. Owing to the specialized materials required, associated costs and the length of the tests, their usage is limited[11]:

(1) University of Pennsylvania smell identification test (UPSIT): a standardized 40-stimulus microencapsulated 'scratch-and-sniff' odor identification test;

(2) Phenyl ethyl alcohol (PEA) test: a forced-choice single-staircase rose-like odor detection threshold test that has little or no intranasal trigeminal stimulation properties at any concentration;

(3) Suprathreshold taste quality identification of sucrose, citric acid, caffeine and sodium chloride;

(4) Taste intensity rating test: uses different concentrations of the tastants mentioned in (3);

(5) Taste threshold test: detects the minimal concentration of detection of the four tastes;

(6) Regional taste quality identification test: identifies unilateral, anterior or posterior tongue deficit that is innervated by different nerves;

(7) Electrogustometric threshold test: differentiates the sensitivity of the two sides of the anterior portion of the tongue to minute electric currents.

Treatment

Currently, no effective treatment for smell dysfunction other than those associated with nasal/sinus disease has been identified. Antibiotics for acute and chronic infection can decrease mucosal inflammation. Nasal decongestants, oral and topical with short-term use, can treat mucosal edema. Topical steroids are frequently used for long-term maintenance of nasal mucosa. Sinonasal surgery may eradicate chronic sinus infection and correct intranasal anatomical anomalies.

For metallic dysgeusia induced by certain medications, most reports indicate quick resolution with termination of the offending agents; but with captopril, it has been reported to persist for months in some patients[28].

IMPACT OF AGING ON SMELL AND TASTE

Age-related decline in both sensory functions demonstrates progressively diminished sensitivity, with that of smell worse than that of taste. These losses begin around age 60 and become more severe at age 70[6]. Such deficits adversely affect nutritional intake, immunological defense and a variety of biochemical measures in the elderly, such as insulin and other pancreatic enzyme secretion. There is no proven pharmacological treatment, and the prognosis for recovery of smell and taste sensation is generally poor[6]. Nevertheless, preventive measures and compensatory methods are available.

Many elderly patients have decreased salivary flow due to dehydration, medication, head and neck irradiation, sialithiasis or vitamin deficiencies. Treating these conditions and ensuring adequate fluid intake may increase saliva flow and help tastants reach taste buds[29]. Sialogogs can be prescribed to stimulate saliva glands if their function is intact.

Tongue brushing twice a day may increase taste acuity by removing thick white mucoid coats on the dorsal tongue[29]. Smoking not only diminishes the taste of food, but also makes flavorful food taste flat and unappetizing[6,29]. Both direct and passive smoking are associated with olfactory loss[16].

Sensory interventions to intensify the taste and odor of food can compensate for certain perceptual loss. It has been shown that sour and bitter are less affected by aging than salty and sweet[6]. To enhance food flavor efficiently, excessive sugar and salt intake should be avoided. Instead, flavoring agents to enhance taste acuity in other aspects should be added, such as vanilla, orange, strawberry, caraway, chilli powder, chives, cinnamon, cloves, curry, garlic (not garlic salt), ginger, lemon juice, mint, dry mustard, peppers, sage, tarragon and vinegar[29].

For patients who complain that 'food doesn't taste the way it used to', i.e. when they were young, elevating concentrations of flavor may offset their loss in smell and taste. For example, adding chicken flavor while cooking chicken may amplify its aroma. Bacon, cheese flavor, tomato and pea can also be added to soups and vegetables[6]. In 13 cancer patients, preferences for food increased from 8–31% to 69–92% after flavoring agents were added[30].

Dietary supplements with zinc, vitamin A or niacin have been tried in the past, but evidence for their effectiveness is not compelling[11].

DIETARY USE OF MONOSODIUM GLUTAMATE

Recent research into monosodium glutamate (MSG) has shown that food intensified with MSG and other flavors increases food acceptance and intake in the elderly, and improves their immune status by enhanced T and B cell levels and immunoglobulin A (IgA) secretion[30].

Monosodium glutamate is the sodium salt of the amino acid, glutamic acid. Its average daily intake is estimated to be 0.3–1.0 g in industrialized countries[31]. Functioning as a flavoring agent, glutamate is added to food during cooking as MSG. Glutamate also occurs naturally in a variety of foods, such as tomatoes, cheese, meat and fish, and in soups where glutamate is released by cellular breakdown and protein hydrolysis, and adds much flavor[32]. Although not widely appreciated in Western culture, glutamate has been a key flavoring ingredient in Asian cuisine for ages. The Chinese call MSG *WeiJing*, the spirit of taste. The Japanese name it *Umami*, distinct from the basic four tastes[33]. A variety of testing techniques have demonstrated that the taste quality of MSG does not fall within the qualitative taste range defined by the traditional four tastes of sweet, sour, salt and bitter[6]. It has been suggested that *Umami*, since Western culture does not have a name for it, is the fifth essential taste[30].

Both central and peripheral actions from glutamate sensors have been identified. After applying MSG to the tongue, selective responding neurons in the hypothalamus, important in appetite control, and the orbital prefrontal cortex, important in taste and smell perception, have been demonstrated[34,35]. There are also glutamate receptors in the oral cavity and small intestine that are found to be capable of inducing a reflex activation of efferent fibers from the brain to the pancreas and elsewhere via the vagus nerve. It is conceivable that glutamate ingestion might facilitate food digestion and nutrient absorption and distribution[36]. Commercially available MSG often contains a mixture of 5´-ribonucleotides including inosine-5´-monophosphate (IMP) and guanosine-5´-monophosphate (GMP). These compounds have potent synergistic effects with MSG, which lower the MSG threshold level[30].

Safety of dietary monosodium glutamate

Once glutamate enters the gut, it is preferentially metabolized by the intestine. Up to half of the energy consumed by the intestine during digestion comes from glutamate[37]. The rest of it participates in a variety of important biochemical pathways in the body, such as gluconeogenesis, transamination and deamination of other amino acids, and hepatic nitrogen elimination via the urea cycle[32]. The fact that a large amount of glutamate is consumed for energy in the gut and as a metabolic substrate in the liver before entering the systemic circulation may help to explain why glutamate concentrations in the blood rise only moderately after large MSG or glutamate doses are ingested by adults, either as MSG added to food or as glutamate contained in food proteins[38].

In 1988 a joint expert committee from the World Health Organization and the Food and Agriculture Organization of the United Nations published its safety evaluation of MSG. The committee noted that intestinal and hepatic metabolism results in elevated levels of MSG in the systemic circulation only after extremely high doses are given by gavage (> 30 mg/kg body weight). The committee allocated an 'acceptable daily intake not specified' to glutamic acid and its salts. The Scientific Committee for Food of the European Commission reached a similar recommendation in 1991[39]. In 1989 the Food and Drug Administration (FDA) affirmed the safety of MSG at levels normally consumed by the general population. In 1991 it again concluded that there is no evidence linking current MSG food use to any serious, long-term medical problems in the general population[39].

The FDA did acknowledge the existence of some evidence of dose-dependent, mild reactions to MSG in a small group of the general population. The 'Chinese-restaurant syndrome' is a complex of symptoms following ingestion of a Chinese meal. It consists of numbness at the back of the neck and arms, weakness, flushing and palpitations[31]. In addition, there have been preliminary reports associating asthma attacks with oral MSG challenge without simultaneous food intake[40]. Nevertheless, double-blind placebo-controlled human studies have failed to confirm an involvement of MSG in Chinese-restaurant syndrome[39]. The existence of MSG-induced asthma, even in patients with a positive history, has not been replicated in well-designed studies[40].

In the mammalian CNS and especially in the retina, glutamate is the principal excitatory neurotransmitter whose extracellular level is tightly regulated. Excessive levels lead to neuroexcitotoxicity, which has been implicated in the pathogenesis of many neurological and ophthalmic diseases, including stroke, trauma, epilepsy, dementia and glaucoma[41]. Under normal conditions, glutamate is stored in neurons and released at neurosynapses for very brief periods in localized areas. Specialized glutamate receptors found in the CNS rapidly transport glutamate back into the intracellular space and thus maintain physiological concentrations. Because functional glutamate transporters should timely restore its homeostatic levels, glutamate transporter malfunction has been strongly implicated in glutamate receptor-mediated neuroexcitotoxicity. In fact, transient release of glutamate is found to be not associated with a significant elevation in extracellular glutamate in some neurological diseases mentioned above, and a decreased level of glutamate transporters is identified in human glaucoma with retinal ganglion cell death[41].

More evidence will emerge over the next decade about the safety of MSG in humans. At present, moderate use of MSG as a food-flavoring agent should be considered safe. In the neonatal mouse the oral effective dose (ED_{50}) for producing noticeable lesions in the hypothalamus where there is a lack of blood–brain barrier is ~ 500 mg MSG/kg body weight by gavage, whereas the largest palatable dose for humans is ~ 60 mg/kg body weight. In a 70-kg man this is about 12 teaspoons or four tablespoons of MSG – with higher doses causing nausea. Thus, voluntary ingestion should not exceed this level[39].

CONCLUSIONS

Smell and taste dysfunction can impact substantially on our psychological well-being, impede performance in some occupations and lead to nutritional deficiency. It may render patients vulnerable to hazardous environments, toxic fumes and spoiled food. The elderly are at greater risk, as smell and taste acuity declines naturally with age. Although treatment options for olfactory impairment remain limited, especially in sensorineural loss, thorough evaluation is needed, particularly with regard to safety issues and other related conditions such as depression and nutritional deficit. Adding food-flavoring agents and monosodium glutamate are proven methods to improve oral intake and immune status in the elderly.

References

1. Schiffman SS. Taste and smell in disease. *N Engl J Med* 1983;308:1275–9, 1337–43

2. Doty RL. A review of olfactory dysfunctions in man. *Am J Otolaryngol* 1979;1:57–79

3. Jones N, Rog D. Olfaction: a review. *J Laryngol Otol* 1998;113:11–24

4. Deems DA, Doty RL, Hummel T, Kratskin IL. Olfactory function and disorders. In Bailey BJ, ed. *Head and Neck Surgery – Otolaryngology*, 2nd edn. Philadelphia: Lippincott-Raven, 1998:317–31

5. Mori K, Yoshihara Y. Molecular recognition and olfactory processing in the mammalian olfactory system. *Prog Neurophysiol* 1995;45:585–619

6. Schiffman SS. Taste and smell losses in normal aging and disease. *J Am Med Assoc* 1997;278:1357–62

7. Wilson-Pauwels L, Akesson EJ, Stewart PA. Olfactory nerve. In Sandoz, ed. *Cranial Nerves – Anatomy and Clinical Comments*. New York: BC Decker, Inc., 1988:

8. Weiffenbach JM, Bartoshuk LM. Taste and smell. *Clin Geriatr Med* 1992;8:543–55

9. Davidson TM, Murphy C. Rapid clinical evaluation of anosmia – the alcohol sniff test. *Arch Otolaryngol Head Neck Surg* 1997;123:591–4

10. Miwa T, Furukawa M, Tsukatani T, *et al.* Impact of olfactory impairment on quality of life and disability. *Arch Otolaryngol Head Neck Surg* 2001;127:497–503

11. Deems DA, Doty RL, Settle GS, *et al.* Smell and taste disorders, a study of 750 patients from the University of Pennsylvania Smell and Taste Center. *Arch Otolaryngol Head Neck Surg* 1991;117:519–28

12. Hendriks APJ. Olfactory dysfunction. *Rhinology* 1988;26:229–51

13. Schiffman SS. Clinical physiology of taste and smell. *Annu Rev Nutr* 1993;13:405–36

14. Cowart BJ, Young IM, Feldman RS, Lowry LD. Clinical disorders of smell and taste. *Occup Med* 1997;12:465–83

15. Mott AE. Disorders of taste and smell. *Med Clin North Am* 1991;75:1321–53

16. Frye RE. Dose related effects of cigarette smoking on olfactory function. *J Am Med Assoc* 1990;263:1233–6

17. Singh N, Grewal MS, Austin JH. Familial anosmia. *Arch Neurol* 1970;22:40–4

18. Leopold DA, Hornung DE, Schwob JE. Congenital lack of olfactory ability. *Ann Otol Rhinol Laryngol* 1992;101:229–36

19. Jesberger JA. Brain output dysregulation induced by olfactory bulbectomy: an approximation in the rat of major depressive disorder in human? *Int J Neurosci* 1988;38:241–65

20. Ward CD, Hess WA, Calne DB. Olfactory impairment in Parkinson's disease. *Neurology* 1983;33:943–6

21. Schiffman SS. Taste and smell losses in normal aging and disease. *J Am Med Assoc* 1997;278:1357–62

22. Nordin S, Murphy C. Odor memory in normal aging and Alzheimer's disease. *Ann NY Acad Sci* 1998;855:686–93

23. Doty R. Olfactory capacities in aging and Alzheimer's disease. *Ann NY Acad Sci* 1991;640:20–7

24. Doty RL, Shaman P, Damm M. Development of the University of Pennsylvania smell identification test: a standardized microencapsulated test of olfactory function. *Physiol Behav* 1984;32:489–502

25. Kveton JF, Bartoshuk LM. Taste. In Bailey BJ, ed. *Head and Neck Surgery – Otolaryngology*, 2nd edn. Philadelphia: Lippincott-Raven, 1998:609–26

26. Bull TR. Taste and the chorda tympani. *J Laryngol Otol* 1965;79:479–93

27. Moon CN, Pullen EW. Effects of chorda tympani section during middle ear surgery. *Laryngoscope* 1963;73:392–405

28. Frank ME, Hettinger TP. The sense of taste: neurobiology, aging, and medication effects. *Crit Rev Oral Biol Med* 1992;3:371–93

29. Winkler S, Garg AK, Trakol M, *et al.* Depressed taste and smell in geriatric patients. *J Am Med Assoc* 1999;130:1759–65

30. Schiffman SS. Intensification of sensory properties of foods for the elderly. *J Nutr* 2000;130:927S–30S

31. Geha RS, Beiser A, Ren C, *et al*. Review of alleged reaction to monosodium glutamate and outcome of a multicenter double-blind placebo-controlled study. *J Nutr* 2000;130:1058S–62S

32. Fernstrom JD. Second international conference on glutamate: conference summary. *J Nutr* 2000;130:1077S–9S

33. Yamaguchi S, Ninomiya K. Umami and food palatability. *J Nutr* 2000;130:921S–6S

34. Nishijo H, Ono T, Uwano T, *et al*. Hypothalamic and amygdalar neuronal responses to various tastant solutions during ingestive behavior in rats. *J Nutr* 2000;130:954S–9S

35. Rolls ET. The representation of umami taste in the taste cortex. *J Nutr* 2000;130:960S–5S

36. Nijima A. Reflex effects of oral, gastrointestinal and hepatoportal glutamate sensors on vagal nerve activity. *J Nutr* 2000;130:971S–3S

37. Reeds PJ, Burrin DG, Stoll B, Jahoor F. Intestinal glutamate metabolism. *J Nutr* 2000;130:978S–82S

38. Tsai PJ, Huang PC. Circadian variation in plasma and erythrocyte glutamate concentrations in adult men consuming a diet with and without added monosodium glutamate. *J Nutr* 2000;130:1002S–4S

39. Walker R, Lupien JR. The safety evaluation of monosodium glutamate. *J Nutr* 2000;130:1049S–52S

40. Stevenson D. Monosodium glutamate and asthma. *J Nutr* 2000;130:1067S–73S

41. Naskar R, Vorwerk CK, Dreyer EB. Concurrent downregulation of a glutamate transporter and receptor in glaucoma. *Invest Ophthalmol Vis Sci* 2000;41:1940–4

Section XI

Skin and hair

Robert A. Norman, DO

During life, the human body goes though many changes. One of the most noticeable places to witness these events is the skin. By studying changes in the skin, we can learn more about the aging process and attempt to prevent, delay, and/or reverse aging. In order to evaluate aging in the skin, we must look at the change in skin function, change in structure (both cellular and molecular), the change in appearance, and the consequences of these skin changes.

The skin functions in many ways. For example, it holds body fluids within its boundaries and protects the underlying tissues from microorganisms, harmful substances, and radiation. The skin also helps in the synthesis of vitamin D, and helps to regulate body temperature. When skin ages, its ability to produce vitamin D declines and it's ability to protect the underlying tissues decreases.

Several structures and physical changes in the skin can be seen with aging. For example, aging skin loses its elasticity secondary to a decrease in collagen and elastin. This loss of elasticity causes the skin to weaken and lose its turgor. In addition to lost elasticity the dermal vascularity tends to decrease with aging. This causes light skinned persons to appear paler. As the skin becomes thinner and loses fat, depigmented patches, known as pseudoscars tend to appear. In addition to these changes, aging skin may show changes at the molecular level due to chromosomal structure abnormalities.

Another important factor to consider in the aging process is the sun and its effect on layers of the skin. The clinical features of photodamaged skin consist of wrinkling, blotchiness, telangiectasia, and a roughened, irregular, 'weather-beaten' appearance. These changes are known as photoaging or dermatoheliosis and with chronically sun-exposed epidermis, there is thickening and morphologic heterogeneity within the basal cell layer. Higher and irregular melanosome content may be present in some keratinocytes, indicating prolonged residence within the basal cell layer. These structural changes may help to explain the leathery texture and blotchy discoloration of sun-damaged skin. The dermal layer is the major site for sun associated chronic damage, manifest as a massive increase in thickened, irregular masses of tangled elastic fibers. Collagen fibers are also abnormally clumped in the deeper dermis. Therefore, one of the major known consequences of chronic skin exposure to sunlight is nonmelanoma skin cancer, such as basal cell and squamous cell carcinoma.

Other changes that are seen with aging skin include actinic purpura, asteatosis, cherry anginomas, seborrheic keratoses, and hair and nail changes. For example, actinic purpuras are well-demarcated, vividly purple macules or patches. These purpuric spots, which will usually fade in two weeks, come from blood that has leaked through poorly supported capillaries and has spread within the dermis. Asteatosis (dry skin) is also a common problem, where the skin is flaky, rough, and often itchy. Many benign lesions also tend to accompany aging. These benign lesions include cherry angiomas, (which often appear early in adulthood), seborrheic keratoses, and actinic lentigines or 'liver spots' along with pre-cancerous actinic keratoses. Aging can also affect the nails of older adults and result in a loss of luster along with yellowing and thickening, seen most commonly on the toenails. One other area affected by aging is hair. The hair's loss of pigment results in graying.

Treatment for aging skin is a rapidly growing and exciting area of exploration. For example, retinoic acid, which is the main ingredient of a well-known cream used successfully in treating acne, has been shown to improve the surface texture of the skin, reduce irregular pigmentation, and increase dermal collagen. It is currently the only treatment approved by the FDA as safe and effective for reversing some of the effects of sun damage. Another product on the market is α–hydroxy acid, which is also showing promise in reversing some of the effects of sun damage. In addition to retinoic and α–hydroxy acid, 'dermal fillers' are being used to correct ones' skin irregularities such as creases and wrinkling due to frowning and squinting. Botulism toxin can also be used in tiny doses to relax the muscles and thus eliminate fixed expression lines like frown markers. Although none of these remedies can guarantee eternally youthful skin, they certainly help fight the battle. We hope that by understanding the pathophysiological causes of skin damage, we can help to delay the skin aging process at an earlier stage.

49 Dermatological problems of men

Murad Alam, MD

INTRODUCTION

In men, dermatologic complaints tend to be age-specific. Adolescent boys may feel socially stigmatized by the eruption of disfiguring acne. Psoriasis and seborrheic dermatitis (including 'dandruff') may also become troublesome early in life. As men become sexually active, they may develop genital warts or orogenital herpes. Dark-skinned and black men who have beard growth are particularly at risk for pseudofolliculitis barbae and acne keloidalis nuchae. Workers who are exposed to chemical and industrial materials, or who perform outdoor work, frequently present with occupational contact dermatitis. Older men are perhaps the most affected by dermatologic concerns. Xerosis (dry skin), calluses and corns, leg ulcers, rosacea, androgenetic alopecia (male pattern-baldness), onychomycosis (nail fungal infection), lipoatrophy, and other visible signs of aging are exceedingly common in late miidle-aged and elderly men. Skin cancer is a problem for all fair-skinned men, in whom it increases in incidence with age. Melanoma, the most deadly skin cancer, differs in that it has a bimodal age distribution, affecting most often elderly men and men in their third and fourth decades.

With the exception of skin cancer, common skin problems in men seldom culminate in dire outcomes. Rather, they are troublesome, itchy, scaly, red, or painful. Visible to the patient as well as friends and acquaintances, these skin lesions are also embarrassing. The psychological consequences of disfiguring and/or persistent dermatologic complaints should not be underestimated. Since many treatments exist to alleviate these conditions, patients can be reassured that simple regimens may often markedly reduce their signs and symptoms.

DRY SKIN (XEROSIS)

Older persons are particularly predisposed to dry skin, or xerosis, which is the most common cause of pruritus (itch) in the aged[1,2]. Xerotic skin is most often seen in the winter, during periods of low humidity. Frequent or prolonged bathing with deodorant soaps and hot water can worsen the condition. Etiologically, the dryness is linked to increased transepidermal water loss caused by the impaired barrier function of damaged skin.

Xerosis in combination with scaliness is referred to as xerotic eczema, winter itch, eczema craquele or asteatotic eczema. Focally, the skin may be red, with fine or coarse scaling, fissures and cracks. Sites most likely to be affected are the anterior lower calves, extensor surfaces of the arms and the flanks.

Xerosis and xerotic eczema can be treated by reducing skin dehydration and promoting rehydration. Moisturizers or bath oils applied immediately after bathing form a protective layer relatively impervious to evaporation. In extreme cases, it may be beneficial for the patient to soak in a tub of warm water for up to 30 min prior to the application of a thick moisturizer such as aquaphor or petrolatum. Preparations containing urea and lactic acid are potent moisturizers. Ammonium lactate, in the 12% preparation, is highly effective for managing xerosis but should only be used after other bland emollients (for example, petrolatum) have already resulted in improved skin integrity, since the former emollient can cause burning and stinging when applied to fissured areas. Severe inflammation, including redness and weeping, may be effectively mitigated by the use of topical corticosteroids. Once xerosis is appropriately treated, the concomitant pruritus also typically diminishes.

CALLUSES AND CORNS

Calluses[3] are small thickened areas of skin caused by persistent rubbing or pressure. They occur on body parts overlying bony prominences, with the palms and soles the most common sites. Occupation may predispose to callus development. For instance, runners and some musicians may have calluses in particular areas, such as under the left chin in violinists. Calluses are frequent in the elderly owing to structural changes of the foot and leg that occur with aging. Replacement of poorly fitting shoes with better shoes can lead to the spontaneous disappearance of calluses. Padding to reduce pressure over bony surfaces, paring of thickened areas, and the application of skin exfoliating chemicals such as salicylic acid and ammonium lactate can improve calluses.

Corns are similar to calluses but are more severely thickened, are conical in shape and have a central core. Hard corns occur on the soles or under the toes, and soft corns are macerated by sweat and emerge between the toes. Like calluses, corns arise in response to pressure or friction. Weight-bearing activities may induce intense pain when the core of the corn

compresses the underlying nerves. A bony spur may underly the corn. Improved footwear improves corns as it does calluses. Unlike calluses, corns are less likely to remit spontaneously after such modifications. Soaking, paring and the application of chemical paring agents is usually required, possibly in combination with the extirpation of any residual bony spur.

LEG ULCERS

Leg ulcers[4-6] can be caused by multiple factors and are difficult to treat. Stasis dermatitis, a red–brown, scaly, shiny, thickening of the skin of the lower legs, has been implicated in the formation of up to 90% of all leg ulcers. Venous insufficiency, the primary cause of stasis dermatitis, is often a result of congestive heart failure or other conditions that cause lower-extremity edema. The lower medial leg is the most common location for venous ulcers. Arterial insufficiency, often in the presence of chronic hypertension or arteriosclerotic disease, can also lead to ulcer formation. Arterial ulcers occur on the lateral ankles or digits and tend to be exquisitely painful. Another major cause of leg ulcers is diabetes. Diabetics with long-standing disease may have paresthesias that increase the likelihood that they will inadvertently injure their legs; subsequently, small-vessel disease associated with diabetes may permit only slow healing or the enlargement of the initial abrasion into an ulcer. Collagen vascular diseases such as lupus erythematosus, rheumatoid arthritis, scleroderma and dermatomyositis are among the less common causes of leg ulcers.

Leg ulcers can be improved by treating their cause. Venous ulcers require leg elevation and the continuous use of compression stockings, which are the mainstay of treatment. Emolliation with moisturizers and the application of topical corticosteroids should be restricted to the red, inflamed skin around the ulcer, not the ulcer itself. If inflammation is suggestive of infection, a culture should be obtained, and a broad-spectrum oral antibiotic may be considered. A vascular surgeon should be consulted regarding ulcers that may have an arterial component. Large non-healing ulcers are a serious problem that may lead to severe morbidity or mortality. For such ulcers, a complicated management regimen, best overseen by a specialist physician, is required.

CONTACT DERMATITIS

Contact dermatitis is a skin eruption caused by substances that come in contact with the skin[7–9]. The two types of contact dermatitis are irritant dermatitis, caused by a substance that elicits such a reaction in most people, and allergic dermatitis, caused by a substance to which a given individual has developed a sensitivity, usually through prior exposure. An immense number of different chemicals and materials can cause contact dermatitis.

Irritant contact dermatitis accounts for the vast majority of cases of contact dermatitis. Common contact irritants are acids, bases, some metal salts, fiberglass, solvents, insecticides, chlorinated compounds, hot peppers and noxious gases, such as tear gas or mustard gas. Diligent review of a patient's recent history of exposures to potential irritants can reveal the likely cause of a dermatitis.

Allergic contact dermatitis can typically be traced to a smaller subset of chemicals (allergens). The patch test is used to detect skin hypersensitivity to these substances. In the patch test, dilute solutions of allergens are applied to a patient's back and the reactions at each site are monitored for several days. Excessive redness, blistering and oozing indicate a positive reaction. A photopatch test is a variant of the patch test in which the patched areas are exposed to ultraviolet light to see whether the patient has an allergy that is mediated by sun exposure (photoallergy). The standard patch test includes about 20 chemicals, and each of these may be present in thousands of common commercial products. Patients may have contact allergies to substances present in plants, clothing, shoes, metals, rubbers, adhesives, resins, cosmetics, preservatives and medications.

Workers in particular occupations are prone to dermatitis from certain irritant and allergic agents. Some workers susceptible to specific types of contact dermatitis are: agricultural workers, airplane workers, artists, bakers, barbers, carpenters, compositors, cooks, dentists, diesel engine workers, dyers, electroplaters, exterminators, foresters, furriers, gardeners, hairdressers, jewelers, masons, metal polishers, milliners, newspaper workers, nurses, painters, photographers, physicians, printers, sculptors, soap makers, surgeons and tanners.

Contact dermatitis is treated by identifying the causative agent and then educating the patient to avoid this agent and products that contain it. Sometimes it may not be possible to find the causative agent.

ACNE

Acne vulgaris is a chronic inflammatory disease that affects the hair follicles and the sebaceous glands associated with them[10–12]. Manifestations include whiteheads and blackheads (comedones) as well as red bumps, with or without drainage or prurulence, that may be of various sizes (papules, pustules, cysts, nodules). The face, neck, upper trunk and upper arms can be involved. Acne is a disease of adolescents, of whom 90% will be affected to some degree. Scarring and hyperpigmentation, or dark spots, can be associated with acne and are the result of prior acne lesions. There is a familial tendency to develop acne, and the metabolic activity of a resident anaerobic bacterium, *Propionibacterium acnes*, has been implicated in the etiology. Androgen secretion in puberty typically triggers acne. Severe cystic acne, acne congoblata, can be a disfiguring disease with profound psychosocial consequences.

Acne is a highly treatable disease. Given the potential psychological distress associated with untreated acne in adolescence, there is seldom any reason not to treat. Topical treatments include topical antibiotics, such as erythromycin, clindamycin and sulfur, as well as benzoyl peroxide preparations. Tretinoin, a topical retinoid, is particularly effective against comedonal acne. Systemic treatments for acne include oral antibiotics, such as the tetracyclines, erythromycin, sulfonamides and clindamycin. Severe cystic acne may necessitate treatment with isotretinoin (Accutane®), a vitamin A analog that frequently results in a permanent remission of acne. Accutane is associated with numerous potential side-effects, including teratogenicity and hypertriglyceridemia. Appropriate management of acne entails a treatment plan tailored to the type and extent of a patient's acne. All acne medications can be drying, and not all patients may be able to tolerate aggressive regimens.

ROSACEA

Rosacea[13,14] is a chronic inflammatory skin disorder that usually affects the mid-face, especially the nose and cheeks. Clinical features include redness, acne-like lesions, fine superficial capillaries (telangiectasia) and enlargement of the sebaceous glands. Mild rosacea entails slight flushing of the central face. As the process progresses, more capillaries and acne-like lesions appear, and the area becomes a chronic deep red or purple color. Burning and stinging in the eye can develop, with severe ocular rosacea requiring the care of an ophthalmologist. The most severe cases of rosacea occur in men.

The manifestations of rosacea may be mitigated by long-term use of oral tetracycline. Topical metronidazole is also safe and effective, as are topical treatments similar to those used for acne. Rosacea is not curable at present, and treatments need to be administered for the duration of the condition.

Extreme hypertrophy of the sebaceous glands in rosacea may culminate in rhinophyma,

a large red mass and hugely dilated follicles on the distal nose. Rhinophyma occurs almost exclusively in men over age 40. This disfiguring condition is best treated surgically. Electrosurgery, with a surgical cutting current, wire-brush surgery or laser ablation are effective at removing the redundant tissue.

PSORIASIS

Psoriasis is a common, chronic inflammatory disease of the skin[15,16]. Red, thick, well-demarcated areas of skin with silvery overlying scale can be seen at various body sites. The scalp, nails, extensor surfaces of the arms and legs, elbows, knees, and umbilical and sacral areas are most likely to be affected. Inverse psoriasis is a variant which selectively involves skin folds and flexor surfaces, most notably the axilla, groin, palms and soles. In guttate psoriasis, a type associated with streptococcal pharyngitis, numerous very small lesions erupt over much of the body. Psoriasis can be accompanied by psoriatic arthritis, a mutilating form that can be widespread but typically affects mostly the joints of the hands. Patients with psoriasis and psoriatic arthritis can suddenly erupt with pustular psoriasis, with intense skin redness and lakes of pus. This is a severe, potentially life-threatening form.

Psoriasis can be induced by drugs, such as beta-blockers, lithium and antimalarials. Stress exacerbates the manifestations of psoriasis.

Management of psoriasis is difficult since the lesions are intermittently recurrent over a patient's lifetime. Treatment regimens may be topical, systemic or both. Topical treatments include corticosteroids, tars, anthralin, tazarotene (a topical retinoid), vitamin D analogs, ultraviolet light, and ultraviolet light in combination with psoralens. Systemically, steroids, methotrexate, cyclosporin, mycophenolate mofetil and retinoids (acitretin) may be employed. Over time there is a tendency for treatments gradually to lose their effectiveness. Sun exposure has been shown to be beneficial, and psoriatics frequently improve in the summer months. Like acne, psoriasis can be emotionally burdensome for the patient. Since the disease is typically not associated with medical morbidities, the patient's preferences should be heavily weighed when selecting treatments.

SEBORRHEIC DERMATITIS (DANDRUFF)

Seborrheic dermatitis[17,18] is a common, superficial skin disorder affecting 2–5% of the population. Most often, seborrheic dermatitis is localized to the scalp, eyebrows, eyelids, creases between the cheeks and nose, lips, ears, mid-chest, axilla, submammary folds, umbilicus, groin or buttocks. Fine, greasy scale, white to yellow in color, is characteristic. The most common form occurs on the scalp as the powdery scale of dandruff. Lesions of seborrheic dermatitis may be associated with redness and itch. Sometimes lesions may resemble those seen in psoriasis and may be described as sebopsoriasis.

Seborrheic dermatitis is a nuisance. Scalp involvement can be controlled by the use of over-the-counter antidandruff shampoos, which should be rotated for optimal effectiveness. Ketoconazole (Nizoral®) cream and corticosteroid creams are effective in reducing facial seborrheic dermatitis.

GENITAL WARTS

The most common sexually transmitted disease, genital warts are caused by infection with human papillomavirus (HPV). Genital warts, or condylomata acuminata, are typically associated with HPV types 6 and 11, which are not implicated in genital dysplasias or cervical cancer. In immunocompetent men, genital warts occur anywhere on the penis or around the anus, with scrotal lesions being much rarer. Warts appear as cauliflower-like lobulated masses and may be malodorous. Intra-anal warts are usually seen in patients practicing receptive anal intercourse. Since genital warts are sexually transmitted, other sexually transmitted diseases may occur concurrently in presenting patients.

No specific antiviral agent exists for the treatment of genital warts. Recurrence is frequent, and possibly due to the persistence of latent or subclinical infection after visible lesions have disappeared. Genital warts may be relatively asymptomatic or be associated with itch, pain, bleeding, malodor or emotional distress. Treatment should be initiated at the patient's request. Topical agents applied by the physician that may be of therapeutic benefit include podophyllin and trichloroacetic acid. Imiquimod®, a local interferon inducer, can be applied by the patient at home. Cryotherapy, and surgical modalities such as excision, electrodesiccation and CO_2 laser[19] are often effective treatments. Genital warts have also been treated with intralesional interferon-α, which is extremely expensive and no more efficacious, on average, than other methods.

ORAL AND GENITAL HERPES

Herpes simplex virus (HSV) infections are typically either perioral (with HSV type 1) or genital (with HSV type 2). Lesions in both cases can be classified as primary infections stemming from initial exposure to the virus or recurrent infections[20,21]. Diagnosis of herpes virus lesions is routinely established by Tzanck smear, culture or fluorescent antibody test.

Lesions on the lips and face, usually caused by HSV-1, present as 'cold sores'. Shallow ulcers or blisters on a red base are the hallmark of this process. Remission is spontaneous and usually without sequelae. Some patients may have herpes outbreaks many times a year. Recurrences are also known to be triggered by sunlight and stress. When outbreaks are severe, attacks may be shortened by commencing treatment with oral acyclovir as soon as prodromal symptoms, such as tingling, itching or burning, are experienced. Patients with frequent recurrences can be treated with a chronic suppressive regimen of low-dose acyclovir.

Genital herpes is generally due to HSV-2. Transmission is typically from sexual contact. Individuals with genital herpes shed virus asymptomatically between outbreaks, and some outbreaks may be subclinical in that they occur without visible lesions. Primary infection with genital herpes can present as a severe febrile illness with extensive lymphadenopathy. HSV-2 infection results in recurrences much more frequently than infection with HSV-1. Recurrent lesions often occur at the same anatomical site, can be extremely tender, and heal without scarring in the absence of superinfection. Primary and recurrent genital herpes, like perioral herpes, can be treated with acyclovir, famciclovir or valaciclovir. Intermittent therapy for severe outbreaks or chronic suppressive therapy for frequent recurrences can be implemented as appropriate. Genital herpes is a significant disease because of the associated social stigma, and patients may require counseling and reassurance. A sexual history and examination should also be obtained to rule out the simultaneous presence of other sexually transmitted diseases. New-onset genital herpes in women during pregnancy can have deleterious effects on the fetus, and men with primary infections should be advised appropriately.

PSEUDOFOLLICULITIS BARBAE

Pseudofolliculitis barbae[22-24] occurs when hairs grow out and then curve back and pierce the skin again to form ingrown hairs. The resulting painful red bumps may drain purulent material and may scar. Most often localized to the beard distribution, Pseudofolliculitis is seen in more than 50% of black men. Close shaving of curly hair increases the likelihood that pseudofolliculitis will develop. In Caucasians, shaving of the pubic hair can result in the disorder.

Prevention is the best management strategy for pseudofolliculitis. Not shaving alleviates the condition. If hairs must be removed, clippers or chemical depilatories should be used. Laser hair removal may be of particular help since it requires only a few minutes to administer, works well on dark hairs, and can decrease the number and coarseness of hairs in the target area. New lasers are being developed that may have a lower associated risk of hyperpigmentation, or skin darkening. Antibiotics and topical steroids may be used to decrease inflammation in exacerbated cases of pseudofolliculitis.

ACNE KELOIDALIS NUCHAE

Acne keloidalis is a persistent folliculitis of the back of the neck that presents as painful red bumps and pustules[25-27]. The progression of disease can result in the formation of sinus tracts and thickened scars or keloids. Young black or Asian men are commonly affected. The condition is not associated with medical complications but can be very unattractive and painful. Scarring associated with acne keloidalis can result in hair loss at the occipital scalp, and this further limits the patient's ability to camouflage the acne keloidalis lesions.

Treatment is difficult. Intralesional corticosteroid injections can decrease inflammation and thin scars. Long-term antibiotic therapy with drugs such as oral tetracyclines may be required in addition. Severely affected areas may be removed surgically.

ANDROGENETIC ALOPECIA (MALE-PATTERN BALDNESS)

Hair loss is a major concern for young and middle-aged men. In fact, remedies for hair loss are the cosmetic treatments most often discussed and advertised in magazines targeted to this population[28-31]. Male-pattern baldness, or androgenetic alopecia, begins in the 20s and 30s, with gradual hair loss at the top and front of the scalp and over the temples. The forehead becomes high as the hairline recedes. Over time, the entire front and top of the scalp may become hairless. Rates of hair loss vary among individuals. Both heredity and androgen stimulation at a particular age mediate the process of androgenetic alopecia.

Treatments for androgenetic alopecia have improved in recent years. Topical solutions of minoxidil (Rogaine®) are more effective at retarding further hair loss than stimulating new hair growth. Minoxidil, if effective, must be used indefinitely to maintain the benefit. Oral finasteride may help in the regrowth of hair to cosmetically appreciable extents, but is less effective at the temples and also must be continued in the long term. Hair transplantation techniques have been refined. Transplantation with up to several thousand grafts of one to several hairs each can recreate a natural frontal hairline. Since the transplanted hairs are from the same patient who is the recipient, and since they are harvested from areas known to be less susceptible to androgenetic alopecia, the transplants typically persist in the long term without rejection or loss.

ONYCHOMYCOSIS

Onychomycosis[32] is infection of the nail by fungus. This is relatively more common in older individuals, who may have developed anatomical changes of their feet, toes and nails that predispose to infection. Etiological agents include dermatophytes, which are fungi that preferentially infect the hair, skin and nails, as well as yeasts and other non-dermatophytic molds. Nails of the toes are more commonly affected than those of the fingers. A thickened, brittle, yellow–white nail with underlying and overlying debris is the typical presentation. Multiple nails tend to be infected. Infection with yeasts manifests

differently, as nails may remain hard and glossy, surrounding skin may become red and drain pus, and the nails may separate from the nail beds. Diagnosis is made by culture or by microscopic examination of nail debris in a preparation of potassium hydroxide (KOH preparation). Nail shavings may also be submitted for histological evaluation with special stains.

Topical antifungal medications are of use in treating athlete's foot (tinea pedis) and fungal infections of the skin of the feet, but are of almost no efficacy in treating onychomycosis. Systemic antifungal agents, including terbinafine, itraconazole and fluconazole, may be effective in clearing onychomycosis if administered for several months, either continuously or in pulses. Hepatoxicity and liver function test elevations may occur if oral medications are used. Treatment relapses are common and treatment may be deferred if the patient so desires.

LIPODYSTROPHY AND LIPOATROPHY

With advancing age, individuals may notice redistribution of subcutaneous fat to certain areas and diminution of fat in other areas. In men, fat accumulation may localize to the bilateral flanks ('love handles') and lower mid-abdomen. Maintenance of ideal total body weight through appropriate diet and exercise may not be sufficient to reduce these focal fatty accumulations. Conversely, despite good general health, some middle-aged men may experience cosmetically significant thinning of facial fat pads. Since facial fat is perceived as a marker of youth and vitality, patients may complain that others see them as tired or relatively old. Human immunodeficiency virus (HIV) or autoimmune deficiency syndrome (AIDS) patients are susceptible to various types of lipodystrophies ('crix belly', 'protease paunch', 'buffalo hump'), including very marked facial atrophy.

Men who are disturbed by the usually medically benign changes of fat redistribution or atrophy may seek cosmetic surgical correction[33,34]. Liposuction is a safe and effective procedure for reducing focal fat pockets. In dermatology, liposuction uses tumescent anesthesia, a mixture of dilute lidocaine and epinephrine that permits this out-patient procedure to be performed without general anesthesia. Lipoatrophy, including depressions and deep lines of the face, can be corrected with specially formulated filler substances. Bovine and human collagen derivatives, available in various types and viscosities, can fill defects for up to several months before requiring replenishment. Autologous fat, harvested from another site on the same patient, can also be used. Permanent, removable inert materials (such as Goretex®) may be implanted alone or in combination with other fillers. Facial lipoatrophy in HIV disease is a treatment challenge that typically responds to a large volume of fillers.

VISIBLE SIGNS OF AGING

Aging results in other visible changes, which are usually most noticeable on the face. Fine wrinkles may develop around the mouth, eyes and nose. Frowning or smiling may reveal other dynamic creases of the forehead, nasal bridge and lateral orbital areas that are not evident when the face is at rest. Accumulated skin damage from sunlight can also result in brown spots (lentigos). Small capillaries (telangiectasias) may become more prominent, especially on the nose and cheeks. Rough, discrete pink to yellow-brown areas of skin that appear stuck-on (seborrheic keratoses) can erupt over much of the body. While none of these changes are abnormal, some men may opt to have them treated for personal or professional reasons[35-38].

Brown spots can be treated with cryotherapy (liquid nitrogen spray), electrodesiccation (unipolar or bipolar cautery) or Q-switched lasers. The family of Q-switched lasers (ruby, alexandrite or neodymium : yttrium–aluminum–garnet (Nd : YAG)) fire for extremely brief intervals, and so destroy pigment without damaging surrounding cells or causing scarring. Q-switched lasers are also the treatment of choice for tattoo removal. Small capillaries can be effectively treated by lasers, such as the pulsed-dye laser, that selectively target vascular structures. Dynamic creases can be injected with medical-grade botulinum toxin, each administration of which inhibits visible frown and smile lines for several months. Patients with severe diffuse wrinkling and sun damage would probably benefit from laser resurfacing. This entails ablating the superficial layers of the facial skin with a CO_2 or erbium : YAG laser and then allowing new, less damaged skin to grow. Laser resurfacing is equivalent to deep chemical peels, which may provide the same effect but be more operator-dependent. Fine wrinkles around the eyes and mouth may be reduced more after laser resurfacing than after a face-lift (rhytidectomy). Still, patients with copious sagging and excess skin may consider combining a resurfacing procedure with a face-lift. Seborrheic keratoses can be frozen with liquid nitrogen, burnt with electrocautery or removed by curettage.

NON-MELANOMA SKIN CANCER: BASAL CELL CARCINOMA

Basal cell cancer[39,40] is the most common cancer of any type among Caucasians. Small, pink, waxy, translucent bumps, sometimes described as 'pearl-like', are the characteristic finding. Lesions may have a central depression, bleed with slight manipulation, and be overlayed by small blood vessels (telangiectasia). Often they are initially noticed by the patient when they develop into shallow, non-healing ulcers or erosions. Most tumors are entirely asymptomatic. Metastatic spread is vanishingly rare, but untreated lesions will grow locally, and may eventually invade adjacent structures. Head and neck lesions constitute the vast majority of basal cell carcinomas, with the nose being a particularly common area of involvement. Unlike actinic keratoses and squamous cell cancers (see below), basal cell cancers are seldom found on the dorsal hands and arms. Diagnosis is made by confirming clinical suspicion with a shave or punch skin biopsy. Risk factors for basal cell cancer include excessive sunlight exposure, exposure to ionizing radiation, chemical carcinogens, genetic predisposition, immunosuppression and certain skin diseases. Sun exposure is probably the most important cause, and basal cell cancers are seen usually in light-skinned middle-aged and elderly people, especially those residing in sunny regions. Occupational exposure to sun can increase the chance of developing basal cell cancers, as well as other skin cancers. Importantly, organ transplant recipients typically develop numerous, rapidly growing basal cell carcinomas after their surgeries.

Tumor and host characteristics must be considered in selecting a treatment for a given basal cell cancer. The goal of treatment is complete cure with good cosmetic results. Small lesions may be entirely removed by an initial biopsy. Surgical excision, electrosurgery and cryotherapy are other commonly used modalities. Mohs micrographic surgery is the treatment of choice for high-risk lesions, particularly large, recurrent and histologically invasive lesions, which have potential for impinging on structures of the face that are important for function or cosmesis. In Mohs procedures, tumor removal is continued in stages until surgical margins are verified intraoperatively by frozen section. Mohs is thus a tissue-sparing modality that offers the surgeon microscopic margin control. Prevention and patient education are the most important methods for reducing the incidence of all skin cancers, including basal cell cancers. Limiting sun exposure among fair-skinned individuals reduces the risk.

NON-MELANOMA SKIN CANCER: CUTANEOUS SQUAMOUS CELL CANCER

Squamous cell cancer[41-43] can develop on the hair-bearing skin or on mucosal surfaces. Cutaneous squamous cell carcinoma, the second most common skin cancer, may arise from red, rough patches of sun-damaged skin called actinic keratoses. Unlike basal cell cancers, squamous cell cancers are more likely to occur on the hands than on the face. Different clinical appearances are possible, with squamous cell cancers typically more scaly, crusted or ulcerated than basal cell cancers. As with basal cell cancers, the main risk factor for squamous cell cancers is the ultraviolet light in sunshine. In addition to the other risk factors mentioned for basal cell cancers, squamous cell cancers are associated with some HPV subtypes and chronic wounds and scars. Metastatic risk, dependent on the tumor's anatomical location and size, is from 0.5% to greater than 5%. Tumors of the lips, ears and scars are at high risk for metastasis. Prognosis of metastatic lesions and lesions with perineural spread is dismal. Among solid organ transplant recipients who tolerate their grafts, metastatic squamous cell carcinoma may be the most common cause of mortality.

Treatment of squamous cell cancer is similar to that of basal cell cancer. Since squamous cell cancer has an associated risk of metastasis, tumors must be treated definitively as soon as possible to minimize morbidity and mortality.

MELANOMA

Melanoma is the most deadly skin cancer[44-48]. During the past 50 years, the world-wide incidence has steadily increased. As with other skin cancers, melanoma is uncommon among darker-skinned people. Young people in their 20s and 30s as well as elderly people are at highest risk. Irregular moles can develop into malignant melanomas over time, and suspicious lesions should be examined carefully to ascertain whether they require biopsy for definitive diagnosis. Screening of moles is possible by application of the 'ABCD' criteria, with melanomas more likely to display *asymmetry, border* irregularity, *color* variation and large *diameter* (greater than 6 mm).

Biopsy-proven melanomas must be promptly excised with appropriate margins. Deeper melanomas are much more likely to undergo local recurrence and regional and distal spread. Surgical removal is usually sufficient to cure melanomas permanently if they are less than 0.75 mm thick. Metastatic disease is often unresponsive to treatment and bears a dismal prognosis. Epidemiological management of melanoma entails the aggressive removal of malignant lesions when they are still thin, and patient education to encourage sun avoidance and self-examination. Fair-skinned patients, or those with many atypical moles or a family history of melanoma, should carefully examine their entire body surfaces at least every month. Primary-care physicians who are not confident of their ability to detect and biopsy suspicious lesions should consider referral to a dermatologist.

References

1. Savin JA. How should we define itching? *J Am Acad Dermatol* 1998;38:268–9
2. Greaves MW, Wall PD. Pathophysiology of itching. *Lancet* 1996;348:938–40
3. Verbov JL, Monk CJE. Tallar callosity – a little recognized common entity. *Clin Exp Dermatol* 1991;16:118–20
4. Miller OF III. Essentials of pressure ulcer treatment. *J Dermatol Surg Oncol* 1993;19:759–63
5. Samson RH, Showalter DP. Stockings and the prevention of recurrent venous ulcers. *Dermatol Surg* 1996;22:373–6
6. Fletcher A, Cullum N, Sheldon TA. A systematic review of compression treatment for venous leg ulcers. *Br Med J* 1997;315:576–80
7. Nurse DS. Industrial dermatitis. *Int J Dermatol* 1987;26:434–5
8. Mathias CGT. Occupational dermatoses. *J Am Acad Dermatol* 1988;19:1107–14
9. Nethercott JR, Holness DL. Disease outcome in workers with occupational skin disease. *J Am Acad Dermatol* 1994;25:569–74
10. Shalita AR. Acne revisited. *Arch Dermatol* 1994;30:363–4
11. Leyden JJ. Therapy for acne vulgaris. *N Engl J Med* 1997;336:1156–62
12. Goulden V, Clark SM, McGeown C, Cinliffe WJ. Treatment of acne with intermittent isotretinoin. *Br J Dermatol* 1997;137:106–8
13. Wilkin JK. Rosacea. *Arch Dermatol* 1994;130:359–62
14. Bleicher PA, Charles JH, Sober AJ. Topical metronidazole therapy for rosacea. *Arch Dermatol* 1987;123:609–14
15. Gupta AK. The Psoriasis Life Stress Inventory: a preliminary index of psoriasis-related stress. *Acta Dermatol Venereol* 1996;75:240
16. Ruzicka T. Psoriatic arthritis. *Arch Dermatol* 1996;132:215
17. Binder RL, Jonelis FJ. Seborrheic dermatitis in neuroleptic-induced Parkinsonism. *Arch Dermatol* 1983;119:473–5
18. Green CA, Farr PM, Shuster S. Treatment of seborrhoeic dermatitis with ketoconazole: II. Response of seborrhoeic dermatitis of the face, scalp, and trunk to topical ketoconazole. *Br J Dermatol* 1987;116:217–21
19. Kauvar ANB, McDaniel DH, Geronemus RG. Pulsed dye laser treatment of warts. *Arch Fam Med* 1995;4:1035–40
20. Brown TJ, Yen-Moore A, Tyring SK. An overview of sexually transmitted diseases, Part 1. *J Am Acad Dermatol* 1999;41:511–29
21. Conant MA, Berger TG, Coates TJ, *et al.* Genital herpes: an integrated approach to management. *J Am Acad Dermatol* 1996;35:601–5

22. Halder RM. Pseudofolliculitis barbae and related disorders. *Dermatol Clin* 1988;6: 407–12

23. Brown LA Jr. Pathogenesis and treatment of pseudofolliculitis barbae. *Cutis* 1983;32: 373–5

24. Coquilla BH. Management of pseudofolliculitis barbae. *Milit Med* 1995;160:263–9

25. Kantor GR, Ratz JL, Wheeland RG. Treatment of acne keloidalis nuchae with carbon dioxide laser. *J Am Acad Dermatol* 1986;14:263–7

26. Dinehart SM, Herzberg AJ, Kern BJ, Pollack SV. Acne keloidalis: a review. *J Dermatol Surg Oncol* 1989;15:642–7

27. Knable AL, Hanke CW, Gonin R. Prevalence of acne keloidalis nuchae in football players. *J Am Acad Dermatol* 1997;37:570–4

28. Unger WP. *Hair Transplantation*, 3rd edn. New York: Marcel Dekker, 1995

29. Sawaya ME. Clinical updates in hair. *Dermatol Clin* 1997;15:37–43

30. Kaufman KD, Olsen EA, Whiting D, *et al.* Finasteride in the treatment of men with androgenetic alopecia. *J Am Acad Dermatol* 1998;39:578–89

31. Price VH, Menefee E, Strauss PC. Changes in hair weight and hair count in men with androgenetic alopecia, after application of 5% and 2% minoxidil, placebo, or no treatment. *J Am Acad Dermatol* 1999;41:717–21

32. Gupta AK, Scher RK, De Doncker P. Current management of onychomycosis. *Dermatol Clin* 1997;15:121–35

33. Cook WR Jr, Cook KK. *Manual of Tumescent Liposculpture and Laser Cosmetic Surgery*. Philadelphia: Lippincott Williams & Wilkins, 1999

34. Coleman WP III, Hanke CW, Alt TH, Asken S. *Cosmetic Surgery of the Skin*, 2nd edn. St. Louis: Mosby, 1997

35. Dover JS, Arndt KA, Geronemus RG, Alora MBT. *Illustrated Cutaneous and Aesthetic Laser Surgery*, 2nd edn. Stamford, CT: Appleton & Lange, 2000

36. Brody HJ. *Chemical Peeling and Resurfacing*, 2nd edn. St. Louis: Mosby, 1997

37. Usatine RP, Moy RL, Tobinick EL, Siegel DM. *Skin Surgery*. St. Louis: Mosby, 1998

38. Ratz JL, Geronemus RG, Goldman MP, *et al.* *Textbook of Dermatologic Surgery*. Philadelphia: Lippincott-Raven, 1998

39. Randle HW. Basal cell carcinoma. Identification and treatment of the high risk patient. *Dermatol Surg* 1996;22:255–61

40. Goldberg LH. Basal cell carcinoma. *Lancet* 1996;347:663–7

41. Goldman GD. Squamous cell carcinoma: a practical approach. *Semin Cutan Med Surg* 1998;17:80–95

42. Johnson TM, Rowe DE, Nelson BR, Swanson NA. Squamous cell carcinoma of the skin (excluding lip and oral mucosa). *J Am Acad Dermatol* 1992;26:467–84

43. Kwa RE, Campana K, Moy RL. Biology of cutaneous squamous cell carcinoma. *J Am Acad Dermatol* 1992;26:1–26

44. Hall HI, Miller DR, Rogers JD. Update on the incidence and mortality from melanoma in the United States. *J Am Acad Dermatol* 1999; 40:35–42

45. Johnson TM, Yahanda AM, Chang AE, *et al.* Advances in melanoma therapy. *J Am Acad Dermatol* 1998;38:731–41

46. Berwick M, Begg CB, Fine JA, *et al.* Screening for cutaneous melanoma by skin self-examination. *J Natl Cancer Inst* 1996;88: 17–23

47. Gross EA. Initial evaluation of melanoma. *Arch Dermatol* 1998;134:623–4

48. Arbiser JL. Melanoma. Lessons from metastases. *Arch Dermatol* 1998;134:1027–8

50 Hair disorders

Janet L. Roberts, MD

INTRODUCTION

There are some hair and scalp conditions that are almost unique to males, and others that are not gender specific, but deserve discussion in the context of the treatment of hair and scalp disorders. One thing that is constant, however, is the societal and psychological significance of hair loss[1-3]. Hair loss can be devastating at any age and affects both men and women with serious societal and pyschologic implications. Hair loss is frequently the most traumatic side-effect for cancer patients[3]; scalp hair can be a source of pride or pain at any age.

HAIR GROWTH CHARACTERISTICS

There are different types of hair shafts. Terminal hairs are large and pigmented. Small, unpigmented hairs, lacking an arrector pili muscle, are called vellus hairs and there are hairs intermediate in caliber and length between the two types called indeterminate hairs. A brief review of hair cycling, which all hair follicles continue throughout the lifetime of an individual, will aid in conceptualizing several scalp hair disorders discussed in this section.

Hair follicle activity is intermittent and characterized by a growth phase (anagen), followed by a brief transition phase (catagen) and a resting phase (telogen). Normally 90% or more of scalp hair is in the anagen phase at any given time, 8–10% is in the telogen phase and less than 1% is in the catagen phase (Figure 1). Anagen phase is determined genetically and is unique to each individual, but averages 2–4 years in duration.

The duration of anagen phase determines the natural length to which an individual's hair will grow and tends to remain stable unless pathologic alterations intervene. Telogen hairs are also retained for defined periods of time and are then shed. On the scalp telogen hairs are held for 2–3 months before they are shed. The follicles in different anatomic sites vary in duration of anagen and telogen phases, which gives hair its growth characteristics by site. Those areas with long anagen cycles and a short telogen phase, such as scalp hair, produce a long hair fiber. A short anagen growth phase coupled with a prolonged telogen phase produces the shorter, stable hairs of the eyebrows and eyelashes, and the terminal hairs on the extremities. Scalp hair grows at approximately one centimeter a month, although the growth rate slows down with advancing age and in some pathologic states such as hypothyroidism.

Hair shafts and root sheaths are of ectodermal derivation. The dermal papillae that nourish the follicles are mesodermal in origin. Because hair follicles are self-renewing, they contain a population of slow-cycling stem cells. The stem cells of hair follicles are thought to be located at the 'bulge' region in the outer root sheath near the insertion of the arrector pili muscle[4]. It has been suggested that the anagen phase is initiated when stem cells are activated by signals from the dermal papilla. This has implications in cicatricial versus non-cicatricial hair conditions, which will be addressed in the following sections. Scalp hair loss can result

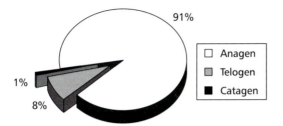

Figure 1 Approximate percentage of time spent in each phase of hair growth. Hair cycles continuously from anagen phase to catagen phase to telogen phase and back to anagen phase throughout the lifespan of an individual

from disturbance of hair cycling, scarring or permanent destruction of the follicles (cicatricial alopecias) and changes in follicular architecture.

MALE PATTERN HAIR LOSS (ANDROGENETIC ALOPECIA)

Clinical presentation

The most prevalent type of scalp hair loss in males is male pattern hair loss (MPHL), also known as androgenetic alopecia. MPHL is caused by a combination of genetic and hormonal influences. It results from long-term changes in follicular architecture and alterations of growth cycles. MPHL is the androgen-dependent manifestation of miniaturization of the hairs of the crown of the scalp, a reflection of progressive diminishing size and pigmentation of the hairs, ultimately rendering them cosmetically insignificant. This is a culmination of three changes in the hair cycle: (1) shortening of the anagen or growing phase, which is ordinarily three or more years in duration, down to months and, ultimately, to weeks, thus shortening the length to which the hairs grow; (2) maintaining the telogen or rest phase stable at three months and increasing the latency period between the telogen and new anagen phase; and (3) a decrease in the volume of matrix cells which reduces the caliber of the hair shaft[5,6].

Males tend to exhibit miniaturization in genetically predetermined patterns of vertex hair loss classified by Hamilton[7] and later

modified by Norwood[8] (Figure 2). Approximately 20% of Caucasian males at age 20 show signs of male pattern hair loss, with the incidence increasing by 10% each decade thereafter, until about 50% of Caucasian males at age 50 are affected. Approximately 5% of males have a diffuse type of thinning over the scalp vertex with retention of the frontal hairline more typical of the female phenotype, but the mechanism is thought to be the same (Figure 3)[9]. It is now felt that hair loss in some individuals over 60 years of age may not necessarily be a result of the hormonal influences discussed below, but may be a response to progressive follicular failure.

Pathophysiology

Hair follicles are capable not only of responding to androgens, but also of participating in the metabolism of androgens. This peripheral metabolism of hormones contributes significantly to the overall endocrine system. Testosterone is the major androgen precursor of dihydrotestosterone in men. Facial, pubic, axillary and body hair follicles in different regions are variably responsive to androgens. Pubic and axillary hair transforms from vellus to terminal hair in response to modest levels of testosterone. Facial and body hair growth requires the 5-α reduced product of testosterone, dihydrotestosterone, for expression[10]. For unknown reasons dihydrotestosterone has the opposite effect on scalp hair in genetically prone males, by converting terminal hairs to vellus-like hairs, termed miniaturized hairs (Figure 4).

Historically, Hamilton first demonstrated that androgens are a prerequisite for the expression of MPHL, although it had long been observed that males at an early age did not go bald.[6] He devised a classification system, later revised by Norwood (Figure 5). Testosterone is converted to dihydrotestosterone by the enzyme 5α-reductase (5-α R) of which there are two subtypes, designated isoenzymes type I and type II. In the 1970s observations of male pseudohermaphrodites genetically lacking the

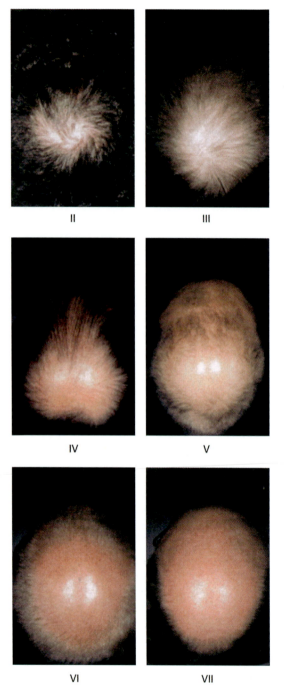

II   III

IV   V

VI   VII

Figure 2 Hamilton–Norwood classification of males with androgenetic alopecia

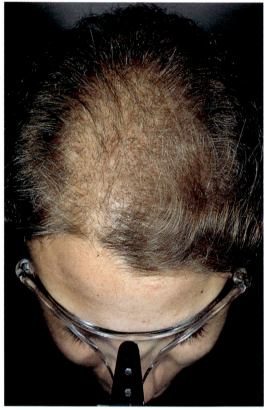

Figure 3 Male with androgenetic alopecia demonstrating female pattern of hair loss with diffuse vertex thinning and retention of frontal hairline

Putative effects of androgens on scalp hair in male pattern hair loss

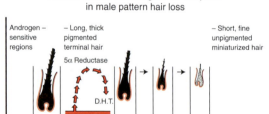

Figure 4 Miniaturizing effect of androgens on scalp hair. Figure reproduced with permission from Wade M, Sinclair R. Disorders of hair. In Parish LC, Brenner S, Ramos-e-Silva M, eds. *Women's Dermatology*. London: Parthenon Publishing, 2000;137. DHT, dihydrotestosterone

type II 5α-reductase enzyme further defined the role of hormones in the development of MPHL. These individuals, who do not develop MPHL, demonstrated that dihydrotestosterone, rather that testosterone, is the hormone responsible for the development of MPHL[11]. The essential role of dihydrotestosterone in the

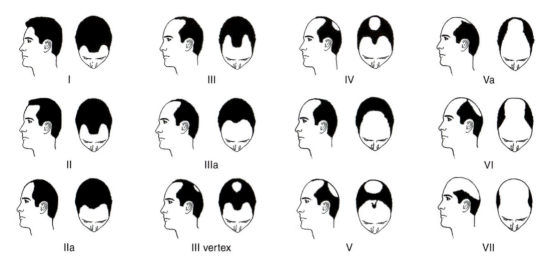

Figure 5 Hamilton–Norwood scale for androgenetic alopecia in males. Figure reproduced with permission from Roberts JL. Geriatric hair and scalp disorders. In Norman RA, ed. *Geriatric Dermatology*. London, UK: Parthenon Publishing, 2001:35–64

manifestation of MPHL was further defined by studies using finasteride, a pure inhibitor of type II 5-α reductase, to treat MPHL.

Diagnosis

The diagnosis of MPHL can be made clinically by examining the entire scalp, noting the Hamilton–Norwood pattern and decreased density secondary to miniaturization of hairs over the vertex. Look for signs of patchy hair loss, inflammation or evidence of scarring, which may signal a different diagnosis.

Treatment

Two medical therapies for MPHL are currently available:

Minoxidil

The mechanism of action of minoxidil, first formulated as an oral antihypertensive agent, on hair follicles is not clearly understood. Hypertrichosis was an unanticipated and serendipitous side-effect. Minoxidil is a vasodilator that works on vascular smooth muscle by opening potassium channels. Uno and colleagues[12] have done extensive research with minoxidil on the stump-tailed macaque monkey, a primate that

has long served as the primary animal model for androgenetic alopecia. They observed early on that minoxidil both grossly and microscopically enlarges vellus follicles to the size of mid-sized and terminal follicles (regrowth) and maintains terminal follicles in prebalding scalps (prevention); the earlier treatment was instituted the better the response to therapy. They further showed that minoxidil enhances DNA synthesis in follicular but not epidermal keratinocytes[12] and causes proliferation and differentiation of the matrix cells in the hair bulb[13].

Two-percent minoxidil has been available for a number of years for the treatment of males under 49 years of age with MPHL[14]. A 5% topical solution of minoxidil (Rogaine Extra Strength for Men®) was granted FDA approval in 1997. The efficacy of topical minoxidil has not been evaluated in males over 50 years of age. However, therapeutic trial in individuals over 50 years is warranted because of the anecdotal observation of hair regrowth following the use of oral minoxidil.

Finasteride

Recent double-blind, placebo-controlled studies on men aged 18–41 exhibiting Hamilton-Norwood patterns II–IV using 1 mg finasteride, a pure type II 5-α reductase inhibitor, have been shown to increase or maintain hair counts from baseline in 83% of men at 24 months in an ongoing 5-year clinical study. At the same time point, 72% of men taking placebo showed a decrease in hair counts[15]. By global photographic assessment, 99% of finasteride patients were rated as having either increased hair growth or no visible loss, and 1% rated as decreased. Sixty-seven per cent of placebo patients were rated as having no further hair loss and 33% rated as decreased[15]. Unpublished 5-year data show a continued benefit in the improvement and/or prevention of further hair loss by global photography. These men showed an average of 0.2 ng/ml decrease in prostate-specific antigen (PSA). Earlier studies on older men treated for benign prostatic hypertrophy showed an approximately 50% decline in serum PSA. Therefore, men over 50 years being treated with finasteride should have PSA values doubled after six months of therapy. Furthermore, it has been demonstrated that finasteride does not mask the detection of prostate cancer[16]. Finasteride reduces serum dihydrotestosterone by 71% and scalp dihydrotestosterone by 65%[17].

Finasteride (Propecia®) was approved by the FDA in the USA in early 1998 for the treatment of men aged 18–41 years with MPHL. The effect of finasteride in males 41–60 years old with androgenetic alopecia is currently being evaluated as are men aged 18–41 years having more advanced MPHL. A specific method of counting anagen hairs showed a 26% net improvement in the anagen hair counts over baseline at 48 weeks of treatment with 1 mg finasteride compared to placebo-treated subjects[18]. Another method of testing finasteride used hair weight as a method to integrate increases in hair caliber, hair length and growth rate. There was a 36% net improvement in hair weight at week 96 as compared to placebo patients observed over the same interval.

Hair transplantation

Refinements in hair transplantation methods are yielding superior results if patients are adequately screened for suitability, including hair quality and degree of hair loss, age considerations, and experience and skill of the surgeon performing the transplanting procedure. In this procedure hairs harvested from the occipital region of the scalp are carefully redistributed to the vertex or frontal hairline utilizing large numbers of very small 'transplants', i.e. follicular units or multiples of individual hairs, giving a more natural appearance. Transplantation can be combined with the use of oral finasteride or topical minoxidil to supplement existing hair density.

Clinical correlations

The possible correlation between baldness and coronary artery disease has been explored in a number of epidemiological studies on men[19–24]. In 1993 Trevisan and colleagues[22] reported on 872 factory workers in southern Italy, comparing cholesterol levels and blood pressure with type of balding. They looked at those men who had no balding, frontotemporal recession only (M-shaped resculpting in post-adolescent males) with men who had frontotemporal and vertex loss. A positive correlation was found with the more severe phenotype and elevated cholesterol and younger age. The relationship became weaker in older individuals. There was no correlation between age and balding and blood pressure. Results indicate that the vertex pattern of baldness is associated with an elevated coronary heart disease risk profile, and the relationship between age and serum cholesterol differs in younger and older men. In the same year Lesko and co-workers[25] reported on a case–control, hospital-based study of 655 men between the ages of 21 and 54 who were experiencing their first myocardial infarction. They were age-matched for patients admitted to the hospital for non-cardiac related illnesses with no prior history of any cardiac disorder. They found that frontal balding was not associated with an increased risk of myocardial infarction while vertex balding was associated with an increased risk, and that this risk increased with the extent of balding. There was an almost 3-fold risk with severe vertex balding (1.3 versus 3.4). In 1997 Ford and colleagues[20] reported similar findings on 2932 men who were rated as having none, minimal, moderate and severe balding. The cohort was followed for 14 years. For men under age 55 at baseline, there was a positive correlation between severe baldness and ischemic heart disease and mortality providing support for earlier studies demonstrating such an association. There was a somewhat less convincing association between the incidence of ischemic heart disease and less severe male-pattern balding in men under 55. The authors hypothesized that there may be some mechanistic relationship between male pattern balding and ischemic heart disease.

The Framingham study, reported by Herrera and colleagues[21] in 1995, followed a cohort of males for up to thirty years. They looked at the progression of balding for new coronary heart-related death, cardiovascular disease and death from any cause. Extent of baldness was not associated with any outcome. Progression of balding pattern, however, was associated with the occurrence of coronary heart disease, mortality and all-cause mortality, indicating that rapid hair loss may be a marker for coronary heart disease.

Two studies finding no associated risk between coronary artery disease and baldness are worthy of note. Halim and co-workers[23] studied 48 men who had recovered from myocardial infarction and age-matched controls. No evidence relating myocardial infarction to androgenic stimulation was noted, as assessed by plasma testosterone, muscle thickness, sebum excretion rate, androgenetic alopecia or density of terminal hair on the body. There was a slight increase in muscle and bone thickness. Cooke[24] studied 478 male in-patient Caucasians, finding no correlation with coronary artery disease and male pattern alopecia[24]. Men who had hypertension, diabetes mellitus or elevated cholesterol were excluded from this study.

Recent publications have suggested that men with early onset MPHL (younger than 35 at onset) have an increased risk for obesity, hypertension and dyslipidemia compared with age-matched controls, suggesting that this phenotype could be a marker for insulin resistance, perhaps the genetic equivalent of polycystic ovarian syndrome in women[26]. A retrospective study on 22 071 males with none, frontal or vertex balding, aged 40–84, related coronary heart disease with degree of MPHL[27]. Adjusting for hypertension, diabetes, smoking and elevated levels of cholesterol, there was a positive correlation between the degree of balding and coronary heart disease.

Histopathology

The first pathologic change noted in early biopsies of androgenetic alopecia is degeneration of the lower third of the connective tissue sheath around the growing or anagen hair follicles. As the condition becomes more severe, the histology mirrors the clinical picture: that of progressive miniaturization of affected terminal hair follicles in a mosaic pattern[28]. The diminution of the follicle size is accompanied by shortening of the anagen phase[13]. The connective tissue sheath is replaced by 'streamers' underneath the miniaturized follicles. The miniaturized anagen hairs retain the arrector pili muscle in contradistinction to true vellus hairs, which are also found in increased numbers. Likewise, the percentage of telogen hairs increases, probably as a result of shortening of the anagen phase. Young and colleagues[29] reported granular immune complex deposits of IgM or C3 or both at the basement membrane of 96% of specimens from involved scalps as well as porphyrins, possibly from the action of UV radiation on *Propionibacterium acnes* around the follicles. Lattanand and Johnson[30] found a moderate amount of chronic inflammatory cells surrounding capillaries and adnexal structures. Both of these authors believe that androgenetic alopecia is an inflammatory process[29,30], though Maguire and Kligman[28] noted no such association in

Table 1 Follicular density by age

Age	Approximate number of hairs/cm^2
Birth	1135
1 year	795
15 years	615
30 years +	485
80 years	435

Table reproduced with permission from Olsen E. *Disorders of Hair Growth, Diagnosis and Treatment*. New York: McGraw Hill

1962. However, Jaworsky, Kligman and Murphy[31] in 1992 examined the ultrastructural changes in alopetic scalp skin, noting progressive fibrosis of the perifollicular sheath associated with mast cell degranulation and fibroblast activation, predated by T-cell infiltration of follicular stem cell epithelium. Injury to follicular stem cell epithelium and/or thickening of the advential sheaths may impair normal hair cycling and lead to hair loss.

SENESCENT ALOPECIA

Etiology

Follicular density decreases with age (Table 1)[32]. This process is called senescent or involutional alopecia and is defined as global or diffuse hair thinning without vertex accentuation after age 50 years. Vertex and occipital regions are similarly affected. It is considered different from MPHL. It results from reduction in follicle size and/or follicular dropout, which are not scarring processes but rather processes in which hair follicles gradually cease to produce a hair shaft. This may be a result of exhaustion of the allocated anagen–telogen cycles within an individual's life span, perhaps genetically predetermined, and appears to be highly variable. Life events which 'use up' or accelerate these cycles may alter the age of onset and extent of senescent alopecia. Some octogenarians have remarkably dense hair. Other individuals demonstrate an obvious global decrease in hair density in the sixth decade.

Histopathology

Histopathology shows an increase in numbers of telogen follicles and a decrease in follicle size, perhaps reflecting a decrease in volume of actively dividing matrix cells in the hair bulb[33,34].

Diagnosis

The diagnosis can generally be made clinically by evaluating the density of hair over the entire scalp. If the density is diminished globally with no patchy hair loss or evidence of scarring, a presumptive diagnosis can be made. The part width on the vertex and occiput should be compared; in senescent alopecia they are the same or nearly so.

Treatment

There are no available data on therapy for senescent alopecia. Anecdotal reports of the regrowth of scalp hair in elderly individuals using oral minoxidil provide a rationale for the trial of topical minoxidil. (See treatment section of androgenetic alopecia for details.) Much remains to be clarified regarding the incidence, etiology and pathophysiology of senescent hair loss.

GRAYING OF HAIR

Another aspect of senescence is the gradual loss of pigment in the hair shaft, which is also a genetically determined trait. Graying can result from the gradual loss of tyrosinase activity resulting in a hybrid of colors, often referred to as 'salt and pepper hair'. Alternatively melanocytes can stop pigment production altogether, resulting in white hair. There have been two recent reports assessing the correlation between early graying and morbidity and mortality. In the prospective Copenhagen City Heart Study, studying a random sample of 20 000 people over a sixteen-year period, no correlation was found between mortality and the extent of graying[35]. A second report of office and autopsy reports showed no correlation of early death or increased morbidity with early graying[36].

TELOGEN EFFLUVIUM

Hair matrix cells are among the most rapidly proliferating cells in the body, second only to bone marrow cells and cells lining the gastric mucosa. Consequently numerous physiologic insults may result in an increase in the premature transformation of the anagen phase to the telogen phase, a process called telogen effluvium. This results in increased numbers of telogen hairs shed daily two to three months following the physiologic insult. Telogen hairs have a small, white club-shaped end and are easily identified on gross examination[37]. On the normal scalp 50–100 hairs are shed daily and fall relatively unnoticed by the individual. 'Effluvium' is a Latin word meaning 'to flow out' and aptly describes the fall of telogen hairs. Hair is shed diffusely from all over the scalp, although the temples and anterior hairline tend to be more severely affected[37]. Regrowth follows the cessation of trauma and resumption of normal follicular cycling. Normal density is regained provided senescent alopecia or MPHL is not unmasked. The incidence of telogen effluvium increases as the number of physiologic insults increase with aging, such as surgery, acute[38] and chronic illnesses, and the increasing numbers of medications to treat them[39]. Some causes of telogen effluvium, such as iron deficiency, are not as prevalent in males because they do not suffer from recurring menstrual blood loss (unpublished data, JL Roberts). Also, fewer males undergo the stresses of protein deprivation due to unusual dietary habits or rapid weight loss due to intentional 'crash dieting', although males may suffer from unintentional weight loss caused by various illnesses. Zinc deficiency and essential free fatty acid deficiency, common in the 1970s and 1980s in patients on total parenteral nutrition, has been largely eliminated in the West as knowledge about nutrition requirements has improved[40–42].

The number of drugs reported to cause telogen effluvium is large[39,43]. The *Physician's Desk Reference* and *Drugs: Facts and Comparisons* .

list alopecia occurring between 1 and 2% of the time for many drugs. These statistics relate to reports of telogen effluvium during clinical trials or post-marketing reporting. In the author's experience, confirmed by literature reports, several drugs are commonly associated with increased hair shedding and deserve special mention. Among these are beta-blockers, both oral and intraocular, antihyperlipemic drugs and non-steroidal anti-inflammatory drugs and anticoagulants (Table 2). Acute or chronic telogen effluvium may unmask or accelerate the expression of MPHL or senescent alopecia in genetically prone individuals.

Evaluation

A careful counting of the telogen hairs shed over a three-day or weekly period will help establish the diagnosis if it averages over 100/day. Physical examination of the scalp and hair should be performed to rule out scarring or patchy hair loss. A light hair-pull test, performed by grasping 40–50 hairs between the thumb and fingers and pulling with enough traction to gently tent up the scalp, is considered positive if 2–3 hairs are retrieved on freshly shampooed hair or 5–6 hairs on unwashed hair. Visualization of the regrowing hair tips will help to determine the length of hairs growing, which can be a helpful clue in determining the onset of shedding. Generally the hair begins to regrow at about the time that shedding begins and grows at a fairly consistent rate of one centimeter/month. A careful health and medication history and physical examination are imperative. Dietary history needs to be assessed to ensure adequate caloric and protein intake. Note should be made of any acute and chronic health problems and medications used, including prescription and over-the-counter medications. The timing of new medications should be noted in relationship to the onset of shedding. Generally the initiation of drug therapy can be timed to the duration of the telogen phase, resulting in a lag period of 2–3 months before the onset of shedding. Cause

Table 2 Drugs that may cause hair loss

Antibiotics	*Antihypertensive agents*	Hydroxyurea	*Histamine (H₂) antagonists*
Ethambutol	Atenolol	Interferon	Cimetidine
Ethionamide	Captopril	Methotrexate	Famotidine
Gentamycin	Enalapril	Radiation	Ranitidine
Nitrofurantoin	Labetalol	Vincristine	
Streptomycin	Metoprolol		*Hormones*
	Minoxidil	*Antipsychotic agents*	Anabolic steroids
Anticoagulants	Nadolol	All tricyclic antidepressants	Clomiphene
Bishydroxycoumarin	Propranolol	Benzodiazepines	Corticosteroids
Coumarin	Verapamil	Buspirone HCl	Danazol
Dextran		Clomipramine HCl	Oral contraceptives
Gemfibrozil	*Intraocular*	Doxepin HCl	Progesterones
Heparin	Betaxolol	Fluoxetine	
Heparinoids	Levobunolol	Fluvoxamine	*Miscellaneous drugs*
	Timolol	Lithium	Acyclovir
Anticonvulsants		Paroxetine HCl	Amphetamines
Carbamazepine	*Anti-inflammatory agents*	Phenothiazines	Boric acid
Clonazopam	Diclofenac	Sertraline HCl	Bromocriptine
Trimethadione	Ibuprofen	Trazodone	Diethylpropion HCl
Valproic acid	Indomethacin		Hydroxychloroquine sulfate
	Naproxen	*Antithyroid drugs*	Levodopa
Antifungal agents	Piroxicam	Carbimazole	Methysergide
Fluconazole	Salicylates	Iodine	Nifedipine
Itraconazole	Sulindac	Methylthiouracil	Pencillamine
Terbinafine		Propylthiouracil	Pyridostigmine
	Antikeratinizing agents		Quinacrine
Antigout agents	Etretinate	*Heavy metals*	Spironolactone
Allopurinol	Isotretinoin	Arsenic	Sulfasalazine
Probenecid	Thallium	Bismuth	Alendronate
Colchicine	Vitamin A	Gold	
		Lead	
Antihyperlipidemic agents	*Anitimitotic agents*	Mercury	
Simvastatin	Alkaloids	Selenium	
Lovastatin	Alkylating drugs		
Pravastatin	Antimetabolites		
Fluvastatin	Colchicine		
Atorvastain	Cyclophosphamide		
Niacin			

and effect of drug therapy should be carefully documented, if possible, with particular attention paid to the onset of shedding. If appropriate, rechallenge with the suspected medication may be helpful. Particular attention should be given to thyroid evaluation and replacement therapy. Patients can shed from over-replacement as well as under-replacement of thyroid.

Laboratory tests should be selected based on the historical findings. Chemical screening will screen for evidence of chronic diseases. Antimitotic drugs usually result in anagen effluvium (see following section), although low doses may cause telogen effluvium. Assess thyroid function by obtaining thyroid stimulating hormone levels and free thyroxine to screen for hypo- and hyperthyroidism, both of which can result in telogen effluvium. Lowered serum albumin may be detected if dietary protein is deficient or the patient is chronically ill. Obtain antinuclear antibody screen if autoimmune disorder is suspected. Iron is an essential element in several enzyme systems related to hair growth. For assessment of adequacy of iron, some clinicians rely on serum iron and percentage saturation. Others prefer to monitor ferritin levels as an indicator of total body iron stores. Because ferritin is an acute phase reactant, it is important to obtain an erythrocyte sedimentation rate (ESR) as well. If ESR is elevated, the ferritin will be artificially elevated. Ferritin levels should be at least 40 ng/dl to ensure adequate stores for hair regrowth. The assessment of hematocrit and hemoglobin is not sufficient, as iron stores may be depleted in the face of normal values of these parameters.

Treatment

The prognosis for spontaneous hair regrowth is good if the underlying causes are addressed, provided senescent and/or androgenetic alopecia is not unmasked or accelerated. In the older age groups, however, chronic diseases and illnesses of aging make chronic telogen effluvium more common. Any dietary deficiencies should be corrected. Iron replacement is necessary in those individuals deficient on testing. Thyroid replacement therapy should be finely tuned. At times it is not possible to substitute for a drug that will not cause shedding. This is particularly true of hyperlipemic drugs, many of which may cause shedding. Beta-blockers, used orally for hypertension and intraocularly for glaucoma, present another therapeutic dilemma, as most of the drugs in this class have been reported to cause shedding[44–46]. The anticoagulants heparin and coumadin have both been implicated in shedding, leaving little choice but to tolerate their side-effects[47]. Bisphosphonates used to treat osteoporosis have been reported to cause telogen effluvium.

ANAGEN EFFLUVIUM

Anagen effluvium is the shedding of anagen or growing hairs following common therapeutic doses of chemotherapeutic drugs, used for the treatment of cancer. Ninety per cent or more of scalp hair is typically in the anagen phase at any given time. This, coupled with the fact that hair matrix cells divide every 9–12 hours, makes them highly vulnerable to the effects of toxic drugs. Up to 90% of hair may be lost as the hair shafts are attenuated by the abrupt interference with or cessation of mitosis in the hair matrix cells. Shedding generally begins within days to a few weeks after therapy as the attenuated hair shafts reach the surface of the scalp. The 10% of hairs not lost in the immediate 2–3 weeks post-therapy period are likely to be telogen hairs that will be shed as a natural event, rendering the loss of scalp hair virtually complete in many patients. If the insult is temporary, as in the case of intermittent or episodic therapy, regrowth should be virtually complete because the bulge area has not been subjected to injury. As discussed in the introduction, this may be the most traumatic side-effect that cancer patients endure.

Treatment

No treatment is necessary for hair regrowth once therapy is terminated.

SCARRING ALOPECIA

Scarring or permanent alopecia can present a confusing clinical picture. Early diagnosis and treatment are essential. Scarring is the result of destruction of the stem cells at the region of the bulge. Once a hair follicle has been destroyed, it is irretrievably lost. Patients presenting with patchy or ill-defined hair loss should be examined thoroughly for any signs of scarring as manifested by patchy hair loss, obliteration of follicular orifices, erythema, telangiectasias, follicular hyperkeratosis or pigmentary changes. The remainder of the skin, mucous membranes and nails should be examined, looking for signs of lichen planus or discoid lupus erythematosus.

If scarring is present or suspected, early biopsy is important, and ideally should include two 4 mm biopsies, one for vertical and one for horizontal sectioning, stained with hematoxylin and eosin. If an autoimmune disease such as lupus erythematosus is suspected, a biopsy for immunofluorescent evaluation is recommended[48,49]. A periodic acid-schiff (PAS) stain may be helpful to examine basement membrane thickening, which may be noted in lupus erythematosus. Scarring or permanent alopecias can be divided into those

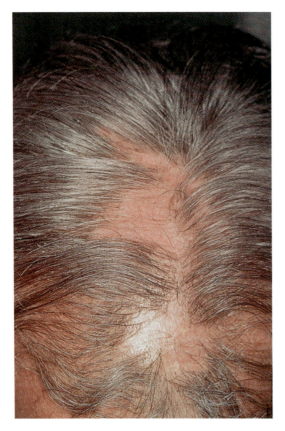

Figure 6 Scarring alopecia (lichen planopilaris). Figure reproduced with permission from Roberts JL. Geriatric hair and scalp disorders. In Norman RA, ed. *Geriatric Dermatology*. London, UK: Parthenon Publishing, 2001: 35–64

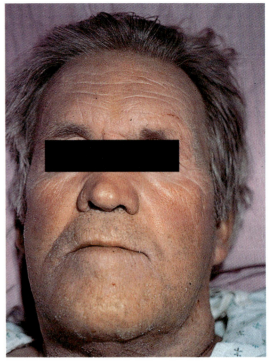

Figure 7 Seborrheic dermatitis in male with involvement of hairline, eyebrows, nasolabial folds and beard areas. Figure reproduced with permission from Roberts JL. Geriatric hair and scalp disorders. In Norman RA, ed. *Geriatric Dermatology*. London, UK: Parthenon Publishing, 2001:35–64

due to inflammatory and those due to non-inflammatory causes[50].

Inflammatory scarring alopecia

Inflammatory scarring alopecias include discoid lupus erythematosus, lichen planopilaris, folliculitis decalvans and infectious processes. End-stage scarring in several conditions may appear similar with white, round to oval patches of smooth bare scalp without evidence of the underlying pathologic process (Figure 6).

Treatment

Topical corticosteroids in a liquid, gel, spray or foam vehicle may be applied once to twice daily to suppress inflammatory processes. Plaquenil, 100–200 mg daily, may be useful in treating discoid lupus erythematosus and lichen planopilaris. For the neutrophilic folliculitis, folliculitis decalvans, not infrequently either primarily or secondarily colonized with *Staphylococcus aureus*, oral antibiotics may be beneficial. Minocycline 100–200 mg daily may be effective, for both its anti-inflammatory and its antibacterial properties. Rifampin, combined with either dicloxicillin or clindamycin, may be useful in patients repeatedly culture positive for *S. aureus*.

Non-inflammatory scarring alopecia

Non-inflammatory causes of scarring alopecia include hereditary and developmental origin,

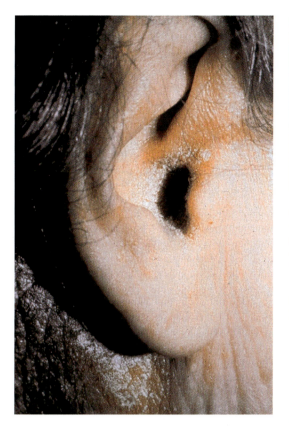

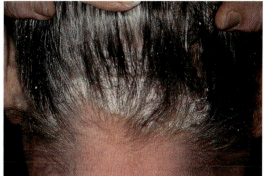

Figure 9 Thick psoriatic plaques in occipital scalp with extension on to posterior neck. Figure reproduced with permission from Roberts JL. Geriatric hair and scalp disorders. In Norman RA, ed. *Geriatric Dermatology*. London, UK: Parthenon Publishing, 2001:35–64

patients are to be found in the kidney and lung. Papillary thyroid carcinoma metastasizing to the scalp is commonly reported in the literature. There are many reports in the literature of a multiplicity of different common and rare malignant tumors presenting initially as scalp nodules. Any lesion that is new, rapidly growing or unfamiliar in appearance should be biopsied.

Treatment

Treatment should address the underlying neoplastic process.

INFLAMMATORY SCALP DISORDERS

Three inflammatory scalp disorders deserve discussion: psoriasis, seborrheic dermatitis and dermatomyositis. Psoriasis of the scalp and seborrheic dermatitis are both common and present in males and females equally.

Seborrheic dermatitis

Greasy, yellowish scales distributed diffusely over the scalp characterize seborrheic dermatitis. Areas of predilection include hairline, retroauricular and posterior neck, beard, nasolabial folds, eyebrows, sternum and groin (Figure 7). It is accompanied by variable degrees of inflammation. When severe, seborrheic dermatitis may

Figure 8 Psoriatic plaques in retroauricular region and external auditory canal. Figure reproduced with permission from Roberts JL. Geriatric hair and scalp disorders. In Norman RA, ed. *Geriatric Dermatology*. London, UK: Parthenon Publishing, 2001:35–64

and neoplastic tumors, both benign and malignant. Of these, those causes that are developmental and hereditary will most likely be expressed, and hence diagnosed, before adulthood. Neoplastic lesions can be either primary to the scalp or metastatic to the scalp. Of the malignant tumors that are primary to the scalp, basal call carcinoma and squamous cell carcinomas are common. Malignant melanoma and malignant hamartomas can be primary to the scalp. Both B-cell and T-cell lymphomas may occur on the scalp. Cutaneous T-cell lymphoma (CTCL) may exhibit a tendency to affect the follicles preferentially. Alopecia mucinosa occurs, either in association with CTCL, or primary to the scalp. Of lesions metastatic to the scalp, the most common primaries in male be accompanied by mild to moderate telogen effluvium. The incidence and severity may be increased in patients with Parkinson's disease, cerebrovascular accidents[51], head trauma and epilepsy[52–54]. These neurologic disorders may be implicated in exacerbating seborrheic dermatitis by increasing sebum excretion rates, although there is no direct correlation between sebum production and seborrheic dermatitis.

Etiology

Pityrosporum ovale may contribute to the pathogenesis of seborrheic dermatitis[55,56]. The density of *P. ovale* organisms has been correlated with the clinical severity. The metabolism of *P. ovale*-generated free fatty acids may contribute to the inflammatory process, though cause and effect are uncertain. Literature reports support the assumption that strong colonization with *P. ovale* in seborrheic dermatitis is due to altered cellular immunity, which may be induced by increased secretion of interleukin-10 (IL-10)[55].

Histopathology

The stratum corneum shows focal parakeratosis. The epidermis shows mild to moderate acanthosis and spongiosis with mononuclear cells contained within the spongiotic areas. There is a mild mononuclear infiltrate in the dermis.

Treatment

Treatment must be directed towards removal of scale, reduction of inflammation and reduction of *P. ovale* organisms. Frequency of shampooing is important with daily to alternate daily shampooing ideal. Tar shampoos address the scale formation secondary to epidermal proliferation; they are, however, a mechanism for applying medication and should not necessarily be considered cleansing shampoos. A keratolytic shampoo containing salicylic acid, and/or cleansing shampoo of preference can be used before or after the application of tar shampoos. Zinc pyrithione, selenium sulfide, sulfur and salicylic acid shampoos are antimitotic. Ketoconazole, selenium sulfide and zinc pyrithione can reduce *P. ovale* colonization[57–60]. All shampoos should be left on for the recommended time period. A corticosteroid solution or spray may be applied to the scalp following shampooing. There have been reports of oral ketoconazole[60] and topical terbinafine solution[61] in the treatment of seborrheic dermatitis. Rotation of shampoos to prevent tachyphylaxis is important and the continued use of shampoos on a rotational basis should be implemented for maintenance therepy. All other grooming aids, such as conditioner, gels, mousses and hair sprays may be used concomitantly.

Scalp psoriasis

The scalp is a site of predilection for psoriasis and scalp psoriasis occurs in 50% of patients with psoriasis[62]. Runne and Kroneisen-Wiersma[63] noted that scalp involvement was the inaugural event in 66% of their series and in 36% it was exclusively involved. More specifically, the sites of predilection can be similar to those of seborrheic dermatitis with post-auricular, external auditory canal and eyebrows the favored sites (Figure 8). Plaques may extend well beyond the hairline, but the edges, in general, remain very sharply marginated (Figure 9). The psoriatic scale is thick and 'silvery' with more defined plaques of involvement compared to those of seborrheic dermatitis. The degree of inflammation also tends to be greater. Itching and scaling are the symptoms most distressing to patients[64]. Excessive manipulation of the plaques from scratching or sharp-edged combs may provoke worsening psoriasis, a phenomenon called Knoebnerization. The constant attention required to treat psoriasis can be frustrating.

Hair loss may be associated with acute and chronic psoriasis. The erythrodermic form may be associated with telogen effluvium because of systemic side-effects. The hair shafts overlying psoriatic plaques often appear dry and lusterless and break easily[65]. Tufts or clumps of hair may be lost as the adherent scale is removed[63]. There is an anagen to telogen shift in hairs within the plaques with resultant increased shedding of telogen hairs and reduced hair density[65,66]. Runne and Kroneisen-Wiersma reported on hair loss in 47 patients and found telogen counts increased by up to 25–86%. Hair loss was reported as acute in 51%, chronic in 36% and chronic-recurrent in 13%. Alopecia was patchy (75%) or diffuse (25%). With control after therapy, complete regrowth was noted in all but five patients, who showed residual thinning or scarring. Scarring in longstanding scalp psoriasis has been reported[67].

Etiology

The thickened scales are a result of proliferation of the keratinocytes, which demonstrate an increased labeling index. The external root sheath, but not the hair bulb, may share this phenomenon, so the rate of hair growth is normal. Activated T-cells, interacting with antigen presenting cells in the dermis and epidermis, play an integral role in the pathogenesis of psoriasis. Once activated, T-cells release cytokines, which induce hyperproliferation of keratinocytes and further stimulation of T-cells.

Treatment

Consistent adherence to a treatment regimen is necessary to control scalp psoriasis[68]. As in seborrheic dermatitis, treatment consists of removal of the scale and medication of the underlying skin. Compliance may prove difficult for patients with this chronic and frustrating condition. Removal of scale is the first step. Hydration of the scalp by shampooing, soaking the scalp, or wrapping with hot towels will help to improve the effectiveness of medications. Several means may be helpful in loosening the scales. Oils (vegetable oils) with or without a corticosteroid may be left on overnight with occlusion and shampooed out the following morning using a rotation of medicated shampoos (discussed in the previous section). One

such oil and corticosteroid product is Derma-Smoothe FS® containing peanut oil and fluocinolone 0.01%. Another is Baker's P & S Liquid® containing phenol and saline. Keratolytic and antimitotic agents such as oils containing tars (T-Derm®, Sebucare®, Estar®, Psorigel®) aid in loosening the adherent scales.

After daily shampooing, corticosteroids in the form of sprays (Kenalog Spray®, AeroSeb Dex®) and short-term high potency[69,70], or long-term mid-strength topical solutions can be used safely without scalp atrophy[71]. A series of Grenz treatments may be helpful in the acute phase[72]. Grenz ray is a soft X-ray, intermediate between ultraviolet light and conventional X-rays, capable of bypassing hair to penetrate approximately 4 mm deep. Application of UV light with a special combing device may be useful and suitable for home use[73]. Calcipotriol (Devonex®) scalp solution is effective in treating the hyperproliferation of psoriasis by its potent growth inhibiting effects[74]. Calcipotriol may be used in conjunction with topical corticosteroids, either sequentially or in pulse fashion. Salicylic acid reduces the potency of calcipotriol and these two agents should not be combined together. Tazarotene gel, 0.05% and 0.1% (Tazorac®) is a topical retinoid compound, which can be useful for the treatment of glabrous skin lesions around the hairline. Combination with topical steroids can reduce the irritancy potential of this compound. Anthralin, 0.25% and 0.1%, which comes in a scalp preparation (Dritho-Scalp Cream®), may be used with short-contact therapy, applied for 10–20 minutes, increasing duration as tolerated. All topical preparations have more potential to cause irritation on the scalp because of the occlusive effects of overlying hair, and should be applied with caution. Oral diflucan and itraconazole have been helpful in severe cases[75]. Oral treatment with methotrexate, acitretin and cyclosporin is rarely indicated for scalp psoriasis unless patients have severe psoriasis elsewhere. Secondary infections should be treated with appropriate antibiotics.

Histology

There are four features of early involvement of the skin and follicles with follicular plugging: enlargement of the follicular ostium, follicular parakeratosis, mild acanthosis and irregular hyperkeratosis. The outer root sheath and hair matrix are not affected. Other common findings include sebaceous gland atrophy, reduction of follicular size and decrease in hair shaft diameter[76]. Scarring can occur in severe psoriasis caused by inflammatory destruction of the follicle[67].

Dermatomyositis

Dermatomyositis is a rare, inflammatory myopathy manifested by progressive proximal muscle weakness, either isolated (polymyositis) or in combination with a constellation of skin manifestations: erythema of forearms and upper back, painful scaly erythematous papules over the joints (Grotron's papules), edema and heliotrope discoloration on the upper eyelids and scalp involvement characterized by atrophic, scaly, erythematous plaques mimicking psoriasis or seborrheic dermatitis. It can be classified as adult idiopathic, juvenile, or amyopathic as well as being associated with internal malignancy[77]. Although the disease occurs in childhood, peak incidence occurs in the fifth and sixth decades (Figure 10).

In one study of 17 consecutive patients, 14 had scalp involvement at the time of diagnosis; 6 of the 14 had hair loss[78]. McDonald and Smith[79] reported on scalp scaling and dermatomyositis in the pediatric population as well. Various reports indicate 12–34% association with internal malignancies, with the majority of these individuals over 40 years old[78,80–83]. The sources of the malignancies in the male patient are gastrointestinal, lung and melanoma. In the literature from Japan[80] and Singapore[82] nasopharyngeal carcinoma predominates; 31% of malignancies addressed in Singapore originated

in the nasopharynx[82]. Wong[84] reported that 75% of malignancies in 23 cases in a Chinese population originated in the nasopharynx. Koh and colleagues[81] reported an older age (mean 61.8 years) and higher percentage of associated malignancy in patients with dermatomyositis compared with those with polymyositis[81]. Recognition of scalp involvement is important as it may be the presenting complaint in some patients with dermatomyositis. Early diagnosis will alert the treating physician to evaluate patients for possible associated malignancies.

INFECTIOUS SCALP DISORDERS

Tinea capitis

In North America *Trichophyton tonsurans* is becoming the most common causative agent of tinea capitis, followed by *Microsporum canis*. *Microsporum audouinii*, formerly the most common cause of tinea capitis in the USA, typically occurred in prepubertal children and cleared spontaneously in adolescence. Tinea capitis caused by *T. tonsurans* may persist into adulthood and may affect multiple generations. In Europe, *Trichophyton violaceum* and *Microsporum canis* have replaced *Trichophyton schoenleinii* as the most frequent etiologic agents. Tinea capitis is becoming more prevalent in all age groups and should be looked for in all patients with unusual or unresponsive scalp conditions. Any dermatophyte-causing disease in children can cause tinea capitis in adults[85]. When present, lesions are variable and often atypical. It is more common in adult and elderly women than men for unexplained reasons, although styling differences between men and women may play a role[85–87].

The presence of asymptomatic carriers is becoming increasingly important. One survey demonstrated that 30% of adults exposed to a child infected with *T. tonsurans* were colonized[88]. In another study, it was estimated that half of the children infected with *T. tonsurans* had at least one adult contact that was culture

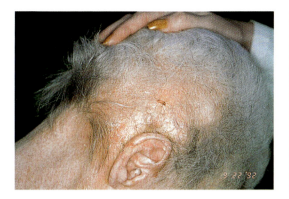

Figure 10 Dermatomyositis of scalp showing erythema and atrophic scaling (Photograph courtesy of JP Callen)

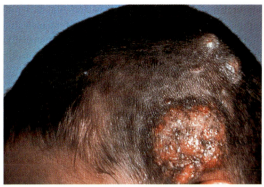

Figure 12 Severely inflammatory tinea capitis with boggy, edematous mass called a kerion

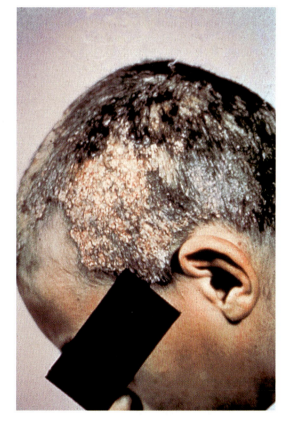

Figure 11 Tinea capitis with inflammatory, adherent scale crust

Clinical presentation

As discussed above, the asymptomatic carrier may have little evidence of infection other than non-inflammatory scaling. The signs of infections may be variable and unusual. Diffuse or patchy alopecia, folliculitis, pustules and/or crusting may be seen in those with more inflammatory infections (Figure 11). A localized, very severe inflammatory reaction presenting as a raised, boggy mass is known as a kerion (Figure 12).

Diagnosis

Direct microscopic examination of infected hairs and/or scales, which have been prepared with 20% KOH solution, will show the hyphal elements in scales or the spores in infected hairs. The spores may be external to the hair shaft as in *Microsporum canis* (ectothrix infection) or inside the hair shaft itself as in *Trichophyton tonsurans* (endothrix infection). Diagnosis can be confirmed by culture on appropriate mycology medium.

Treatment

Oral therapy is generally necessary for treatment of tinea capitis. Griseofulvin has been the standard therapy for decades. Long-term treatment is necessary to achieve cure, which can

positive[89]. Adult individuals who live with or have frequent contact with infected children, especially in crowded conditions, should be considered at risk.

potentially be a deterrent to therapy. Newer oral agents have shown promise in treatment. The azole antifungals fluconazole and itraconazole, and the allylamine antifungal terbinafine have all been examined in comparative studies[90]. Intraconazole (Sporonox™) has been evaluated in multiple studies for the treatment of tinea capitis[91-93]. Several favorable reports using fluconazole in the treatment of tinea capitis have been published[94]. A pulse dosing regimen, using once weekly 8 mg/kg, showed promise[95].

Terbinafine (Lamisil™) has superior penetration into the epidermis, is concentrated in hair and sebum and is effective against all dermatophytes[96], but less so for *Mircosporum* infections[97,98]. Terbinafine is significantly more economical than itraconazole and fluconazole for short courses of therapy and less expensive than griseofulvin used in standard dosage regimens. Safety and tolerability of itraconazole, fluconazole and terbinafine are good. Adjunctive therapy with 2% ketoconazole or 2.5% selenium sulfide shampoo, allowed to remain on the scalp for five minutes three times weekly, should be added to oral therapy to aid in the eradication of infection[99].

Syphilis

Clinical presentation

Syphilis is a systemic disease caused by the spirochete *Treponema pallidum* which, if untreated, may progress through three stages of infection: primary, secondary and tertiary. Loss of scalp hair does not occur in primary syphilis unless a primary lesion is localized to the scalp. Hair loss is not uncommon in the secondary and tertiary stages of syphilis. In its classic form the hair loss in secondary syphilis is an irregular 'moth-eaten' loss of hair scattered throughout the scalp, resembling in some cases a diffuse and patchy alopecia areata. The eyebrows may be shed and there may be a patchy alopecia noted in the beard and other hair-bearing areas

of the body. A second presentation in secondary syphilis is diffuse hair loss resembling that seen in telogen effluvium. A third form of hair loss is associated with the nodulo-ulcerative cutaneous lesions found in patients with lues maligna[100,101]. This nodulo-ulcerative or papulo-pustular presentation of secondary syphilis may affect the scalp as well as other areas of the body. It presents as a papular eruption, becomes generalized, and develops numerous cutaneous ulcerations. Histologically, it is a necrotizing vasculitis[102]. The pleomorphic lesions may be pustular or ulcerative and occur more frequently in immunocompromised hosts. There seems to be a correlation between the papulo-pustular type and the development of neurosyphilis[103,104]. In tertiary syphilis hair loss occurs in the area overlying a gumma.

Histology

Microscopic examination of an area of patchy or diffuse alopecia in a patient with syphilis reveals an inflammatory, non-scarring alopecia. Follicular changes include a decrease in the percentage of hairs in the anagen phase and a corresponding increase in catagen and telogen hairs. There tends to be a sparse, predominantly peribulbar, lymphocytic, superficial perivascular infiltrate with scattered plasma cells and fibrous tract formation. In most cases, even when using special stains, spirochetes are rarely demonstrated in the tissue. This is in contrast to the histology of the scalp alopecia in the nodulo-ulcerative form (secondary stage variant) of syphilis. In the latter specimens, the entire dermis shows a perivascular, lymphohistiocytic infiltrate with epithelioid histiocytic granulomata. In the center of the dermis there is a zone of degenerated collagen and an infiltrate consisting of lymphocytes, histiocytes, neutrophils and fragmented nuclear particles. This pattern follows vessels that show varying degrees of degeneration and necrosis of vessel walls. Throughout the whole inflammatory reaction, plasma cells are predominant and the Warthin–Starry stain demonstrates many spirochetes[101,105].

Epidemiology

Between 1986 and 1990 an epidemic of syphilis occurred throughout the USA paralleling the use of crack cocaine[106]. In 1991 the number of reported cases of primary and secondary syphilis began to decline for the first time since 1985 and have steadily declined since. In 1999 there were 7000 reported cases of primary and secondary syphilis in the USA, almost a 90% decrease in cases from the peak epidemic in 1990[107]. Rates of infection were highest in the south (6.6 cases per 100 000) followed by the midwest (2.0), northeast (1.1) and west (1.0)[106].

Despite the increase in the incidence of secondary syphilis between 1986 and 1990, there was not a substantial increase in the number of patients noted with hair loss as part of the clinical presentation of their disease. Acute hair loss is probably a common manifestation of secondary syphilis, but it tends to be overlooked by both the patient and the physician. Careful inspection of a group of patients with secondary syphilis revealed that 48% had acute hair loss at the time of presentation[108].

Diagnostic procedures

Dark field examination and direct fluorescent antibody tests of lesion exudates or tissue are the definitive methods for distinguishing early syphilis from chancre. A presumptive diagnosis may be made with the use of serologic tests. In secondary syphilis the rapid plasma reagin (RPR) is more reliable[101]. An RPR may be negative in active secondary syphilis owing to an extremely high antibody titer (prozone reaction), but this can be detected by quantitation and serial dilution of the patient's serum. Non-treponemal-test (VDRL and RPR) antibody titers usually correlate with disease activity. The antibody response in patients infected with human immunodeficiency virus (HIV), particularly in the later stages of acquired immunodeficiency syndrome (AIDS), may be compromised and thus the diagnosis obscured[109,110]. Treponemal tests (fluorescent treponemal antibody absorption test (FTA-ABS) and microhemaglutination assay for *Trepomena pallidum* (MHA-TP)) can be confirmatory if clinically warranted.

Treatment

The current Centers for Disease Control (CDC) treatment recommendation for all stages of syphilis is a weekly intramuscular injection of benzathine penicillin G of 2.4 million units with the length of treatment dependent on the stage and clinical manifestation of the disease. Alternative treatments for patients with AIDS and for those who are allergic to penicillin are available in the CDC brochure on syphilis (Division of Sexually Transmitted Diseases, Centers for Disease Control, Atlanta, GA). Patients with early syphilis who are successfully treated have a characteristic pattern of serological response. The RPR titer declines approximately four-fold in 3 months and eight-fold by 6 months. In patients who are immunocompromised owing to HIV infection, these titers should be evaluated at one, two, three, six, and twelve months to assure a continued decline and, therefore, adequate therapeutic response. A Jarisch–Herxheimer reaction – an acute febrile reaction – may occur within the first 24 hours after any treatment for syphilis. This reaction can usually be controlled with corticosteroids or indomethacin[105] but there are no proven methods of prevention.

Herpes zoster

The herpes zoster virus can involve the scalp when the ophthalmic branch of the trigeminal nerve becomes involved. Diagnosis can be made clinically and by Tzank smear. It presents as grouped vesicles along a dermatomal distribution. The vesicles can evolve into crusts and occasionally ulcerations (Figure 13). Pain may be severe. It is estimated that 300 000 new cases of herpes zoster are seen in the USA each year[111]. Several factors influence the incidence, with increasing age being the most consistent[111]. Post-herpetic neuralgia is the number one cause of intractable, debilitating pain in the elderly and is the leading cause of suicide in chronic pain patients over the age of 70 years[111]. Incidence increases with age, particularly after 50 years[112]. The onset of herpes zoster is often preceded by a prodrome consisting of pain, itching and paresthesias. Patients over 50 years old more commonly experience prodromal pain, pain during acute phase infection and post-herpetic neuralgia[113]. Comorbidity symptoms such as insomnia are common[113].

Post-herpetic neuralgia is a serious consequence of herpes zoster and occurs more commonly and lasts longer in patients over 60 years old[112,114]. It is often severe and refractory to treatment. More than 50% of patients over 60 years of age will develop post-herpetic neuralgia, which may persist for months or even years[112]. It is more common in those with trigeminal involvement. Involvement of the cornea is considered a medical emergency as it may cause keratoconjunctivitis, uveitis and ocular motor paralysis[115]. Hair loss and eventual scarring may occur in areas of ulceration.

Treatment

Acute herpes zoster antiviral treatment has changed rapidly in recent years. The efficacy of valacyclovir, the prodrug of acyclovir, and famciclovir[116], the prodrug of penciclovir, has been documented in large clinical trials[117,118]. Both drugs are effective on herpes zoster-associated pain and in shortening the course of the disease. Development of resistance to acyclovir and the nucleoside analogs in the treatment of

immunocompetent individuals has not become a problem. Famciclovir and valacyclovir allow for less frequent daily dosing and higher concentrations of serum drug. Initiation of therapy as soon as possible is advised. Famciclovir, 500 mg t.i.d. for one week, and valacyclovir, 1 gram t.i.d. for one week, are the recommended dosages. Prednisone in cases of trigeminal involvement has been shown to be beneficial[119,120].

TRICHOTILLOMANIA

Trichotillomania (TTM) is a form of traction alopecia characterized by an irresistible compulsion to pull out or twist and break off one's own hair. It represents a complex behavioral pattern of uncertain origins and is associated with biologic and perhaps biochemical brain abnormalities. In this section TTM will include significant hair pulling not occurring in the context of psychosis. It is now recognized that many patients with TTM exhibit compulsive behavior patterns, and TTM is now categorized either as belonging on the obsessive–compulsive disorder (OCD) spectrum[121–123], or as an impulse control disorder[124]. There has been renewed interest in treatment strategies because of the advances in the understanding of associated biochemical abnormalities and the recent availability of medications specifically addressing these abnormalities.

Epidemiology

Trichotillomania is relatively common, with an estimated incidence of up to 1 million Americans, although the exact prevalence is difficult to determine because of dissimilarities in survey methods and the secretiveness of those with this disorder[125].

Clinical features

Two types of trichotillomania (TTM) are recognized. A benign form occurs in early childhood, which is typically of short duration with a 3 : 2

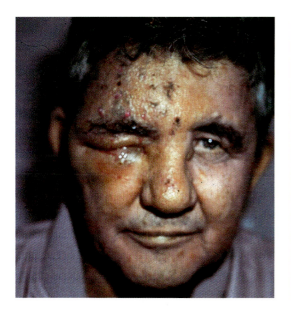

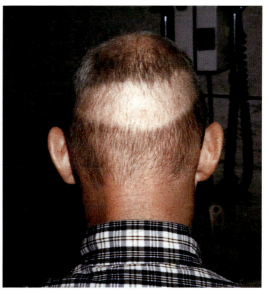

Figure 13 Herpes zoster involving ophthalmic branch of trigeminal nerve. Figure reproduced with permission from Roberts JL. Geriatric hair and scalp disorders. In Norman RA, ed. *Geriatric Dermatology*. London, UK: Parthenon Publishing, 2001:35–64

Figure 15 Trichotillomania in adult male with unusual pattern of hair loss

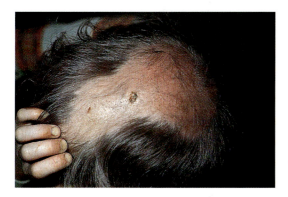

Figure 14 Trichotillomania in young male showing bizarre geometric pattern of self-induced hair loss.

male : female ratio[125,126]. The second type is a more severe form with onset typically at puberty, characterized by a chronic course. There is a 9 : 1 female : male ratio, although it can certainly be seen in male children and adult males (Figures 14 and 15).

Single or multiple areas of the scalp, especially in the parietal and vertex regions, are commonly involved in TTM. The tonsorial pattern of scalp hair is generally spared,

perhaps because it is more painful to pluck hair from this region of the scalp. Although scalp hair is the most commonly affected area, any hair-bearing areas may be affected including (in descending order) the eyelashes, eyebrows, pubes, face and extremities[125,127]. The patches of alopecia are of variable size and are usually irregular, asymmetrical and bizarre geometric shapes. Involvement of eyebrows and eyelashes may be seen in as many as a quarter of affected patients. Telogen hairs in the involved areas are plucked with relative ease and hence are generally plucked out by the roots. Anagen hairs may be plucked out or twisted and broken at various lengths from the otherwise normal, non-inflammatory skin. Patients may complain of associated sensory disturbances. Tactile sensations associated with hair pulling are common, with hairs feeling large, sensitive or otherwise attracting attention. Hair pulling is often associated with activities in which the mind is occupied and the hands are idle, including reading, studying, watching television, driving or lying in bed at night before falling asleep[127,128]. The broken hairs often show blunt frayed distal ends owing to chronic manipulation. The traumatically avulsed anagen hairs leave behind the internal root sheath and appear as dark dots on the scalp. The overall effect is irregular patches with hairs broken at differing lengths and visual evidence of the retained root sheaths. Clinically, the incomplete nature of the hair loss, the bizarre geometric patterns and the absence of underlying scalp inflammation or scale can distinguish TTM from other causes of patchy, non-scarring hair loss. The broken hairs do not resemble the 'exclamation-mark' hairs of alopecia areata, and the sparseness of hair in the involved area is unusual for a hair shaft disorder. Usually, no hairs are obtained in a hair pull from the involved areas because the patient has already plucked out all the telogen hairs.

Diagnostic procedures

Examination of the distal ends of plucked hairs reveals an unusual combination of broken hairs with ends blunted by manipulation, and tapered ends of new anagen growth. KOH examination and fungal culture are negative. In cases where the child or family member insists that the hair 'just won't grow', a 'hair window' with occlusion of the clipped area should be performed. The hair window should be done in an area that the patient cannot see. Removal of the occlusion in 1 to 3 weeks should show the proportional 1 cm per month hair growth typical for the normal scalp.

Histopathology

In classic cases the histopathology is quite distinctive, although changes can be subtle. In areas of active involvement plucking induces a sudden shift into the resting phases: catagen phase briefly, followed by telogen phase. Because catagen hairs make up only approximately 1% of the scalp hairs, finding two to three catagen hairs in a biopsy specimen is suggestive of the diagnosis. Catagen hairs, some of which may be morphologically abnormal, are more commonly found in this hair disorder than any other. There are follicular plugs with hair cast remnants, a characteristic feature found in approximately 60% of biopsies. These are usually located in the isthmus or infundibular area of the follicle, representing clumps of melanin and keratinaceous debris. Trichomalacia, evidenced by clumped, plicated, amorphous, corkscrew terminal hairs contained within the traumatized follicle, is uncommon but is thought to be specific for TTM[129,130]. Characteristically, normal follicles are found among involuted, damaged or empty follicles. Perifollicular hemorrhages may be located between the inner and outer root sheath or between the outer root sheath and the connective tissue sheath near the hair bulb[130]. Although inflammation of the hair bulb is generally absent, mild perifollicular or perivascular lymphocytic folliculitis may occasionally be noted. Rarely in advanced cases, a perifollicular, fibrotic-type reaction localized to the hair papillae has been noted in the deep dermis and subcutis[129–131].

Treatment

In the 1980s, researchers became interested in the neurobiology of TTM following observations that obsessive–compulsive disorders (OCD) were more responsive to the new class of drugs called serotonin reuptake inhibitors (SSRIs) than to tricyclic antidepressant drugs such as desipramine[132–134]. Serotonin metabolism has been hypothesized to play a role in TTM for various reasons. Fluoxetine, clomipramine and desipramine have all been used with some benefit. Care must be used when prescribing these medications, which should be done under the supervision of a psychiatrist experienced in the treatment of OCD and related disorders.

In the author's experience, the profile of patients seeking help with TTM has changed in the past decade. The increasing acceptance and public knowledge that TTM is probably a manifestation of a biochemical disorder reassures patients of their 'sanity' and increases their comfort in seeking treatment. A national organization, the Trichotillomania Learning Center, is an important resource for patients and parents of patients with TTM[135]. The Trichotillomania Learning Center is dedicated to education, support and research. In turn, they have lists of community resources for different geographic locations in the USA, including mental health professionals experienced in treating TTM, and for the growing number of local support groups for patients. Many adult patients are now seeking care directly from these professionals, bypassing the dermatologic community entirely, or eagerly accepting referrals by the dermatologist to these professionals. Children represent a different challenge, as the parents are perplexed and the child often unwilling to admit to the self-induced nature of this hair loss. Frequently, scalp biopsies do help convince the parents of children with this disorder of the nature of the problem. The problem may then be addressed frankly with the parents and child, offering information on the biochemical nature of the disorder, eliminating culpability, instead stressing the need for a co-operative approach between the family, child, dermatologist and mental health professional.

Other treatments for TTM include psychotherapy, behavior-modification therapy and habit reversal training, as well as trials of SSRIs, alone or in combinations with antidepressant or anti-anxiety medications as discussed above[136,137]. Readers are referred to a recently published comprehensive book on all clinical and treatment facets of TTM[137].

ALOPECIA AREATA

Alopecia areata is an inflammatory, non-scarring form of hair loss characterized by round or oval patches of complete hair loss; the incidence in males and females is equal. Any hair-bearing area can be affected, including the beard (Figure 16). The condition can progress to loss of all scalp hair (alopecia totalis) or complete loss of all hair on the body (alopecia universalis) (Figure 17). There are several distinctive forms. It affects between 0.1 and 0.2% of the population[138], including more than 4 million people in the USA[139]. Twelve per cent of cases initially present in patients over the age of 50 years. Patients may present with patchy, ophiasis, reverse ophiasis, reticulate, diffuse, totalis and universalis patterns and/or extent. Figure 18 demonstrates loss of pigmented hair in the reverse ophiasis distribution, with retention of pigment and density in the ophiasis distribution.

Etiology

The etiology of alopecia areata is unknown, although an autoimmune pathogenesis has been frequently proposed. Support for this hypothesis is provided by the increased association with other autoimmune disorders such as hyper- and hypothyroid disorders, vitiligo, lupus erythematosus, discoid lupus erythematosus, rheumatoid arthritis, pernicious anemia, and ulcerative colitis. There is a high prevalence of auto-antibodies against thyroid, gastric parietal cells, nuclear constituents and rheumatoid factors[140,141]. Forty per cent of patients with alopecia areata have an atopic diathesis including allergic rhinitis, asthma or atopic dermatitis[142]. Between 10 and 27% of patients have a family history of alopecia areata[143]. Melanocytes are suspected to be one target of the immune attack. It is well known that the pigmented hairs are affected preferentially and that the senile white or gray hairs may be spared. There is also an increased association with vitiligo[144].

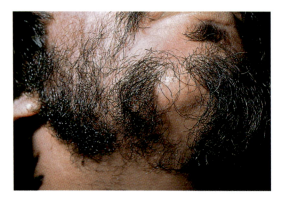

Figure 16 Alopecia areata showing patchy hair loss in beard

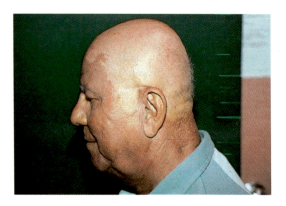

Figure 17 Late onset alopecia areata universalis with vitiligo. Figure reproduced with permission from Roberts JL. Geriatric hair and scalp disorders. In Norman RA, ed. *Geriatric Dermatology*. London, UK: Parthenon Publishing, 2001:35–64

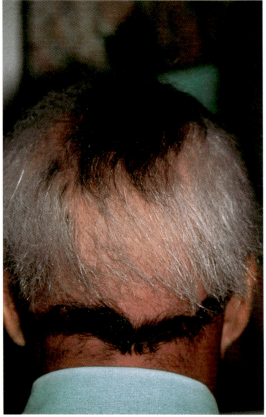

Figure 18 Unusual pattern of hair loss in alopecia areata. Retention of peripheral hair is termed reverse ophiasis. Only pigmented hairs were lost in the remainder of the scalp (ophiasis distribution)

Treatment

Treatment can be divided into immunomodulators (oral, intralesional, intramuscular corticosteroids, cyclosporin, ultraviolet light with or without PUVA), immunostimulants (topical squaric acid dibutyl ester, diphenylcyclopropenone, anthralin) and non-specific hair follicle growth promoters (minoxidil). Corticosteroids require careful monitoring whether administered by the oral, intralesional or intramuscular routes, because of the potential for serious side-effects. These include causing or potentiating cataracts, glaucoma, hypertension, hyperglycemia and osteoporosis.

In the author's experience, alopecia areata is no less devastating to male patients than to females, although they may choose to deal with it cosmetically in a different manner. Males are less likely to wear hair prostheses or to choose permanent cosmetic application (tattooing) of eyebrows and eyelashes, although in capable hands it can be a satisfactory alternative. Some males opt for intralesional injections of eyebrows with Kenalog 5–10 mg/ml, one ml injected into each brow on a monthly or bimonthly basis in order to provide a 'frame' for the features of the face.

References

1. Freedman TG. Social and cultural dimensions of hair loss in women treated for breast cancer. *Cancer Nurs* 1994;17(4):334–41

2. Cash TF, Price VH, Savin RC. Psychological effects of androgenetic alopecia on women: comparisons with balding men and with female control subjects. *J Am Acad Dermatol* 1993;29(4):568–75

3. Pickard-Holley S. The symptom experience of alopecia. *Semin Oncol Nurs* 1995;11(4):235–8

4. Cotsarelis G, Sun TT, Lavker RM. Label-retaining cells reside in the bulge area of pilosebaceous unit: implications for follicular stem cells, hair cycle and skin. *Cell* 1990;61(7):1329–37

5. Courtois M, Loussouarn G, Hourseau C, Grollier JF. Ageing and hair cycles. *Br J Dermatol* 1995;132(1):86–93

6. Roberts JL. Androgenetic alopecia in men and women: an overview of cause and treatment. *Dermatol Nurs* 1997;9(6):379–86

7. Hamilton JB. Patterned loss of hair in man: types and incidence. *Ann NY Acad Sci* 1951;53:708–28

8. Norwood OT. Male pattern baldness: classification and incidence. *South Med J* 1975;68:1359–65

9. Olsen EA. Androgenetic alopecia. In Olsen EA, ed. *Disorders of Hair Growth, Diagnosis and Treatment*. McGraw-Hill, New York 1994:257–83

10. Ebling FJ. The biology of hair. *Dermatol Clin* 1987;5(3):467–81

11. Imperato-McGinley J, Guerrero L, Gautier R, Peterson RE. Steroid 5α reductase deficiency in man: an inherited form of male pseudohermaphroditism. *Science* 1974;186:1213–15

12. Uno H, Cappas A, Brigham P. Action of topical minoxidil in the bald stump-tailed macaque. *J Am Acad Dermatol* 1987;16(3 pt 2):657–68

13. Headington JT. Hair follicle biology and topical minoxidil: possible mechanism of action. *Dermatologica* 1987;175(Suppl 2):19–22

14. Roberts JL. Androgenetic alopecia: treatment results with topical minoxidil. *J Am Acad Dermatol* 1987;1(3):705–10

15. Data available on request from Professional Services, WP1-27, Merck & Co., Inc., West Point, PA 19486. Please specify information package DA-PRP6(1)

16. Andriole GL, Guess HA, Epstein JI, *et al*. Treatment with finasteride preserves usefulness of prostate-specific antigen in the detection of prostate cancer: results of a randomized, double-blind, placebo-controlled clinical trial. PLESS Study Group. Proscar long-term Efficacy and Safety Study. *Urology* 1998;52(2):195–201; discussion 201–2

17. Drake L, Hordinsky M, Fiedler V, *et al*. The effects of finasteride on scalp skin and serum androgen levels in men with androgenetic alopecia. *J Am Acad Dermatol* 1999;41(4):550–4

18. Van Neste D, Fuh V, Sanchez-Pedreno P, *et al*. Finasteride increases anagen hair in men with androgenetic alopecia. *Br J Dermatol* 2000;143(4):804–10

19. Lesko SM, Rosenberg L, Shapiro S. A case-control study of baldness in relation to myocardial infarction in men. *J Am Med Assoc* 1993;269(8):998–1003

20. Ford ES, Frudman DS, Byers T. Baldness and ischemic heart disease in a national sample of men. Comment in: *Am J Epidemiol* 1997;145(7):670–1

21. Herrera R, D'Agostino RB, Girstman BB, *et al*. Baldness and coronary heart disease in men from the Framingham study. *Am J Epidemiol* 1995;142(8):828–33

22. Trevisan M, Farinaro E, Krogh V, *et al*. Baldness and coronary heart disease risk factors. *J Clin Epidemiol* 1993;46(10):1213–18

23. Halim MM, Meyrick G, Jeans WD, *et al*. Myocardial infarction, androgens and the skin. *Br J Dermatol* 1978;98:63–8

24. Cooke NT. Male pattern alopecia and coronary heart disease in men. *Br J Dermatol* 1979;101:455–8

25. Lesko SM, Rosenberg L, Shapiro S. A case-control study of baldness in relation to

myocardial infarction in men. *J Am Med Assoc* 1993;269(8):998–1003

26. Matilainen V, Koskela P, Keinanen-Kuikaaniemi S. Early androgenetic alopecia as a marker of insulin resisitance. *Lancet* 2000;356(9236):1165–6

27. Lotufo P, Chae C, Ajani A, *et al*. Male pattern baldness and coronary artery disease: the physicians health study. *Arch Intern Med* 2000;160:165–71

28. Maguire HC Jr, Kligman AM. The histopathology of common male baldness. *Excerta Medica Foundation* 1962;55:1438–9

29. Young JW, Conte ET, Leavitt ML, *et al*. Cutaneous immunopathology of androgenetic alopecia. *J Am Osteopath Assoc* 1991;91(8):765–71

30. Lattanand A, Johnson WC. Male pattern alopecia: a histopathologic and histochemical study. *J Cutan Pathol* 1975;2:58–70

31. Jaworsky C, Kligman AM, Murphy GF. Characterization of inflammatory infiltrates in male pattern alopecia: implications for pathogenesis. *Br J Dermatol* 1992;127(3):239–46

32. Abell E. Embryology and anatomy of the hair follicle. In Olsen EA, ed. *Disorders of Hair Growth: Diagnosis and Treatment*. McGraw-Hill, New York 1994:7

33. Kligman A. The comparative histopathology of male-pattern baldness and senescent baldness. *Clin Dermatol* 1988;6(4):108–18

34. Pinkus H. Alopecia: clinicopathologic correlations. *Int J Dermatol* 1980;19(5):245–53

35. Schnohr P, Lange P, Nyboe J, *et al*. Gray hair, baldness, and wrinkles in relation to myocardial infarction, the Copenhagen City Heart Study. *Am Heart J* 1995;130(5):1003–10

36. Glasser M. Is early onset of gray hair a risk factor? *Med Hypothesis* 1991;36(4):404–11

37. Rebora A. Telogen effluvium. *Dermatology* 1997;195(3):209–12

38. Bernstein GM, Crollick JS, Hassett JM. Post febrile telogen effluvium in critically ill patients. *Crit Care Med* 1988;16(1):98–9

39. Broden MB. Drug-related alopecia. *Dermatol Clin* 1987;5(3):571–9

40. Kay RG, Tasman Jones C. Acute zinc deficiency in man during intravenous alimentation. *Aust NZ J Surg* 1975;45:325–30

41. Tucker SB, Schroeter AL, Brown PW, McCall JT. Acquired zinc deficiency. *J Am Med Assoc* 1976;235:2399–402

42. Weismann K, Wadskov S, Mikkelsen HI, *et al*. Acquired zinc deficiency dermatosis in man. *Arch Dermatol* 1978;114:1509–11

43. Tosti A, Mesciali C, Peroccini BM, *et al*. Drug induced hair loss and hair growth. Incidence, management and avoidance. *Drug Safety* 1994;10(4):310–17

44. Graeber CW, Lapkin RA. Metoprolol and alopecia. *Cutis* 1981;28:633–4

45. Fraunfelder FT, Meyer SM, Menacker SJ. Alopecia possibly secondary to topical ophthalmic β-blockers. *J Am Med Assoc* 1990;263(11):1493–4

46. Martin CM, Southwick EG, Maibach HI. Propranolol induced alopecia. *Am Heart J* 1973;86(2):236–7

47. Miki Y. Alopecia from heparin. *Med J Osaka Univ* 1960;11:315–23

48. Smith WB, Grabski WJ, McCollough ML, Davis TL. Immunofluorescence findings in lichen planopilaris. A contrasting experience (letter). *Arch Dermatol* 1992;128:1405–6

49. Ioannides D, Bystryn JC. Immunofluorescence abnormalities in lichen planopilaris. *Arch Dermatol* 1992;128:214–16

50. Elston DM, Bergfeld WF. Cicatricial alopecia (and other causes of permanent alopecia). In Olsen EA, ed. *Disorders of Hair Growth: Diagnosis and Treatment*. McGraw-Hill, New York 1994:285–313

51. Tarkowski E, Jensen C, Ekholm S, *et al*. Localization of the brain lesions affects the lateralization of T-lymphocyte dependent cutaneous inflammation. Evidence for immunoregulatory role of the right frontal cortex-putamen region. *Scand J Immunol* 1998;47(1):30–6

52. Martignoni E, Godi L, Pacchetti C, *et al*. Is seborrhea a sign of autonomic impairment in Parkinson's disease? *J Neural Transm* 1997;104(11–12):1295–304

53. Binder RL, Jonelis FJ. Seborrheic dermatitis in neuroleptic-induced Parkinsonism. *Arch Dermatol* 1983;119(5):473–5

54. Flint A. The skin in Parkinson's disease. *Prim Care* 1977;4(3):475–80

55. Neuber K, Kroger S, Grusek E, *et al*. Effects of *Pityrosporum ovale* on proliferation,

immunoglobulin (IgA, G, M) synthesis and cytokine (IL-2, Il-10, IFN gamma) production of peripheral blood mononuclear cells from patients with seborrheic dermatitis. *Arch Dermatol Res* 1996;288(9):532–6

56. Bergbrant IM. Seborrhoeic dermatitis and *Pityrosporum* yeasts. *Curr Top Med Mycol* 1995;6:95–112

57. Peter RU, Richarz-Barthauer U. Successful treatment and prophylaxis of scalp seborrheic dermatitis and dandruff with 2% ketoconazole shampoo. *Br J Dermatol* 1995;132 (3):441–5

58. Nenoff P, Huastein UF, Munzberger C. *In vitro* activity of lithium succinate against *Malassezia furfur*. *Dermatology* 1995;190 (1):48–50

59. Danby FW, Maddin WS, Margesson J, Rosenthal D. A randomized, placebo-controlled trial of ketoconazole shampoo versus selenium 2.5% shampoo in the treatment of moderate to severe dandruff. *J Am Acad Dermatol* 1993;29(6):1008–12

60. Faergemann J. *Pityrosporum* infections. *J Am Acad Dermatol* 1994;31(3 pt 2):S18–S20

61. Faergemann J, Jones JC, Hettler O, *et al*. *Pityrosporum ovale* (*Malassezia furfur*) as the causative agent in seborrheic dermatitis: new treatment options. *Br J Dermatol* 1996; 134(Suppl 46):12–15; discussion, 38

62. Farber EM, Nall L. Natural history and treatment of scalp psoriasis. *Cutis* 1992;49(6): 396–400

63. Runne U, Kroneisen-Wiersma P. Psoriatic alopecia; acute and chronic hair loss in 47 patients with scalp psoriasis [published erratum appears in *Dermatology* 1993;187 (3):232] *Dermatology* 1992;185(2):82–7

64. van de Kerkhof PC, de Hoop D, de Korte J, Kuipers MV. Scalp psoriasis: clinical presentations and therapeutic management. *Dermatology* 1998;197(4):326–34

65. Stanimirovic A, Skerlev M, Stipic T, *et al*. Has psoriasis its own characteristic trichogram? *J Dermatol Sci* 1998;17(2):156–9

66. Kuijpers-AL, van-Baar HM, van Gasselt MW, van de Kerkhof PC. The hair root pattern after calcipotriol treatment for scalp psoriasis. *Acta Derm Venereol* 1995;75(5): 388–90

67. Wright AL, Messenger AG. Scarring alopecia in psoriasis. *Acta Derm Venereol* 1990;70(2): 156–9

68. Boyd AS. Scalp psoriasis. *Am Fam Physician* 1988;38(4):163–70

69. Olsen EA, Cram DL, Ellis CN, *et al*. A double-blind, vehicle-controlled study of clobetasol propionate 0.05% (Temovate) scalp application in the treatment of moderate to severe scalp psoriasis. *J Am Acad Dermatol* 1991;24(3):443–7

70. Katz HI, Lindholm JS, Weiss JS, *et al*. Efficacy and safety of twice-daily augmented betamethasone dipropionate lotion versus clobetasol propionate solution in patients with moderate-to-severe scalp psoriasis. *Clin Ther* 1995;17(3):390–401

71. Prakash A, Benfield P. Topical mometasone. A review of its pharmacological properties and therapeutic use in the treatment of dermatological disorders. *Drugs* 1998;55(1):145–63

72. Johannesson A, Lindelof B. Additional effect of Grenz rays on psoriasis lesions of the scalp treated with topical corticosteroids. *Dermatologica* 1987;175(6):290–2

73. Caccialanza M, Piccinno R, Cappio F, *et al*. Phototherapy of psoriasis of the scalp. Results in 21 patients treated with a special portable ultraviolet rays lamp. *G Ital Dermatol Venereol* 1989;124(11–12):LXI–LXV

74. Klaber MR, Hutchinson PE, Pedvis-Leftick A, *et al*. Comparative effects of calcipotriol solution (50 micrograms/ml) and betamethasone 17-valerate solution (1 mg/ml) in the treatment of scalp psoriasis. *Br J Dermatol* 1994;131(5):678–83

75. Faergemann J. Treatment of sebopsoriasis with itraconazole. *Mykosen* 1985;28(12): 612–8

76. Wilson CL, Dean D, Lane EB, *et al*. Keratinocyte differentiation in psoriatic scalp: morphology and expression of epithelial keratins. *Br J Dermatol* 1994;131(2):191–200

77. Maoz CR, Langevitz P, Leyneh A, *et al*. High incidence of malignancies with dermatomyositis and polymyositis: an 11-year analysis. *Semin Arthritis Rheum* 1998;27(5): 319–24

78. Kasteler JS, Callen JP. Scalp involvement in dermatomyositis. Often overlooked or

misdiagnosed. *J Am Med Assoc* 1994;272 (24):1939–41

79. McDonald LL, Smith ML. Diagnostic dilemmas in pediatric/adolescent dermatology: scaly scalp. *J Pediatr Health Care* 1998;12 (2):80–4

80. Hatada T, Aoki I, Ikeda H, *et al*. Dermatomyositis and malignancy: case report and review of the Japanese literature. *Tumori* 1996;82(3):273–5

81. Koh ET, Seow-Ong B, Ratnyopal P, *et al*. Adult onset polymyositis/dermatomyositis: clinical and laboratory features in 75 patients. *Ann Rheum Dis* 1993;52(12):857–61

82. Peng JC, Sheen TS, Hsu MM. Nasopharyngeal carcinoma dermatomyositis: analysis of 12 cases. *Arch Otolaryngol Head Neck Surg* 1995;121(11):1298–301

83. Davis MD, Ahmed I. Ovarian malignancy in patients with dermatomyositis and polymyositis: a retrospective analysis of 14 cases. *J Am Acad Dermatol* 1997;37(5 pt 1): 730–3

84. Wong KO. Dermatomyositis: a clinical investigation of twenty-three cases in Hong Kong. *Br J Dermatol* 1969;81(7):544–7

85. Teragni L, Lasagni A, Oreoni A. Tinea capitis in adults. *Mycoses* 1989;32(9):482–6

86. Pursley TV, Raimer SS. Tinea capitis in the elderly *Int J Dermatol* 1980;19:220–22

87. Ridely CM. Tinea capitis in an elderly woman. *Clin Exp Dermatol* 1979;4(2):247–9

88. Williams JV, Honig PJ, McGinley KJ, Leyden JJ. Semiquantitative study of tinea capitis and the asymptomatic carrier state in inner-city school children. *Pediatrics* 1995;96(2 pt 1): 265–7

89. Babel DE, Baughman SA. Evaluation of the adult carrier state in juvenile tinea capitis caused by *Trichophyton tonsurans*. *J Am Acad Dermatol* 1989;21(6):1209–12

90. Gupta AK, Sauder DN, Shear NH. Antifungal agents: an overview. Part II. *J Am Acad Dermatol* 1994;30(6):911–33

91. Elewski BE. Treatment of tinea capitis with itraconazole. *Int J Dermatol* 1997;36:539–42

92. Elewski BE. Tinea capitis: Itraconazole in *Trichophyton tonsurans* infection. *J Am Acad Dermatol* 1994;31:65–7

93. Legendre R, Esola-Macre J. Itraconazole in the treatment of tinea capitis. *J Am Acad Dermatol* 1990;23:559–60

94. Mercurio MG, Silverman RA, Elewski BE. Tinea capitis: Fluconazole in *Trichophyton tonsurans* infections. *Pediatr Dermatol* 1998;15:29–32

95. Montero GF. Fluconazole in the treatment of tinea capitis. *Int J Dermatol* 1998;37:870–1

96. Haroon TS, Hussain I, Mahmood A, *et al*. An open clinical pilot study of the efficacy and safety of oral terbinafine in dry non-inflammatory tinea capitis. *Br J Dermatol* 1992;126(Suppl 39):47–50

97. Mock M, Monod M, Baudraz-Rosselet F. Tinea capitis dermatophytes: Susceptibility to antifungal drugs tested *in vitro* and *in vivo*. *Dermatology* 1998;197(4):361–7

98. Krafchik B. An open label study of tinea capitis in 50 children treated with a 2-week course of oral terbinafine. *J Am Acad Dermatol* 1999;41(1):60–3

99. Allen HB, Honig PJ, Leyden JJ, McGinley KJ. Selenium sulfide: adjunctive therapy for tinea capitis. *Pediatrics* 1982;69(1):81–3

100. Parisu H. Precocious noduloulcerative cutaneous syphilis. *Arch Dermatol* 1975;111: 76–7

101. Shulkin D, Tripoli L, Akell E. Lues maligna in a patient with human immunodeficiency virus infection. *Am J Med* 1998;85:425–7

102. Petrozzi JW, Lockskin NA, Berger BJ. Malignant syphilis. *Arch Dermatol* 1974; 109:387–9

103. Stokes JH, Beerman H, Ingraham NR. *Modern Clinical Syphilology*, 3rd edn. Philadelphia: WB Saunders Co., 1944:250

104. Mikhail GR, Chapel TA. Follicular papulopustular syphilid. *Arch Dermatol* 1969;100: 471–3

105. Skeetal S, Weatherhead L. Extensive nodular secondary syphilis. *Arch Dermatol* 1989; 125:1666–9

106. From the Centers for Disease Control: Primary, secondary syphilis: U.S., 1981–1990. *J Am Med Assoc* 1991;265:2940

107. Koplan J. From the CDC; Syphilis elimination: history in the making – opening remarks. *Sex Trans Dis* 2000;27(2):63–5

108. Lee Y-YJ, Hsu M-L. Alopecia syphilitica, a simulator of alopecia areata: histopathology and differential diagnosis. *J Cutan Pathol* 1991;12:87–92

109. Tramont EC. Syphilis in the AIDS era. *N Engl J Med* 1987;316(2):1600–1

110. Hicks CB. Seronegative secondary syphilis in a patient infected with the human immunodeficiency virus (HIV) with Kaposi sarcoma: a diagnostic dilemma. *Ann Intern Med* 1987;107:492–4

111. Hess TM, Lutz LJ, Nauss LA, Lamer TJ. Treatment of acute herpetic neuralgia. A case report and review of the literature (see comments). *Minn Med* 1990;73(4):37–40

112. Gershon AA. Epidemiology and management of post herpetic neuralgia. *Semin Dermatol* 1996;15(2 Suppl 1):8–13

113. Goh CL, Khoo L. A retrospective study of the clinical presentation and outcome of herpes zoster in a tertiary dermatology outpatient referral clinic. *Int J Dermatol* 1997;36(9):667–72

114. Higa K, Mori M, Hirata K, *et al*. Severity of skin lesions of herpes zoster at the worst phase rather than age and involved region most influences the duration of acute herpes zoster pain. *Pain* 1997;69(3):245–53

115. Schoenlaub P, Grange F, Nasica X, Guillaume JC. *Ann Dermatol Venereol* 1997; 125(5):401–3

116. Tyring SK. Efficacy of famciclovir in the treatment of herpes zoster. *Semin Dermatol* 1996;15(2 Suppl 1):27–31

117. Wutzler P. Antiviral therapy of herpes simplex and varicella zoster virus infections. *Intervirology* 1997;40(5–6):343–56

118. Erlich KS. Management of herpes simplex and varicella-zoster virus infections. *West J Med* 1997;166(3):211–15

119. Lycka BA. Postherpetic pain neuralgia and systemic corticosteroid therapy. *Int J Dermatol* 1990;29(7):523–7

120. Post BT, Philbrick JT. Do corticosteroids prevent postherpetic neuralgia? A review of the evidence. *J Am Acad Dermatol* 1988; 18(3):605–10

121. Tynes LL, White K, Steketee GS. Toward a new nosology of obsessive compulsive behavior. *Compr Psychiatry* 1988;31: 465–80

122. Stein DJ, Hollander E, Simeon D, *et al*. Neurological soft signs in female trichotillomania patients, obsessive-compulsive disorder patients, and healthy control subjects. *J Neuropsychiatry Clin Neuro Sci* 1994;6: 184–7

123. Stein DJ, Simeon D, Cohen LJ, *et al*. Trichotillomania and obsessive-compulsive disorders. *J Clin Psychiatry* 1995;56: 28–35

124. American Psychiatric Association: Diagnostic and Statistical Manual of Mental Disorders, 4th edn. Washington, DC: American Psychiatric Association, 1994

125. Swedo SE, Leonard HL. Trichotillomania: an obsessive spectrum disorder? *Psychiatr Clin North Am* 1992;15:777–90

126. Winchel RM. Trichotillomania: presentations and treatment. *Psychiatric Annuals* 1992;22: 84–9

127. Mansueto CS. Typography and phenomenology of trichotillomania. Presented at the annual convention of the Association for the Advancement of Behavior Therapy, San Francisco, CA, November 1990

128. Schlosser S, Black DW, Blum N, *et al*. The demography, phenomenology, and family history of 22 persons with compulsive hair pulling. *Ann Clin Psychiatry* 1994;6: 147–52

129. Muller SA. Trichotillomania: A histopathologic study in sixty-six patients. *J Am Acad Dermatol* 1990;23:56–62

130. Whiting DA. Traumatic alopecia. *Int J Dermatol* 1999;38(1):34–44

131. Mehregan AM. Trichotillomania: a clinicopathologic study. *Arch Dermatol* 1970;102: 129–33

132. Swedo SE, Leonard HL, Rapoport JL, *et al*. A double-blind comparison of clomipramine and desipramine in the treatment of trichotillomania (hair pulling). *N Engl J Med* 1989;321:497–501

133. Zohar J, Insel TR. Obsessive-compulsive disorder: pyschobiological approaches to diagnosis, treatment, and pathophysiology. *Biol Psychiatry* 1987;22:667–87

134. Leonard HL, Swedo SE, Rapoport JL, *et al*. Treatment of obsessive-compulsive disorder with clomipramine and desipramine in children and adolescents: a double-blind crossover comparison. *Arch Gen Psychiatry* 1989;46:1088–92

135. Trichotillomania Learning Center, 1215 Mission Street, Santa Cruz, CA 95060

136. Azrin NH, Nunn RG. Habit reversal: a method of eliminating nervous habits and tics. *Behav Res Ther* 1973;11:619–28

137. Stein DJ, Christenson GA, Hollander E, eds. *Trichotillomania*. Washington, DC: American Pyschiatric Press, Inc, 1999

138. Safavi K. Prevalence of alopecia areata in the First National Health and Nutrition Examine Survey. *Arch Dermatol* 1992;128:702

139. National Alopecia Areata Foundation, PO Box 150760 San Rafael, CA 94915–0760

140. Friedmann PS. Alopecia areata and auto-immunity. *Br J Dermatol* 1981;105(2):153–7

141. Schenk EA, Schneider P, Brown AC. Autoantibodies in alopecia and vitiligo. In Brown AC, Crounse RG eds. *Hair, Trace Elements and Human Illness*. New York: Praeger, 1980:334–43

142. Young E, Bruns HM, Berrens L. Alopecia areata and atopy: a clinical study. *Dermatologica* 1984;156:306–8

143. Suader DN, Bergfeld WF, Krakauer T. Alopecia areata: an inherited autoimmune disease. In Brown AC, Crounse RG eds. *Hair, Trace Elements and Human Illness*. New York: Praeger, 1980:343–5

144. Messenger AG, Bleehan SS. Alopecia areata: light and electron microscopic pathology of the regrowing white hair. *Br J Dermatol* 1984;110(2):155–62

51 Hormone treatments and preventive strategies in aging men; who to treat, when to treat and how to treat

Louis Gooren, MD, PhD, Alvaro Morales, MD, and Bruno Lunenfeld, MD

The therapeutic area of hormonal alterations in the aging male is attracting increasing interest in the medical community and the public at large. Simultaneously, industry has realized the growing importance and enormous potential of the impact of a rapidly mounting population of men over the age of 50 years, which will be positioned for special health needs in the near future. Among these needs, hormone replacement therapy (HRT) for men rates high, as it has for postmenopausal women over the last 25 years.

It is recognized that the endocrine changes associated with male aging are not limited to sex hormones. Indeed, profound changes occur in other hormones such as growth hormone (GH), dehydroepiandrosterone (DHEA) and melatonin. For a long time it has been controversial whether men show a decline of testosterone (T) at all levels with aging. The first studies were performed in men attending clinics for various reasons, and their clinical conditions may explain the lower than normal T levels. More recent methodologically-sound studies in healthy men show that T levels, particularly free bioactive levels of T, do decline with aging, although there is considerable inter-individual variation[1-5].

It is increasingly realized that androgens have a large number of non-reproductive effects, they are important anabolic factors in the maintenance of muscle and bone mass and in non-sexual psychological functioning. The latter are important constituents of well-being in old age. Not only gonadal androgen production declines with aging, but also the secretion of GH and adrenal androgens diminishes. The biological actions of androgens and GH are largely intertwined. Some anabolic effects of androgens have GH-related factors as intermediaries. A small portion of secreted androgens in the male are aromatized to estrogenic hormones. There are recent insights that these estrogens fulfil a significant role in the male body.

Strategies have to be devised to let the aging male benefit from new medical insights into the aging process. Up to the present day there is a considerable misuse of hormonal preparations in the medical care of aging men. The following contribution will address a number of pertinent issues. Only on the basis of sound scientific data will a consensus be reached on this controversial subject.

QUANTITATIVE ASPECTS OF THE DECLINE OF ANDROGEN LEVELS IN AGING

Several cross-sectional[1-3] and longitudinal studies[4,5] have documented a statistical decline in plasma T by approximately 30% in healthy men between the ages of 25–75 years. Since plasma levels of sex hormone-binding globulin (SHBG)[3] increase with aging, free plasma T levels decrease by about 50% over that period. Studies in twins have shown that genetic factors account for 63% of the variability of plasma T levels and for 30% of the variability of SHBG levels[6]. Systemic diseases, increasing with age, are a cause of declining plasma levels of T[7]. While it has now been shown that plasma T, and in particular free T, decline with aging it remains uncertain what percentage of men actually become T-deficient with aging. Stringent criteria for diagnosing T deficiency have not been formulated. Vermeulen and colleagues[3] studied 300 healthy men (age range 20–100 years) with a T reference range set at 11–40 nmol/l. They found one man with subnormal T in the age group of 20–40 years, but more than 20% in the age group of over 60 years, while 15% of men above the age of 80 years still had T values above 20 nmol/l. The implication is that only a certain proportion of men have lower than normal T values in old age. It is a group that is difficult to identify. It has not become clear whether two different criterias for T deficiency should be established: one for aging men and another for younger men. T has a number of physiological functions in the male. In adulthood it is responsible for maintenance of reproductive capacity and of secondary sex characteristics, it has positive effects on mood and libido, anabolic effects on bone and muscle, and it affects fat distribution and the cardiovascular system. Threshold plasma values of T for each of these functions have not been firmly established nor whether these threshold values change over the life cycle. Theoretically it is possible that in old age androgen levels suffice for some but not for all androgen-related functions. Male sexual functioning in adulthood, for example, can be maintained with lower than normal values[8,9]. But there are indications that the threshold required for behavioral effects of T increases with aging[10]. For lean body mass there is some quantitative information in young subjects. T deprivation in young adult male-to-female transsexuals led to an average loss of 4.1 kgs in lean body mass, while female-to-male transsexuals treated with parenteral T esters in a dose of 250 mg/2 weeks gain the same amount. These data compare very well with the findings of Bhasin and colleagues[11] studying the effects of androgen replacement with similar dosages in hypogonadal men.

For androgen deficiency it is difficult to rely on clinical symptoms. In adults who have previously been eugonadal, symptoms of T deficiency emerge only gradually, therefore, only long-standing T deficiency will be clinically recognized. Laboratory reference values of T and free T show a wider range than those for most other hormones (for example thyroid hormones) which makes it difficult to establish whether measured values of T in patients are normal or abnormal. Is a patient whose plasma T levels have fallen from the upper to the lower range of normal T levels (which may constitute a drop of as much as 50%) T deficient? Levels may well remain within the reference range. In thyroid pathophysiology, plasma thyroid stimulating hormone (TSH) proves to be a better criterion of thyroid hyper/hypofunction than plasma thyroxine (T_4) or triiodothyronine (T_3), but it is uncertain whether plasma luteinizing hormone (LH) is a reliable indicator of male hypogonadism. There is another complicating factor. With aging there are reductions in LH pulse frequency and amplitude. Several studies have found that LH levels are elevated in response to the decline of T levels with aging, but less so than is observed in younger men with similarly decreased T levels[2,12]. This may be due to a shift in the set point of the negative feedback of T on the hypothalamic pituitary unit resulting in an enhanced negative feedback action, which leads to a relatively lower LH output. A recent study found that serum LH levels increase with age in independently living elderly men and correlate inversely with a variety of indicators of frailty. The observed relation between LH and frailty, independent of T, suggested that LH reflects serum androgen activity in a different way than T, possibly reflecting more closely the combined feedback effect of estrogen and androgen[13]. This observation would argue for using LH as a parameter for evaluating the quality of health in old age.

Another variable that might be significant to assess the androgen status in old age is plasma level of SHBG. Its levels increase with aging possibly due to a decrease in GH production and an increase of the ratio of free estradiol (E_2) over free T[3]. The same authors[14] have demonstrated that the free T value calculated by total T/SHBG as determined by immunoassay appears to be a rapid, simple and reliable indicator of free T, comparable to T values obtained by equilibrium dialysis. Another indicator of the androgenic status of aging men is the level of so-called bioavailable T, which is total T minus T bound to SHBG. So, without solid criteria for T deficiency, determination of values of T together with LH and SHBG might provide a reasonable index of the androgen status of an aging person.

There are still a number of questions open: *Are there reliable clinical signs of androgen deficiency? Can reliable criteria of androgen deficiency in old age be formulated? Are there unequivocal laboratory criteria, i.e. levels of total and non-bound T, SHBG and LH? If yes, do we know threshold values for the diverse biological actions of T?*

TARGET TISSUES OF ANDROGENS IN AGING MEN

While it can statistically be shown that plasma T levels drop with aging, the actual decrease is often only moderate and does not affect all men to the same degree. Set against the characteristics of aging reminiscent of androgen deficiency, such as loss of muscle and bone mass, plasma levels of androgens are often not correspondingly low. It must be remembered that the plasma levels of a hormone merely provides information on the strength of the signal and not about receptor and postreceptor events, i.e. how this hormonal signal will be translated into biological action. It could be hypothesized that aging is associated with a decrease in androgen action in the presence of rather normal plasma androgen levels. A significant decrease in both T and dihydrotestosterone (DHT) concentrations has been found in different tissues with aging[15], which could support this assumption. Aging might result in a reduction in androgen effect through a loss of sensitivity of target tissues to T via, for instance, alterations in receptor number or affinity, or in postreceptor mechanisms (for example, the androgen receptor number and affinity are decreased in many organs of the aging rat)[16]. In human pathophysiology a certain parallel might be drawn with X-linked spinal and bulbar muscular atrophy (Kennedy's disease) which is an abnormality of the androgen receptor. This genetic error of the androgen receptor manifests itself usually not earlier than the ages of 20–40 years but sometimes as late as 60. These patients frequently show glucose intolerance or diabetes mellitus. The number of CAG triplets coding for glutamines in the androgen receptor, normally between 11–33, is approximately doubled in patients suffering from this condition[17]. That properties of the androgen receptor may be involved in the age-related decline of plasma androgen levels was recently documented. It was demonstrated that the CAG repeat length was significantly associated with plasma T, albumin-bound T, and free T, when controlled for age, baseline hormone levels and anthropometrics. Follow-up levels of androgen measurements decreased per CAG repeat elements[18].

If target organ sensitivity to androgens does diminish with age, this would limit the potential benefit which androgen supplementation in aging men could have. Whether higher than normal dosages of androgens would be effective, as is the case in partial androgen sensitivity[19,20], remains to be investigated.

Questions: *Do plasma levels of androgens reliably reflect a subject's androgenic status, particularly in old age? Is there an impairment of the accumulation of androgens in target tissues or of the transcription of androgen action?*

A PRAGMATIC APPROACH TO THE ISSUE OF ANDROGEN DEFICIENCY IN ELDERLY MEN

The previous section has outlined the many unresolved questions as to the verification of deficiencies in the biological action of androgens in aging men and what plasma T levels conclusively represent androgen deficiency. Consequently, a pragmatic approach to this issue must be taken in order to let aging androgen-deficient men benefit from replacement therapy. This question has recently been authoritatively reviewed by Vermeulen[21]. He argues that there is no generally accepted cut-off value of plasma T for defining androgen deficiency, and in the absence of convincing evidence for an altered androgen requirement in elderly men, he considers the normal range of (F) T levels in young males are also valid for elderly men. In his healthy male, non-obese population age 20–40 years ($n = 150$), the mean of log transformed early morning T levels was 21.8 nmol/l (627 ng/dl); the mean minus 2 SD was 12.5 nmol/l (365 ng/dl) and minus 2.5 SD

11 nmol/l (319 ng/dl). For FT, measured by equilibrium dialysis or calculated from T and SHBG levels[14], the mean was 0.5 nmol/l (14 ng/dl), minus 2 SD 0.26 nmol/l (7.4 ng/dl) and minus 2.5 SD 0.225 nmol/l (6.5 ng/dl). If one takes the lowest normal limit and threshold of partial androgen deficiency, a conservative value of 11 nmol/l for T and 0.225 nmol/l for FT, which represent the lower 1% value of healthy young males, then it appears that more than 30% of men over 75 years old have subnormal (F)T levels. Most authors report rather similar values[22-25].

It should be mentioned that direct FT assays using a T analog, do not yield a reliable estimate of FT[14]. The age associated decline in (F) T levels has both a testicular (decreased Leydig cell number) and central origin, the latter being characterized by a decrease in the amplitude of LH pulses in elderly men. Hence, many elderly men have normal LH levels and an increase in LH levels is unlikely to be required for the diagnosis of hypogonadism in elderly men[12].

As already mentioned, in the absence of a reliable, clinically useful biological parameter of androgen action, these criteria of hypogonadism of the aging man are somewhat arbitrary but for the time being are the best to provide guidance.

The treatment aims at restoring hormone levels to the normal range of young adults and, more importantly, at alleviating the symptoms suggestive of the hormone deficiency. The ultimate goals, however, are to maintain or regain the highest quality of life, to reduce disability, to compress major illnesses into a narrow age range and to add life to years.

ANDROGENS AND CARDIOVASCULAR DISEASE

Traditionally it is thought that the relationship between sex steroids and cardiovascular disease (CVD) is predominantly determined by the relatively beneficial effects of estrogens and by the relatively detrimental effects of androgens on lipid profiles. Recent research shows that this view is too limited and that the effects of sex steroids on other biological systems, such as fat distribution, endocrine/paracrine factors produced by the vascular wall (such as endothelial factor, nitric oxide), blood platelets and coagulation, must also be considered. It is now generally accepted that premenopausal women, in comparison to men, are protected against CVD. It is then paradoxical that in cross-sectional studies of men, elevated levels of estrogens and relatively low levels of T[26–29] appear to be associated with coronary disease and myocardial infarction. Some studies in aging men have shown results that seem to contradict the overall notion that androgens, by their action on lipid profiles, increase the risk for coronary artery disease. In a study of geriatric male patients who had suffered a myocardial infarction it was found that these patients had low T levels in a threshold manner[28]. These studies suggest the intriguing possibility that, in spite of the overall negative effects of androgens on lipid profiles, a lower than normal androgen level in aging men is associated with an increase of atherosclerotic disease. The explanation may lie in the fact that a complex of risk factors for CVD, termed syndrome X or the metabolic syndrome (comprising hypertension, insulin resistance, hypertriglyceridemia and visceral obesity), is associated with low T levels. Whether T supplementation in aging men can reverse these cardiovascular risks is an interesting question (for review see reference 29).

The first results of studies wherein T was actually administered to mildly hypogonadal aging men were comforting. In a double-blind, placebo-controlled, crossover study, Tenover[22] found that administering T enanthate (100 mg per week) for 3 months to 13 healthy elderly men (with low serum total and non-SHBG bound T levels) decreased total and low density lipoprotein (LDL) cholesterol without affecting levels of high density lipoprotein (HDL) cholesterol. Results of a study by Morley and co-workers[23] are in agreement with these findings; administration of 200 mg of T enanthate every 2 weeks for 3 months decreased total cholesterol without affecting HDL cholesterol levels.

PROSTATE DISEASE AND ANDROGEN SUPPLEMENTATION IN OLD AGE

An immediate concern of androgen supplementation in old age is the development and/or progression of prostate diseases such as benign prostate hyperplasia (BPH) and prostate carcinoma. It is widely accepted that both conditions do not develop without T exposure early in life, up to early adulthood. The present position of experts in the field is that androgens do not truly cause BPH or prostate carcinoma but that they have a 'permissive' role, evidenced by the beneficial effects of treatment aiming to reduce the biological effects of androgens on both conditions[30].

Several studies have found that the prevalence of microscopic prostate cancer and its precursor lesions increases strongly with aging, with a prevalence of 33–50% found in men between 60 and 70 years of age[31]. However, only a small subset of these men (4–5%) will go on to develop clinically detectable carcinomas[30]. The results of the Massachussets Male Aging Study showed convincingly that sex steroids only account for 11% of our current understanding of prostate cancer risks, 30% is related to nutrition and 40% for other factors largely not subject to change, such as height, weight and family history[32].

There is presently no conclusive evidence that those who do go on to develop carcinomas have higher androgen levels[33]. While the prevalence of microscopic prostate cancer is similar in different parts of the world, the progression to clinical cancer varies strongly, with the highest prevalence in those parts with a Western lifestyle. Thus it is probable that lifestyle factors, such as nutrition, might play a role. With regard to BPH, there is no evidence that androgen administration to hypogonadal[34,35] or to eugonadal men[36] increases the incidence of BPH over that observed in control eugonadal men. A number of studies of androgen supplementation in elderly men who were not hypogonadal, have shown that, in the short term there is only a modest increase in size and in levels of prostate specific antigen (PSA)[34,36,37]. So, it would seem that non-obstructive BPH is no contraindication against androgen administration but obstructive BPH is.

Tissue concentrations of T and DHT in the prostate are substantially higher than serum concentrations, it could be that a modest increase in androgens in the peripheral circulation, as would be the aim of androgen supplementation in old age, has no large effect on prostate androgen levels. As to how far an androgen, that can be aromatized to E_2 but cannot be reduced to DHT by 5α-reductase, signifies progress with regard to safety for the prostate, remains to be determined[38]. Thus, even if there are no reasons for immediate concern, T administration should be administered to aging men with caution. The following recommendations were formulated with regard to safety of androgen administration to aging men by Snyder[39], at the Second International Androgen Workshop (Long Beach, California, 17–20 February, 1995). Investigators conducting trials of T treatment should screen the men for prostate cancer before entering them in a study and monitor those who enter the study for possible development of prostate cancer, because prostate cancer is, to some extent, T dependent. Screening should include a digital rectal examination and a PSA test. The detection of a prostate nodule should prompt for a urological consultation. Subjects who have an elevated PSA should be excluded. Using a PSA value of 4.0 ng/ml as the upper limit would be conservative, alternatively, an age-adjusted range of (normal or PSA density) could be used. The latter was documented in a recent publication[40]. This paper argued convincingly for age-specific and race-specific PSA values to be applied for the early detection of prostate cancer. For subjects being studied, an annualized rate of change of >0.75 ng/ml/year (or the so-called PSA velocity) for 2 years should lead to urological evaluation and prostate biopsy[39]. Such guidelines allow clinical studies to be carried out or for androgens to be administered to individual hypogonadal aging men with due concern for adverse effects on the prostate[40,41].

Other potential side-effects of androgen administration

The stimulatory effect of T on erythropoiesis is well documented. A moderate increase in hematocrit in elderly males is possibly beneficial, but hematocrit values should not go above 51%, which is the case in some studies. Available data suggest that the frequency of this side-effect is related to supraphysiological levels[42]. Oral or transdermal patches yield T levels within the normal range, this may explain the reported lower frequency of polycythemia with this form of treatment, but more experience is required before a definitive opinion.

Whereas sleep apnea has been reported by Matsumoto[43] none of the reports on T supplementation in elderly males mentioned the development of sleep apnea, which itself is often associated with lower T levels[44]. Nevertheless, it is safe to consider obstructive pulmonary disease in overweight persons or heavy smokers as a relative contraindication.

As already discussed, T supplementation in physiological doses does not seem to induce an atherogenic lipid profile, but, as mentioned T has also non lipid mediated effects on the cardiovascular system which might even be beneficial. Water and sodium retention generally do not cause a problem, except in patients with cardiac insufficiency, hypertension or renal insufficiency.

Hepatotoxicity is rare, even after the long-term use of relatively high oral doses of T-undecanoate (TU)[45], but is relatively frequent when synthetic 17-alpha-alkylated anabolic-androgenic steroids are used.

Gynecomastia is a benign complication of androgen supplementation, perhaps more frequent in elderly obese men than in young hypogonadal men. It is the consequence of the aromatization of T into E_2 in peripheral fat and muscle tissue. A rare, but absolute contraindication is mammary carcinoma in the male as well as a prolactinoma, as their growth may be stimulated by HRT. Even after proper treatment men with prolactinomas often do not return to normal T levels and these men may benefit from androgen replacement.

SUITABLE TESTOSTERONE PREPARATIONS

If it turns out that some men benefit from androgen supplements, are there suitable T preparations available to treat them?

The androgen deficiency of the aging male is only partial and consequently only partial substitution will be required. Hormone secretion via the hypothalamic-pituitary axis should not be suppressed and it should leave the residual testicular androgen production intact. However, conventional parenteral T preparations do not meet this requirement, even for young hypogonadal males they are less than ideal, if not obsolete, because plasma T levels fluctuate strongly following administration. The most widely used pharmaceutical forms are the intramuscular (i.m.) administratered hydrophobic long chain T-esters in oily depot, enanthate and the cypionate, at a dose of 200–250 mg/2weeks. They yield transient supraphysiological levels on the first 2–3 days after injection, followed by a steady decline to subphysiological levels just prior to the next injection[46]. These fluctuations in T levels are experienced by some of the patients as unpleasant and accompanied by changes in energy, libido and mood. The transient supraphysiological levels might increase the frequency of side-effects[42]. Preliminary studies with i.m. injection of TU 1000 mg indicate that this treatment might yield physiological T levels

during 6–8 weeks[47]. Longer acting T esters (4–6 months), such as the buciclate are probably not suited for use in elderly males; in case of serious side-effects, a rapid withdrawal of T should be possible.

Oral or transdermal T may be better candidates, although both preparations are associated with high plasma DHT levels following resorption. Orally administered T is almost completely inactivated by its first pass through the liver, the only orally active form is TU in oleic acid which, due its lipophilic side-chain is partly taken up by the lymph and partly escapes hepatic inactivation. The maximal plasma concentration of T is generally observed within 2–3 hours, but after 6–8 hours, levels have returned to pretreatment levels. Hence, TU in oleic acid should be administered 2–3 times daily, preferably with a meal to improve absorption. A dosage of 2–3 × 40 mg, generally provides adequate androgen replacement, yielding T levels within the (low) normal range, whereas DHT levels are moderately increased (2–4 nmol/l)[48]. The absorption is, however, rather variable and the dose required should be determined on the basis of plasma levels and clinical effects. Other orally active, synthetic androgen/anabolic steroids are either only weakly active (mesterolon, fluoxymesterone) or hepatotoxic due to the presence of an alkylgroup in position 17 of the molecule.

Transdermal scrotal or permeation enhanced non-scrotal patches, delivering 4–6 mg of T per day, provide physiological T levels both in young and eldely hypogonadal men[49]. Peak levels are obtained 2–4 hours after application; subsequently levels decrease to two-thirds of peak levels after 22–24 hours, mimicking the normal circadian variation of T levels in young adults. The scrotal patches yield supranormal DHT levels (4–5 nmol/l) whereas with the non-scrotal patches DHT levels are lower but they often cause local skin irritation. With a second generation torso patch (Testoderm[R]) this irritation is reportedly seen less frequently. Besides providing physiological levels in young and elderly hypogonadal men, the patches have the advantage that the therapy can be immediately stopped, when necessary[50].

DHT gel is available (25–50 mg DHT/g)[53] at a dose of 125–250 mg/day which yields plasma DHT levels comparable to physiological T levels. More recently it has been shown that in healthy elderly males, a lower dose of 32–64 mg/day yields comparable levels. DHT cannot be aromatized and, therefore, it will not induce gynecomastia, but it is probably inactive at the bone level. It has been hypothesized that the decrease in E_2 levels by DHT gel treatment may be favorable at the level of the prostate, where estrogens stimulate the proliferation of the stroma[52,53].

Recently a 1% hydro-alcoholic T gel has become available in some countries[54,55]. When administered to hypogonadal men between the ages of 12–68 years, about 9–14% of the T applied was bioavailable and with a daily application of 100 mg/day in 10 g gel, the plasma T levels are in the upper normal quartile, DHT levels being only slightly increased. The gels permit an easy adaptation of the dose to the individual needs. It is not known whether the elevation of plasma DHT with oral or transdermal administration is a cause for concern. The target organs of T, in as far as they convert T to DHT, have high local concentrations of DHT, and plasma levels of DHT might be a reflection of these conversions in target organs, the products of which leak into the circulation. It is currently unknown as to whether elevated plasma levels of DHT are of pathophysiological significance. In any case they are far below local concentrations in target organs. Other T formulations, such as biodegradable T microspheres or cyclodextrin complexed sublingual formulations are under experimentation.

ADRENAL ANDROGENS

While it is now well documented that serum levels of adrenal androgens decline strongly with aging, it has not been definitively established whether this impressive fall of adrenal androgens has any pathophysiological significance. Theoretically, it could be a meaningful mechanism of adaptation to aging. There is no doubt that strong correlations can be established between the declining levels of adrenal androgens and ailments of aging, but whether these statistical associations are causally pathophysiologically interrelated remains to be established. One way of establishing whether there is a relationship between the two is via intervention studies. Suppressing or elevating levels of adrenal androgens and monitoring the subsequent biological effects could provide clues as to whether the falling levels of adrenal androgens with aging are a cause for concern. The effects in laboratory animals are impressive (for review see reference 61). Beneficial effects on processes such as atherosclerosis, type 2 diabetes, obesity, immune function/cancer prevention and brain function have been reported, but it must be noted that laboratory animals, i.e. rats and rabbits, do not physiologically produce adrenal androgens in the same quantities as human species.

So far, studies in humans are limited. While some studies have found correlations between circulating levels of adrenal androgens and age-related ailments, others have not. Intervention studies present an equally sober picture. One study has found a positive effect on well-being[57]. The effects of DHEA replacement on indices of sexual functioning in men and women with complete adrenal insufficiency, who are virtually devoid of adrenal androgens, are convincing[58,59]. It would seem that a total absence of adrenal androgens has negative effects on the female well-being and sexuality. A positive effect on self-esteem and maybe on well-being was found in men[59] and this argues more in favor of an independent effect of DHEA on the brain, since the men were not T-deficient.

A consequence of the conversion of DHEA to androgens and estrogens is that the effects of DHEA administration are not necessarily harmless. They may influence hormone-sensitive diseases such as breast or prostate cancer. So far there are no reports in the literature of any side-effects from self-administration of DHEA, which occurs on a massive scale with DHEA sold as a health product. Well-designed studies, investigating the effects of deficiency of adrenal androgens and the results of replacement therapy in humans are required to resolve the long-term effect of levels of adrenal androgens.

GROWTH HORMONE

Signs associated with aging show a striking similarity with features observed in adults who are GH deficient, and therefore speculation has arisen that (some of) the features of aging must be ascribed to the age-related decline in GH, and can potentially be remedied with GH replacement. The actions of GH and androgens are strongly intertwined; only in the presence of normal GH levels can androgen express its full biological potential, and *vice versa*. It is, therefore, not surprising that the signs and symptoms of GH deficiency and androgen deficiency show a strong overlap.

The interrelationship between sleep and the somatotropic axis is well documented. This relationship is relevant since most aging subjects experience a deterioration of their sleep. During aging, slow wave sleep and GH decline concurrently, raising the possibility that the age-related decline of GH is also a reflection of age-related alterations in sleep–wake patterns[60].

Unlike the situation in androgen physiology it is much more difficult to establish who is GH-deficient in adulthood. The pulsatile nature of GH secretion and the large number of factors determining circulating levels of GH complicate the matter considerably in the sense that a single measurement of GH does not provide meaningful information. A single measurement of insulin-like growth factor (IGF)-1 is a reasonable first indicator of GH status. In subjects over the age of 40 years, a IGF-1 value of 15 nmol/l or higher excludes a deficiency of

GH[61]. The problem lies among patients with values below this level. Surprisingly, some patients with proven GH deficiency (on the basis of extensive testing such as insulin-hypoglycemia, GH releasing hormone (GHRH) and L-dopa stimulation tests) still have normal IGF-1 levels. Another useful index of the GH status is IGF-binding protein (BP)-3. For the time being, the combination of signs and symptoms potentially attributable to GH deficiency and an IGF-1 level and IGFBP-3 in the lowest tertile provides a reasonable indication of (relative) GH deficiency. The starting dose of GH administration is not well established but a dose of 0.05–0.1 U/kg subcutaneously (s.c.) seems reasonable. Once placed on GH administration, individual dose titration must be done on the basis of the IGF-1 levels resulting from GH administration and the occurrence of side-effects. The aim is to produce IGF-1 levels in the normal range or only slightly above normal (0–1 SD above mean levels of IGF-1). Secondly, if side-effects occur (flu-like symptoms, myalgia, arthralgia, carpal tunnel syndrome, edema, impairment of glucose homeostasis) GH dosage is reduced in steps of 25%. Contraindications against GH use include type I diabetes, active (or a history of) cancer, intracranial hypertension, diabetic retinopathy or carpal tunnel syndrome and severe cardiac insufficiency. It seems there is a place for GH administration in aging subjects at this point in time, primarily to gather information as to whether there are groups that might benefit from its supplementation. In view of the narrow dose limits and potential side-effects, it is not advisable at present to administer GH to aging patients outside the framework of a clinical trial that provides intensive guidance and safeguards for patients.

The requirement for daily s.c. injections of recombinant human (r-h) GH is clearly an unattractive feature of the treatment of GH deficiency. The treatment would be more acceptable if injections were less frequent or the mode of administration was more user-friendly. And, indeed, there are some interesting pharmaceutical developments in the area of GH and GHRH, such as slow-release formulations for example, depot formulations Nutropin Depot (Genentech/Alkermes), slow-release r-hGH Granditropin depot (Gandis/Novartis/InfiMed), and a transdermal patch (Transdermal GHRH Theratechnoloy)[1-42].

Future developments also comprise oral secretagogues and downstream intracellular effectors of GH signalling pathway such as protein tyrosine kinases. In the meantime, needle-free injection techniques and a depot formulation of GH offer alternatives to daily s.c. injections.

MELATONIN

Melatonin is mainly synthesized by the pineal gland (both in humans and other animals) and its secretion has a circadian (or 24-hour) rhythm. It is thought to have a function in the sleep–wake rhythm. Levels are high during the night (50–70 pg/ml) and low during the day (<10 pg/ml). The melatonin rhythm is inversely coupled with the rhythm of core body temperature, the high nocturnal melatonin levels correlate with low core body temperature. The production of melatonin is regulated by input from the hypothalamic nucleus suprachiasmaticus that serves as our internal biological clock. The daily secretion of melatonin is governed by the dark-light cycle: activated by darkness and inhibited by light.

Sleep quality in many older people undergoes clinically relevant deterioration, presenting itself as difficulty falling asleep, or more often, frequent and longer-lasting nocturnal awakenings with daytime napping as compensation. Several studies document that nocturnal plasma melatonin levels decline considerably in most people by the sixth and seventh decades of their lives. It has been found that elderly people experiencing good sleep quality do not necessarily have higher nocturnal melatonin levels than those subjects

who experience poor sleep quality. So, the age-related decline in levels of melatonin is not sufficient to disrupt sleep in old age. Melatonin levels can be measured successfully in either saliva or urine. A urine sample taken in the morning can provide an insight into the nocturnal levels of melatonin secreted. The main urinary metabolite of melatonin is 6-sulphatoxymelatonin. Some drugs affect nocturnal melatonin production: β_1-adrenergic receptor blockers such as atenolol and propanol, and prostaglandin synthase inhibitors such as ibuprofen and other antirheumatics, inhibit neurotransmission to the pineal gland and thus impair the production of melatonin.

Insomnia observed in some elderly people can be partially restored by administering melatonin. The dose required to restore sleep in insomniac elderly patients has not been firmly established. In one study doses of 0.1, 0.3 and 3.0 mg were administered. The best effect was observed with the 0.3 mg dose. This raised night-time plasma melatonin levels to those observed in early adult life. Sleep efficiency was also improved with an increase in time spent in bed (when subjects were actually asleep), and a significant decrease seen in nocturnal awakenings and in sleep latency (the time between going to bed and actually falling asleep). From this study it seems that the optimal dose is around 0.3 mg, to be given 30 minutes before bedtime. An earlier study addressed dosage requirements: it was found that 2 mg of fast-release melatonin effectively induced sleep while 2 mg slow-release was effective for sleep maintenance. The use of 1 mg slow-release melatonin over 2 months produced satisfactory results with no signs of tolerance being developed. Few side-effects of melatonin have been reported, even though it is widely used as an over-the-counter drug in the USA.

THYROID DISEASE IN ELDERLY MEN

The clinical presentation of thyroid diseases in the elderly differs from the typical clinical manifestation in the younger population. Laboratory test results should be interpreted with the age of the patient in mind. The use of drugs and the frequent occurrence of non-thyroidal illness (NTI), consisting of lowered T_3 and an insignificant reduction in T_4, in the elderly are factors in these age-related changes of laboratory parameters of thyroid function. The treatment of thyroid dysfunction in the elderly also requires more caution than in younger patients.

In elderly subjects there is a decrease in production of T_4 with a concomitant decrease in T_4 clearance, so circulating levels do not change significantly. Basal TSH levels do not change very much in old age but the response to thyrotropin-releasing hormone (TRH) may be somewhat decreased as a sign of the aging process of the pituitary.

Drugs may alter the profiles of thyroid hormone levels, which is relevant since the elderly subjects often take some form of medication over long periods[62]. Long-term therapy with lithium may lead to hypothyroidism and patients should be screened for this complication. The iodine-containing cardiac drug, amiodarone, may produce both hyper- and hypothyroidism. Glucocorticoids inhibit the conversion of T_4 to T_3. Conversely, a state of hyper- or hypothyroidism affects the half-lives of certain drugs. In hypothyroidism the plasma half-lives of digoxin, morphine, glucocorticoids and insulin are increased, with the consequence of a lower than normal maintenance dosage of these drugs. The reverse pattern is observed in hyperthyroidism.

Hypothyroidism may be overlooked in the elderly since the symptoms may be less apparent. The symptoms themselves are often attributed to the aging process with its associated asthenia, effects of drug use and loss of agility. These symptoms range from weakness, chronic fatigue and decreased heart rate, to dry skin, hoarseness and slower tendon reflexes. Intolerance to cold and weight gain may be less pronounced in the elderly. Hypothyroidism should

be suspected if there are occurrences of unexplained high levels of cholesterol and creatinine phosphokinase, severe constipation, congestive heart failure with cardiomyopathy and unexplained macrocytic anemia. Loss of weight due to anorexia may occur. Lethargy, memory loss and depression may be the presenting symptoms. Long-term hypothyroidism will result in irreversible psychic symptoms.

The prevalence of hypothyroidism in the elderly lies somewhere between 1–7% for the full-fledged disease and 5–16% for subclinical hypothyroidism. Patients who have been treated surgically with radioactive iodine may tip over to hypothyroidism later in their lives.

The best diagnostic test for primary hypothyroidism is an increased serum TSH level, although TSH levels in the elderly who have hypothyroidism are lower than in younger patients with the same disease. Levels of both T_4 and free T_3 are a less helpful indicator, since they are lower in cases of NTI.

Treatment of hypothyroidism in the elderly involves substitution with T_4, the guiding principle being the normalization of TSH levels. An abrupt increase in circulating levels of T_4 may provoke cardiac symptoms, therefore replacement should be carried out in a stepwise fashion.

Hyperthyroidism in the elderly may have a different presentation than in younger hyperthyroid patients. Patients with atrial fibrillation should be suspected of hyperthyroidism since the likelihood of thyroid hyperfunction is approximately three times higher. Conventional treatment of cardiac disease is less successful if hyperthyroidism lies at the basis of cardiac symptoms. Another complication of long-standing hyperthyroidism is osteoporosis. Bone resorption is increased, particularly in subjects with other etiological factors. Unexplained osteoporosis must be a reminder of possible hyperthyroidism.

The prevalence of hyperthyroidism is estimated to be 1–2% of the aging population, with higher rates observed in women. The etiology is identical to that in younger subjects: Graves' disease, toxic multi-adenoma, toxic adenoma and thyroiditis, and often thyroid hormone replacement therapy that is poorly monitored. Treatment with amiodarone or iodine-containing radiocontrast agents, as mentioned, may also evoke hyperthyroidism in the elderly. The diagnosis is based essentially on elevated levels of T_4 and free T_3, and suppressed levels of TSH. Occasionally only free T_3 levels are elevated (T_3 thyrotoxicosis). Radioactive iodine is the optimal treatment of hyperthyroidism in elderly patients, providing a definitive solution and posing less risks than surgical treatment.

ERECTILE DYSFUNCTION

It is obvious that aging *per se* is associated with a deterioration of the biological functions mediating erectile function: hormonal, vascular and neural processes. This is not rarely aggravated by intercurrent disease in old age, such as diabetes mellitus, cardiovascular disease and use of medical drugs. There is still uneasiness with the aging population when it comes to sexual dysfunction. It is essential that physicians make sexuality a conversation topic in their interaction with aging patients and provide an opportunity for patients to discuss the quality of their sex lives. It is a fact of life that lots of physicians are themselves not comfortable with bringing up these issues in their contact with patients and this conspiracy of silence is non-verbally communicated to patients. If embarrassment arises in a conversation on sexuality the doctor must give the patient 'permission' to use vernacular expressions to describe sexual complaints.

The advent of effective treatment methods of erectile dysfunction (ED) with oral preparations such as peripherally acting inhibitors of cGMP phosphodiesterase (sildenafil, or newer cGMP phosphodiesterase inhibitors under investigation such as IC351, BAY 38-9456) or central acting dopaminergic agents such as 'apomorhine', or intracavernous (i.c.) injection

therapy has improved our therapeutical arsenal greatly. Sildenafil, has been shown to be an effective and well-tolerated oral agent for treating ED with a wide range of causes in the general population of adult men (a starting dose of 25 mg or 50 mg, with an option to increase the dose to 100 mg, or to decrease it to 25 mg depending on efficacy and tolerability). The most commonly experienced adverse events are headache, flushing, and dyspepsia, which occur in about 17%, 13% and 8%, respectively[63]. Although sildenafil is clearly a reliable treatment option for the majority of elderly patients with ED, extensive information about other therapeutic modalities including intracavernous injection therapy, intraurethral drug therapy and placement of penile implants should be given to the aging ED patients. Libido in men is linked to T, and when T is replaced in hypogonadal men there is increase in sexual thoughts and sexual desire[64,65]. The use of androgens in the treatment of ED, either alone or in combination with phosphodiesterase inhibitors in the aging male should be reserved for men with proven hypogonadism.

Though oral therapy is a major step forward, it has made clear at the same time that many patients have attributed their unfulfilled sexual situation almost exclusively to their ED. Restoration of erectile function has often not brought the happiness that patients anticipated. For example, because the communication with their partner has been neglected for many years while the patient's erectile difficulties were developing, and resuming sexual activity may not be as unquestionable and unequivocal as it might have seemed. For others the demands for sexual performance are unrealistic.

A fulfilling sex life is part of a good life. We need to educate our patients that like any other human endeavour, human sexuality is not exempt from problems for which solutions must be and can often be found. We have to tell our patients that aging has its impact on life and on sexuality, but it should not and need not defeat men. Erection and ejaculation become less dependable but there are also non-coital forms of sexual expression providing enjoyment and satisfaction. Sexual creativity is a must! The latter requires an open and playful relationship with one's own sexuality and one's sexual partner.

As indicated above, erectile potency is physiologically a complex interaction of vascular, neural, metabolic, endocrine and, last but not least, psychological factors. Erectile difficulties often provide a window into the presence of pathology of these areas. But precisely the advent of successful treatment modalities of erectile difficulties have led to a concept of erectile failure as an entity in itself, rather than an expression of underlying pathology of its constituents. In other words, it has opened the door to view diagnosis and treatment of underlying pathology of erectile failure as not necessary. A holistic approach to the aging male requires, however, that all aspects of health are addressed and complaints of erectile difficulties provide an opportunity for a more thorough evaluation of health problems of the aging man who will find motivation to work on these health issues if the reward is an improvement of his sex life.

NUTRITION AND THE EPIDEMIC OF OBESITY

In industrialized countries outright nutritional deficiencies are rare nowadays except cases of severe gastrointestinal pathology or psychiatric disturbance. The very old may show deficient calcium intake or vitamin D deficiencies. A simple rule for healthy eating is to ensure that the meal size is commensurate with energy expenditure, that fats, in particular animal fat, are avoided in the diet, and that there is a substantial fiber and fruit content to the daily food intake. A major problem is the management of obesity. Obesity is a condition that is reaching epidemic proportions in both the developed and the developing world. In the United States,

63% of men and 55% of women are classified as overweight, of these, 22% are deemed grossly overweight, with a body mass index above 30 kg/m^2, and the consequences of this rapid increase are serious. Approximately 80% of obese adults suffer from at least one, and 40% from two or more of the diseases associated with obesity, such as type 2 diabetes, hypertension, CVD, gallbladder disease, cancers and diseases of the locomotor system, such as arthrosis. Genetics play a significant role in the development of obesity, with studies in identical twins showing that 60–70% of overweight can be ascribed to genetic factors, with just 30–40% attributable to environmental influences[66].

The pathophysiology of obesity is poorly understood. In simple terms, obesity is a discrepancy between food intake and energy expenditure. However, the physiological mechanisms involved and how these can be influenced to redress obesity, are not known completely.

In recent years it has been demonstrated that the lipid cell functions as an endocrine cell, producing and secreting molecules with regulatory potential. The discovery of the hormonal signal of the lipid cell termed leptin, was an important step in a better understanding of obesity. The main target of leptin is the central nervous system. By modulating neurotransmitters in the hypothalamus it increases energy expenditure and inhibits appetite and weight gain. Leptin influences neuropeptides affecting appetite and anorexia. The question has arisen whether obesity is an abnormality of leptin physiology. Indeed, both animals and humans with abnormalities of the gene involved in the production of leptin are very obese. In animals this could be partially corrected by the administration of exogenous recombinant leptin. Most obese subjects have high circulating levels of leptin interpreted as a state of leptin insensitivity which is not well understood, rather than a state of leptin deficiency. It may be a deficient transport of leptin into the brain or deficient receptor or postreceptor mechanisms of leptin making its action less efficient. Current research is focused on finding out if the administration of exogenous leptin will aid weight reduction.

The treatment of obesity is not simple, even more difficult is the maintenance of a reduced weight in the long term (after successful weight loss). It is evident that a combination of reduced caloric intake and an increase in energy expenditure will lead to a reduction in weight. However, when placed on a calorie-restricted diet, the body responds by developing countermeasures to minimize the loss of weight, a system which evolved to enhance an individual's chance of survival during prolonged times of famine. Recent studies indicate that a weight loss of just 5–10% leads to clinically significant reductions in the risk factors associated with obesity, even if the 'ideal' weight is not reached[67]. A reduction of 10% of weight in 6 months to 1 year can be considered good progress, however, it is estimated that over 80% of those who lose weight will gradually regain it[68]. The addition of various pharmacotherapies to a weight reducing diet can increase the degree of success. However, it is difficult, even with pharmacotherapy to achieve a weight reduction of more than 6–8% of initial body weight. Considering the amount of investment and expenditure directed towards weight reduction each year, the fight against obesity is largely unsuccessful. Indeed, it may be a difficult, if not impossible battle to win in the setting of clinical medicine. Eating patterns are very resistant to change. It will require extensive public health campaigns educating populations to eat sensibly and to be more physically active from an early age. The food industry may play a significant role in view of the increasing consumption of convenience food. Marketing techniques of healthy food may have a large impact.

The current lack of success in the battle against obesity can lead to frustration for both patients and physicians alike. The medical profession has little to offer the obese patient in terms of efficacious treatment. The physician is then inclined to leave full responsibility for loss of weight to the patient himself, implying more or less that the patient lacks willpower. Thus the battle against the epidemic of obesity cannot easily be won.

EXERCISE AND PHYSICAL FITNESS

Technological and socioeconomic developments have made a quantum leap in recent history in relation to the amount of physical exercise and energy expenditure required from our bodies on a daily basis. There are strong parallels with the situation of nutrition in modern times. These developments are very appealing to almost everyone and must be considered as irreversible, durable products of western civilization. The inevitable consequence is that many people are overfed and physically unfit. Men should be advised to perform regular physical exercise (aerobic for maintaining cardiac function, anaerobic – targeted to specific muscle groups as well as stretching). These exercises have to be performed on a regular basis and tailored to 'the biological age' and condition of the person. Similar to the situation of obesity, people are of good will but lack the stamina to implement physical exercise in their daily lives much beyond an initial period of fresh determination. There are apparently in the lives of most people too many intervening circumstances prompting one to give up regular exercise. The demands of daily life cause fatigue which can in fact be remedied by recreational exercise if people could only muster the energy to do it. Again, similar to the situation with obesity, education seems to be a major factor and small steps must be encouraged. Working out, albeit moderately, in the work place, or with a group of friends may bolster tenacity of purpose. Nutrition and physical exercise with fitness as an outcome are pivotal for the health situation of the aging male and his quality of life, and therefore deserve a more prominent place in the medical curriculum.

Their implementation can be left to health workers with a focus on exploring individual motivations and opportunities for a healthier lifestyle for which there is no substitute.

CONCLUSION

Physicians who are educated about the value that preventative health care can play in prolonging life span and quality of life will be more likely to participate in health screening. Men are not likely to consult a doctor until they have an acute illness. Therefore the physician should take that opportunity to also consider the family history, body constitution, life style and risk factors and advise the patient on preventive strategies or refer him to consult the appropriate specialist. We hope that the next few years will enrich us with greater understanding of the aging process in men. Thus, permit us to help improve the quality of life, prevent the preventable, and postpone and decrease the pain and suffering of the inevitable.

References

1. Gray A, Feldman A, McKinlay JB, Longcope C. Age, disease, and changing sex hormone levels in middle-aged men: results of the Massachusetts Male Aging Study. *J Clin Endocrinol Metab* 1991;73:1016–25

2. Kaufman JM, Vermeulen A. Declining gonadal function in elderly men. *Bailliere's Clin Endocrinol* 1997;11:289–98

3. Vermeulen A, Kaufman JM, Giagulli VA. Influence of some biological indices on sex hormone binding globulin and androgen levels in aging and obese males. *J Clin Endocrinol Metab* 1996;81:1921–27

4. Pearson UJD, Blackman MR, Metter EJ. Effect of age and cigarette smoking on longitudinal changes in androgens and SHBG in healthy males. Abstracts of the 77th Annual Meeting of the Endocrine Society 1995;129

5. Morley JE, Kaiser FE, Perry HM, *et al.* Longitudinal changes in testosterone, luteinizing hormone, and follicle-stimulating hormone in healthy older men. *Metabolism* 1997;46:410–3

6. Meikle AW, Bishop DT, Stringham JD, West DW. Quantitating genetic and nongenetic factors that determine plasma sex steroid variation in normal male twins. *Metabolism* 1986;35:1090–5

7. Handelsman DJ. Testicular dysfunction in systemic disease. *Endocrinol Metab Clin North Am* 1994;23:839–56

8. Gooren LG. Androgen levels and sex functions in testosterone treated hypogonadal men. *Arch Sex Behav* 1987;16:463–73

9. Bagatell CJ, Heiman JR, Rivier JE, Bremner WJ. Effects of endogenous testosterone and estradiol on sexual behavior in normal young men. *J Clin Endocrinol Metab* 1994;78:1520

10. Schiavi RC, White D, Mandeli J, Schreiner-Engel P. Hormones and nocturnal penile tumescence in healthy aging men. *Arch Sex Behav* 1993;22:207–15

11. Bhasin S, Storer TW, Berman N, *et al.* Testosterone replacement increases fat-free mass and muscle size in hypogonadal men. *J Clin Endocrinol Metab* 1997;82:407–13

12. Deslypere JP, Kaufman JM, Vermeulen T, *et al.* Influence of age on pulatile luteinizing hormone release and responsiveness of the gonadotrophs to sex hormone feedback in men. *J Clin Endocrinol Metab* 1987;64:69–73

13. Van den Beld A, Huhtaniemi IT, Pettersson KS, *et al.* Luteinizing hormone and different genetic variants, as indicators of frailty in healthy elderly men. *J Clin Endocrinol Metab* 1999;84:1334–9

14. Vermeulen A, Verdonck L, Kaufman JM. A critical evaluation of simple methods for the estimation of free testosterone in serum. *J Clin Endocrinol Metab* 1999;84:3666–72

15. Deslypere JP, Vermeulen A. Influence of age on steroid concentrations in skin and striated

muscle in women and cardiac muscle and lung tissue in men. *J Clin Endocrinol Metab* 1985;60:648–53

16. Greenstein BD. Androgen receptors in the rat brain, anterior pituitary glands and ventral prostate gland: effects of orchiectomy and aging. *J Endocrinol* 1979;81:75–81

17. Fischbeck KH, Lieberman A, Bailey CK, *et al.* Androgen receptor mutation in Kennedy's disease. *Philos Trans R Soc Lond B Biol Sci* 1999;354:1075–8

18. Krithivas K, Yurgalevitch SM, Mohr BA, *et al.* Evidence that the CAG repeat in the androgen receptor gene is associated with the age-related decline in serum androgen levels in men. *J Endocrinol* 1999;162:137–42

19. Tincello DG, Saunders PT, Hodgins MB, *et al.* Correlation of clinical, endocrine and molecular abnormalities with in vivo responses to high-dose testosterone in patients with partial androgen insensitivity syndrome. *Clin Endocrinol* 1997;46:497–506

20. Weidemann W, Peters B, Romalo G, *et al.* Response to androgen treatment in a patient with partial androgen insensitivity and a mutation in the deoxyribonucleic acid-binding domain of the androgen receptor. *J Clin Endocrinol Metab* 1998;83:1173–6

21. Vermeulen A. Androgen replacement therapy in the aging male- a critical evaluation. *J Clin Endocrinol Metab* 2001;86:2380–90

22. Tenover JS. Effects of testosterone supplementation in the aging male. *J Clin Endocrinol Metab* 1992;75:1092–8

23. Morley JE, Perry HM, Kaiser FE, *et al.* Effect of testosterone replacement therapy in old hypogonadal males: a preliminary study. *J Am Geriatr Soc* 1993;41:149–52

24. Snyder PJ, Peachy H, Hannoush P, *et al.* Effect of testosterone treatment on body composition and muscle strength in men over 65 years of age. *J Clin Endocrinol Metab* 1999;84:2647–53

25. Wang C, Swerdloff RS, Iranmanesh A, *et al.* The testosterone gel study group. Transdermal testosterone gel improves sexual function, mood, muscle strength, body composition parameters in hypogonadal men. *J Clin Endocrinol Metab* 2000;85:2839–53

26. Barrett-Connor E. Lower endogenous androgen levels and dyslipidemia in men with non-insulin dependent diabetes mellitus. *Ann Int Med* 1992;117:807–11

27. Phillips GB, Pinkernell BH, Jing TY. The association between hypotestosteronemia with coronary artery disease in men. *Arteriosclerosis and Thrombosis* 1994;14:701–6

28. Swartz CA, Young MA. Low serum testosterone and myocardial infarction in geriatric male inpatients. *J Am Ger Soc* 1987;35:39–44

29. Vermeulen A, Kaufman JM. Androgens and cardiovascular disease in men and women. *The Aging Male* 1998;1:35–50

30. Marcelli M, Cunningham GR. Hormonal signaling in prostatic hyperplasia and neoplasia. *J Clin Endocrinol Metab* 1999;84:3463–8

31. Sakr WA, Grignon DJ, Crissman JD, *et al.* High grade prostatic intraepithelial neoplasia (HGPIN) and prostate adenocarcinoma between the ages of 20–69: an autopsy study of 249 cases. *In Vivo* 1994;8:439–43

32. Kleinman KJP, McKinlay JB. Prostate cancer: how much do we know and how do we know it? *The Aging Male* 2000;3:115–23

33. Carter HB, Pearson JD, Metter EJ, *et al.* Longitudinal evaluation of serum androgen levels in men with and without prostate cancer. *Prostate* 1995;27:25–31

34. Behre HM, Bohmeyer J, Nieschlag E. Prostate volume in testosterone-treated and untreated hypogonadal men in comparison to age-matched normal controls. *Clin Endocrinol* 1994;40:341–9

35. Sasagawa I, Nakada T, Kazama T, *et al.* Volume change of the prostate and seminal vesicles in male hypogonadism after androgen replacement therapy. *Int Urol Nephrol* 1990;22:279–84

36. Wallace EM, Pye SD, Wildt SR, Wu FC. Prostate specific antigen and prostate gland size in men receiving exogenous testosterone for male contraception. *Int J Androl* 1993;16:35–40

37. Holmäng S, Marin P, Lindstedt G, Hedelin H. Effect of long-term oral testosterone undecanoate treatment on prostate volume and serum prostate specific antigen in eugonadal middle-aged men. *Prostate* 1993;23:99–106

38. Sundaram K, Kumar N, Bardin CW. 7α-methyl-nortestosterone (MENT): the optimal androgen for male contraception. *Ann Med* 1993; 25:199–205

39. Snyder PJ. Development of criteria to monitor the occurrence of prostate cancer in testosterone clinical trials. In Bhasin S, Gabelnick HL, Swerdloff RS, Wang C, eds. *Pharmacology, Biology, and Clinical Applications of Androgens*. Wiley-Liss: New York, 1996;143–50

40. Morgan TO, Jacobsen SJ, McCarthy WF, *et al*. Age specific reference ranges for prostate specific antigen in black men. *N Engl J Med* 1996;335:304–10

41. Morales A. Andropause, androgen therapy and prostate safety. *The Aging Male* 1999; 2:81–7

42. Dobs AS, Meikle AW, Arver S, *et al*. Pharmacokinetics, efficiency and safety of a permeation enhanced testosterone transdermal system in comparison with bi-weekly injections of testosterone-enanthate for the treatment of hypogonadal men. *J Clin Endocrinol Metab* 1999;84:3469–78

43. Matsumoto AM, Sandblom RE, Schoene RB, *et al*. Testosterone replacement in hypogonadal men: effect on obstructive sleep apnoea, respiratory drives and sleep. *Clin Endocrinol Metab* 1985;22:713–21

44. Santamaria JD, Prior SC, Fleetham JA. Reversible reproductive dysfunction in men with obstructive sleep apnea. *Clin Endocrinol* 1988;28:461–70

45. Gooren LJG. A ten year safety study of the oral androgen, testosterone-undecanoate. *J Androl* 1994;15:212–15

46. Nieschlag E, Cuppers HJ, Wieglmann W, Wickings ES. Bioavailability and LH suppressive effects of different testosterone preparations in normal and hypogonadal men. *Horm Res* 1976;7:134–41

47. Zhang Gy, Gu Yq, Wang XH, *et al*. A pharmaco kinetic study of injectable testosterone-undecanoate in hypogonadal men. *J Androl* 1998;19:761–8

48. Davidson DW, O'Carroll RO, Bancroft J. Increasing circulating androgens with testosterone-undecanoate in eugonadal men. *J Ster Biochem* 1987;26:713–16

49. Snyder PJ, Peachey H, Hannoush P, *et al*. Effects of testosterone treatment on bone mineral density in men over 65 years old. *J Clin Endocrinol Metab* 1999;84: 1966–72

50. Meikle AW, Mazer NA, Moellmer JD, *et al*. Enhanced transdermal delivery across non scrotal skin produces physiological concentrations of testosterone and its metabolites in hypogonadal men. *J Clin Endocrinol Metab* 1992;74:623–8

51. Vermeulen A, Deslypere JP. Longterm transdermal dihydrotestosterone therapy: effects on pituitary gonadal axis and plasma lipoproteins. *Maturitas* 1985;7:281–7

52. Wang C, Iranmanesh A, Berman V, *et al*. Compararative pharmacokinetics of three doses of percutaneous dihydrotestosterone gel in healthy elderly men. A clinical research center study. *J Clin Endocrinol Metab* 1998; 83:2749–57

53. Swerdloff ES, Wang C. Dihydrotestosterone: a rationale for the use of a non aromatizable androgen replacement therapeutic agent. *Bailliére's Clin Endocrinol Metab* 1998;12: 501–6

54. Wang C, Berman C, Longstreth JA, *et al*. Pharamacokinetics of transdermal testosterone gel in hypogonadal men: application of gel at one site versus four sites. A general clinical research center study. *J Clin Endocrinol Metab* 2000;85:964–9

55. Swerdloff RS, Wang C, Cunningham G, *et al*. The testosterone gel study group. Long term pharmacokinetics of transdermal testosterone in hypogondal men. *J Clin Endocrinol Metab* 2000;85:4500–10

56. Nippoldt TB, Nair KS. Is there a case for DHEA replacement? In Bhasin S ed. The therapeutic role of androgens. *Bailliere's Clin Endocrinol Metab* 1998;12:507–20

57. Morales AJ, Nolan JJ, Nelson JC, Yen SS. Effects of replacement dose of dehydroepiandrosterone in men and women of advancing age. *J Clin Endocrinol Metab* 1994; 78:1360–7

58. Arlt W, Callies F, Van Vlijmen JC. Dehydroepiandrosterone replacement in women with adrenal insufficiency. *N Engl J Med* 1999;341:1013–20

59. Hunt PJ, Gurnell EM, Huppert FA, *et al.* Improvement in mood and fatigue after dehydroepiandrosterone replacement in Addison's disease in a randomised double blind trial. *J Clin Endocrinol Metab* 2000;85:4650–6

60. Van Cauter E, Leproult R, Plat L. Age related changes in slow wave sleep and REM sleep and relationship with growth hormone and cortisol levels in healthy men. *J Am Med Ass* 2000;284:861–8

61. Span JP, Pieters GF, Sweep CG, *et al.* Plasam IGF-1 is a useful marker of growth hormone deficiency in adults. *J Endocrinol Invest* 1999; 22:446–50

62. Surks MI, Sievert R. Drugs and thyroid function. *N Engl J Med* 1995;333:1688–94

63. Montorsi F, McDermott TED, Morgan R. Efficacy and safety of fixed-dose oral sildenafil in the treatment of erectile dysfunction of various etiologies. *Urology* 1999,53:1011–18

64. Davidson JM, Kwan M, Greenleaf WJ. Hormonal replacement and sexuality. *Clin Endocrinol Metab* 1882;11:599–614

65. Kwan M, Greenleaf WJ, Mann J. The nature of androgen on men sexuality: A combined laboratory/self reported study on hypogonadal men. *J Clin Endocrinol Metab* 1983:57:557–61

66. Sorensen TI, Echwald SM. Obesity genes. *Br Med J* 2001;322:652–3

67. Mertens IL, Van Gaal LF. Overweight, obesity, and blood pressure: The effects of modest weight reduction. *Obes Res* 2000;8:270–8

68. National Heart, Lung, and Blood Institute's Obesity Education Initiative: Expert Panel on the Identification, Evaluation, and Treatment of Overweight in Adults. Clinical guidelines on the identification, evaluation, and treatment of overweight and obesity in adults: Executive summary. *Am J Clin Nutr* 1998; 68:899–917

Index

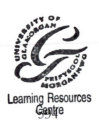